KT-545-079

Head and Neck Imaging

Editors

RICHARD H. WIGGINS III
ASHOK SRINIVASAN

RADIOLOGIC CLINICS OF NORTH AMERICA

www.radiologic.theclinics.com

Consulting Editor
FRANK H. MILLER

January 2015 • Volume 53 • Number 1

ELSEVIER

1600 John F. Kennedy Boulevard • Suite 1800 • Philadelphia, Pennsylvania, 19103-2899

http://www.theclinics.com

RADIOLOGIC CLINICS OF NORTH AMERICA Volume 53, Number 1
January 2015 ISSN 0033-8389, ISBN 13: 978-0-323-34184-4

Editor: John Vassallo (j.vassallo@elsevier.com)
Developmental Editor: Donald Mumford

Radiologic Clinics of North America (ISSN 0033-8389) is published bimonthly by Elsevier Inc., 360 Park Avenue South, New York, NY 10010-1710. Months of issue are January, March, May, July, September, and November. Periodicals postage paid at New York, NY and additional mailing offices. Subscription prices are USD 460 per year for US individuals, USD 709 per year for US institutions, USD 220 per year for US students and residents, USD 535 per year for Canadian individuals, USD 905 per year for Canadian institutions, USD 660 per year for international individuals, USD 905 per year for international institutions, and USD 315 per year for Canadian and foreign students/residents. To receive student and resident rate, orders must be accompanied by name of affiliated institution, date of term and the signature of program/residency coordinatior on institution letterhead. Orders will be billed at individual rate until proof of status is received. Foreign air speed delivery is included in all *Clinics* subscription prices. All prices are subject to change without notice. **POSTMASTER:** Send address changes to *Radiologic Clinics of North America*, Elsevier Health Sciences Division, Subscription Customer Service, 3251 Riverport Lane, Maryland Heights, MO63043. **Customer Service: Telephone: 1-800-654-2452** (U.S. and Canada); **1-314-447-8871** (outside U.S. and Canada). **Fax: 1-314-447-8029. E-mail: journalscustomerservice-usa@elsevier.com** (for print support); **journalsonlinesupport-usa@elsevier.com** (for online support).

Reprints. For copies of 100 or more of articles in this publication, please contact the Commercial Reprints Department, Elsevier Inc., 360 Park Avenue South, New York, New York 10010-1710. Tel.: +1-212-633-3874; Fax: +1-212-633-3820; E-mail: reprints@elsevier.com.

Radiologic Clinics of North America also published in Greek Paschalidis Medical Publications, Athens, Greece.

Radiologic Clinics of North America is covered in *MEDLINE/PubMed (Index Medicus), EMBASE/Excerpta Medica, Current Contents/Life Sciences, Current Contents/Clinical Medicine, RSNA Index to Imaging Literature, BIOSIS, Science Citation Index,* and *ISI/BIOMED.*

Printed in the United States of America.

Contributors

CONSULTING EDITOR

FRANK H. MILLER, MD
Chief, Body Imaging Section and Fellowship Program and GI Radiology; Medical Director MRI; Professor, Department of Radiology, Northwestern University, Feinberg School of Medicine, Northwestern Memorial Hospital, Chicago, Illinois

EDITORS

RICHARD H. WIGGINS III, MD, CIIP, FSIIM
Director of Head and Neck Imaging; Professor, Departments of Radiology, Otolaryngology, Head and Neck Surgery, and BioMedical Informatics, University of Utah Health Sciences Center, Salt Lake City, Utah

ASHOK SRINIVASAN, MBBS, MD
Associate Professor and Director of Neuroradiology, Department of Radiology, University of Michigan Health System, Ann Arbor, Michigan

AUTHORS

TRAVIS A. ABELE, MD
Department of Radiology, University of Utah, Salt Lake City, Utah

JUSTIN L. BRUCKER, MD
Head and Neck Imaging, Department of Neuroradiology, University of Wisconsin Hospital, University of Wisconsin, Madison, Wisconsin

J. LEVI CHAZEN, MD
Assistant Professor, Department of Radiology, Weill Cornell Medical College, New York-Presbyterian Hospital, New York, New York

LAURA B. EISENMENGER, MD
Departments of Radiology and Biomedical Informatics, University of Utah, Salt Lake City, Utah

P. LEO GALVIN, MD
Department of Radiology, Duke University Medical Center, Durham, North Carolina

CARYN GAMSS, MD
Clinical Fellow, Department of Radiology, Weill Cornell Medical College, New York-Presbyterian Hospital, New York, New York

LINDELL R. GENTRY, MD
Head and Neck Imaging, Department of Neuroradiology, University of Wisconsin Hospital, University of Wisconsin, Madison, Wisconsin

CHRISTINE M. GLASTONBURY, MBBS
Professor of Radiology and Biomedical Imaging, Otolaryngology–Head and Neck Surgery and Radiation Oncology, University of California, San Francisco, San Francisco, California

JULIUS GRIAUZDE, MD
Department of Radiology, University of Michigan Health System, Ann Arbor, Michigan

AJAY GUPTA, MD
Assistant Professor, Department of Radiology, Weill Cornell Medical College, New York-Presbyterian Hospital, New York, New York

GARY L. HEDLUND, DO
Director, Pediatric Neuroimaging, Department of Pediatric Medical Imaging, Primary Children's Hospital, Intermountain Healthcare, Salt Lake City, Utah

JENNY K. HOANG, MBBS
Department of Radiology; Department of Radiation Oncology, Duke University Medical Center, Durham, North Carolina

DAVID LANDRY, MD, FRCPC, B.Eng
Fellow in Neuroradiology, Department of Radiology and Biomedical Imaging, University of California, San Francisco, San Francisco, California

JUSTIN K. LAPLANTE, MD, MS
Department of Neuroradiology, University of Utah, Salt Lake City, Utah

INDU REKHA MEESA, MD, MS
Department of Radiology, University of Michigan Health system, Ann Arbor, Michigan; Summit Radiology, Fort Wayne, Indiana

DANIEL E. MELTZER, MD
Associate Professor of Radiology, Icahn School of Medicine, Mount Sinai Health System; Roosevelt Division, Mount Sinai Hospital, New York, New York

MEGAN K. MILLS, MD
Department of Radiology, University of Utah, Salt Lake City, Utah

XUAN V. NGUYEN, MD, PhD
Department of Radiology, The Ohio State University Wexner Medical Center, Columbus, Ohio

JORGE D. OLDAN, MD
Department of Radiology, Duke University Medical Center, Durham, North Carolina

C. DOUGLAS PHILLIPS, MD, FACR
Professor of Radiology; Director of Head and Neck Imaging, Department of Radiology, Weill Cornell Medical College, New York-Presbyterian Hospital, New York, New York

NICHOLAS S. PIERSON, MD
Department of Neuroradiology, University of Utah, Salt Lake City, Utah

BRUNO A. POLICENI, MD
Clinical Associate Professor, Department of Radiology, University of Iowa Hospitals and Clinics, Iowa City, Iowa

LUBDHA M. SHAH, MD
Department of Radiology, University of Utah, Salt Lake City, Utah

WENDY R.K. SMOKER, MD
Professor Emeritus, Department of Radiology, University of Iowa Hospitals and Clinics, Iowa City, Iowa

JULIE A. SOSA, MD, MA
Division of Surgical Oncology, Department of Surgery, Duke University Medical Center, Durham, North Carolina

ASHOK SRINIVASAN, MBBS, MD
Associate Professor and Director of Neuroradiology, Department of Radiology, University of Michigan Health system, Ann Arbor, Michigan

RICHARD H. WIGGINS III, MD, CIIP, FSIIM
Director of Head and Neck Imaging; Professor, Departments of Radiology, Otolaryngology, Head and Neck Surgery, and BioMedical Informatics, University of Utah Health Sciences Center, Salt Lake City, Utah

Contents

Preface: Head and Neck Imaging xi

Richard H. Wiggins III and Ashok Srinivasan

Imaging of the Skull Base: Anatomy and Pathology 1

Bruno A. Policeni and Wendy R.K. Smoker

The skull base is a critical landmark, separating intracranial from extracranial structures. This intricate anatomic structure has several foramina and crossing structures, which can be a challenge for novices. Comprehensive anatomic knowledge is critical for narrowing the differential diagnosis of lesions that may affect the skull base. These lesions can be divided into major categories to help in a systematic approach for skull base pathology evaluation.

Imaging of the Temporal Bone 15

Travis A. Abele and Richard H. Wiggins III

A variety of congenital, infectious, inflammatory, vascular, and benign and malignant neoplastic pathology affects the temporal bone. Knowledge of normal temporal bone anatomy and space-specific differential diagnoses is key to imaging interpretation of temporal bone. Correlation with clinical history and physical examination is vital to making the correct diagnosis or providing an appropriate differential. Computed tomography and magnetic resonance imaging are complementary imaging modalities in the evaluation of temporal bone abnormalities.

Orbital Imaging: A Pattern-Based Approach 37

Daniel E. Meltzer

Providing a concise and relevant differential diagnosis for clinicians who order imaging studies can be difficult for the interpreting radiologist. The myriad disease processes that occur in the orbit have overlapping features both clinically and at imaging. However, these disease entities can be categorized into a small set of relatively distinct patterns. In conjunction with careful consideration of the clinical history, a pattern-based approach to the interpretation of cross sectional imaging studies of the orbit can help the radiologist provide a list of possible causes for the computed tomography and magnetic resonance imaging findings.

Squamous Cell Carcinoma of the Upper Aerodigestive Tract: A Review 81

David Landry and Christine M. Glastonbury

Squamous cell carcinoma (SCCa) is the most common head and neck malignancy. The radiologist has several roles in the long-term management of patients with SCCa, the first of which is determining the extent of local disease spread and the presence of nodal metastases. The most widely used tumor staging system is the American Joint Committee on Cancer tumor node metastasis system, which creates the initial staging of SCCa patients. In this review the relevant reportable findings of pharyngeal SCCa are explored, and each subsite of the pharynx and larynx is addressed, from the nasopharynx to the hypopharynx.

Common Pediatric Head and Neck Congenital/Developmental Anomalies 181

Justin K. LaPlante, Nicholas S. Pierson, and Gary L. Hedlund

Pediatric head and neck neuroradiology is a broad and complex topic. This article focuses on several of the common and sometimes challenging pediatric head and neck congenital/developmental anomalies physicians may encounter in clinical practice. Although some diagnoses may be evident on physical examination, others may present a diagnostic dilemma. Patients may initially present with a variety of secondary findings. Imaging serves an important role in making a diagnosis, guiding referral, and in some cases even providing treatment options through interventional radiology. Key diagnostic criteria and critical points of interest for each diagnosis are presented.

Imaging of Vascular Lesions of the Head and Neck 197

Julius Griauzde and Ashok Srinivasan

The diagnosis of vascular lesions of the head and neck should be directed by classifying the lesions as tumors or malformations and by determining their flow characteristics. Location of the lesion is key when differentiating between vascular neoplasms. Ultrasonography is an appropriate screening tool; MRI is often used to confirm the diagnosis. Computed tomography can be used for further characterization of the lesion, particularly when there is bony involvement. In many cases, vascular lesions grow to be extensive. In these cases, percutaneous sclerotherapy or embolization therapy can be employed to aid in surgical resection.

Imaging of Head and Neck Emergencies 215

Justin L. Brucker and Lindell R. Gentry

The anatomy of the head and neck contains very few structures that could be considered expendable and, consequently, is exceptionally intolerant to infection, inflammation, and injury. Acute pathologic processes in this body region, therefore, tend to result in significant suffering, functional impairment, or life endangerment if the diagnosis is missed or treatment is delayed. Many emergent processes within the cervical region also need to be considered for their possible impact on structures within the head and chest, into which there are many routes for potential communication.

Index 253

PROGRAM OBJECTIVE

The objective of the *Radiologic Clinics of North America* is to keep practicing radiologists and radiology residents up to date with current clinical practice in radiology by providing timely articles reviewing the state of the art in patient care.

TARGET AUDIENCE

Practicing radiologists, radiology residents, and other health care professionals who provide patient care utilizing radiologic findings.

LEARNING OBJECTIVES

Upon completion of this activity, participants will be able to:

1. Review considerations in imaging of the head and neck including during emergency treatment.
2. Discuss considerations in pediatric head and neck imaging.
3. Review suprahyoid and infrahyoid neck imaging.

ACCREDITATION

The Elsevier Office of Continuing Medical Education (EOCME) is accredited by the Accreditation Council for Continuing Medical Education (ACCME) to provide continuing medical education for physicians.

The EOCME designates this enduring material for a maximum of 15 *AMA PRA Category 1 Credit*(s)™. Physicians should claim only the credit commensurate with the extent of their participation in the activity.

All other health care professionals requesting continuing education credit for this enduring material will be issued a certificate of participation.

DISCLOSURE OF CONFLICTS OF INTEREST

The EOCME assesses conflict of interest with its instructors, faculty, planners, and other individuals who are in a position to control the content of CME activities. All relevant conflicts of interest that are identified are thoroughly vetted by EOCME for fair balance, scientific objectivity, and patient care recommendations. EOCME is committed to providing its learners with CME activities that promote improvements or quality in healthcare and not a specific proprietary business or a commercial interest.

The planning committee, staff, authors and editors listed below have identified no financial relationships or relationships to products or devices they or their spouse/life partner have with commercial interest related to the content of this CME activity:

Travis A. Abele, MD; Justin L. Brucker, MD; J. Levi Chazen, MD; Laura B. Eisenmenger, MD; P. Leo Galvin, MD; Caryn Gamss, MD; Lindell R. Gentry, MD; Christine M. Glastonbury, MBBS; Julius Griauzde, MD; Ajay Gupta, MD; Gary L. Hedlund, DO; Kristen Helm; Jenny K. Hoang, MBBS; Brynne Hunter; David Landry, MD, FRCPC, B.Eng; Justin K. LaPlante, MD, MS; Sandy Lavery; Indu Rekha Meesa, MD, MS; Daniel E. Meltzer, MD; Frank H. Miller, MD; Megan K. Mills, MD; Xuan V. Nguyen, MD, PhD; Jorge D. Oldan, MD; C. Douglas Phillips, MD, FACR; Nicholas S. Pierson, MD; Bruno A. Policeni, MD; Lubdha M. Shah, MD; Wendy R.K. Smoker, MD; Julie A. Sosa, MD, MA; Ashok Srinivasan, MBBS, MD; Karthikeyan Subramaniam; John Vassallo; Richard H. Wiggins III, MD, CIIP, FSIIM.

The planning committee, staff, authors and editors listed below have identified financial relationships or relationships to products or devices they or their spouse/life partner have with commercial interest related to the content of this CME activity:

UNAPPROVED/OFF-LABEL USE DISCLOSURE

The EOCME requires CME faculty to disclose to the participants:

1. When products or procedures being discussed are off-label, unlabelled, experimental, and/or investigational (not US Food and Drug Administration [FDA] approved); and
2. Any limitations on the information presented, such as data that are preliminary or that represent ongoing research, interim analyses, and/or unsupported opinions. Faculty may discuss information about pharmaceutical agents that is outside of FDA-approved labelling. This information is intended solely for CME and is not intended to promote off-label use of these medications. If you have any questions, contact the medical affairs department of the manufacturer for the most recent prescribing information.

TO ENROLL

To enroll in the *Radiologic Clinics of North America* Continuing Medical Education program, call customer service at 1-800-654-2452 or sign up online at http://www.theclinics.com/home/cme. The CME program is available to subscribers for an additional annual fee of USD 315.

METHOD OF PARTICIPATION

In order to claim credit, participants must complete the following:

1. Complete enrolment as indicated above.

2. Read the activity.
3. Complete the CME Test and Evaluation. Participants must achieve a score of 70% on the test. All CME Tests and Evaluations must be completed online.

CME INQUIRIES/SPECIAL NEEDS

For all CME inquiries or special needs, please contact elsevierCME@elsevier.com.

RADIOLOGIC CLINICS OF NORTH AMERICA

FORTHCOMING ISSUES

March 2015
Coronary Artery Disease and the Myocardial Ischemic Cascade
U. Joseph Schoepf and James C. Carr, *Editors*

May 2015
Advanced MR Imaging in Clinical Practice
Hersh Chandarana, *Editor*

July 2015
Emergency Radiology
Savvas Nicolaou, *Editor*

RECENT ISSUES

November 2014
Update in Ultrasound
Leslie M. Scoutt, *Editor*

September 2014
Iatrogenic Conditions of the Chest, Abdomen, and Pelvis
Gabriela Gayer and Douglas S. Katz, *Editors*

July 2014
Adult Body MR
Frank H. Miller, *Editor*

ISSUE OF RELATED INTEREST

Neuroimaging Clinics, August 2014 (Vol. 24, No. 3)
Craniofacial Trauma
Deborah R. Shatzkes, *Editor*

Preface
Head and Neck Imaging

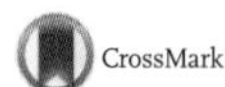

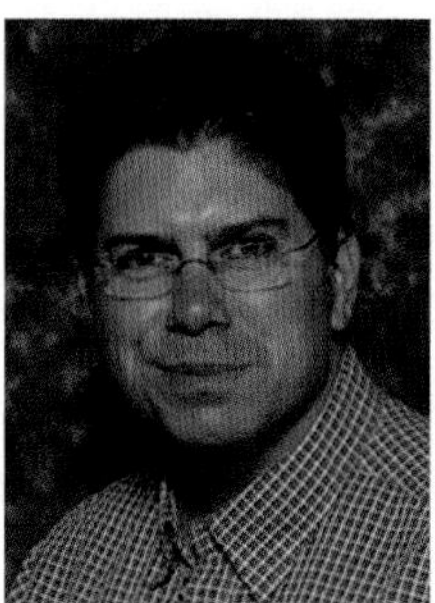

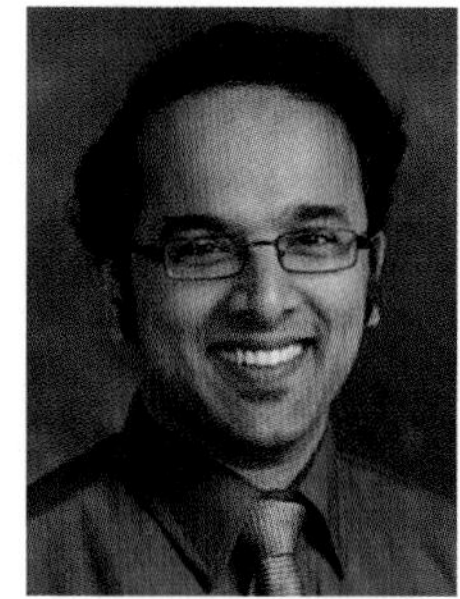

Richard H. Wiggins III, MD, CIIP, FSIIM Ashok Srinivasan, MBBS, MD
Editors

Hello, fellow intrepid head and neck imagers.

We are pleased to bring forth this issue of *Radiologic Clinics of North America* focusing on head and neck imaging. Even in the era of increasing subspecialization, the general radiologist continues to serve as the face of Imaging in the enterprise, and it is increasingly difficult for imagers to accurately evaluate complex head and neck studies. This issue covers a variety of head and neck imaging issues, from basic imaging anatomy to complex pathology, including new and advanced imaging techniques. We hope that this will help imagers learn and revise the fundamentals of head and neck imaging, and to break down the perceived complexity of the head and neck anatomic landscape by approaching sections and compartments in a systematic manner.

These articles have been organized by anatomical regions, pathologic entities, and clinical presentations, highlighting the importance of clinical information on interpreting these difficult cases. Each article provides a refresher of the cross-sectional anatomy and focuses on the clinical and imaging manifestations of the common pathologies likely to be encountered in general practice. Rare and uncommon conditions are also discussed when appropriate. Each article is also rich with "take-home messages" with numerous illustrations to reinforce the teaching points. There is enough material for both the reader who is looking for a quick reference and the enthusiast interested in widening their knowledge base. The ability to critically analyze cross-sectional imaging and to recognize the strengths and weaknesses of CT and MRI to arrive at the correct diagnosis is discussed from these different viewpoints in the issue's articles.

We wish to thank all the expert authors for their invaluable contributions and attention to detail in their articles, which are critical to the success of any journal. Last, we would like to thank the publisher, for giving us the honor of editing this issue, and our families, for the time to devote to this task.

Sincerely,

Richard H. Wiggins III, MD, CIIP, FSIIM
Departments of Radiology, Otolaryngology, Head and Neck Surgery, and BioMedical Informatics
University of Utah Health Sciences Center
30 North, 1900 East, #1A071
Salt Lake City, UT 84132–2140, USA

Ashok Srinivasan, MBBS, MD
Department of Radiology
University of Michigan Health System
1500 E Medical Center
Ann Arbor, MI 48109, USA

E-mail addresses:
Richard.Wiggins@hsc.utah.edu (R.H. Wiggins)
ashoks@med.umich.edu (A. Srinivasan)

Radiol Clin N Am 53 (2015) xi
http://dx.doi.org/10.1016/j.rcl.2014.10.001
0033-8389/15/$ – see front matter

Imaging of the Skull Base
Anatomy and Pathology

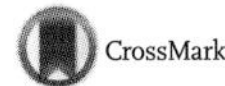

Bruno A. Policeni, MD*, Wendy R.K. Smoker, MD

KEYWORDS

• Skull base anatomy • Skull base pathology • Foramina • Cranial nerves • CT • MR imaging

KEY POINTS

- The skull base is divided into anterior, middle, and posterior sections with specific anatomic landmarks in each of them.
- Disorders affecting the skull base can be categorized as congenital, traumatic, infectious, tumor-like, and neoplastic.
- Imaging plays an important role in the diagnosis of skull base lesions.

INTRODUCTION

The skull base (SB) is a major landmark that acts as a divider for the intracranial and the extracranial compartments. The anatomy of this area can be a challenge for novices given the several communication pathways along with the crossing structures (**Box 1**). The SB is mainly formed by bone; however, disorders can also arise from the crossing structures (ie, nerves, vessels, and so forth) as well as the adjacent soft tissues. The surgical approach has evolved, with several of these disorders currently approached through endoscopic surgery, making presurgical imaging characterization, as well as anatomic localization, critical. Approaching these lesions from an imaging perspective requires comprehensive knowledge of anatomic landmarks (**Box 2**), communicating foramina, and imaging characteristics of common disorders to allow precise description and anatomic localization. Surgical approach selection relies on several imaging findings, including location of the lesion and involvement of adjacent structures.[1]

SKULL BASE ANATOMY

The SB forms the floor of the intracranial compartment and serves as the pathway for most of the critical structures that connect the central nervous system with the extracranial compartment. It is divided anatomically into 3 main segments: anterior, middle, and posterior (**Fig. 1**).

Anterior Skull Base

The anterior cranial fossa (ACF) is formed by the orbital plates of the frontal bone laterally and the cribriform plate (CP) of the ethmoid bone in the midline, which also includes the crista galli. It is formed posteriorly by the lesser sphenoid wing as well as the anterior part of the greater sphenoid wing. The frontal sinuses, ethmoid sinuses, nasal cavity, and orbits are just inferior to the ACF. The frontal lobes and meninges are just superior to the ACF. The CP forms the roof of the nasal cavity and contains numerous small foramina that transmit the olfactory folia from the nasal mucosa to the olfactory bulbs.[2] The fovea ethmoidalis (FE) is located more superiorly than the CP and is formed by the medial extension of the orbital plates. The lateral lamella connects the CP with the FE. The height difference between the CP and the FE was classified by Keros as type I if it measured 1 to 3 mm, type 2 if it measured 4 to 7 mm, and type III if it measured more than 8 mm.[3] The foramen cecum is located in the midline, posterior to

Disclosure: The authors have nothing to disclose.

Department of Radiology, University of Iowa Hospitals and Clinics, 200 Hawkins Drive, Iowa City, IA 52246, USA
* Corresponding author.
E-mail address: bruno-policeni@uiowa.edu

Radiol Clin N Am 53 (2015) 1–14
http://dx.doi.org/10.1016/j.rcl.2014.09.005

Box 1
Communication pathways and crossing structures

ACF

- Foramen cecum: emissary veins to the superior sagittal sinus
- Foramina of cribriform plate: olfactory fibers bundles (I)
- Optic canal: optic nerve (II) and ophthalmic artery

Middle cranial fossa:

- Superior orbital fissure: ophthalmic (V1), oculomotor (III), trochlear (IV), and abducens (VI) nerves; superior and inferior ophthalmic veins
- Vidian canal: vidian nerve and artery
- Foramen rotundum: maxillary nerve (V2)
- Foramen ovale: mandibular nerve (V3)
- Foramen spinosum: middle meningeal artery

Posterior cranial fossa:

- Internal auditory canal: facial (VII) and vestibular-cochlear (VIII) nerves

  Labyrinthine artery
- Jugular foramen: glossopharyngeal (IX), vagus (X), and spinal accessory nerve (XI)

  Inferior petrosal sinus and sigmoid sinus
- Hypoglossal canal: hypoglossal nerve (XII)
- Foramen magnum: medulla oblongata

  Anterior and posterior spinal arteries and vertebral artery
- Stylomastoid foramen: facial (VII) nerve

  Stylomastoid artery

Box 2
Important anatomic landmarks

ACF

- Cribriform plate
- Crista galli
- Fovea ethmoidalis
- Lateral lamellae
- Foramen cecum
- Planum sphenoidale

Middle cranial fossa

- Tuberculum sellae
- Sella turcica
- Pterygopalatine fossa
- Foramen rotundum
- Vidian canal
- Foramen ovale
- Foramen spinosum
- Anterior clinoid process
- Optic canal
- Superior orbital fissure
- Carotid canal
- Foramen lacerum

Posterior cranial fossa

- Foramen magnum
- Internal auditory canal
- Vestibular aqueduct
- Jugular foramen
- Hypoglossal canal

the nasal bones; it is typically obliterated by a fibrous structure.[4] The anterior ethmoidal artery travels through the roof of the anterior ethmoid sinus as it goes from the orbit to the anterior SB (ASB) and can be a potential area of risk for surgical damage during endoscopic sinus surgery.[5]

Middle Skull Base

The middle SB (MSB) is mainly formed by the sphenoid bone and the temporal bone anterior to the petrous ridge.[6] The sphenoid bone is composed of a central body and, laterally, the greater and lesser wings, and inferiorly there are also the pterygoid processes. The MSB is an intricate anatomic structure with several foramina that transmit nerves and vessels coursing between the intracranial and extracranial compartments allowing disorders to spread between compartments.

The anterior portion of the sphenoid body articulates centrally with the CP where it has a smooth central surface named the planum sphenoidale. Also in the body are the tuberculum sellae and sella turcica, which are, respectively, posterior to the planum sphenoidale. The sella turcica harbors the pituitary gland. The dorsum sella constitutes the posterior part of the sella turcica.[7]

The greater wing of the sphenoid laterally constitutes most of the MSB. It forms the posterior wall of the pterygopalatine fossa where the V2 ganglion is located. The maxillary nerve (V2) traverses the SB within the foramen rotundum and the vidian nerve traverses the skull base in the vidian canal. The posterolateral wall forms the

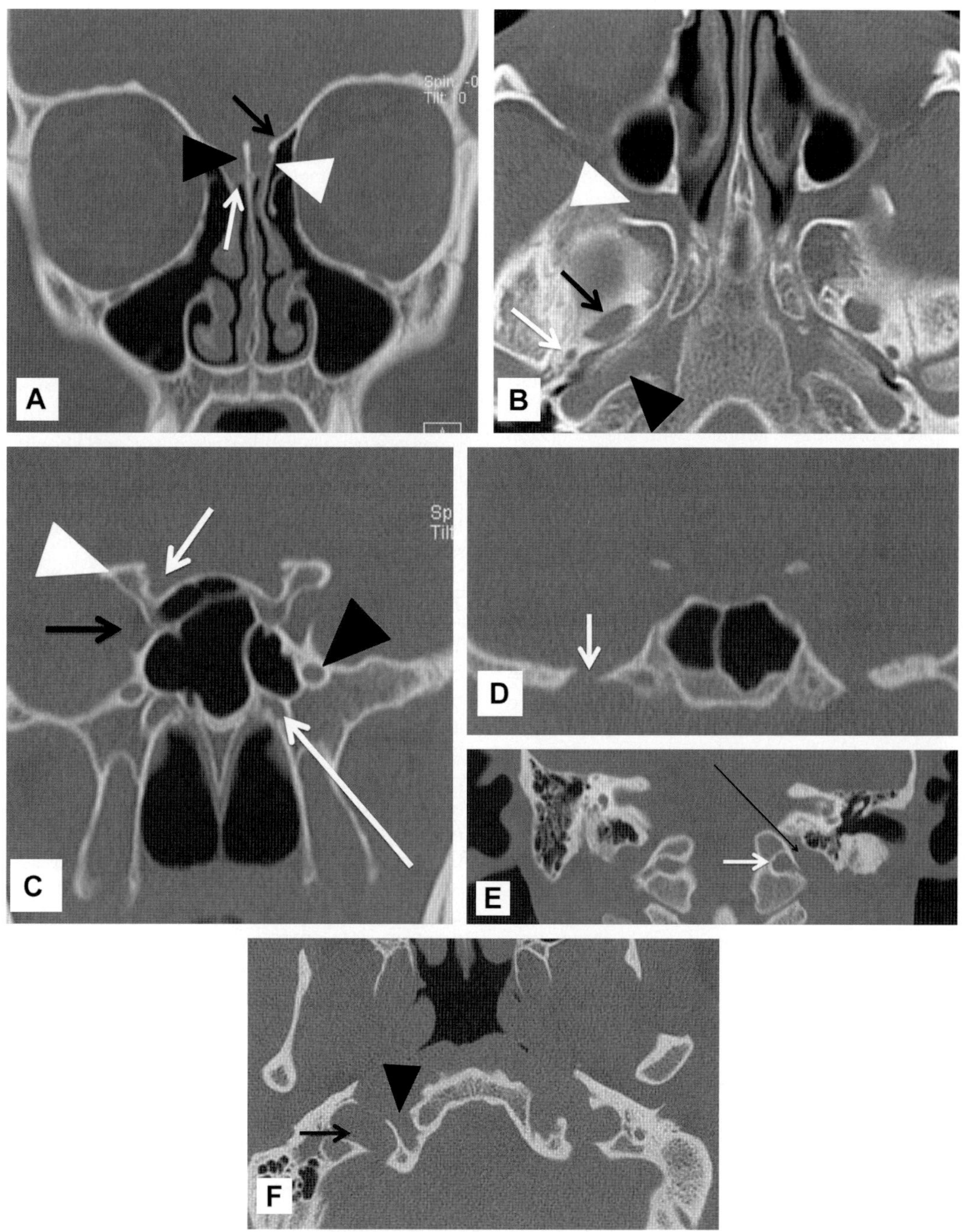

Fig. 1. SB anatomy. (*A*) Cribriform plate (*white arrow*), fovea ethmoidales (*black arrow*), crista galli (*black arrowhead*), lateral lamellae (*white arrowhead*). (*B*) Foramen spinosum (*white arrow*), foramen ovale (*black arrow*), pterygopalatine fossa (*white arrowhead*), carotid canal (*black arrowhead*). (*C*) Optic canal (*short white arrow*), superior orbital fissure (*black arrow*), foramen rotundum (*black arrowhead*), anterior clinoid (*white arrowhead*), vidian canal (*long white arrow*). (*D*) Foramen ovale (*white arrow*). (*E*) Hypoglossal canal (*white arrow*), jugular foramen (*black arrow*). (*F*) Hypoglossal canal (*arrowhead*), jugular foramen (*arrow*).

inferior border of the superior orbital fissure (SOF), which serves as a pathway for cranial nerves (CNs) III (oculomotor), IV (trochlear), VI (abducens), and V1 (ophthalmic), as well as the ophthalmic vein. The SOF is also bordered by the lesser sphenoid wing superiorly. The anterior clinoid is an anatomic landmark that separates the SOF from the optic canal, which transmits the optic nerve. The foramen ovale and foramen spinosum are the 2 other important foramina located in the greater sphenoid wing. The foramen ovale is located more anteromedially and serves as the pathway for the mandibular nerve (V3) into the masticator space. Through the foramen spinosum, located more posterolaterally, courses the middle meningeal artery.

Posterior Skull Base

The posterior SB (PSB) is formed by the occipital bone and parts of the temporal and sphenoid bones. The sphenoid and occipital bones form the clivus (basisphenoid plus basiocciput) located in the midline posterior to the dorsum sella. The occipital bone fuses laterally with the temporal bone. The foramen magnum is the largest SB foramen and is located in the midline PSB, through which transverse the medulla oblongata/spinal cord.

The internal auditory canal, located in the posterior surface of the petrous temporal bone, transmits CN VII (facial) and CN VIII (vestibulocochlear) to the geniculate ganglion and inner ear structures, respectively. The vestibular aqueduct is also located in the temporal bone, posterior to the internal auditory canal, and contains the endolymphatic sac.

The jugular foramen is bordered by the occipital and temporal bones. It is divided by an incomplete fibrous or bony septum into 2 parts: the anteromedial pars nervosa contains CN IX (glossopharyngeal) and the inferior petrosal sinus, whereas the posterolateral pars vascularis contains CN X (vagus) and CN XI (accessory) as well as the jugular vein, located laterally to the nerves.[8]

The hypoglossal canal is located in the occipital bone, anteromedial to the jugular foramen and superior to the occipital condyle, serving as the pathway for CN XII (hypoglossal). The hypoglossal canal lies in close proximity to the jugular foramen[9] and it is common to encounter disorders involving both.

DISORDERS

Given the difficult access to physical examination, imaging has a primary role in the work-up of patients with suspected SB disorders. The list of disorders (**Table 1**) is extensive and can be divided into major categories, including congenital, traumatic, infectious, tumorlike, and neoplastic.

Congenital

An encephalocele, which is a herniation of meninges with cerebral spinal fluid that may or may not contain brain tissue, shows a direct intracranial communication. These lesions typically show high T2 signal because of cerebrospinal fluid (CSF) surrounding the herniated brain parenchyma when it is present within the herniation (**Fig. 2**). Nasal encephaloceles are categorized as frontoethmoidal (sincipital) and basal. The frontoethmoidal encephalocele presents as a facial mass at the root of the nose (nasofrontal) or causes proptosis and displacement of the eye (nasoethmoidal),[10] with the intracranial connection typically anterior to the CP. Basal encephaloceles may cause nasal obstruction with the connection either at or posterior to the CP.

Areas of arrested pneumatization (**Fig. 3**) may occur, typically involving the basisphenoid. These areas are usually incidentally noted and should be treated as do-not-touch lesions. They are nonexpansile, fat-containing, geographic lesions with internal curvilinear calcification and a peripheral sclerotic margin.[10]

Traumatic

The anterior cranial fossa (ACF) (**Fig. 4**) is the most common SB location for CSF leak, typically posttraumatic in origin. However, this can also occur in the middle cranial fossa (MCF) and PCF. Most (80%) are a result of nonsurgical trauma. Surgical procedures resulting in trauma to the ACF (16%) and nontraumatic causes (4%) comprise the remaining 20%.[11] Most patients with nonsurgical trauma present within the first week, typically with unilateral rhinorrhea. The watery rhinorrhea can be tested for beta-2 transferrin to confirm the CSF origin. Thin-section computed tomography (CT) is the imaging of choice to detect the bone defect.

Infectious

In the MCF and posterior cranial fossa (PCF), osteomyelitis is typically initiated by ear infection in elderly diabetic patients (**Fig. 5**). The typical pathogen is *Pseudomonas aeruginosa*. This condition has been called malignant otitis because of its mortality and poor response to treatment.[12] Evaluation with imaging typically initiates with CT. However, initially soft tissue inflammation is the only finding, associated with mastoid effusion because 30% of the affected bone needs to be demineralized to appear eroded on CT.[13] MR imaging better shows the soft tissue abnormality. Atypical SB osteomyelitis that is centered in the sphenoid and occipital bone, rather than the temporal bone, may also occur.[14] This is a challenging diagnosis because most of these patients present with isolated headache without cranial neuropathy.

Table 1
SB disorders

Common SB Lesions	CT	MR Imaging
Sinonasal tumor (ACF)	Soft tissue mass with bone destruction	Best to evaluate brain parenchyma and meningeal invasion
Encephalocele (ACF of MCF)	Bone defect	Direct intracranial communication High T2 signal caused by CSF surrounding herniated brain parenchyma when that is present within the herniation
Chordoma (MCF)	Midline soft tissue mass with lytic, expansile pattern	High T2 signal Small foci of increased T1 signal Honeycomb pattern enhancement
Chondrosarcoma (MCF)	Off midline (sphenopetroclival and petroclival, petrous bone) Bone destruction with punctuate areas of chondroid matrix	High T2 signal Mild peripheral and septal enhancement
Invasive pituitary adenoma (MCF)	SB invasion with bone destruction	Nonidentification of a normal pituitary Soft tissue mass
Nasopharyngeal cancer (MCF)	Nasopharyngeal soft tissue with bone erosion (best appreciated on MR imaging)	Nasopharyngeal mass Precontrast T1W images show replacement of the marrow corresponding with tumor invasion
Paraganglioma (PCF)	Permeative erosion	Salt-and-pepper appearance
Meningioma (ACF, MCF, and PCF)	Hyperostosis Intrinsic calcification	Extra-axial mass, isointense to cortex on T1 and T2 Avid postcontrast enhancement
Schwannoma (ACF, MCF, and PCF)	Scalloping Remodeling	Cystic component Dumbbell shape
Fibrous dysplasia (ACF, MCF and PCF)	Ground-glass appearance	T2 signal is variable Postcontrast enhancement
Metastatic disease (ACF, MCF, and PCF)	Lytic, sclerotic, or permeative lesion	Precontrast T1W images show replacement of normal fatty marrow

Abbreviations: ACF, anterior cranial fossa; CSF, cerebrospinal fluid; MCF, middle cranial fossa; PCF, posterior cranial fossa.

Tumorlike

Fibrous dysplasia

Fibrous dysplasia (FD) is a developmental abnormality that can affect any bone and is characterized by a highly disorganized mixture of immature fibrous tissue and fragments of immature trabecular bone.[15] FD is termed monostotic if it presents with 1 lesion or polyostotic when it has a widespread distribution with multiple lesions that affect many bones. FD is usually an isolated skeletal finding but can sometimes occur as a component of McCune-Albright syndrome, which is also associated with precocious puberty. The skull and facial bones are the affected sites in 10% to 25% of patients with monostotic FD and in 50% of patients with polyostotic FD.[15] FD can be a challenging diagnosis on MR imaging and may mimic a tumor because of the amount of fibrous tissue that shows avid contrast enhancement. The T2 signal is variable. Some lesions with a highly mineralized matrix show correspondingly low T2 signal intensity, whereas lesions with high fibrous tissue content and cystic spaces show high T2 signal intensity. Unlike mature scar tissues that show low signal intensities on all imaging sequences, the fibrous tissues in FD are metabolically active, thus accounting for the high signal intensities on T2-weighted images.[15] CT typically shows a ground-glass appearance.[16] Fibrous dysplasia usually shows nonspecific increased uptake of radiotracer on bone scans (**Fig. 6**).[17]

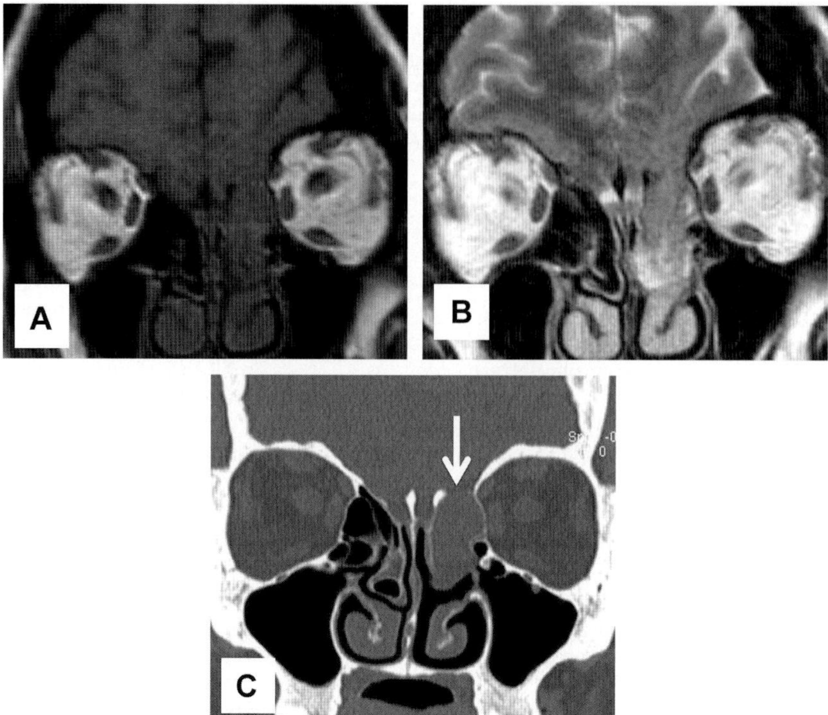

Fig. 2. Ethmoid encephalocele. Coronal T1-weighted (T1W) (*A*) and T2-weighted (T2W) (*B*) MR images show a mass in the left ethmoid cavity, directly connected to the brain parenchyma and surrounded by CSF. Coronal computed tomography (CT) (*C*) shows the bone defect in the FE (*arrow*).

Neoplastic

Sinonasal tumors

In the ASB paranasal sinus and nasal cavity lesions can involve adjacent bone and brain parenchyma.[18] Imaging is an important part of the diagnostic evaluation, defining lesion extent, which is critical for accurate presurgical planning. Involvement of adjacent structures, such as the orbits and brain parenchyma/meninges, is important for the surgeon to know in order to decide whether the tumor is surgically resectable.[2] SB and orbital involvement are major prognostic factors for sinonasal tumors.[19] MR imaging is the best technique to evaluate meningeal, parenchymal, and orbital involvement. Meningeal and brain parenchymal involvement is defined by nodular enhancement of the meninges and intraparenchymal enhancement as well as brain edema (**Fig. 7**).

Nasopharyngeal carcinoma

This malignant tumor is different from the other head and neck squamous cell carcinomas. It originates in the nasopharynx (typically the lateral recess) and is caused by an interaction of genetic susceptibility, environmental factors (such as exposure to chemical carcinogens), and infection

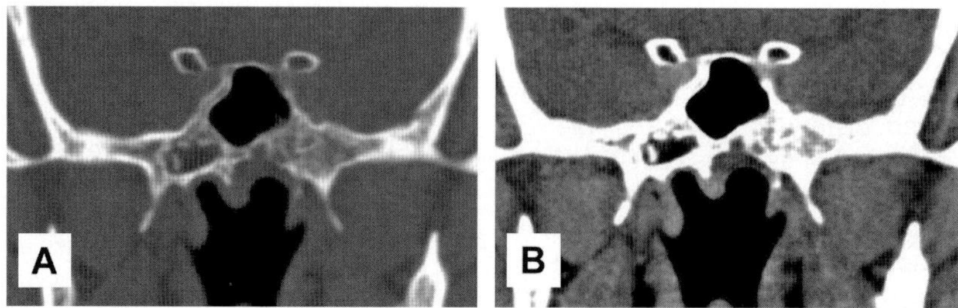

Fig. 3. Arrested pneumatization. Coronal CT bone (*A*) and soft tissue windows (*B*) show a nonexpansile, fat-containing lesion with internal curvilinear calcifications in the right basisphenoid.

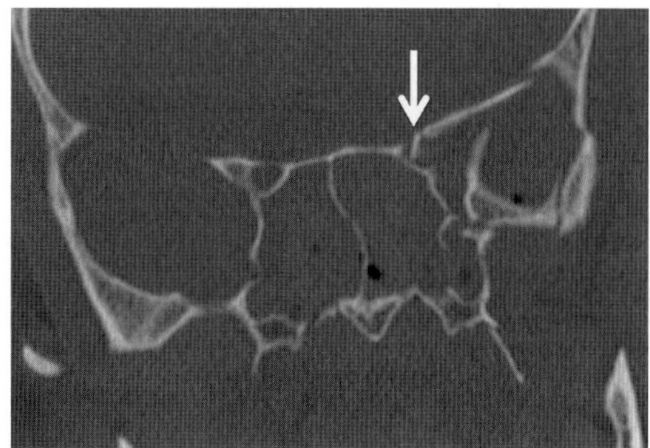

Fig. 4. Trauma. Coronal CT shows multiple SB fractures. Note bone fragment in left optic canal (*arrow*).

with the Epstein-Barr virus[20]; however, its cause is not completely understood. The incidence is 2-fod to 3-fold higher in men than in women.[21]

MR imaging is the study of choice to evaluate bone involvement of nasopharyngeal carcinoma (NPC), with the T1-weighted precontrast sequence best showing replacement of marrow corresponding with tumor invasion (**Fig. 8**). The clivus, pterygoid bones, body of the sphenoid, and apices of the petrous bones are most commonly involved.[20] MR imaging is also useful to show retropharyngeal lymph node involvement. Patients who have received radiation treatment may present a diagnostic conundrum attempting to differentiate tumor recurrence from radiation necrosis. In these cases MR imaging, CT, and PET can be equivocal and surgical sampling may be necessary.

Invasive pituitary adenoma

Pituitary adenoma is the most common pituitary tumor in adults. These lesions can be classified as microadenomas when smaller than 1 cm, or macroadenomas when larger than 1 cm. Macroadenomas most commonly show suprasellar extension, but, on rare occasions, infrasellar and SB invasion can also be seen (**Fig. 9**). SB invasion with bone destruction can pose a challenging diagnosis because these lesions may not have a suprasellar component and only invade the bone. Most of these patients are imaged with MR imaging, which shows a soft tissue mass with bone destruction. The nonidentification of a normal pituitary gland suggests a tumor that is originating from the pituitary gland. There are reports of pure ectopic pituitary adenomas, which are thought to originate from the craniopharyngeal duct. Most of these lesions have been reported in the sphenoid sinus, cavernous sinus, or nasopharynx.[22]

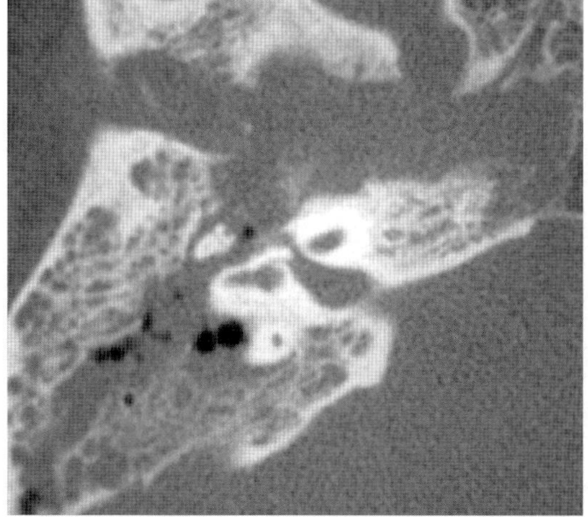

Fig. 5. Malignant external otitis. Axial temporal bone CT shows opacification with erosion of the right mastoid air cells and temporal bone.

Metastases

Osseous metastatic disease (**Fig. 10**) can affect any of the 3 SB compartments. Most primary tumors are breast, lung, and prostate carcinomas.[23] Clinical presentations vary. Some patients may initially be asymptomatic and only start to show symptoms once the metastatic lesion grows and compresses adjacent structures, and symptoms vary depending on lesion location.[24] The imaging characteristics are nonspecific. These lesions can be detected on CT, MR imaging, and bone scan. MR imaging, without and with contrast, is the most comprehensive imaging study to detect and define adjacent structural involvement by these lesions. In particular, T1-weighted precontrast imaging is most useful to show replacement of normal fatty marrow and diffusion-weighted imaging shows restriction caused by the typical increased tumor cellularity. Radiotherapy is typically the first line of treatment; a few patients may be treated surgically, including those with unknown primary tumors or resectable large solitary metastases, and patients on palliative radiotherapy with progressive neurologic deficit.[25]

Meningioma

SB meningiomas (**Fig. 11**) account for 20% to 30% of all intracranial meningiomas.[26] These lesions can be located in several sites along the SB, including the olfactory groove, tuberculum sella and sphenoid wing in the ACF, cavernous sinus, petroclival junction in the MCF, and jugular foramen or foramen magnum in the PCF. Most meningiomas are benign and show a slow growth pattern; however, some recur after treatment and show aggressive behavior.[27] An SB location does not contribute to increased mortality or morbidity compared with other intracranial

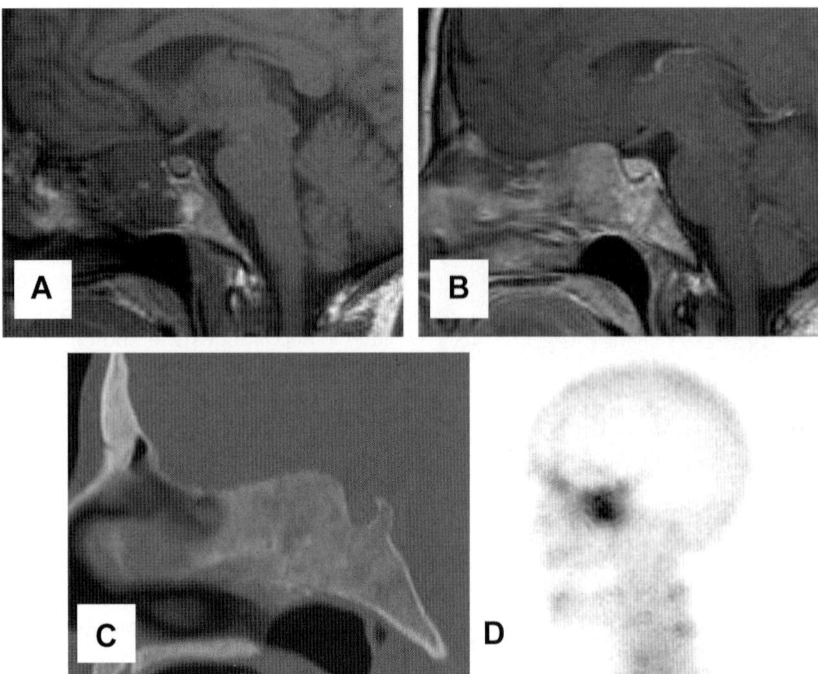

Fig. 6. FD. Sagittal T1W precontrast (*A*) and postcontrast (*B*) MR images show a mass with low signal intensity in the clivus with avid enhancement. Sagittal CT (*C*) shows typical ground-glass appearance. Bone scan (*D*) shows uptake in the lesion.

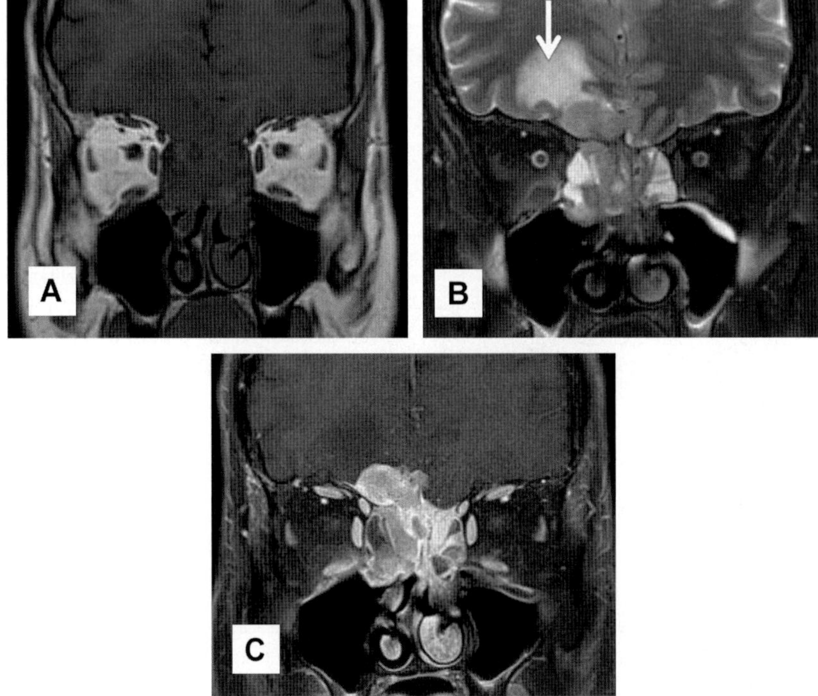

Fig. 7. Sinonasal undifferentiated carcinoma. Coronal precontrast T1W (*A*), postcontrast T1W (*B*), and T2W (*C*) MR images show a heterogeneous enhancing soft tissue mass in the nasal cavity/ethmoid air cells with invasion of the SB and brain parenchyma. Note associated brain edema (*arrow*).

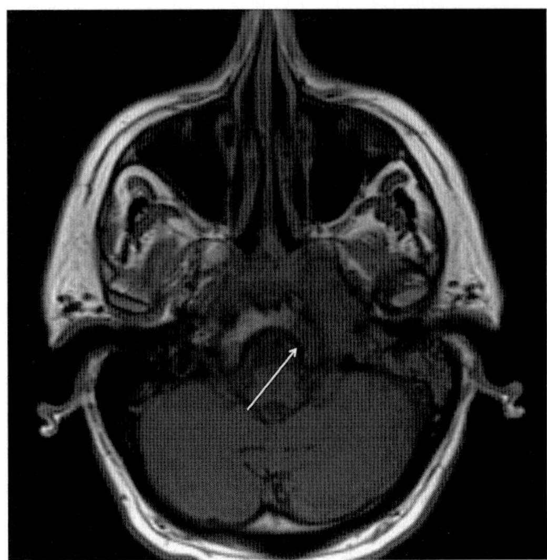

Fig. 8. NPC. Axial T1W MR without contrast shows a left nasopharyngeal mass with involvement of the left clivus (*arrow*).

locations.[28] Most meningiomas present on imaging as extra-axial masses with isointense signal to the cortex on T1-weighted and T2-weighted images and avid postcontrast enhancement. The dural tail is a feature of these lesions, which represents dural infiltration versus reactive vascularity. These lesions can show intrinsic calcification, which is best appreciated on CT. Associated bone changes are seen in some of these lesions, consistent with hyperostosis. Primary jugular foramen meningiomas are characterized by extensive bone infiltration, which can extend into the middle ear cavity, internal auditory canal, hypoglossal canal, clivus, carotid canal, and/or posterior fossa.[29] This appearance is different from other lesions that arise in the jugular foramen, as described in this article.

Nerve sheath tumors

Nerve sheath tumors (NSTs) of the cranial nerves can occur along the SB. These lesions accounts

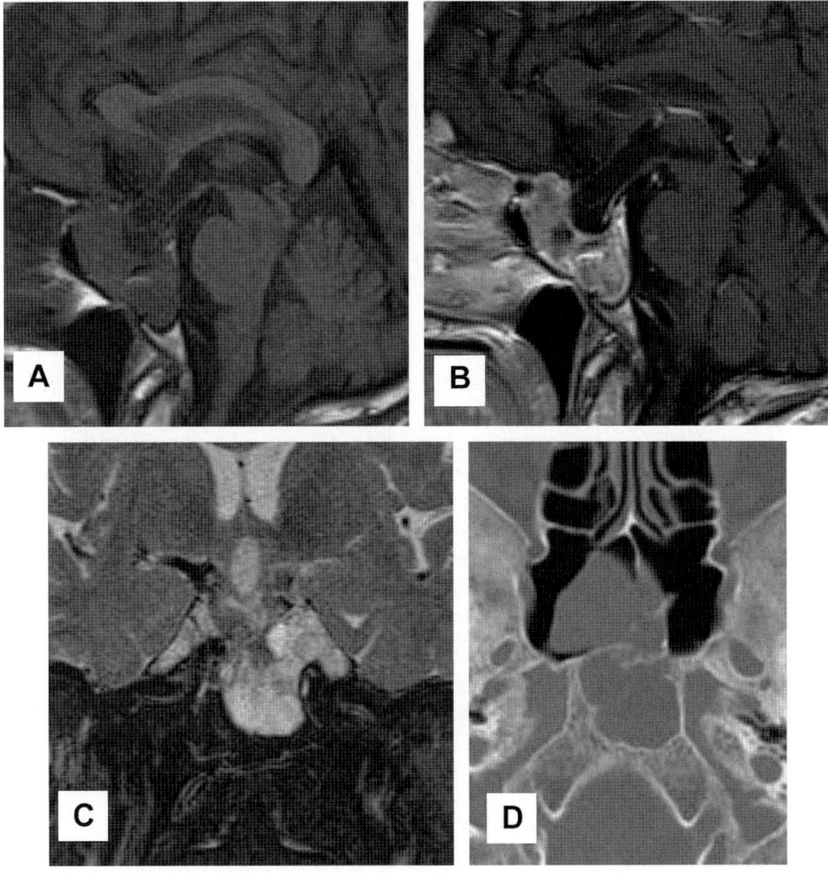

Fig. 9. Invasive pituitary adenoma. Sagittal T1W precontrast (*A*), postcontrast (*B*), and coronal T2W (*C*) MR images show a sella mass with infrasellar extension. A normal pituitary gland is not identified. Axial CT (*D*) shows the bone erosion in the clivus.

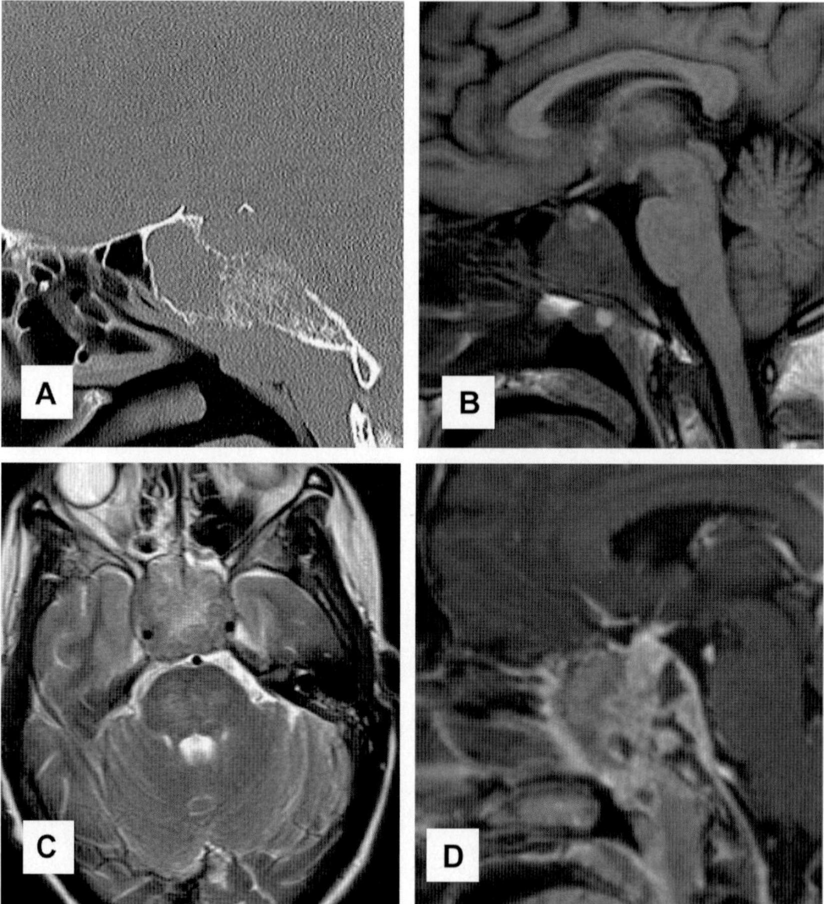

Fig. 10. Metastatic lung cancer. Sagittal CT (*A*) shows a permeative lytic lesion in the clivus. Sagittal T1W (*B*) and axial T2W (*C*) MR images show replacement of the clivus marrow with expansion. Two-month follow-up sagittal T1W postcontrast (*D*) MR image shows heterogeneous enhancement with enlargement of the clivus mass consistent with refractory disease.

for 5% to 10 % of all intracranial neoplasms.[30] Vestibular schwannoma is the most common, followed by the trigeminal NST.[31] NSTs can also occur in the jugular foramen (CNs IX, X, and XI) (**Fig. 12**) and the hypoglossal canal (CN XII). Imaging shows an enhancing tubular mass along the pathway of the parent nerve with a dumbbell shape where it transverses the foramen. On MR imaging the T2-weighted sequence can show cystic components within these lesions. CT is the best technique to show associated smooth bone erosion and foraminal widening as the lesion extends through the SB foramen.

Paragangliomas

Paragangliomas are neuroendocrine neoplasms that occur in different body sites. In the head and neck they occur in 4 main sites: the carotid bifurcation (carotid body tumor), high carotid space (vagal paraganglioma), jugular foramen (jugular paraganglioma), and cochlear promontory (tympanicum paraganglioma). The jugular paraganglioma (**Fig. 13**) is most pertinent for this discussion, given its location in the jugular foramen. Imaging shows a soft tissue mass in the jugular foramen. MR may show a salt-and-pepper appearance if the lesion is large enough, with the "pepper" thought to represent flow voids and the "salt" thought to represent slow flow or hemorrhagic foci within the lesion.[8] Large lesions may extend to the middle ear cavity and are called jugulotympanic paragangliomas.[32] Given the infiltrative pattern, CT is the best technique to show the patchy destruction of adjacent bone.

Chordoma

Chordoma is a rare tumor that originates from the notochord and is most commonly seen in the sacrum and spheno-occipital regions.[33] These lesions are usually centrally located. CT typically

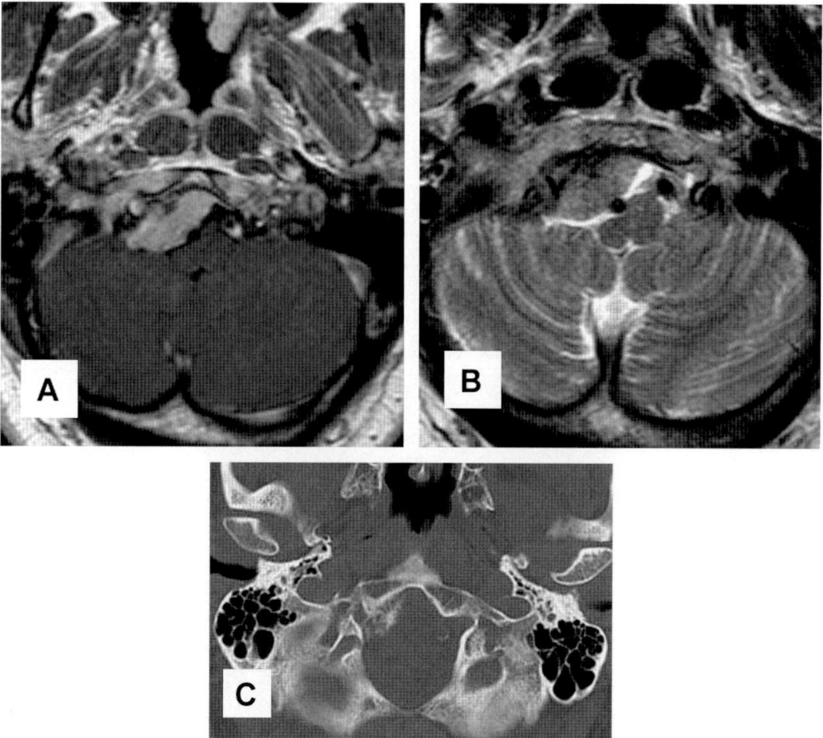

Fig. 11. Meningioma. Axial T1W postcontrast (*A*) and T2W (*B*) MR images show an extra-axial enhancing lesion adjacent to the clivus. Axial CT (*C*) shows calcification within the mass.

shows a midline soft tissue mass with a lytic, expansile pattern. Small, irregular, intratumoral calcifications may be seen and likely represent residual fragments from bone destruction, as opposed to dystrophic calcification. There is a chondroid variant of these tumors that is more likely to show real intratumoral calcification.[34] MR imaging is superior in defining the intrinsic characteristics of the soft tissue mass as well as surrounding structural involvement. The T2-weighted sequence manifests characteristic high signal intensity within the mass, which likely correlates with increased water content. The T1-weighted sequence can show small foci of increased signal, related to intratumoral blood. Postcontrast imaging shows a septated, ill-defined enhancement, which has been defined as having the appearance of honeycomb (**Fig. 14**).[34]

Chondrosarcoma

Chondrosarcoma is a malignant bone tumor with a chondroid matrix. The tumor is slow growing with a

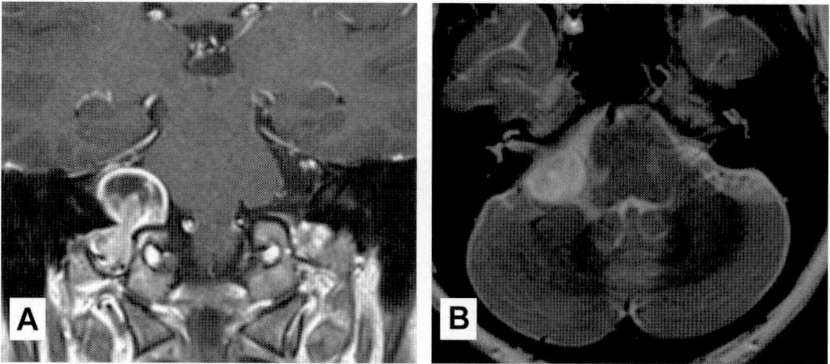

Fig. 12. Schwannoma. Coronal T1W postcontrast (*A*) and axial T2W (*B*) MR images show an enhancing dumbbell-shaped mass traversing the right jugular foramen with high T2 signal.

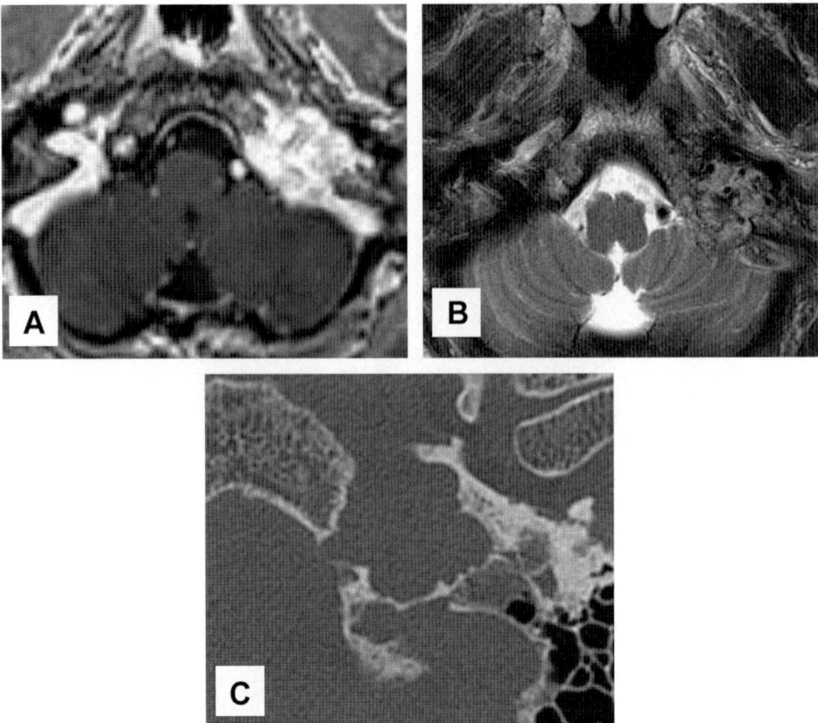

Fig. 13. Jugular paraganglioma. Axial T1W postcontrast (*A*) and T2W (*B*) MR images show an avidly enhancing mass in the left jugular foramen with flow voids, best seen on T2. Axial CT (*C*) shows the permeative destruction of the jugular foramen.

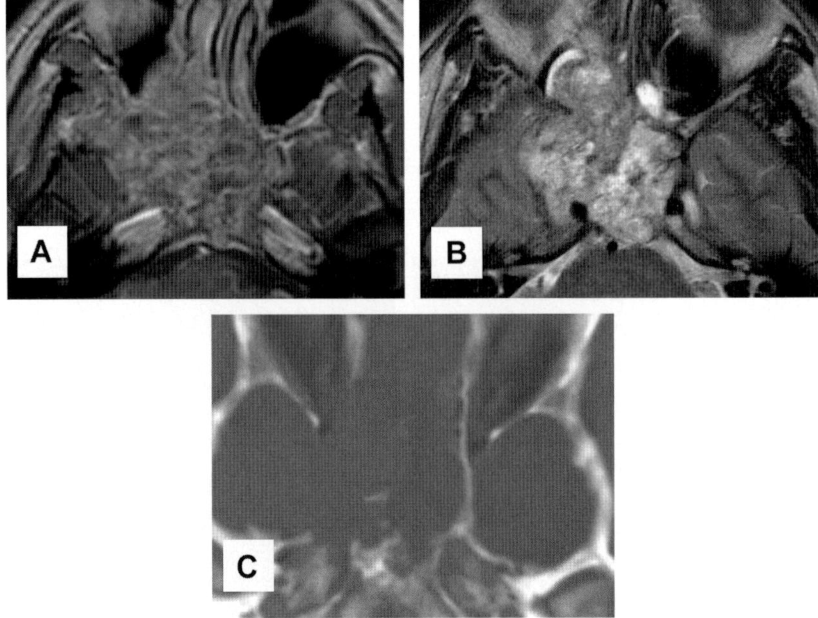

Fig. 14. Chordoma. Axial T1W postcontrast (*A*) and T2W (*B*) MR images show a midline heterogeneous enhancing mass with high T2 signal eroding the clivus. Axial CT (*C*) shows the associated clivus destruction.

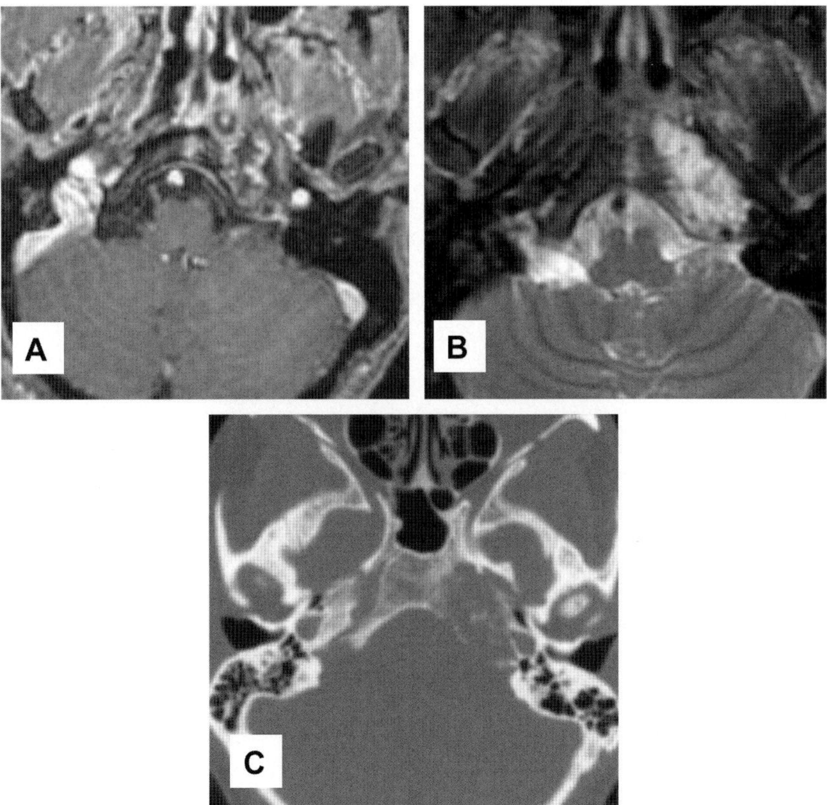

Fig. 15. Chondrosarcoma. Axial T1W postcontrast (*A*) and T2W (*B*) MR images show an off-midline heterogeneous enhancing mass with high T2 signal at the left petroclival synchondrosis. Axial CT (*C*) shows the chondroid matrix associated with this lesion.

high local recurrence rate, and is the second most common malignant bone tumor after osteosarcoma. The most common site is the pelvis. The head and neck account for only 1% to 12 % of cases, with most of these tumors originating from the jaw, paranasal sinus, nasal cavity, maxilla, and cervical spine.[35] In the SB these lesions are typically located off midline in the sphenopetroclival and petroclival regions or the adjacent petrous bone.[36] CT and MR imaging show bone destruction with areas of chondroid matrix, best seen on CT. The areas that are not mineralized have a characteristic high T2 signal because of the high water content. Postcontrast imaging shows mild peripheral and septal enhancement, which corresponds with the decreased vascularity of these tumors, helping to differentiate them from more vascular tumors such as meningiomas and skull metastases (**Fig. 15**).[37]

SUMMARY

Knowledge of anatomy is critical when evaluating lesions that affect the SB. Given the remote location and difficulties of physical examination, imaging plays an important role in defining the extent of disorders and allowing the interpreter to narrow the diagnosis to a specific anatomic region. Separating disorders into major categories also allows helps clinicians to provide a differential diagnosis.

REFERENCES

1. de Divitiis E, Laws ER Jr. The transnasal versus transcranial approach to lesions of the anterior skull base. World Neurosurg 2013;80(6):728–31.
2. Parmar H, Gujar S, Shah G, et al. Imaging of the anterior skull base. Neuroimaging Clin N Am 2009; 19(3):427–39.
3. Erdem G, Erdem T, Miman MC, et al. A radiological anatomic study of the cribriform plate compared with constant structures. Rhinology 2004;42(4): 225–9.
4. Rahbar R, Resto VA, Robson CD, et al. Nasal glioma and encephalocele: diagnosis and management. Laryngoscope 2003;113(12):2069–77.
5. Simmen D, Raghavan U, Briner HR, et al. The surgeon's view of the anterior ethmoid artery. Clin Otolaryngol 2006;31(3):187–91.

6. Borges A. Imaging of the central skull base. Neuroimaging Clin N Am 2009;19(3):441–68.
7. Laine FJ, Nadel L, Braun IF. CT and MR imaging of the central skull base. Part 1: techniques, embryologic development, and anatomy. Radiographics 1990;10(4):591–602.
8. Caldemeyer KS, Mathews VP, Azzarelli B, et al. The jugular foramen: a review of anatomy, masses, and imaging characteristics. Radiographics 1997;17(5):1123–39.
9. Karasu A, Cansever T, Batay F, et al. The microsurgical anatomy of the hypoglossal canal. Surg Radiol Anat 2009;31(5):363–7.
10. Hoving EW. Nasal encephaloceles. Childs Nerv Syst 2000;16(10–11):702–6.
11. Prosser JD, Vender JR, Solares CA. Traumatic cerebrospinal fluid leaks. Otolaryngol Clin North Am 2011;44(4):857–73, vii.
12. Illing E, Zolotar M, Ross E, et al. Malignant otitis externa with skull base osteomyelitis. J Surg Case Rep 2011;5(6):1–4.
13. Sreepada GS, Kwartler JA. Skull base osteomyelitis secondary to malignant otitis externa. Curr Opin Otolaryngol Head Neck Surg 2003;11(5):316–23.
14. Chang PC, Fischbein NJ, Holliday RA. Central skull base osteomyelitis in patients without otitis externa: imaging findings. AJNR Am J Neuroradiol 2003;24(7):1310–6.
15. Chong VF, Khoo JB, Fan YF. Fibrous dysplasia involving the base of the skull. AJR Am J Roentgenol 2002;178(3):717–20.
16. Arana E, Marti-Bonmati L. CT and MR imaging of focal calvarial lesions. AJR Am J Roentgenol 1999;172(6):1683–8.
17. Fitzpatrick KA, Taljanovic MS, Speer DP, et al. Imaging findings of fibrous dysplasia with histopathologic and intraoperative correlation. AJR Am J Roentgenol 2004;182(6):1389–98.
18. Vrionis FD, Kienstra MA, Rivera M, et al. Malignant tumors of the anterior skull base. Cancer Control 2004;11(3):144–51.
19. Suarez C, Llorente JL, Fernandez De Leon R, et al. Prognostic factors in sinonasal tumors involving the anterior skull base. Head Neck 2004;26(2):136–44.
20. Abdel Khalek Abdel Razek A, King A. MRI and CT of nasopharyngeal carcinoma. AJR Am J Roentgenol 2012;198(1):11–8.
21. Chang ET, Adami HO. The enigmatic epidemiology of nasopharyngeal carcinoma. Cancer Epidemiol Biomarkers Prev 2006;15(10):1765–77.
22. Bhatoe HS, Kotwal N, Badwal S. Clival pituitary adenoma with acromegaly: case report and review of literature. Skull Base 2007;17(4):265–8.
23. Greenberg HS, Deck MD, Vikram B, et al. Metastasis to the base of the skull: clinical findings in 43 patients. Neurology 1981;31(5):530–7.
24. Laigle-Donadey F, Taillibert S, Martin-Duverneuil N, et al. Skull-base metastases. J Neurooncol 2005;75(1):63–9.
25. Chamoun RB, Suki D, DeMonte F. Surgical management of cranial base metastases. Neurosurgery 2012;70(4):802–9 [discussion: 809–10].
26. Lefkowitz MA, Hinton DR, Weiss MH, et al. Prognostic variables in surgery for skull base meningiomas. Neurosurg Focus 1997;2(4):e2.
27. Mendenhall WM, Friedman WA, Amdur RJ, et al. Management of benign skull base meningiomas: a review. Skull Base 2004;14(1):53–60 [discussion: 61].
28. Nanda A, Vannemreddy P. Recurrence and outcome in skull base meningiomas: do they differ from other intracranial meningiomas? Skull Base 2008;18(4):243–52.
29. Macdonald AJ, Salzman KL, Harnsberger HR, et al. Primary jugular foramen meningioma: imaging appearance and differentiating features. AJR Am J Roentgenol 2004;182(2):373–7.
30. Eldevik OP, Gabrielsen TO, Jacobsen EA. Imaging findings in schwannomas of the jugular foramen. AJNR Am J Neuroradiol 2000;21(6):1139–44.
31. Srinivas D, Somanna S, Ashwathnarayana CB, et al. Multicompartmental trigeminal schwannomas: management strategies and outcome. Skull Base 2011;21(6):351–8.
32. Rao AB, Koeller KK, Adair CF. From the archives of the AFIP. Paragangliomas of the head and neck: radiologic-pathologic correlation. Armed Forces Institute of Pathology. Radiographics 1999;19(6):1605–32.
33. Soo MY. Chordoma: review of clinicoradiological features and factors affecting survival. Australas Radiol 2001;45(4):427–34.
34. Erdem E, Angtuaco EC, Van Hemert R, et al. Comprehensive review of intracranial chordoma. Radiographics 2003;23(4):995–1009.
35. Koch BB, Karnell LH, Hoffman HT, et al. National cancer database report on chondrosarcoma of the head and neck. Head Neck 2000;22(4):408–25.
36. Cho YH, Kim JH, Khang SK, et al. Chordomas and chondrosarcomas of the skull base: comparative analysis of clinical results in 30 patients. Neurosurg Rev 2008;31(1):35–43 [discussion: 43].
37. Murphey MD, Walker EA, Wilson AJ, et al. From the archives of the AFIP: imaging of primary chondrosarcoma: radiologic-pathologic correlation. Radiographics 2003;23(5):1245–78.

Imaging of the Temporal Bone

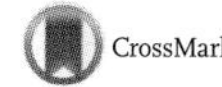

Travis A. Abele, MD[a], Richard H. Wiggins III, MD, CIIP, FSIIM[a,b,c,*]

KEYWORDS

• Temporal bone • Computed tomography • Magnetic resonance imaging • Acquired • Congenital

KEY POINTS

- Knowledge of normal temporal bone anatomy and space-specific differential diagnoses is key to interpretation of temporal bone imaging.
- Correlation with clinical history and physical examination is vital to making the correct diagnosis or providing an appropriate differential.
- Computed tomography and magnetic resonance imaging are complementary imaging modalities in the evaluation of temporal bone abnormalities.

INTRODUCTION

Interpretation of temporal bone can be a challenging task for the general radiologist and neuroradiologist alike. An understanding of temporal bone anatomy and common abnormalities affecting the individual spaces of the temporal bone facilitates an expert interpretation. Although grouping temporal bone disease into types such as congenital, infectious, neoplastic, traumatic, or vascular can be a helpful memory tool, a space-specific approach is more valuable to the interpreting radiologist who rarely knows the pathologic category beforehand. Like all head and neck radiology, critical diagnostic information is derived from the clinical assessment and otoscopic examination. This article reviews common temporal bone abnormalities in a space-specific fashion with attention to key observations that the referring clinician will wish to know.

IMAGING TECHNIQUES

Computed tomography (CT) is the mainstay imaging modality for evaluation of the temporal bone (**Box 1**). The authors' institutional temporal bone CT protocol acquires noncontrast volumetric CT data of the bilateral temporal bones, and reconstructs the data into 0.6-mm thick axial and coronal planes and 0.6-mm thick planes parallel (Poschl) and perpendicular (Stenver) to the superior semicircular canals. Each plane is reconstructed in a bone algorithm with a field of view centered over each individual temporal bone. Axial 2-mm thick soft-tissue algorithm CT images are also reconstructed with a field of view including both temporal bones to evaluate the soft tissues. Intravenous contrast is only administered if there is clinical concern for abscess in the soft tissues of the external ear, or in cases when magnetic resonance (MR) imaging is not possible.

For MR imaging the authors use both a noncontrast protocol and a contrast-enhanced protocol for imaging of the temporal bone. The noncontrast protocol is a screening study comprising an axial 3-dimensional (3D) T2-weighted Sampling Perfection with Application optimized Contrast using different flip angle Evolutions (SPACE) sequence and a 1.25-mm thick 3D coronal T2 sequence, used to evaluate patients with clinical suspicion

The authors have no disclosures.

[a] Department of Radiology, University of Utah Health Sciences Center, 30 North, 1900 East #1A071, Salt Lake City, UT 84132-2140, USA; [b] Division of Otolaryngology – Head and Neck Surgery, University of Utah Health Sciences Center, 30 North, 1900 East #1A071, Salt Lake City, UT 84132-2140, USA; [c] Department of Biomedical Informatics, University of Utah Health Sciences Center, 30 North, 1900 East #1A071, Salt Lake City, UT 84132-2140, USA
* Corresponding author. Department of Biomedical Informatics, University of Utah Health Sciences Center, 30 North, 1900 East #1A071, Salt Lake City, UT 84132-2140.
E-mail address: Richard.Wiggins@hsc.utah.edu

Radiol Clin N Am 53 (2015) 15–36
http://dx.doi.org/10.1016/j.rcl.2014.09.010

Box 1
Imaging techniques

Computed Tomography

- 0.6-mm thick axial and coronal bone algorithm (each temporal bone)
- 0.6-mm thick Poschl and Stenvers bone algorithm (each temporal bone)
- 2-mm thick axial soft-tissue algorithm (both temporal bones)
- Intravenous contrast administered if concern for soft-tissue abscess

Magnetic Resonance Imaging

Noncontrast protocol

- Axial 3-dimensional (3D) Sampling Perfection with Application optimized Contrast using different flip angle Evolutions (SPACE)
- 1.25-mm thick 3D coronal T2

Contrast-Enhanced Protocol

- Axial 3D SPACE
- 3-mm thick axial and coronal T1 precontrast
- 3-mm thick axial and coronal T1 fat-suppressed postcontrast

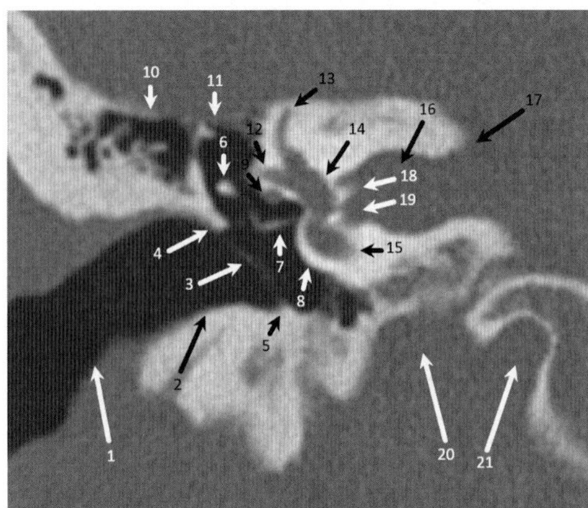

Fig. 1. Anatomy of the temporal bone. Coronal bone algorithm computed tomography (CT) image shows important structures of the external auditory canal (EAC), middle ear, and inner ear. (1) Cartilaginous EAC, (2) osseous EAC, (3) tympanic membrane, (4) scutum, (5) tympanic annulus, (6) incus, (7) stapes, (8) cochlear promontory, (9) tympanic segment of the facial nerve, (10) tegmen mastoideum, (11) tegmen tympani, (12) lateral semicircular canal, (13) superior semicircular canal, (14) vestibule, (15) basal turn of the cochlea, (16) internal auditory canal (IAC), (17) porus acusticus, (18) crista falciformis, (19) cochlear nerve canal, (20) jugular foramen, (21) hypoglossal canal.

for vestibular schwannoma. The T2 SPACE sequence was added to the screening MR imaging protocol to evaluate its utility as a cisternographic fluid-sensitive sequence, similar to constructive interference in steady-state (CISS) but without banding artifact.

For the contrast-enhanced protocol, the authors obtain 3-mm thick axial and coronal T1-weighted precontrast and T1-weighted fat-suppressed postcontrast sequences in addition to the 3D SPACE sequence. This protocol is typically used when there is clinical suspicion for disorder other than vestibular schwannoma.

NORMAL ANATOMY

Temporal bone anatomy can be conceptualized into the following key spaces: external auditory canal (EAC), middle ear and mastoid, inner ear, petrous apex, and facial nerve course. Accurate localization of temporal bone abnormality into one of these spaces is crucial to making the correct diagnosis or providing an appropriate differential.

The EAC (**Fig. 1**) is bordered laterally by the external ear and medially by the tympanic membrane. It is composed of 2 parts: the fibrocartilaginous EAC laterally and osseous EAC medially. The fibrocartilaginous EAC contains inferior fissures (of Santorini), which allow for abnormality in the EAC to pass into the adjacent parotid space inferiorly. The parotid lymph nodes are the first-order lymphatic drainage for the EAC and external ear.

The tympanic membrane (TM) is a 3-layered sound-transducing partition between the EAC and middle ear. Its superior attachment is the scutum, which should always have a sharp medial margin, and the inferior attachment is the tympanic annulus. The TM is divided into the pars flaccida (superior one-third) and the pars tensa (inferior two-thirds), which are demarcated by the attachment of the umbo of the medial malleolus to the TM.

The middle ear (see **Fig. 1**; **Fig. 2**) comprises the hypotympanum, mesotympanum, and epitympanum. An artificial plane between the tympanic annulus and cochlear promontory in the axial plane divides the hypotympanum and mesotympanum. The mesotympanum and epitympanum are divided by an artificial plane extending between the scutum and tympanic segment of the facial nerve. The hypotympanum contains air and no vital structures.

The mesotympanum (see **Fig. 2**) contains all parts of the ossicles with the exception of the head of the malleus and the short process of the

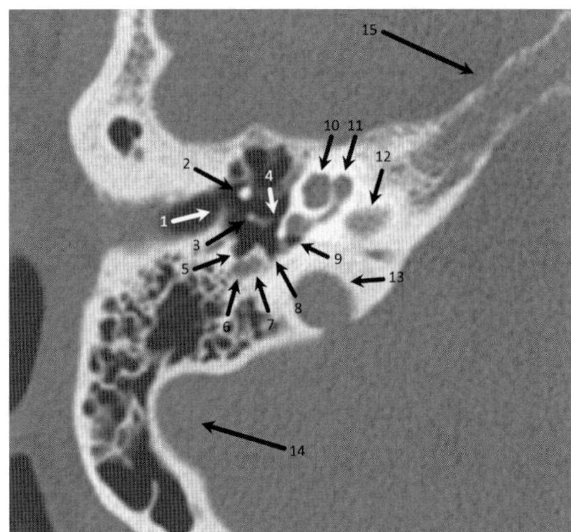

Fig. 2. Anatomy of the middle ear. Axial bone algorithm CT image shows anatomy of the middle ear. (1) Tympanic membrane, (2) malleus neck, (3) incus long process, (4) anterior crus of stapes, (5) facial nerve recess, (6) facial nerve mastoid segment, (7) stapedius muscle within the pyramidal eminence, (8) sinus tympani, (9) round window, (10) middle turn of cochlea, (11) basal turn of cochlea, (12) IAC, (13) jugular bulb (high riding), (14) transverse sinus, (15) petrous apex.

incus. Other important structures include the tensor tympani and stapedius muscles, which insert on the malleus and stapes, respectively, to restrict ossicle movement and dampen transmitted sound. Along the posterior wall of the mesotympanum are 3 recognizable structures (lateral to medial): facial nerve recess (containing mastoid segment of the facial nerve), pyramidal eminence (origin of the stapedius muscle), and sinus tympani. The oval window, where the stapes articulates, and the round window are located on the medial wall of the mesotympanum. For detailed ossicle anatomy, please refer to **Fig. 3**.

In addition to the head of the malleus and short process of the incus, the epitympanum contains the lateral epitympanic space between the malleus and the scutum. The tegmen tympani forms the superior margin of the epitympanum, and posteriorly the aditus ad antrum leads to the mastoid air cells.

The petrous apex is a variably aerated structure of the anteromedial temporal bone over which cranial nerve 6 runs to enter the abducens canal (Dorello canal). The carotid canal is located along the inferomedial temporal bone, and contains the petrous internal carotid artery (ICA). The jugular foramen is located within the inferoposterior temporal bone, and contains the jugular bulb of the internal jugular vein.

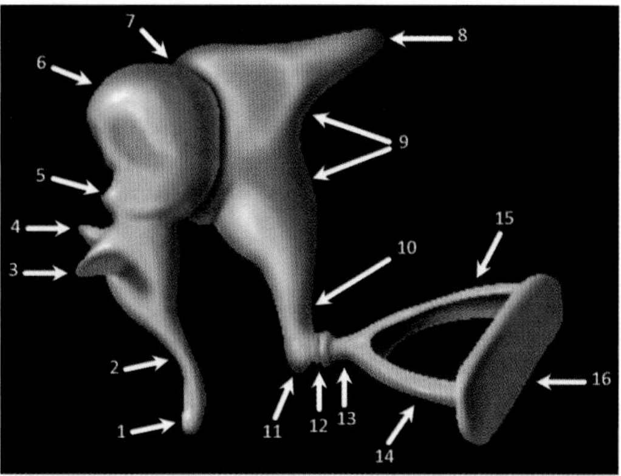

Fig. 3. Middle ear ossicles. Three-dimensional graphic, anterior oblique view, shows key ossicle anatomy. (1) Malleus umbo, (2) manubrium of malleus, (3) malleus anterior process, (4) malleus lateral process, (5) malleus neck, (6) malleus head (7), malleoincudal articulation, (8) short process incus, (9) incus body, (10) incus long process, (11) incus lenticular process, (12) incudostapedial articulation, (13) stapes head, (14) anterior stapes crus, (15) posterior stapes crus, (16) stapes footplate.

The inner ear (**Fig. 4**) has 3 compartments: the osseous labyrinth, the perilymphatic space, and the membranous labyrinth. The osseous labyrinth makes up the bony covering of the vestibule, cochlea, and semicircular canals. The perilymphatic space contains perilymph, which bathes the membranous labyrinth, and is composed of the vestibule, semicircular canals, scala tympani and

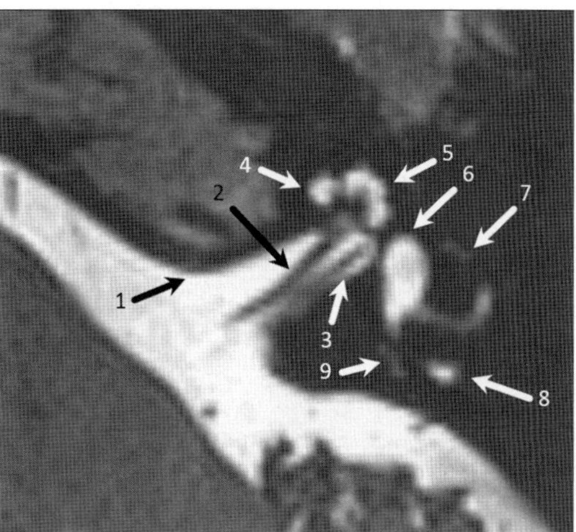

Fig. 4. Anatomy of the inner ear. Axial T2-weighted magnetic resonance (MR) image shows important structures of the inner ear. (1) Porus acusticus of IAC, (2) cochlear nerve, (3) inferior vestibular nerve, (4) basal turn of the cochlea, (5) middle turn of the cochlea, (6) vestibule, (7) lateral semicircular canal, (8) posterior semicircular canal, (9) vestibular aqueduct.

scala vestibuli of the cochlea, and vestibular aqueduct. The membranous labyrinth contains endolymph, and is composed of the saccule and utricle (not resolved on clinical CT and MR imaging) within the vestibule, semicircular ducts, scala media of the cochlea, and endolymphatic duct and sac. The cochlea has 2.5 turns (basal, middle, and apical) and consists of 3 scalar chambers for transducing sound into neural information. The vestibule has superior, lateral, and posterior semicircular canals oriented perpendicular to each other to detect movement in space.

The internal auditory canal (IAC) (**Fig. 5**) is an osseous passageway bordered medially by the porus acusticus and laterally by the IAC fundus. The facial nerve and vestibulocochlear nerves course through the IAC, with the facial nerve in the anterosuperior quadrant, cochlear nerve in the anteroinferior quadrant, and the superior and inferior vestibular nerves in the superoposterior and inferoposterior quadrants, respectively. At the IAC fundus, the vestibular nerves traverse the macula cribrosa to enter the vestibule, and the cochlear nerve crosses the cochlear nerve canal to enter the cochlea.

The facial nerve course is important to evaluate in any temporal bone study to assess pathologic involvement and prevent iatrogenic injury during surgical treatment. The facial nerve's functions are to facilitate motor to the face, parasympathetics to the lacrimal, submandibular, and sublingual glands, and taste from the anterior two-thirds of the tongue. Segments of the facial nerve are as follows: intra-axial (including the facial nerve nuclei within the pons); cisternal segment crossing the cerebellopontine angle; canalicular segment within the IAC; labyrinthine, tympanic, and mastoid segments of the intratemporal facial nerve (**Fig. 6**); and extracranial segment extending through the parotid gland and spreading out over the face.

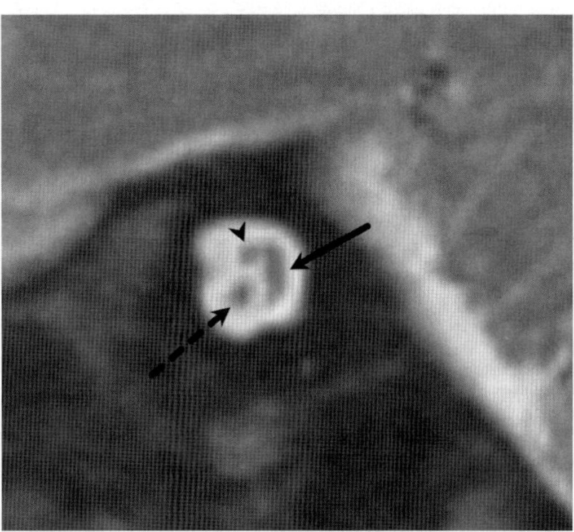

Fig. 5. Anatomy of the IAC. T2-weighted MR image perpendicular to the IAC shows the vestibular nerve (*arrow*) posteriorly just before dividing into the superior and inferior branches. The facial nerve is anterior and superior (*arrowhead*), and the cochlear nerve is anterior and inferior (*dashed arrow*).

IMAGING FINDINGS AND PATHOLOGY

External Auditory Canal

EAC lesions are easily examined and are often diagnosed with direct otoscopy. Radiology is useful for evaluating the extent of disease and invasion of structures that cannot be directly visualized. Common pathologic groups of the EAC include congenital, inflammatory, benign neoplastic, and malignant (**Box 2**).

Congenital EAC atresia encompasses a range of complex congenital dysplasias affecting both the EAC and the middle ear. Potentially dysplastic anatomic structures that must be individually evaluated include the external ear, EAC, TM, size of middle ear, ossicles, mastoid air cells, oval window, round window, course of the facial nerve, and possible presence of a congenital cholesteatoma. The status of these structures prognosticates surgical outcome.[1] Atresia of the EAC can be complete or stenotic and osseous or membranous. The ossicles may be fused, rotated, hypoplastic, or absent, and accompanied by middle ear cavity dysplasia. Subtle cases of EAC atresia may be commonly missed on imaging. In EAC atresia, the tympanic segment of the facial nerve canal shortens, and the mastoid segment may exit more anteriorly into the temporomandibular joint rather than the stylomastoid foramen (**Fig. 7**). In EAC atresia, the inner ear (cochlea, vestibule, and semicircular canal) are not affected because they arise from a different embryologic anlage than the middle ear and EAC.

Cholesteatoma is one of the most common abnormalities encountered in the EAC, although it is more often encountered in the middle ear. EAC cholesteatoma is an erosive lesion composed of keratinizing squamous epithelium that clinically presents with otorrhea and sometimes dull otalgia. EAC cholesteatoma is usually secondary to trauma, surgery, or EAC stenosis, but can also be idiopathic.[2,3] On CT, a soft-tissue mass with erosion of the osseous EAC inferiorly is a common presentation, and approximately 50% will contain osseous fragments within the mass,[3] which can be helpful for distinguishing cholesteatoma from squamous cell carcinoma (**Fig. 8**). It is important to evaluate possible extension into the middle ear and/or facial nerve, which may not be apparent to the otolaryngologist on examination.

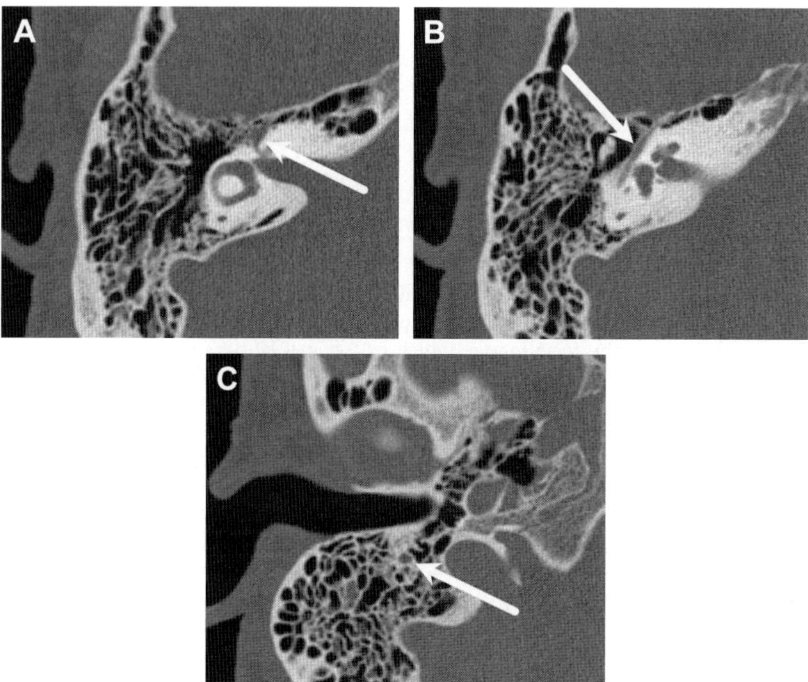

Fig. 6. Intratemporal segments of the facial nerve. Series of axial bone algorithm CT images show the labyrinthine (*A*), tympanic (*B*), and mastoid segments of the facial nerve (*C*) (*arrows*).

EAC squamous cell carcinoma is the most common malignancy of the EAC. It presents as a unilateral soft-tissue mass with bony erosion, which can mimic an EAC cholesteatoma without osseous fragments. Squamous cell carcinoma of the EAC is typically secondary to spread from squamous cell skin cancer of the external ear, and thus clinical examination and careful review of the soft-tissue algorithm on temporal bone CT can be key to this diagnosis (**Fig. 9**).[4] Contrast-enhanced MR imaging is a helpful adjunct in evaluating intracranial and perineural spread or malignant nodes in the parotid space.

Necrotizing external otitis (NEO) is soft-tissue infection of the EAC that can spread through the inferior fissures (of Santorini) into the parotid and soft tissues of the suprahyoid neck. It is invariably caused by *Pseudomonas aeruginosa* and arises most commonly in immunocompromised patients. Mild NEO can be indistinguishable from EAC squamous cell carcinoma on imaging.[5,6] Clues to making the diagnosis of NEO are soft-tissue abscess and clinical presentation, culture positive for *P aeruginosa*, and elevated erythrocyte sedimentation rate. CT or MR imaging will demonstrate radiology findings typical for infection with abnormal soft-tissue thickening, soft-tissue stranding, and enhancement of the EAC and/or the infratemporal soft tissues. Osseous erosion or marrow signal abnormality suggests coexistent osteomyelitis, and rim-enhancing fluid collections favor abscess in the setting of NEO (**Fig. 10**).

> **Box 2**
> **Common external auditory canal (EAC) abnormalities**
>
> - Congenital: EAC atresia
> - Inflammatory: cholesteatoma, necrotizing external otitis
> - Benign neoplasm: osteoma, exostosis
> - Malignant neoplasm: squamous cell carcinoma

Two distinct benign osseous lesions are worth mentioning in any discussion of EAC disease: osteoma and exostoses. EAC osteomas are pedunculated osseous lesions arising at the junction of the cartilaginous and osseous EAC (**Fig. 11**). These lesions are unilateral, covered by normal soft tissue, and of no clinical importance unless they obstruct the canal.[7] EAC exostoses are typically bilateral benign circumferential broad-based osseous lesions covered with normal mucosal soft tissue occurring within the EAC (**Fig. 12**). This entity is also known as “surfer’s ear” owing to its association with exposure to

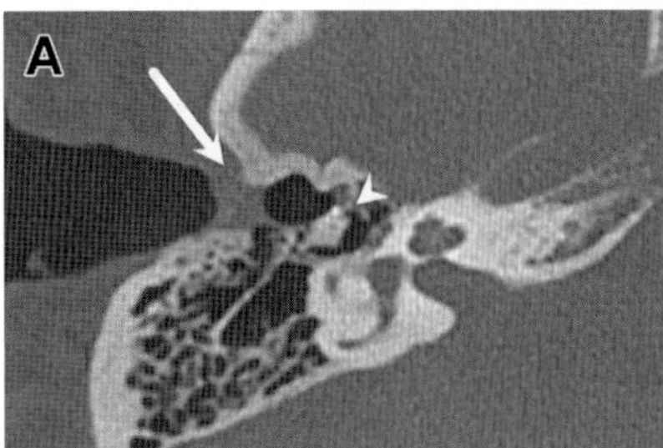

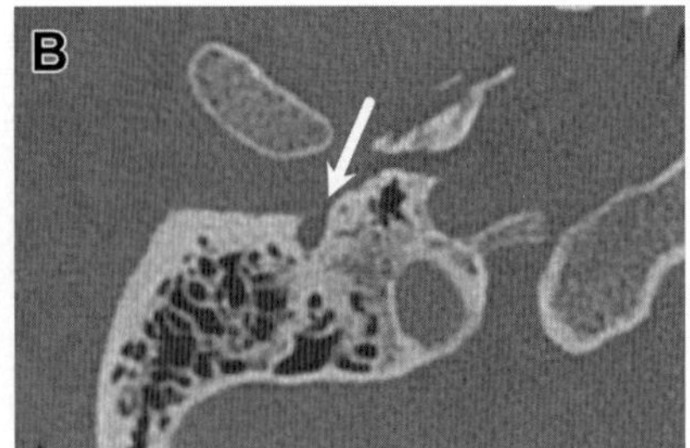

Fig. 7. Right EAC atresia. Axial bone algorithm CT (*A*) shows dysplasia of the malleoincudal articulation (*arrowhead*) and partial cartilaginous atresia of the EAC (*arrow*). Axial bone algorithm CT (*B*) shows anterior displacement of the mastoid segment of the facial nerve, which exits the skull base into the temporomandibular joint (*arrow*) rather than the stylomastoid foramen.

cold water; like EAC osteomas, EAC exostoses are infrequently treated.[8]

Middle Ear and Mastoid Air Cells

The middle ear and mastoid air cells are grouped because of their open connection through the aditus ad antrum. This connection allows for sharing of common malignancies, which include inflammatory, infectious, congenital, and neoplastic diseases (**Box 3**).

Cholesteatomas, one of the most common abnormalities affecting the middle ear and mastoids, are erosive lesions composed of keratinizing squamous epithelium, similar to EAC cholesteatomas. Cholesteatomas can be acquired or congenital, and clinically present as a white mass behind the TM with conductive hearing loss and/or otorrhea. Congenital cholesteatomas make up only 2% of middle ear cholesteatomas, and arise from congenital epithelial rests located anywhere within the temporal bone.[9] Of note, when congenital epithelial rests form tumors elsewhere intracranially they are identified as epidermoid cysts. Acquired cholesteatomas, which include most of the middle ear and mastoid lesions, are thought to arise from retraction pockets or TM perforations. Approximately 80% occur at the pars flaccida extending into Prussak space (an anatomic region between the pars flaccida laterally and the neck of the malleus medially, and the scutum superiorly).[9] On CT a soft-tissue mass lateral to the ossicles in Prussak space with extension superiorly into the lateral epitympanic recess is a common presentation of a pars flaccida cholesteatoma (**Fig. 13**). Approximately 20% occur at the pars tensa and grow medial to the ossicles (**Fig. 14**). Osseous erosion involving the scutum or ossicles is key to distinguishing a cholesteatoma from benign debris or otitis media on CT, although absence of erosion does not exclude cholesteatoma.

Diffusion-weighted MR imaging (DWI) is useful in distinguishing cholesteatoma from other disorders of the middle ear in that cholesteatomas, similar to epidermoid cysts, demonstrate restricted diffusion (**Fig. 15**). Traditional echo-planar DWI may be limited in evaluation of the temporal bone because of osseous susceptibility artifact. Recently, nonecho-planar DWI sequences, which have markedly decreased susceptibility artifact, have proved useful in detection of recurrent postsurgical cholesteatomas, and have even demonstrated utility in primary detection.[10]

Detecting complications of cholesteatoma is often more important to the referring otolaryngologist than the diagnosis, which he or she may have already made on otoscopy. Cholesteatomas can erode anywhere within the middle ear or into nearby structures. Important structures to evaluate and comment on include the ossicles, facial nerve (especially the tympanic segment), tegmen

Fig. 8. EAC cholesteatoma. Coronal bone algorithm CT image shows a soft-tissue attenuation lesion with erosion of the floor of the EAC, containing osseous fragments (*arrowhead*) within the mass.

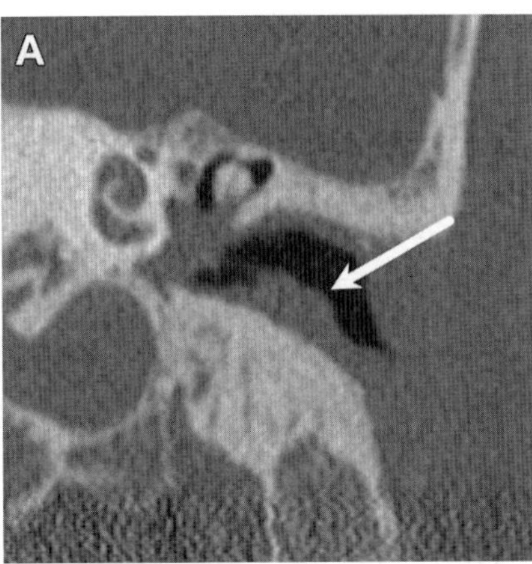

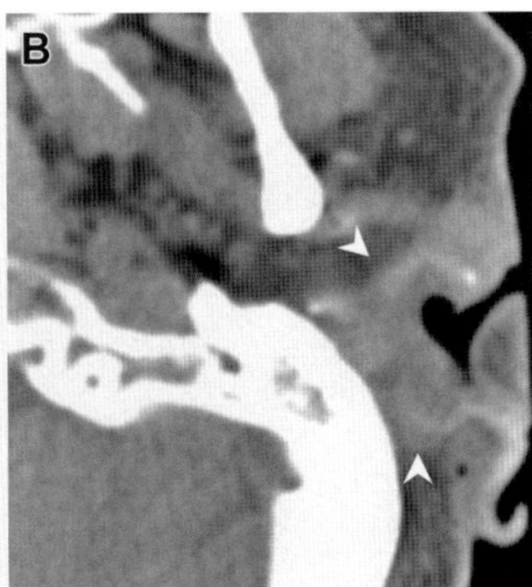

Fig. 9. EAC squamous cell carcinoma. Coronal bone algorithm CT (*A*) shows a nonspecific soft-tissue attenuation lesion along the floor of the left EAC (*arrow*), which could represent debris, infection, neoplasm, or cholesteatoma. Axial soft-tissue algorithm CT (*B*) shows diffuse thickening of the external ear (*arrowheads*), consistent with squamous cell skin cancer that had secondarily spread into the EAC.

tympani and mastoideum (dehiscence can lead to cerebrospinal fluid [CSF] leak or indicate intracranial extension), oval and round windows, and semicircular canals (**Fig. 16**).

Otitis media and otomastoiditis comprise a range of pathologies from coalescent otomastoiditis with abscess to chronic otomastoiditis with tympanosclerosis. Acute otitis media most commonly occurs in children during the first 5 years of life, resulting from infection by *Streptococcus* or *Haemophilus influenzae*, which spread from the upper respiratory tract via the Eustachian tube.[11] Otitis media and otomastoiditis are both clinical diagnoses because they are indistinguishable on imaging from benign effusion in the middle ear and mastoids. Untreated otomastoiditis can eventually erode the mastoid air cells and transform into coalescent otomastoiditis, which is distinguished from a benign effusion or otomastoiditis by air-cell erosion (**Fig. 17**). The radiologist must interrogate for complications of coalescent otomastoiditis, including: (1) subperiosteal abscess, (2) intracranial abscess (see **Fig. 17**), (3) dural venous sinus thrombosis, (4) carotid arteritis, (5) labyrinthitis, or (6) petrous apicitis.

In chronic otomastoiditis, repeated inflammation of the mucous membranes of the middle ear and mastoids leads to reactive bone formation and appearance of underpneumatized mastoid air cells.[12] In contrast to acute otomastoiditis, which is associated with fluid in the middle ear and mastoids, chronic otomastoiditis presents with web-like linear soft-tissue density. Because chronic otomastoiditis is often a clinical diagnosis, the role of the radiologist is to identify postinflammatory sequelae that can exacerbate conductive hearing loss, such as ossicular erosion or tympanosclerosis (**Fig. 18**). Common places to develop tympanosclerotic calcifications include the TM, ossicle surfaces, ossicle ligaments, and muscular

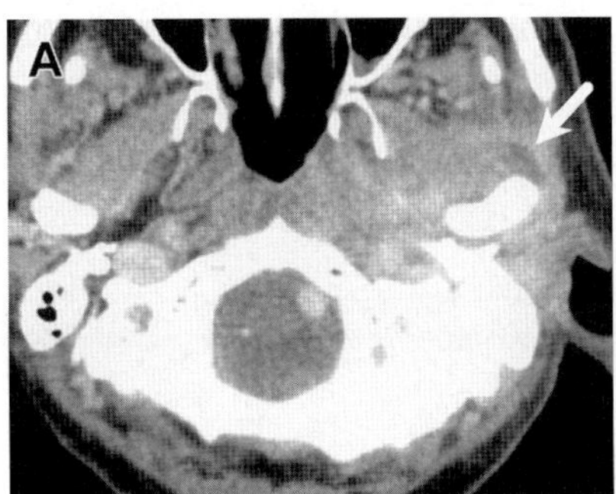

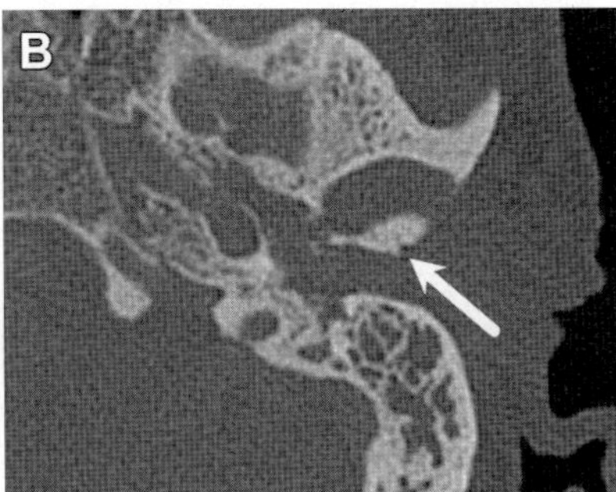

Fig. 10. Necrotizing external otitis. Axial contrast-enhanced axial CT image (*A*) shows asymmetric soft-tissue swelling and hyperenhancement of the inferior left EAC and adjacent masticator space. Hypoattenuating collection (*arrow*) anterior to the mandibular condyle represents abscess. Axial bone algorithm CT zoomed in on the left EAC (*B*) shows small erosions of anterior wall of the EAC (*arrow*), suggestive of osteomyelitis.

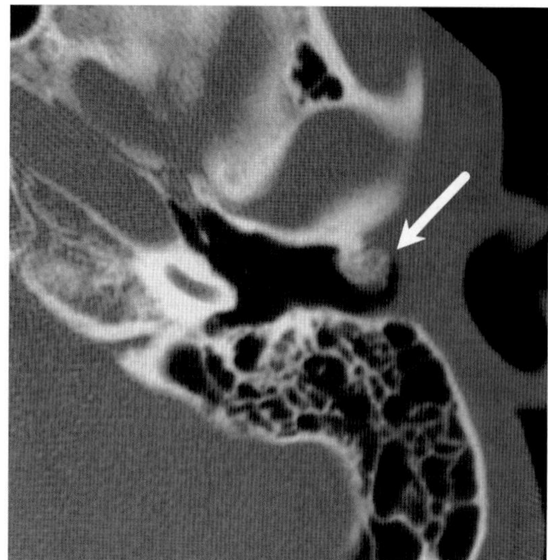

Fig. 11. EAC osteoma. Axial bone algorithm CT shows a nonaggressive pedunculated bony mass (*arrow*) arising at the junction of the osseous and cartilaginous EAC.

tendons. It is important for the imager to remember that fluid within the mastoid air cells is not mastoiditis, even if the fluid is shown to enhance on MR imaging following contrast administration. Mastoiditis is a clinical diagnosis, only made when new osseous destruction is seen on imaging in the correct clinical setting.

Cholesterol granuloma is an inflammatory mass of granulation tissue caused by recurrent hemorrhage that can mimic otomastoiditis or cholesteatoma on CT. On otoscopy, this lesion presents as a blue retrotympanic mass when found within the middle ear. CT features of cholesterol granulomas are nonspecific, with expansile scalloping of the mastoid and middle ear including the ossicles. Cholesterol granuloma can be distinguished from other middle ear lesions on MR imaging by the expansile nature and distinctive T1 and T2 hyperintense signals reflecting hemorrhage and granulation tissue (**Fig. 19**).[13]

Glomus tympanicum and glomus jugulare tumors are benign vascular paragangliomas that arise from glomus bodies along the cochlear promontory and jugular bulb, respectively. On otoscopy, both paragangliomas can present as a red

Box 3
Common middle ear and mastoid abnormalities

- Congenital/vascular: congenital cholesteatoma, aberrant internal carotid artery (ICA), lateralized ICA, dehiscent jugular bulb, high riding jugular bulb, jugular bulb dehiscence
- Inflammatory: acquired cholesteatoma, cholesterol granuloma
- Infectious: acute otomastoiditis, coalescent otomastoiditis, chronic otomastoiditis
- Benign neoplastic: glomus tympanicum, glomus paraganglioma
- Malignant neoplastic: osseous metastases

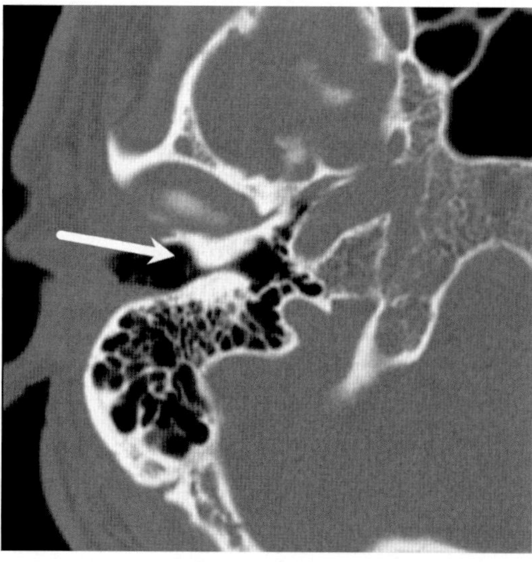

Fig. 12. EAC exostoses. Axial bone algorithm CT image shows broad-based circumferential osseous lesion (*arrow*) near the tympanic annulus, which nearly occludes the EAC.

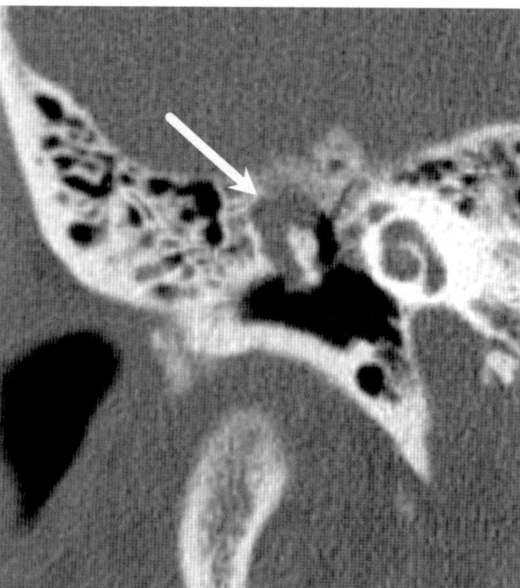

Fig. 13. Pars flaccida cholesteatoma. Coronal bone algorithm CT image shows a soft-tissue attenuation mass within Prussak space and the lateral epitympanic recess (*arrow*), with erosion of the scutum and head of the malleus.

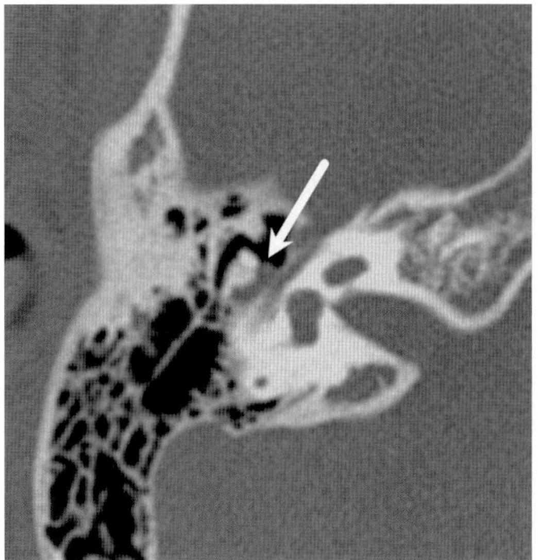

Fig. 14. Pars tensa cholesteatoma. Axial bone algorithm CT shows a soft-tissue mass lateral to the ossicles (*arrow*) without significant erosion that would be difficult to distinguish from benign debris. Characteristic location and symptoms prompted surgery, which confirmed a cholesteatoma.

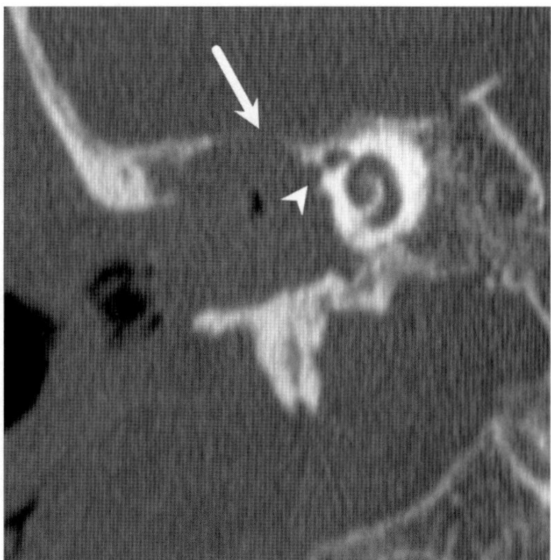

Fig. 16. Complications of middle ear cholesteatoma. Coronal bone algorithm CT shows an erosive, rounded, soft-tissue density mass centered with the middle ear. Important complications to recognize are erosion and absence of the ossicles, tegmen tympanic erosion and dehiscence (*arrow*), and erosion into the tympanic segment of the facial nerve (*arrowhead*).

retrotympanic mass in a patient with pulsatile tinnitus. Thus it is the responsibility of the radiologist to distinguish between the two. On CT the glomus tympanicum tumor appears as a small, circumscribed mass along the cochlear promontory, which is T1 hypointense, T2 hyperintense, and homogeneously enhancing on MR imaging (**Fig. 20**). Tumor may spread within the middle ear, but osseous erosion is atypical.[14] By contrast, glomus jugulare paraganglioma tumors manifest as erosive masses centered within the jugular foramen. On MR imaging, jugular paraganglioma lesions show the classic "salt and pepper" appearance[15] with mixed T1 hypointense signal (vascular flow voids) and less common T1 hyperintense signal (slow flow or hemorrhage), and homogeneous enhancement after gadolinium. Glomus jugulare is characterized by permeative osseous erosion with a vector of spread often extending superolaterally through the floor of the middle ear, clinically mimicking a glomus tympanicum (**Fig. 21**). One must look for multicentric paragangliomas, with possible additional carotid body or

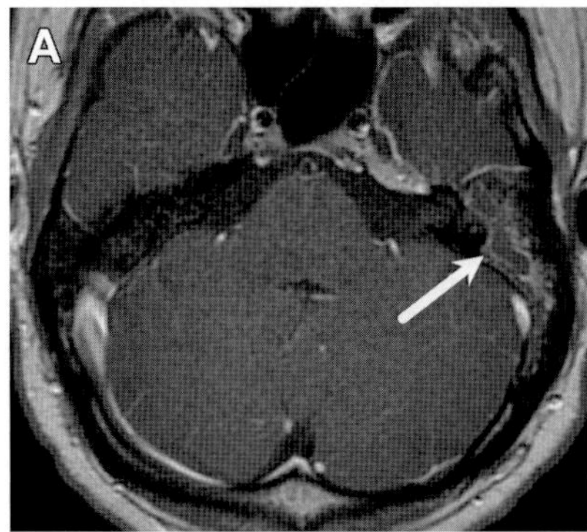

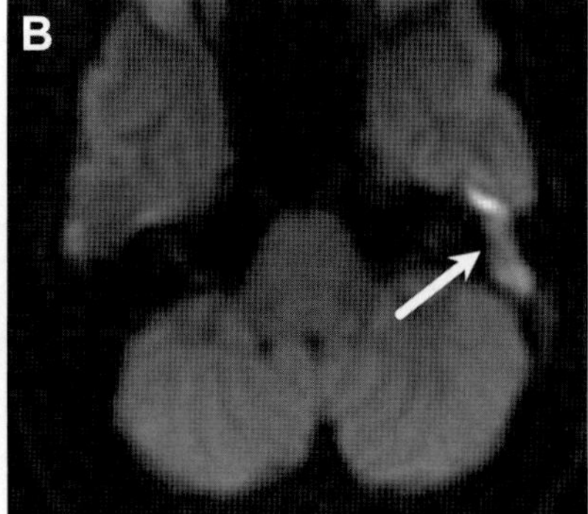

Fig. 15. Mastoid cholesteatoma. (*A*) Axial postcontrast T1-weighted image shows a nonenhancing T1 hypointense mass (*arrow*) within the left middle ear, and mastoid air cells with surrounding hyperintense enhancement of the mastoid air cell mucosa. (*B*) Axial diffusion-weighted MR image shows restricted diffusion within the mass (*arrow*). Apparent diffusion coefficient map (not pictured) showed corresponding hypointense signal.

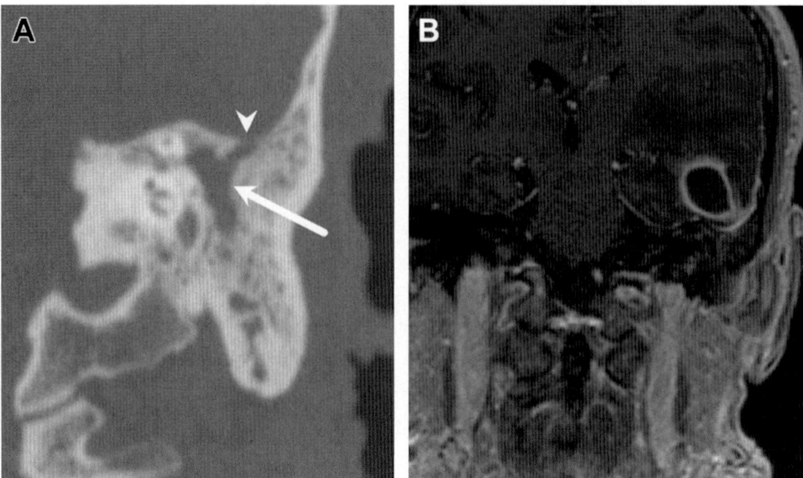

Fig. 17. Coalescent otomastoiditis with intracranial abscess. (*A*) Coronal bone algorithm CT shows coalescence of mastoid air cells (*arrow*) and dehiscence or severe thinning of the tegmen mastoideum (*arrowhead*). (*B*) Coronal postcontrast T1-weighted image shows a peripherally enhancing temporal lobe abscess extending from the tegmen mastoideum.

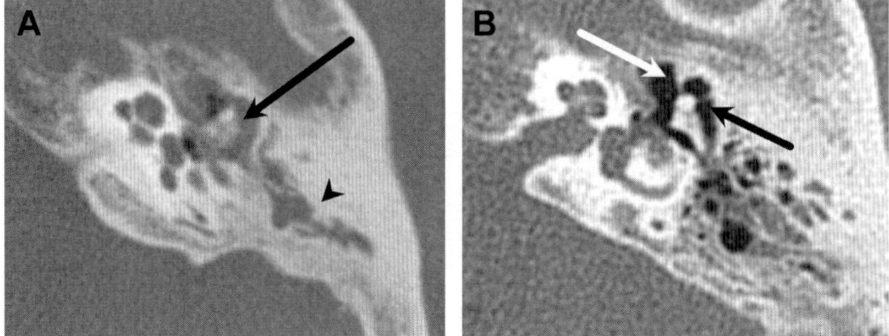

Fig. 18. Two cases of chronic otomastoiditis with tympanosclerosis. (*A*) Underpneumatization of the mastoid air cells (*arrowhead*) is consistent with chronic infection. Severe tympanosclerosis has developed, with calcifications (*arrow*) obscuring the native middle ear ossicles. (*B*) Mild tympanosclerosis is present in a different patient with calcification of the malleolar ligaments (*arrows*).

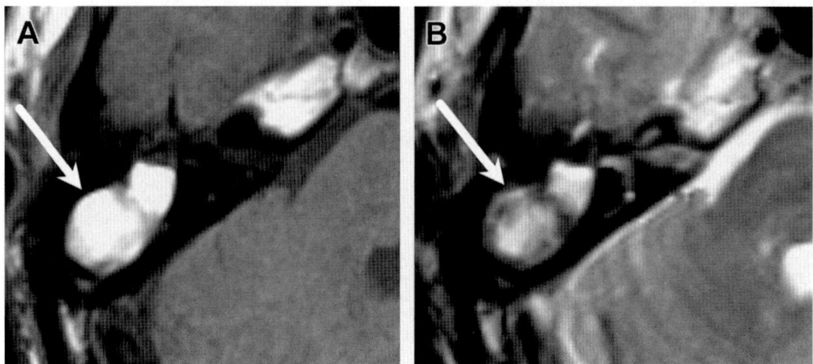

Fig. 19. Mastoid cholesterol granuloma. (*A*) Axial T1-weighted and (*B*) axial T2-weighted MR images show an expansile lesion (*arrows*) within the middle ear, and mastoid air cells with distinctive T1 hyperintense and T2 hyperintense signals.

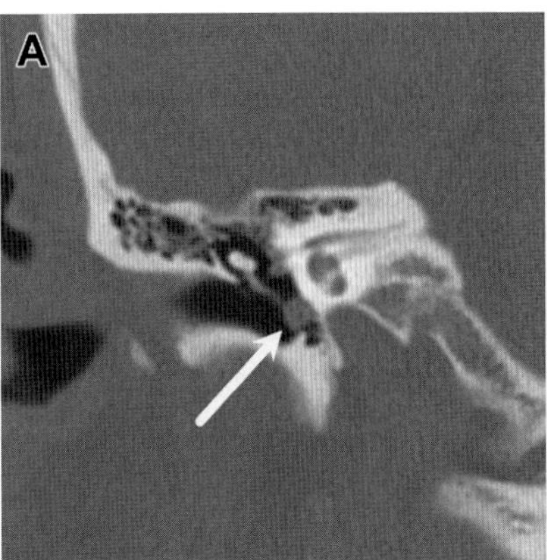

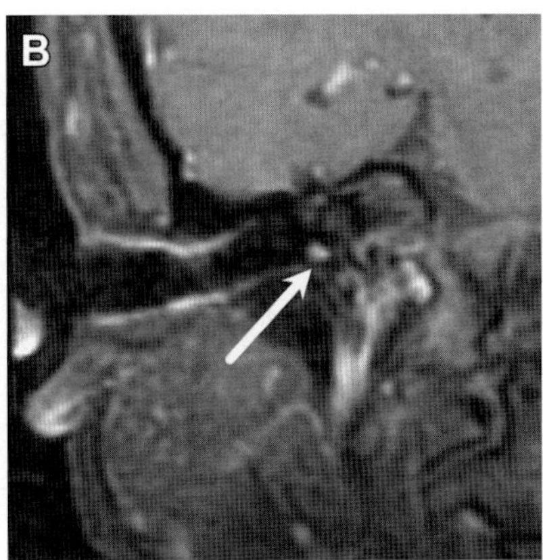

Fig. 20. Glomus tympanicum. (*A*) Coronal bone algorithm CT shows a small, circumscribed, soft-tissue attenuation mass along the cochlear promontory (*arrow*). (*B*) On coronal postcontrast T1-weighted fat-suppressed MR imaging there is enhancement of the mass (*arrow*), confirming the diagnosis.

glomus vagale. Malignant adult middle ear neoplasms are largely osseous metastases.

Common arterial anomalies of the temporal bone include aberrant ICA and lateralized ICA. The aberrant ICA is a congenital variant in which the ICA enters the skull base through the posterior hypotympanum and courses anteriorly along the cochlear promontory to turn medially and enter the normal horizontal carotid canal.[16] This lesion can be confused with a glomus tympanicum because it presents as a retrotympanic mass in a patient with pulsatile tinnitus to the otolaryngologist, and can appear as a soft-tissue mass on the cochlear promontory to the radiologist on CT (**Fig. 22**). The radiologist must be confident about the diagnosis to avoid a disastrous biopsy. The lateralized ICA is a normal variant course of the horizontal petrous ICA that normally enters the skull base posterolaterally (not within the middle ear), and protrudes laterally toward the middle ear cavity with thinned or dehiscent overlying bone (**Fig. 23**). The importance of recognizing this variant is to not confuse it with aberrant ICA and to alert the referring clinician to avoid arterial injury during surgery.[17]

Anatomic variations in the jugular bulb include size asymmetry, jugular bulb dehiscence, high-riding jugular bulb, and jugular bulb diverticulum. Severe asymmetry in jugular bulb size, defined as greater than 20 mm difference in diameter, occurs in approximately 50% of individuals.[18] The combination of venous flow MR signal heterogeneity and differences in jugular bulb size can create a pseudolesion, which should not be mistaken for true abnormality. Concordant asymmetry of the internal jugular veins of the neck can

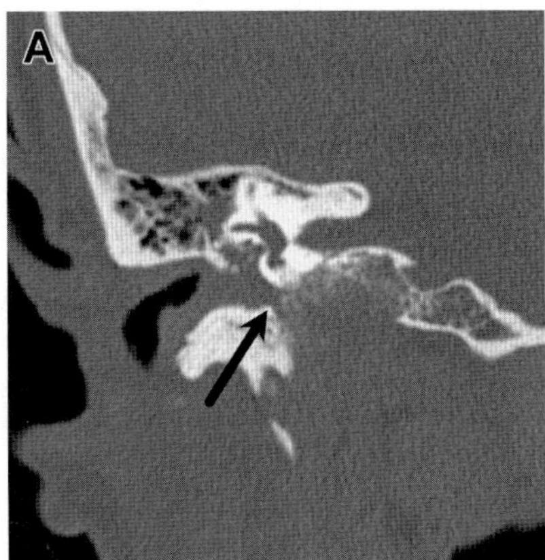

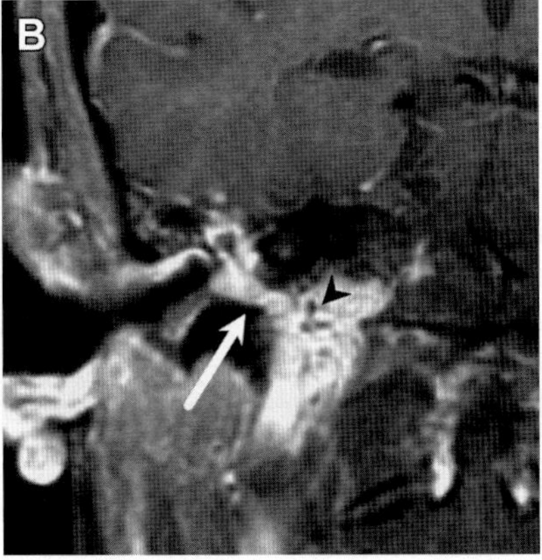

Fig. 21. Glomus jugulare. (*A*) Coronal bone algorithm CT shows a permeative destructive mass centered at the jugular bulb with extension through the sigmoid plate (*arrow*) into the middle ear. (*B*) On coronal postcontrast T1-weighted fat-suppressed MR imaging there is avid enhancement and flow voids (*arrowhead*) within the mass, confirming the diagnosis of a paraganglioma. Note extension into the middle ear (*arrow*).

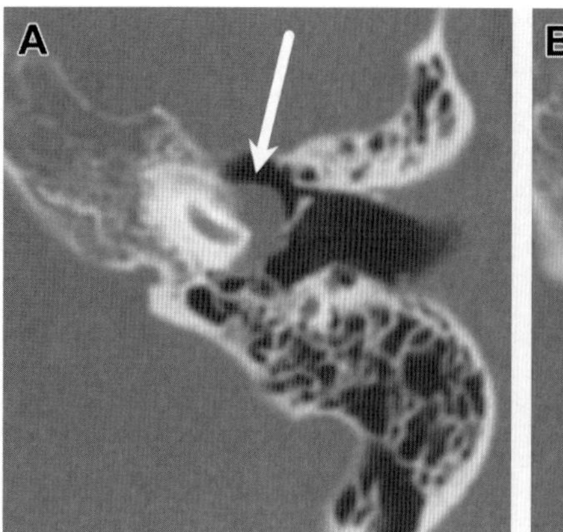

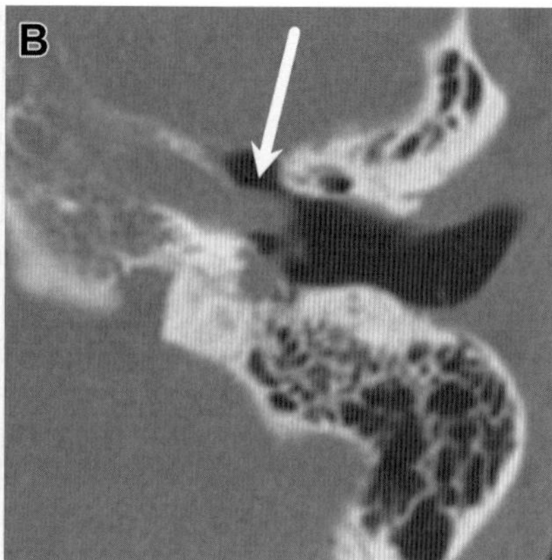

Fig. 22. Aberrant ICA. (*A*) Axial bone algorithm CT shows a soft-tissue attenuation lesion along the cochlear promontory (*arrow*), which on a single image is indistinguishable from a glomus tympanicum. (*B*) More inferior axial bone algorithm CT image shows the lesion to be continuous with the carotid canal (*arrow*), confirming an aberrant ICA.

be reassuring of normal jugular bulb asymmetry rather than a true jugular bulb lesion.

The clinical significance of jugular bulb dehiscence, high-riding jugular bulb, and jugular diverticulum is controversial, especially with respect to pulsatile tinnitus.[19–21] These lesions should be described on imaging studies for surgical planning purposes, but other causes should sought for the cause of clinical pulsatile tinnitus. Jugular bulb dehiscence (**Fig. 24**) can present incidentally to the otolaryngologist as a retrotympanic blue mass.

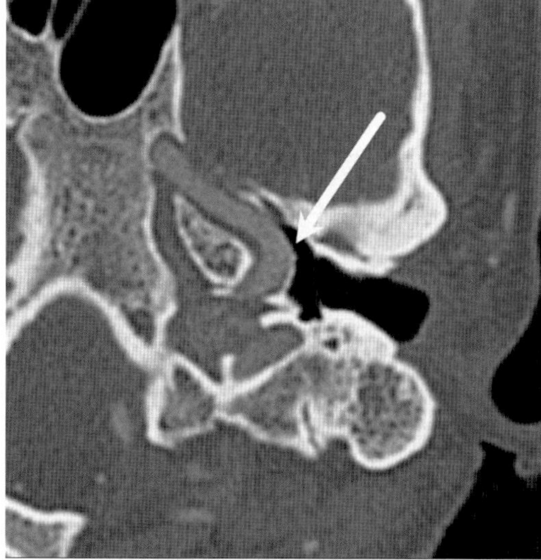

Fig. 23. Lateralized ICA. Axial postcontrast bone algorithm CT image shows protrusion of the ICA into the hypotympanum with thinned overlying bone (*arrow*). The ICA does not enter the middle ear, distinguishing it from an aberrant ICA.

Inner Ear

Inner ear disease is important to assess in any evaluation of a patient with sensorineural hearing loss or vestibular dysfunction (**Box 4**). A complete discussion of the myriad of congenital inner ear dysplasias is beyond the scope of this article. Instead the authors touch on one of the more common congenital inner ear dysplasias, large vestibular aqueduct. Although only 40% of radiologic studies in children with sensorineural hearing loss will be abnormal, by far the most commonly identified malformation is enlarged vestibular aqueduct (also known as large endolymphatic sac anomaly).[22] An enlarged vestibular aqueduct has been defined as a vestibular aqueduct measuring greater than 1.5 mm in greatest diameter at its midpoint and greater than 2.0 mm at the operculum (**Fig. 25**).[23,24] Practically speaking, any vestibular aqueduct with a diameter greater than the nearby lateral semicircular canal is considered abnormal.[25] Large vestibular aqueduct is associated with other inner ear abnormalities, including cochlear anomalies, such as modiolar deficiency and scalar asymmetry (76%) and vestibular anomalies (40%).[26]

Otosclerosis is an idiopathic disease characterized by spongiotic change of the otic capsule that can result in conductive, mixed, or sensorineural hearing loss.[27] The mildest form of otosclerosis is the fenestral form, which presents with conductive hearing loss and manifests as a lucency in the fissula ante fenestram, a small segment of bone located just anterior to the oval window (**Fig. 26**). Some patients with the fenestral form of otosclerosis will progress to the cochlear form, which is characterized by sensorineural or mixed hearing

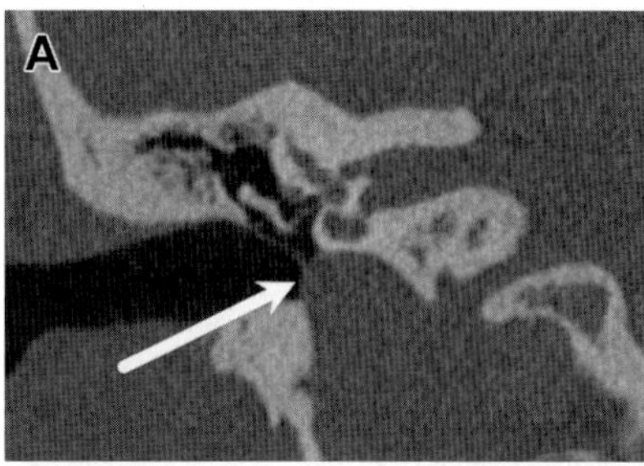

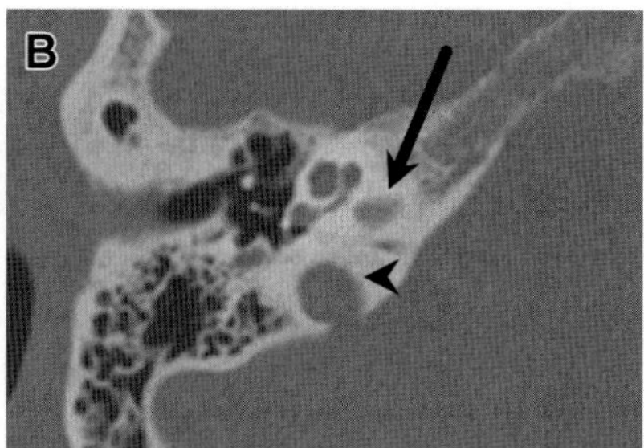

Fig. 24. Jugular bulb variants. (*A*) Coronal bone algorithm CT shows dehiscence of the sigmoid plate and protrusion of the jugular bulb (*arrow*) into the middle ear. (*B*) Axial bone algorithm CT in a different patient shows a high-riding jugular bulb, which is recognized when the superior margin of the jugular bulb (*arrowhead*) is at the level of the IAC (*arrow*).

loss, and shows lucency on CT and/or enhancement on MR imaging surrounding the cochlea (**Fig. 27**). It is important to make the subtle diagnosis of fenestral otosclerosis, as these patients may respond to fluoride treatment rather than require surgery.

Labyrinthitis related to bacterial meningitis is the most common causes of acquired deafness in children.[28] Other causes of labyrinthitis include viral infection and sequelae of trauma or surgery. On MR imaging, labyrinthitis manifests as enhancement of the inner ear structures with preserved T2 or fluid-sensitive signal (**Fig. 28**). Normal inner ear T2 signal distinguishes labyrinthitis from labyrinthitis ossificans, hemorrhage, and intralabyrinthine neoplasm. As sequelae of suppurative bacterial labyrinthitis, the labyrinth may develop progressive fibrosis and ossification, called labyrinthitis ossificans. On MR imaging, labyrinthitis ossificans manifests as decreased hyperintense signal within the labyrinth on T2 or fluid-sensitive sequences, with corresponding ossification and increased density on CT (**Fig. 29**). Early in the course of labyrinthitis ossificans there may be labyrinthine enhancement, but as the labyrinth continues to ossify the enhancement subsides. It is important to make a diagnosis early in the process of labyrinthitis or labyrinthitis ossificans, because as the cochlea becomes more ossified it is less amenable to cochlear implantation.[29]

Primary intralabyrinthine schwannomas were previously thought to be a rare neoplasm; however, with recent advances in high-resolution MR imaging, their prevalence has been reported as 10% of all vestibulocochlear nerve schwannomas.[30] On MR imaging, intralabyrinthine schwannoma presents as an enhancing neoplasm with corresponding circumscribed T2 hypointense filling defect within the affected portion of the labyrinth (**Fig. 30**). Intralabyrinthine schwannomas have been classified into 6 anatomic subtypes: intracochlear, transmodiolar (intracochlear extending to into IAC), intravestibular, transmacular (intravestibular extending into the IAC), vestibulocochlear, and transotic (extending into IAC and middle ear).[31] Surgery is reserved for lesions that extend into the IAC or patients with intractable vertigo.

Endolymphatic sac tumors are rare tumors of early adulthood that are typically unilateral and sporadic, but may be bilateral and associated with von Hippel-Lindau syndrome. The neoplasms are centered in the retrolabyrinthine temporal bone and nearly always show permeative destructive osseous changes, central calcification, and at least a partial posterior rim of calcification on CT. Characteristic MR imaging findings include heterogeneous enhancement and intrinsic T1 hyperintense foci related to hemorrhage or proteinaceous contents (**Fig. 31**). Imaging features and location can reliably distinguish endolymphatic sac tumor from its mimics, including meningioma, schwannoma, paraganglioma, and cholesterol granuloma.[32]

Semicircular canal dehiscence is a frequently suspected pathology on temporal bone imaging because of its myriad of audiovestibular symptoms including autophony, ear blockage, pressure, and sound-induced vertigo (also known as Tullio phenomenon).[33] On CT imaging, a

Box 4
Common inner ear abnormalities

- Congenital: enlarged vestibular aqueduct, semicircular canal dehiscence
- Acquired: otosclerosis
- Infectious: labyrinthitis, labyrinthitis ossificans
- Neoplastic: intralabyrinthine schwannoma, endolymphatic sac tumor

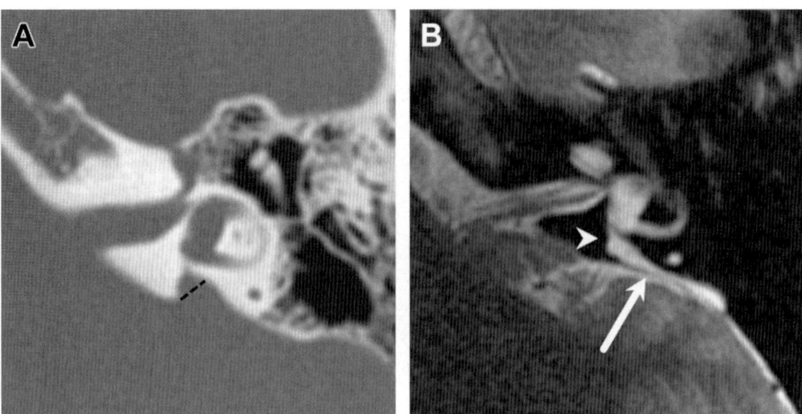

Fig. 25. Enlarged vestibular aqueduct (large endolymphatic sac anomaly). (*A*) Axial bone algorithm CT shows enlargement of the operculum of the vestibular aqueduct greater than 2 mm in diameter (*dashed line*). (*B*) Axial T2-weighted image of the same patient shows enlargement of the vestibular aqueduct (*arrowhead*) greater than the adjacent lateral semicircular canal, and gross enlargement of the endolymphatic sac (*arrow*).

dehiscence measuring 2.5 mm or greater over the superior semicircular canal has a higher association with auditory and vestibular symptoms in comparison with smaller dehiscences.[34] Thus, a conservative criterion for diagnosis of superior or posterior semicircular canal dehiscence would be a defect greater than or equal to 2 mm, as small focal dehiscence can be seen incidentally (**Fig. 32**). Semicircular canal dehiscence can also be suggested on high-resolution coronal T2-weighted MR imaging as absence of the hypointense bony covering.[35] Despite imaging findings, it is important to correlate with clinical symptoms, as CT is known to overdiagnose semicircular canal dehiscence with an 8-times greater prevalence than histologic evaluation.[36]

Petrous Apex

Common petrous apex abnormalities include pseudolesions, cephalocele, petrous apicitis, cholesterol granuloma, and chondrosarcoma (**Box 5**).

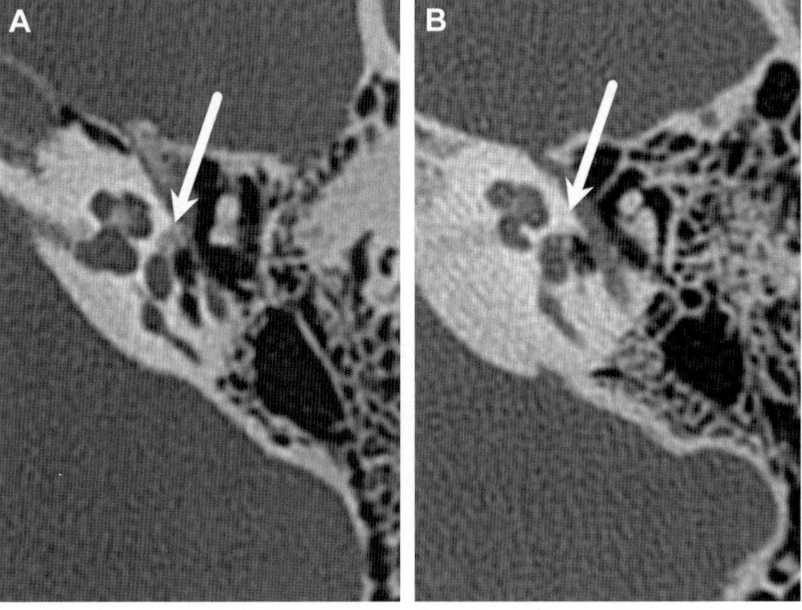

Fig. 26. Fenestral otosclerosis. (*A*) Axial bone algorithm CT shows a small lucency (*arrow*) within the fissula ante fenestram, which is often the only imaging finding of this abnormality on CT. (*B*) Axial bone algorithm CT in a different patient shows normal hyperdense bone within the normal fissula ante fenestram (*arrow*) anterior to the oval window.

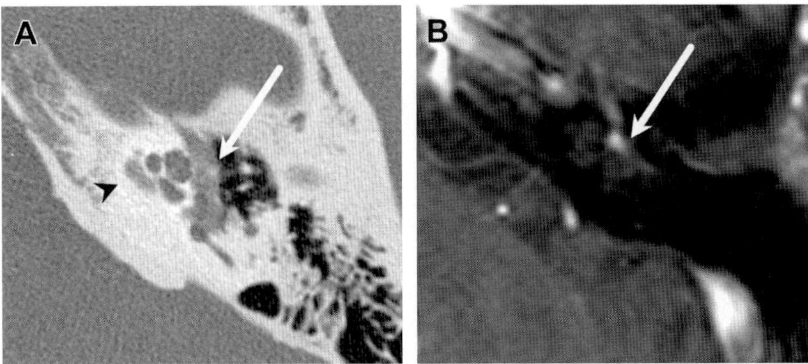

Fig. 27. Cochlear otosclerosis. (*A*) Axial bone algorithm CT shows abnormal lucency within the otic capsule in the region of the oval window and fissula ante fenestram (*arrow*) and also medial to the cochlea (*arrowhead*). (*B*) Axial postcontrast T1-weighted fat-suppressed MR image shows abnormal enhancement within the lateral pericochlear otic capsule (*arrow*).

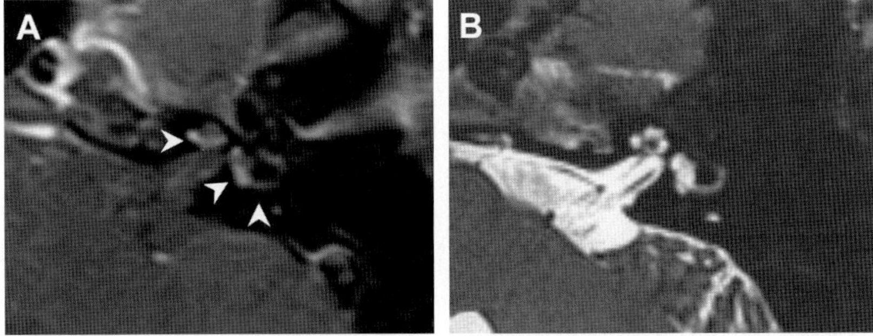

Fig. 28. Labyrinthitis. (*A*) Axial postcontrast T1-weighted fat-suppressed MR image shows abnormal enhancement of the basal turn of the cochlea, vestibule, and lateral semicircular canal (*arrowheads*). (*B*) Axial constructive interference in steady-state (CISS) MR image shows no abnormal hypointense mass within the inner ear, confirming labyrinthitis rather than neoplasm.

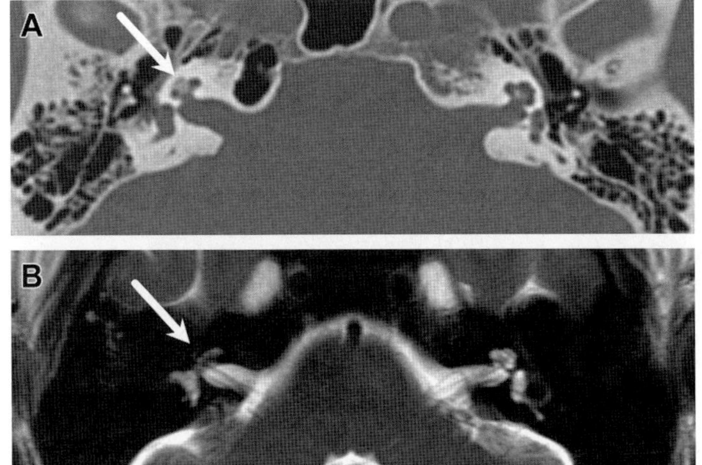

Fig. 29. Labyrinthitis ossificans. (*A*) Axial bone algorithm CT image of the bilateral temporal bones shows asymmetric hyperdensity within the middle turn of the right cochlea (*arrow*). (*B*) On axial T2-weighted imaging there is hypointensity in the middle turn and apex of the cochlea (*arrow*), corresponding to hyperdensity on CT.

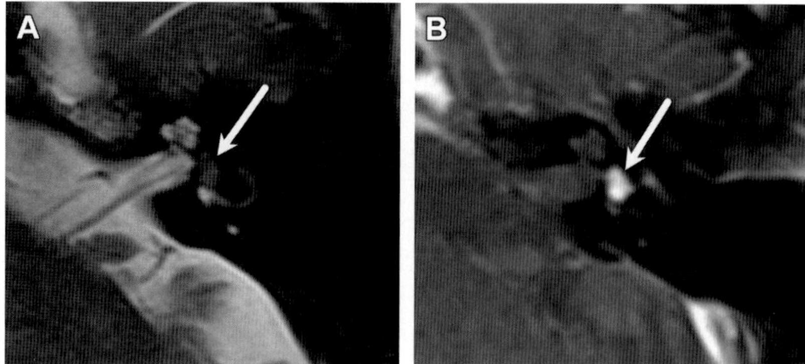

Fig. 30. Intravestibular schwannoma. (*A*) Axial CISS MR image shows circumscribed hypointense signal within the vestibule and adjacent lateral semicircular canal (*arrow*). (*B*) Axial postcontrast T1-weighted fat-suppressed MR image displays corresponding enhancement (*arrow*), confirming an intravestibular neoplasm.

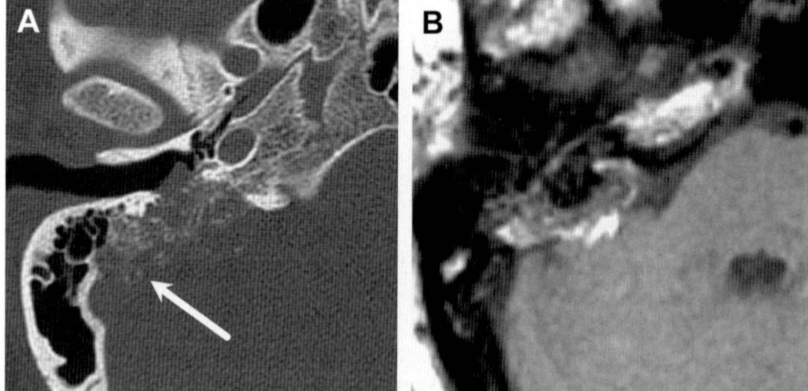

Fig. 31. Endolymphatic sac tumor. (*A*) Axial bone algorithm CT image shows a permeative destructive mass of the posterior temporal bone, which contains central calcification and has a thin rim of peripheral posterior calcification (*arrow*). (*B*) Axial precontrast T1-weighted MR image shows intrinsic T1 hyperintensity within the mass.

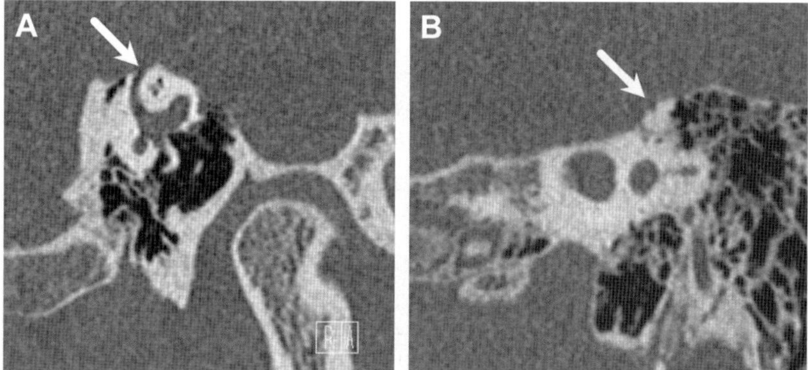

Fig. 32. Semicircular canal dehiscence. (*A*) Poschl view CT image parallel to the superior semicircular canal shows dehiscence (*arrow*) of the superior bony covering of the superior semicircular canal, also known as the arcuate eminence. (*B*) Stenvers view CT image perpendicular to the semicircular canal also shows the bony dehiscence (*arrow*).

Box 5
Common petrous apex abnormalities

- Pseudolesions: asymmetric marrow, benign effusion
- Congenital: cephalocele
- Infectious/inflammatory: petrous apicitis, cholesterol granuloma
- Neoplasm: chondrosarcoma, metastases, any primary osseous lesion

Normal variants of the petrous apex caused by asymmetric marrow or effusion within an aerated petrous apex can result in pseudolesions that may be misinterpreted as pathology. The key to identifying benign marrow is that it follows fat signal on all sequences and suppresses on fat suppression. Benign fluid can have variable signal on T1-weighted and T2-weighted imaging but lacks enhancement or osseous change on CT.[37] Symptoms related to the petrous apex, such as apical petrositis (Gradenigo syndrome), should prompt the radiologist to look for radiologic signs of abnormality, such as expansile bony changes in the setting of cholesterol granuloma or aggressive bony changes and peripheral enhancement in the setting of petrous apicitis.

Petrous apex cholesterol granuloma has pathogenesis and radiologic features similar to those of middle ear cholesteatoma (**Fig. 33**).[38] Fat-suppressed sequences are valuable in distinguishing cholesterol granuloma from asymmetric petrous apex marrow. Petrous apicitis is typically due to infectious spread of otitis media and has similar infectious complications of abscess, sinus thrombosis, and meningitis.[39]

Petrous apex cephaloceles are protrusions of meninges and CSF from the trigeminal cistern (Meckel cave) posteriorly and laterally into the petrous apex. These lesions manifest on MR imaging as CSF isointense collections within the petrous apex that may contain trigeminal neural tissue (**Fig. 34**). On CT, petrous apex cephaloceles are soft-tissue attenuation lesions surrounded by benign bony scalloping.[40] Coronal or sagittal CT or MR imaging often show a direct connection between the cephalocele and CSF. Petrous apex cephaloceles are critical to recognize, because they can be a source of CSF leak or an iatrogenic CSF leak may develop if this lesion is mistaken for neoplasm and resected.

Although various neoplasms can involve the petrous apex, chondrosarcoma have an unparalleled tropism for the petro-occipital fissure and the petrous apex.[41] Because chondrosarcomas arise at the fissure within the paramidline skull base, they can be distinguished by location from

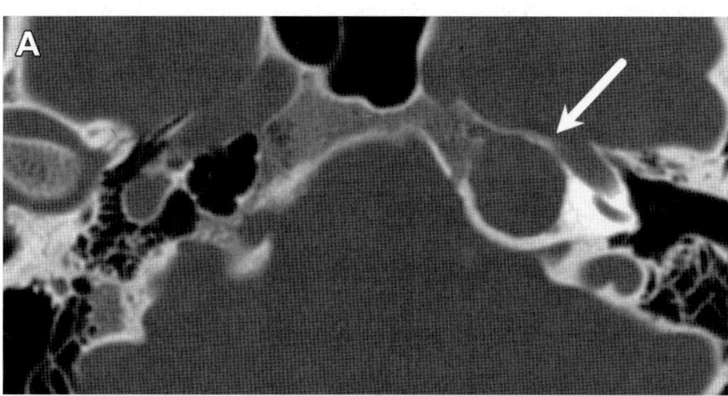

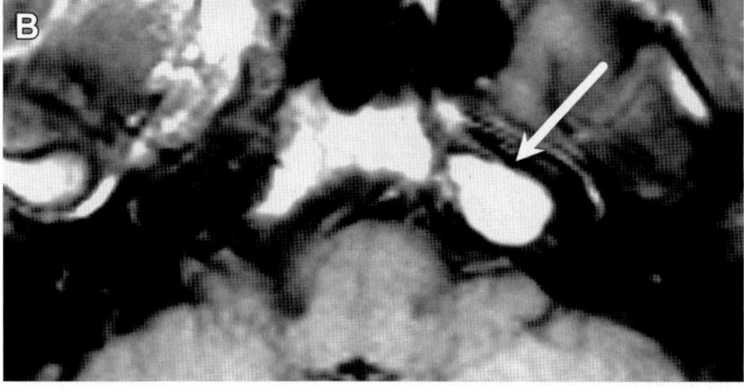

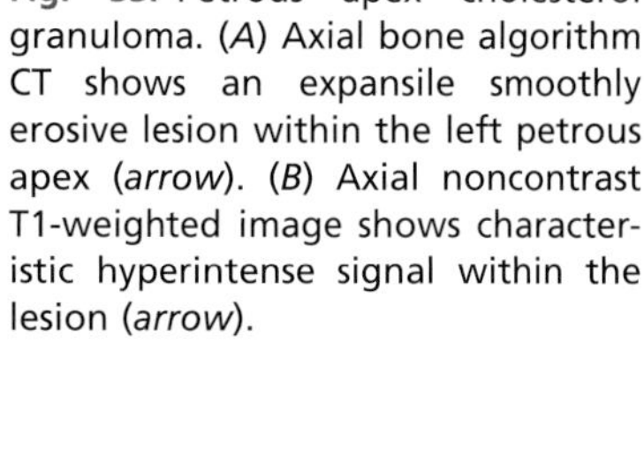

Fig. 33. Petrous apex cholesterol granuloma. (*A*) Axial bone algorithm CT shows an expansile smoothly erosive lesion within the left petrous apex (*arrow*). (*B*) Axial noncontrast T1-weighted image shows characteristic hyperintense signal within the lesion (*arrow*).

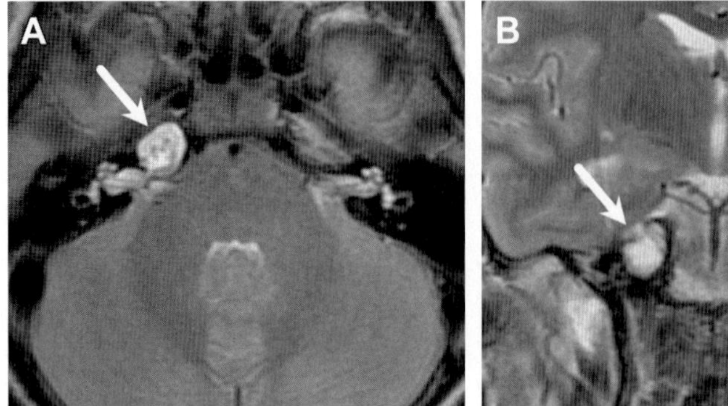

Fig. 34. Petrous apex cephalocele. (*A*) Axial T2-weighted image shows an expansile cerebrospinal fluid (CSF) signal T2 hyperintense lesion (*arrow*) within the right petrous apex, which contains linear hypointense neural elements of the trigeminal nerve. (*B*) Coronal T2-weighted image shows the CSF connection between the cephalocele and the inferior aspect of Meckel cave (*arrow*).

chordomas, which occur midline along the notochordal remnant. On MR imaging, chondrosarcomas are expansile, aggressive, paramidline, enhancing neoplasms with T2 hyperintense signal caused by chondroid matrix (**Fig. 35**).[41,42] On CT, these lesions have permeative destructive margins, and approximately 50% of skull base chondrosarcomas contain calcified chondroid matrix.[42]

Intratemporal Facial Nerve

Common abnormalities affecting the intratemporal facial nerve include schwannoma, herpetic (Bell) palsy, venous malformation, and perineural tumor spread (**Box 6**). The classic imaging presentation of facial nerve schwannoma is tubular enlargement and enhancement of the facial nerve on MR imaging, with corresponding expansion of the facial nerve canal on CT. Schwannomas affecting the IAC and labyrinthine segments of the facial nerve can be mistaken for vestibular nerve schwannomas if extension along the labyrinthine segment is not appreciated (**Fig. 36**). Facial nerve schwannomas involving the geniculate ganglion, tympanic segment, or mastoid segments may have nonclassic imaging features with extension or smooth erosion into the middle cranial fossa, middle ear, or mastoid air cells, respectively.[43] Treatment is typically delayed until the patient develops significant facial nerve palsy because of the risk of injury to the facial nerve during resection.

Herpetic neuralgia (Bell palsy) is thought to be a herpetic viral infection of the facial nerve, resulting in temporary facial nerve palsy that responds to steroids.[44] Imaging is indicated only when symptoms are atypical, so as to exclude any underlying

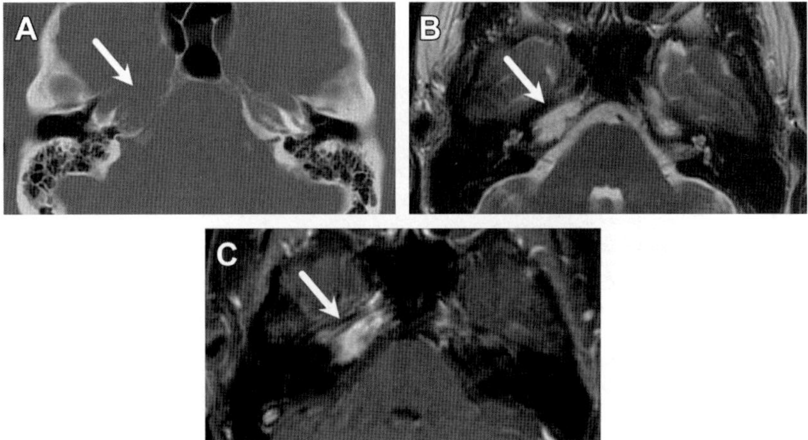

Fig. 35. Petrous apex chondrosarcoma. (*A*) Axial bone algorithm CT image shows a permeative destructive lesion (*arrow*) within the petrous apex centered at the petro-occipital fissure. (*B*) Axial T2-weighted image shows hyperintense signal within the lesion (*arrow*) caused by internal chondroid matrix. (*C*) Axial postcontrast fat-suppressed T1-weighted image shows enhancement within the lesion (*arrow*).

Box 6
Common facial nerve abnormalities

- Congenital: venous malformation
- Inflammatory: Herpetic neuralgia (Bell palsy)
- Neoplasm: facial nerve schwannoma, perineural tumor spread

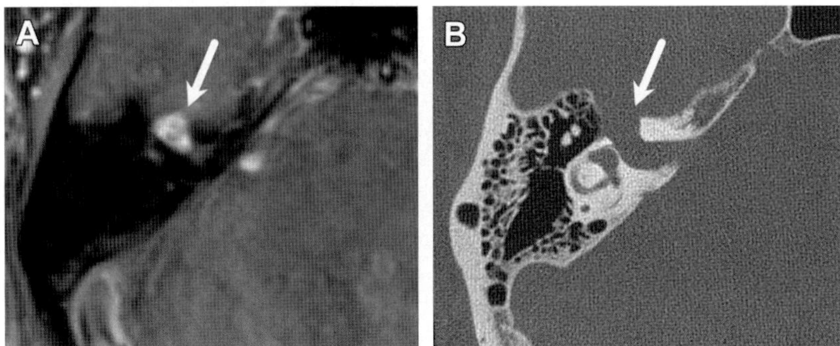

Fig. 36. Facial nerve schwannoma. (*A*) Axial postcontrast fat-suppressed T1-weighted image shows a tubular enhancing mass (*arrow*) involving the IAC segment of the facial nerve within the IAC fundus and the labyrinthine segment and geniculate ganglion. (*B*) Axial bone algorithm CT shows smooth erosion and expansion of the labyrinthine segment of the facial nerve canal and geniculate ganglion fossa (*arrow*).

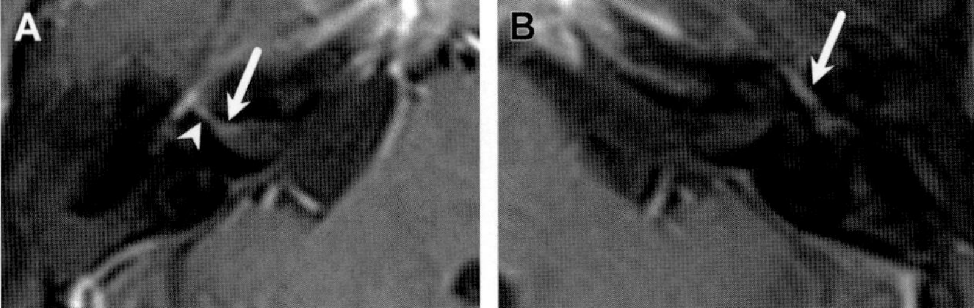

Fig. 37. Herpetic neuralgia (Bell palsy). (*A*) Axial postcontrast fat-suppressed T1-weighted image shows abnormal enhancement (without mass effect) of the IAC segment of the right facial nerve within the IAC fundus (*arrow*) and enhancement of the labyrinthine segment (*arrowhead*). (*B*) Axial postcontrast fat-suppressed T1-weighted image of the patient's normal left ear, which has normal enhancement of the tympanic segment of the facial nerve (*arrow*).

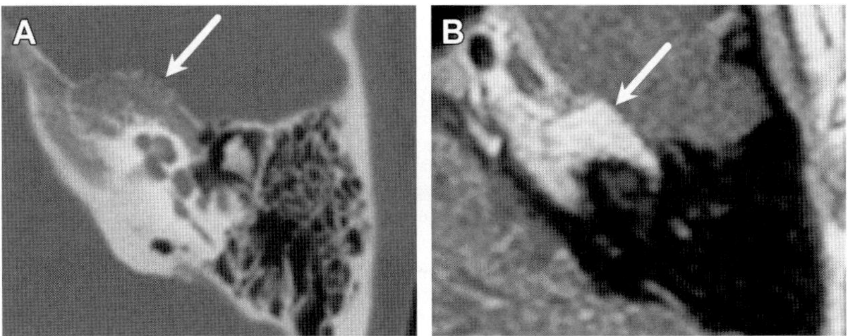

Fig. 38. Facial nerve venous malformation. (*A*) Axial bone algorithm CT shows an irregularly marginated mass (*arrow*) centered at the geniculate ganglion with internal honeycomb-like osseous changes characteristic of this lesion. (*B*) Axial postcontrast T1-weighted image shows avid enhancement within the mass (*arrow*).

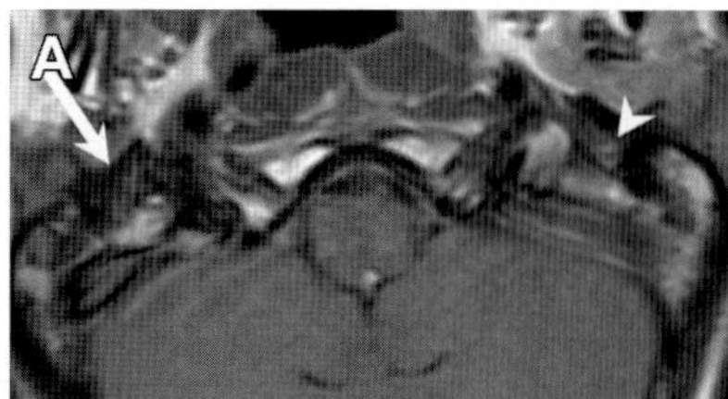

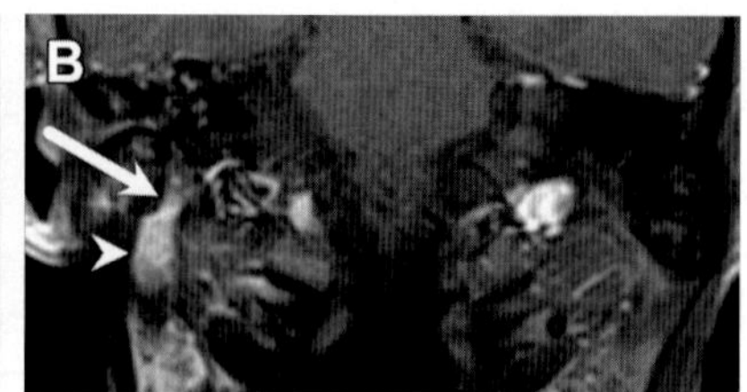

Fig. 39. Facial nerve perineural tumor spread. (*A*) Axial precontrast T1-weighted image shows normal hyperintense fat (*arrowhead*) within the left stylomastoid foramen. The right stylomastoid foramen is effaced by T1 hypointense material (*arrow*). (*B*) Coronal postcontrast fat-suppressed T1-weighted image shows abnormal enhancement and enlargement of the mastoid segment of the right facial nerve (*arrow*) within the stylomastoid foramen. An enhancing adenoid cyst carcinoma (*arrowhead*) within the posterior right parotid gland is the source of perineural tumor spread.

lesion. On MR imaging, herpetic neuralgia shows abnormal enhancement of the facial nerve within the fundus of the IAC and intralabyrinthine facial nerve segment (**Fig. 37**). Abnormal enhancement may extend along the remainder of the intratemporal facial nerve, and the nerve may swell; however, the facial nerve canal is not enlarged on CT (otherwise a neoplasm is suspected). The degree and extent of enhancement inversely correlates with recovery of facial nerve function.[45]

Facial nerve venous malformations are rare lesions formerly known as facial nerve hemangiomas.[46] The lesions are most commonly centered at the geniculate ganglion, but may extend along the labyrinthine or tympanic segments of the facial nerve. On CT, they manifest as a poorly marginated mass with internal hyperattenuating foci and characteristic honeycomb-like osseous changes. On MR imaging, facial nerve venous malformations have avid enhancement with ill-defined margins (**Fig. 38**).[47] Early radiologic diagnosis and treatment is key to preservation of facial nerve function.

Perineural spread of tumor along the facial nerve should be sought in any patient with parotid malignancy (especially adenoid cystic carcinoma) or periauricular skin cancer. Because most perineural tumor spread (PNTS) is asymptomatic, it is often the radiologist's responsibility to make the diagnosis. On MR imaging, an enhancing, enlarged facial nerve from the parotid gland proximal to the brainstem is evident; one should specifically look for preserved fat within the stylomastoid foramen to search for PNTS (**Fig. 39**). CT is helpful in evaluating enlargement of the facial nerve canal, but will otherwise miss spread along the nerve.[48]

SUMMARY

An understanding of temporal bone anatomy and common space-specific abnormality can facilitate an expert interpretation of temporal bone imaging. Communication with the referring otolaryngologist is crucial, as the clinical history and otoscopic examination may be as helpful as the imaging findings in making a radiologic diagnosis.

REFERENCES

1. Jahrsdoerfer RA, Yeakley JW, Aguilar EA, et al. Grading system for the selection of patients with congenital aural atresia. Am J Otol 1992;13(1):6–12.
2. Dubach P, Häusler R. External auditory canal cholesteatoma: reassessment of and amendments to its categorization, pathogenesis, and treatment in 34 patients. Otol Neurotol 2008;29(7):941–8. http://dx.doi.org/10.1097/MAo.0b013e318185fb20.
3. Heilbrun ME, Salzman KL, Glastonbury CM, et al. External auditory canal cholesteatoma: clinical and imaging spectrum. AJNR Am J Neuroradiol 2003; 24(4):751–6.
4. Stambuk HE. EAC skin SCCa. In: Harnsberger HR, editor. Diagnostic imaging: head and neck. 2nd edition. Salt Lake City (UT): Amirsys; 2011. Part 6–Section 2. p. 20–21.
5. Grandis JR, Curtin HD, Yu VL. Necrotizing (malignant) external otitis: prospective comparison of CT and MR imaging in diagnosis and follow-up. Radiology 1995;196(2):499–504.
6. Rubin Grandis J, Branstetter BF, Yu VL. The changing face of malignant (necrotising) external otitis: clinical, radiological, and anatomic correlations. Lancet Infect Dis 2004;4(1):34–9.
7. Yuen HW, Chen JM. External auditory canal osteoma. Otol Neurotol 2008;29(6):875–6. http://dx.doi.org/10.1097/mao.0b013e318161aaf8.
8. Sheard PW, Doherty M. Prevalence and severity of external auditory exostoses in breath-hold divers. J Laryngol Otol 2008;122(11):1162. http://dx.doi.org/10.1017/S0022215108001850.
9. Barath K, Huber AM, Stampfli P, et al. Neuroradiology of cholesteatomas. AJNR Am J Neuroradiol 2011;32(2):221–9. http://dx.doi.org/10.3174/ajnr.A2052.

10. Li PM, Linos E, Gurgel RK, et al. Evaluating the utility of non-echo-planar diffusion-weighted imaging in the preoperative evaluation of cholesteatoma: a meta-analysis. Laryngoscope 2013;123(5):1247–50. http://dx.doi.org/10.1002/lary.23759.
11. Vazquez E, Castellote A, Piqueras J, et al. Imaging of complications of acute mastoiditis in children. Radiographics 2003;23(2):359–72.
12. Mafee MF, Aimi K, Kahen HL, et al. Chronic otomastoiditis: a conceptual understanding of CT findings. Radiology 1986;160(1):193–200. http://dx.doi.org/10.1148/radiology.160.1.3715032.
13. Martin N, Sterkers O, Mompoint D, et al. Cholesterol granulomas of the middle ear cavities: MR imaging. Radiology 1989;172(2):521–5. http://dx.doi.org/10.1148/radiology.172.2.2748835.
14. Rao AB, Koeller KK, Adair CF. From the archives of the AFIP. Paragangliomas of the head and neck: radiologic-pathologic correlation. Armed Forces Institute of Pathology. Radiographics 1999;19(6):1605–32. http://dx.doi.org/10.1148/radiographics.19.6.g99no251605.
15. Olsen WL, Dillon WP, Kelly WM, et al. MR imaging of paragangliomas. AJR Am J Roentgenol 1987;148(1):201–4. http://dx.doi.org/10.2214/ajr.148.1.201.
16. Lo WW, Solti-Bohman LG, McElveen JT. Aberrant carotid artery: radiologic diagnosis with emphasis on high-resolution computed tomography. Radiographics 1985;5(6):985–93.
17. Glastonbury CM, Harnsberger HR, Hudgins PA, et al. Lateralized petrous internal carotid artery: imaging features and distinction from the aberrant internal carotid artery. Neuroradiology 2012;54(9):1007–13. http://dx.doi.org/10.1007/s00234-012-1034-8.
18. Tomura N, Sashi R, Kobayashi M, et al. Normal variations of the temporal bone on high-resolution CT: their incidence and clinical significance. Clin Radiol 1995;50(3):144–8.
19. Remley KB, Coit WE, Harnsberger HR, et al. Pulsatile tinnitus and the vascular tympanic membrane: CT, MR, and angiographic findings. Radiology 1990;174(2):383–9. http://dx.doi.org/10.1148/radiology.174.2.2296650.
20. Weissman JL, Hirsch BE. Imaging of tinnitus: a review. Radiology 2000;216(2):342–9. http://dx.doi.org/10.1148/radiology.216.2.r00au45342.
21. Sonmez G, Basekim CC, Ozturk E, et al. Imaging of pulsatile tinnitus: a review of 74 patients. Clin Imaging 2007;31(2):102–8. http://dx.doi.org/10.1016/j.clinimag.2006.12.024.
22. Mafong DD, Shin EJ, Lalwani AK. Use of laboratory evaluation and radiologic imaging in the diagnostic evaluation of children with sensorineural hearing loss. Laryngoscope 2002;112(1):1–7. http://dx.doi.org/10.1097/00005537-200201000-00001.
23. Valvassori GE, Clemis JD. The large vestibular aqueduct syndrome. Laryngoscope 1978;88(5):723–8.
24. Vijayasekaran S, Halsted MJ, Boston M, et al. When is the vestibular aqueduct enlarged? A statistical analysis of the normative distribution of vestibular aqueduct size. AJNR Am J Neuroradiol 2007;28(6):1133–8. http://dx.doi.org/10.3174/ajnr.A0495.
25. Weissman JL. Hearing loss. Radiology 1996;199(3):593–611. http://dx.doi.org/10.1148/radiology.199.3.8637972.
26. Davidson HC, Harnsberger HR, Lemmerling MM, et al. MR evaluation of vestibulocochlear anomalies associated with large endolymphatic duct and sac. AJNR Am J Neuroradiol 1999;20(8):1435–41.
27. Lee TC, Aviv RI, Chen JM, et al. CT grading of otosclerosis. AJNR Am J Neuroradiol 2009;30(7):1435–9. http://dx.doi.org/10.3174/ajnr.A1558.
28. Fortnum H, Davis A. Hearing impairment in children after bacterial meningitis: incidence and resource implications. Br J Audiol 1993;27(1):43–52.
29. Hegarty JL, Patel S, Fischbein N, et al. The value of enhanced magnetic resonance imaging in the evaluation of endocochlear disease. Laryngoscope 2002;112(1):8–17. http://dx.doi.org/10.1097/00005537-200201000-00002.
30. Tieleman A, Casselman JW, Somers T, et al. Imaging of intralabyrinthine schwannomas: a retrospective study of 52 cases with emphasis on lesion growth. AJNR Am J Neuroradiol 2008;29(5):898–905. http://dx.doi.org/10.3174/ajnr.A1026.
31. Salzman KL, Childs AM, Davidson HC, et al. Intralabyrinthine schwannomas: imaging diagnosis and classification. AJNR Am J Neuroradiol 2012;33(1):104–9. http://dx.doi.org/10.3174/ajnr.A2712.
32. Patel NP, Wiggins RH, Shelton C. The radiologic diagnosis of endolymphatic sac tumors. Laryngoscope 2006;116(1):40–6. http://dx.doi.org/10.1097/01.mlg.0000185600.18456.36.
33. Zhou G, Gopen Q, Poe DS. Clinical and diagnostic characterization of canal dehiscence syndrome: a great otologic mimicker. Otol Neurotol 2007;28(7):920–6.
34. Pfammatter A, Darrouzet V, Gärtner M, et al. A superior semicircular canal dehiscence syndrome multicenter study: is there an association between size and symptoms? Otol Neurotol 2010;31(3):447–54. http://dx.doi.org/10.1097/MAO.0b013e3181d27740.
35. Krombach GA, Di Martino E, Martiny S, et al. Dehiscence of the superior and/or posterior semicircular canal: delineation on T2-weighted axial three-dimensional turbo spin-echo images, maximum intensity projections and volume-rendered images. Eur Arch Otorhinolaryngol 2006;263(2):111–7. http://dx.doi.org/10.1007/s00405-005-0970-x.
36. Sequeira SM, Whiting BR, Shimony JS, et al. Accuracy of computed tomography detection of superior

canal dehiscence. Otol Neurotol 2011;32(9):1500–5. http://dx.doi.org/10.1097/MAO.0b013e318238280c.

37. Moore KR, Harnsberger HR, Shelton C, et al. "Leave me alone" lesions of the petrous apex. AJNR Am J Neuroradiol 1998;19(4):733–8.
38. Greenberg JJ, Oot RF, Wismer GL, et al. Cholesterol granuloma of the petrous apex: MR and CT evaluation. AJNR Am J Neuroradiol 1988;9:1205–14.
39. Koral K, Dowling M. Petrous apicitis in a child: computed tomography and magnetic resonance imaging findings. Clin Imaging 2006;30(2):137–9. http://dx.doi.org/10.1016/j.clinimag.2005.10.007.
40. Moore KR, Fischbein NJ, Harnsberger HR, et al. Petrous apex cephaloceles. AJNR Am J Neuroradiol 2001;22(10):1867–71.
41. Oghalai JS, Buxbaum JL, Jackler RK, et al. Skull base chondrosarcoma originating from the petroclival junction. Otol Neurotol 2005;26(5):1052–60. http://dx.doi.org/10.1097/01.mao.0000185076.65822.f7.
42. Meyers SP, Hirsch WL, Curtin HD, et al. Chondrosarcomas of the skull base: MR imaging features. Radiology 1992;184(1):103–8. Available at: http://pubs.rsna.org/doi/abs/10.1148/radiology.184.1.1609064.
43. Wiggins RH, Harnsberger HR, Salzman KL, et al. The many faces of facial nerve schwannoma. AJNR Am J Neuroradiol 2006;27(3):694–9.
44. Yeo SG, Lee YC, Park DC, et al. Acyclovir plus steroid vs steroid alone in the treatment of Bell's palsy. Am J Otol 2008;29(3):163–6. http://dx.doi.org/10.1016/j.amjoto.2007.05.001.
45. Kress B, Griesbeck F, Stippich C, et al. Bell palsy: quantitative analysis of MR imaging data as a method of predicting outcome. Radiology 2004;230(2):504–9. http://dx.doi.org/10.1148/radiol.2302021353.
46. Benoit MM, North PE, McKenna MJ, et al. Facial nerve hemangiomas: vascular tumors or malformations? Otolaryngol Head Neck Surg 2010;142(1):108–14. http://dx.doi.org/10.1016/j.otohns.2009.10.007.
47. Martin N, Sterkers O, Nahum H. Haemangioma of the petrous bone: MRI. Neuroradiology 1992;34(5):420–2.
48. Parker GD, Harnsberger HR. Clinical-radiologic issues in perineural tumor spread of malignant diseases of the extracranial head and neck. Radiographics 1991;11(3):383–99. http://dx.doi.org/10.1148/radiographics.11.3.1852933.

Orbital Imaging
A Pattern-Based Approach

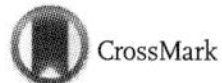

Daniel E. Meltzer, MD

KEYWORDS

• Metastasis • Lymphoproliferative disease • Computed tomography • Magnetic resonance imaging • Intraocular • Intraconal • Extraconal

KEY POINTS

- Several inflammatory and lymphoproliferative diseases are hypointense signal on T2W images, due to the high nuclear to cytoplasmic ratio of their cellular content.
- Dedicated multiplanar thin section images with fat saturation technique is required for diagnostic MRI studies of the orbit. Routine brain imaging is insufficient.
- A pattern-based approach to image interpretation, and consideration of the symptoms, will help the radiologist generate a concise and clinically relevant differential diagnosis.

INTRODUCTION

The imaging modalities most commonly used to evaluate the orbit are ultrasonography, computed tomography (CT), and magnetic resonance (MR) imaging. Ultrasonography is mainly used to evaluate intraocular lesions, and is often performed by ophthalmologists in an outpatient setting. MR and CT frequently provide complementary information, and both may be indicated for evaluating complex disease. CT is often the initial imaging modality for patients presenting with signs and symptoms of infection. CT is also optimal for detecting calcifications and assessing osseous disease of the orbit. MR is the modality of choice for evaluating most retrobulbar disease, including lesions of the optic nerve sheath complex (ONSC). MR is also best for determining the full extent of lesions that have orbital and intracranial components.

For the radiologist interpreting imaging studies of the orbit, it may often be difficult to generate a concise and targeted differential diagnosis for the ordering clinician. There are a wide variety of diseases that can occur within the orbit, many of which may affect one or multiple orbital structures. Several of these entities, such as idiopathic orbital inflammatory syndrome and lymphoproliferative disease, can have various presentations both clinically and at imaging and may mimic other disease processes. A well-known approach to differential diagnosis is to divide disease processes into categories such as neoplastic, inflammatory, infectious, traumatic, developmental, and so forth. However, in the orbit, many specific entities from each of these general classifications of disease may manifest with similar imaging findings. Consequently, strictly adhering to this method may lead to long lists of possible causes, which do not help the clinician direct their diagnostic efforts.

Despite the myriad potential causes of a given imaging abnormality in the orbit, there are a limited number of patterns that the findings can comprise. This limitation is related to the constraints of the anatomy of the orbit and its adjacent structures, and the relatively few organs that comprise this region of the body. Therefore, a pattern-based approach can be useful for generating a concise list of differential diagnoses that help the clinician direct further diagnostic or therapeutic efforts. Clinical findings such as the patient's age, duration of symptoms, presence or absence of pain, and whether the process is unilateral or bilateral are crucial. For example,

Mount Sinai Hospital, Roosevelt Division, 1000 Tenth Ave, Suite 4B–14, New York, NY 10019, USA
E-mail address: dmeltzer@chpnet.org

Radiol Clin N Am 53 (2015) 37–80
http://dx.doi.org/10.1016/j.rcl.2014.09.004
0033-8389/15/$ – see front matter

unilateral rapid onset of pain brings infection and inflammation to the top of the list of potential diagnoses. Rapid onset of painless clinical findings may indicate a malignant or vascular cause. A painless indolent course raises the possibility of benign neoplasm or developmental anomalies, or possibly metabolic disease.

This article is divided into 6 sections, each section focusing on a basic imaging pattern of orbital disease: ONSC lesions, intraconal lesions, extraconal lesions, extraocular muscle enlargement, infiltrative disease, and intraocular lesions. Within each section, there is a description of 5 to 7 important pathologic processes to be considered for the differential diagnosis of a particular imaging pattern, from various etiologic categories. Certain diseases, such as lymphoproliferative disease, metastases, sarcoidosis, and idiopathic orbital inflammation (IOI), may present with many of the imaging patterns explored in this article, and are discussed only briefly in some sections to avoid redundancy. Ample figures are provided to show their appearance on CT and MR imaging. In addition, the reader may refer to the anatomic illustrations of the orbit (**Figs. 1–3**).

OPTIC NERVE SHEATH COMPLEX LESION

Optic Neuritis

When imaging a patient to assess for disease of the ONSC, especially optic neuritis, CT has virtually no role, and proper MR image acquisition is paramount for accurate diagnosis. The normal ONSC is only about 4 to 5 mm thick throughout most of its orbital course, and therefore, 5-mm axial sections used in routine protocols for postcontrast MR imaging of the brain are not adequate, because the ONSC is subject to a volume-averaging artifact. A reasonable protocol includes 3-mm axial images, and 4-mm coronal images. Fat saturation is paramount, because this technique renders abnormal enhancement or T2 signal in the ONSC more conspicuous on postcontrast T1 or short tau inversion recovery (STIR) imaging

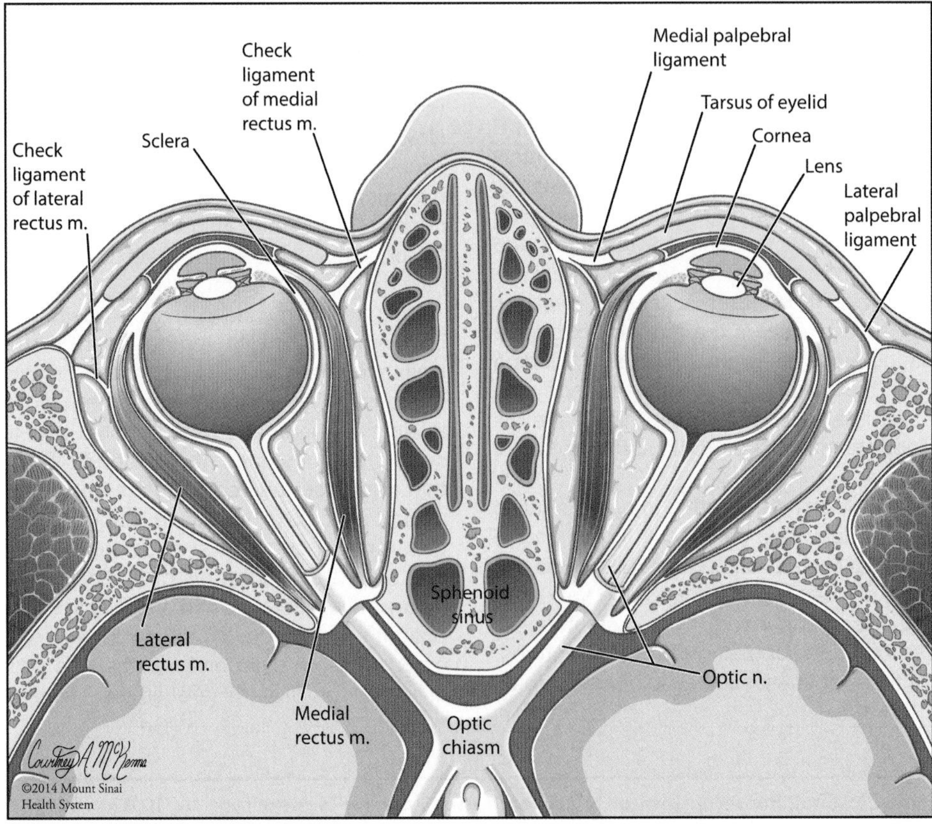

Fig. 1. Axial anatomy. m., muscle; n., nerve. (Illustration created by Courtney McKenna © Mount Sinai Health System, New York, NY. Used with permission.)

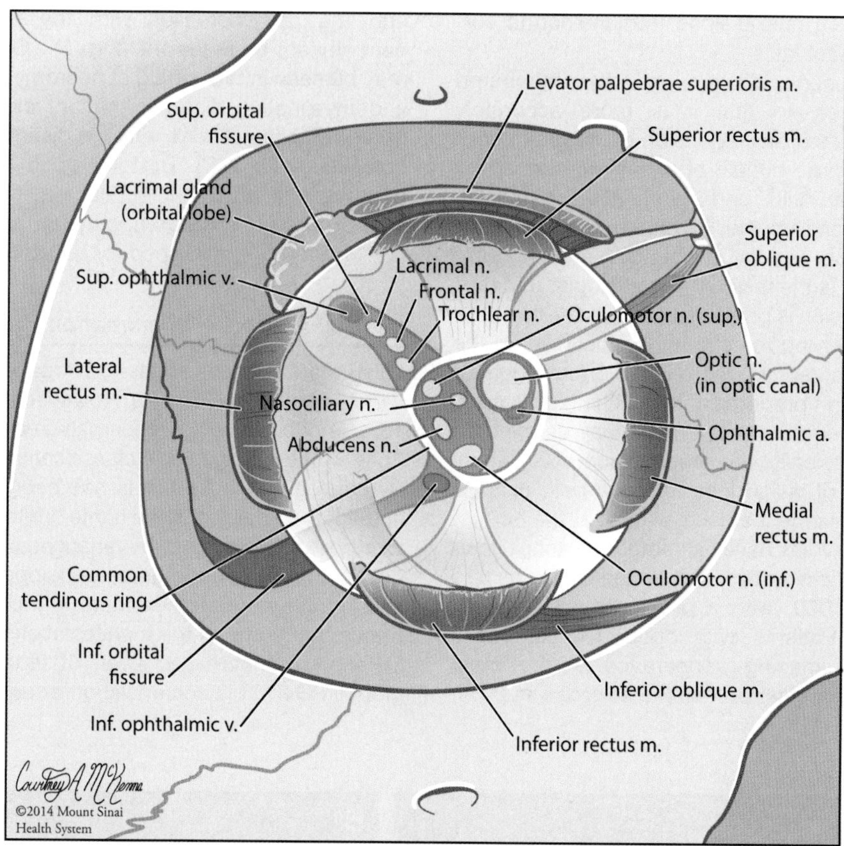

Fig. 2. Coronal anatomy. a., artery; Inf., inferior; m., muscle; n., nerve; Sup, superior; v., vein. (Illustration created by Courtney McKenna © Mount Sinai Health System, New York, NY. Used with permission.)

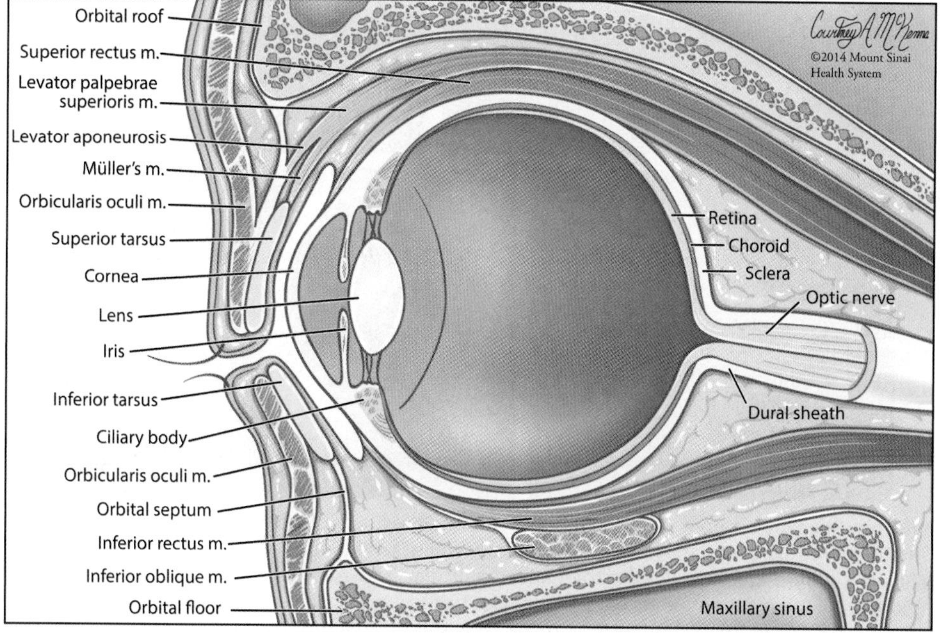

Fig. 3. Sagittal anatomy. m., muscle. (Illustration created by Courtney McKenna © Mount Sinai Health System, New York, NY. Used with permission.)

respectively, by nulling signal from the normal surrounding orbital fat.

The optic nerve is unlike the other numbered cranial nerves, in that it is more accurately described as a direct extension of the brain, consisting of a large bundle of axons surrounded by cerebrospinal fluid and meninges. Frequently, abnormal signal in the ONSC seems to involve both the nerve and the surrounding sheath at imaging, and it is the task of the radiologist to determine if the lesion is primarily involving the nerve, or primarily involving the sheath (perineuritis). In the case of optic neuritis, there is abnormal signal or enhancement predominantly within the optic nerve. Any segment of the nerve may be affected (**Fig. 4**). Classically, the presentation of unilateral rapid onset of vision loss and eye pain exacerbated by movement aids in arriving at the correct diagnosis. Studies have estimated the annual incidence of optic neuritis in the United States as 5 to 6.4 per 100,000, with a prevalence of 115 per 100,000.[1,2] Patients with optic neuritis and a normal MR imaging appearance of the brain have a 15-year risk for multiple sclerosis of 25%, and the risk increases with the presence of concomitant brain lesions (**Fig. 5**).[3] Optic neuritis may be seen in the setting of neuromyelitis optica, a demyelinating disorder that attacks the optic nerves and spinal cord, which is distinct from multiple sclerosis (MS). Bilateral optic neuritis has been associated with infectious cause, such as a viral prodrome in children, although the association is not well established for adults (**Fig. 6**).[4]

Idiopathic Orbital Inflammation

Inflammatory disease of the orbit may be seen in a variety of distinct diseases. However, about 5% to 13% of cases have no discernable cause after biopsy[5,6] and fall under the classification of IOI. The terminology of these cases has been varied and subject to debate, with the name orbital pseudotumor being widely used, or variations such as idiopathic orbital pseudotumor or idiopathic orbital inflammatory syndrome. There is increasing evidence that some of the manifestations of IOI may be related to increased levels of serum immunoglobulin G4.[6] This accumulation of data may lead

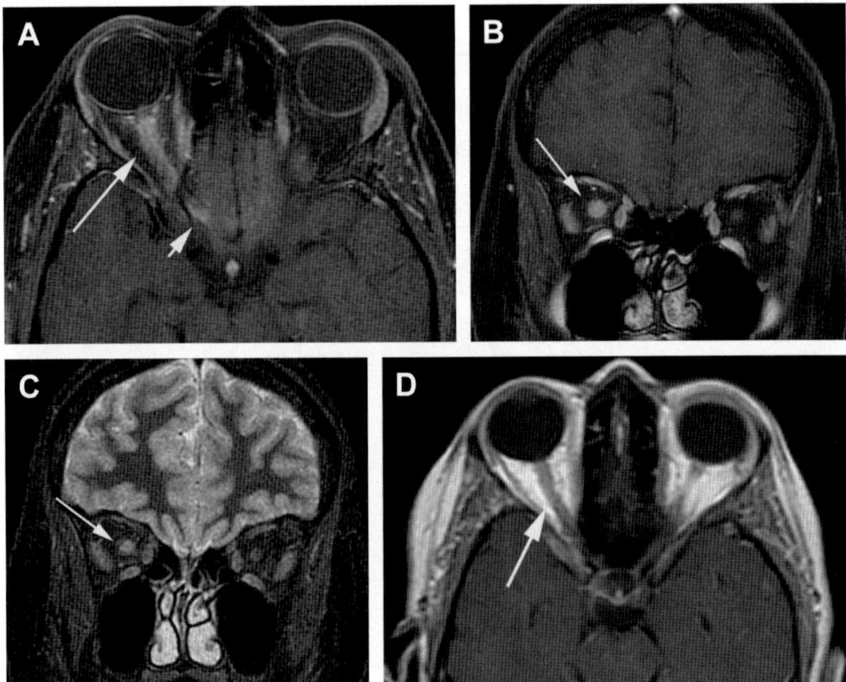

Fig. 4. Optic neuritis whole nerve. A 25-year-old woman with acute right orbital pain and vision loss. (*A*) Axial postcontrast T1-weighted image shows abnormal enhancement of the right optic nerve along nearly the entirety of its course, including the orbital (*long arrow*) and canalicular (*short arrow*) segments. (*B*) Coronal postcontrast T1-weighted image again shows abnormal enhancement of the right ONSC, predominantly involving the nerve (*arrow*), and (*C*) a corresponding coronal STIR image shows abnormal signal in the nerve consistent with edema (*arrow*). (*D*) Routine 5-mm axial postcontrast T1-weighted image does not clearly show the abnormal findings seen on the thin section fat-saturated images (*arrow*).

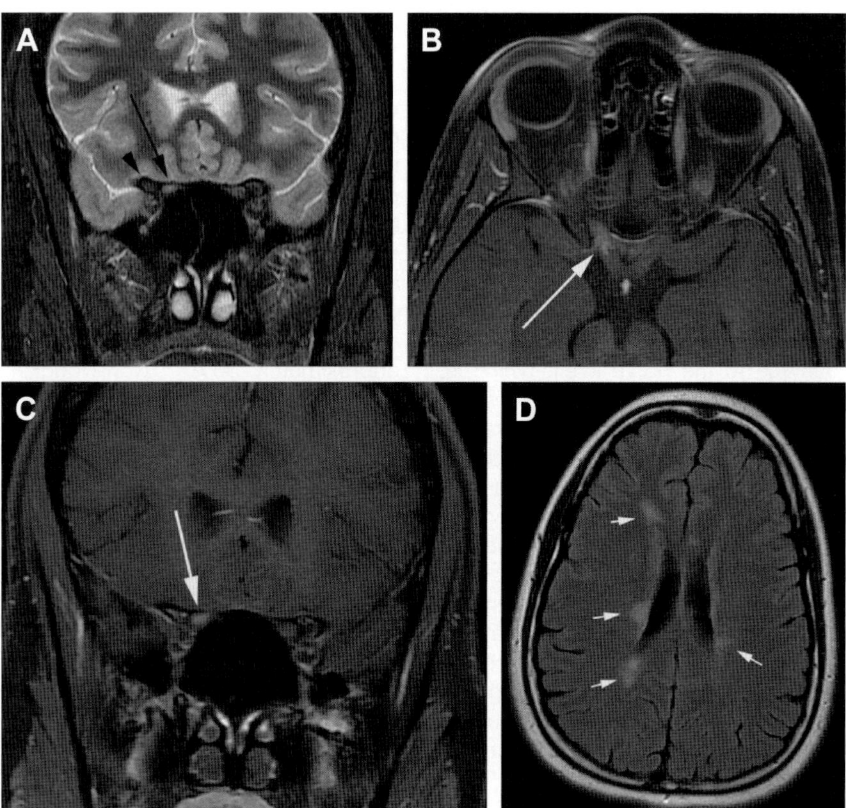

Fig. 5. Optic neuritis with multiple sclerosis. A 27-year-old woman with acute right orbital pain and vision loss. (*A*) Coronal STIR image shows abnormal signal hyperintensity in the canalicular segment of the right optic nerve (*arrow*). The adjacent anterior clinoid process (*arrowhead*) is a good anatomic landmark. (*B*) Axial and (*C*) coronal postcontrast fat-saturated T1-weighted images show corresponding abnormal enhancement of the canalicular segment of the right optic nerve (*arrows*). (*D*) Axial fluid-attenuated inversion recovery image of the brain shows abnormal signal intensity in the periventricular white matter (*arrows*), in a pattern commonly seen in the setting of multiple sclerosis.

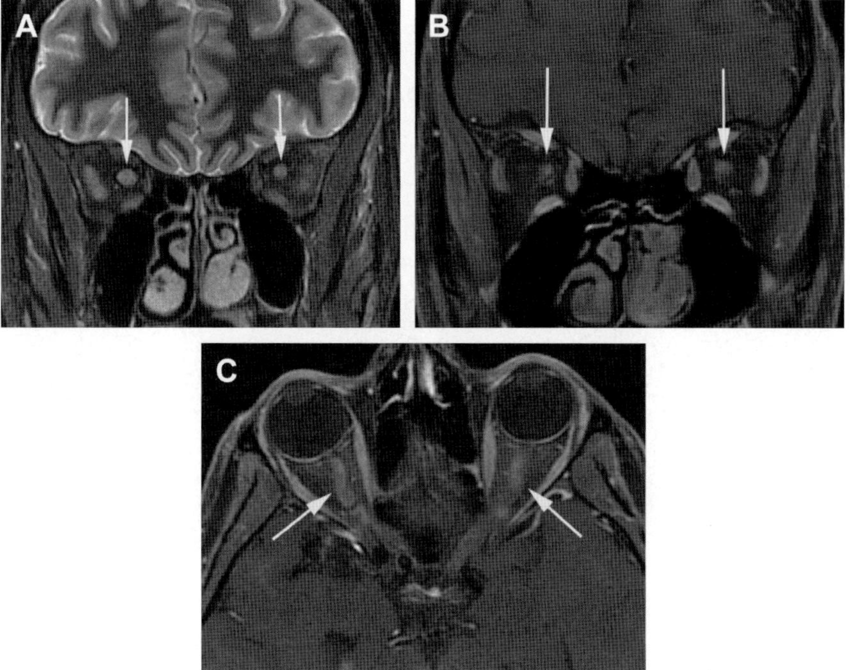

Fig. 6. Optic neuritis bilateral postviral. A 26-year-old man with acute bilateral orbital pain and vision loss. (*A*) Coronal STIR image shows abnormal signal hyperintensity in the bilateral optic nerves (*arrows*). (*B*) Corresponding coronal postcontrast T1-weighted image shows abnormal enhancement of the bilateral optic nerves (*arrows*). (*C*) Axial postcontrast T1-weighted image shows abnormal enhancement of the orbital segments of the bilateral optic nerves (*arrows*).

to reclassification of some forms of IOI. However, for the time being, IOI has been described as the third most common disease process of the orbit in adults, behind thyroid orbitopathy and lymphoproliferative disorders.[7]

When occurring in the ONSC, IOI predominantly involves the sheath, in contradistinction to optic neuritis, in which the nerve is mainly affected (**Fig. 7**). Nevertheless, the inflammation can cause permanent damage to the nerve itself, which is clinically evident and which may also manifest on imaging as atrophy of the optic nerve. The retrobulbar fat surrounding the ONSC may be involved to varying degrees, and there may be concurrent involvement of the extraocular muscles or lacrimal gland (**Fig. 8**). The classic clinical presentation is rapid onset of pain and possibly diplopia; less often, vision loss. The symptoms are usually unilateral, although some patients present with bilateral disease, more commonly children.[8] The rapidly progressive painful onset may help to distinguish IOI from lymphoproliferative disease or sarcoidosis, which often appear similar to IOI at imaging.

Lymphoproliferative Disease

Lymphoproliferative disorders include lymphoma, lymphoid hyperplasia and atypical lymphoid hyperplasia, and ocular adnexal lymphoma. Of these disorders, malignant lymphoma is the most common, accounting for 67% to 90% of orbital lymphoproliferative tumors and 24% of all space-occupying orbital tumors in patients older than 60 years.[9,10] Orbital disease may be a manifestation of systemic lymphoma or may arise primarily in the orbit. Many patients who initially present with an orbital lymphoproliferative tumor develop systemic lymphoma within the next 10 years, approximately 30%.[10] Non-Hodgkin lymphoma, specifically the mucosa-associated lymphoid tissue (MALT) form, is the most common subtype of primary orbital lymphoma.[9] On MR imaging, lymphoproliferative disease of the ONSC may be indistinguishable from sarcoidosis or IOI (**Fig. 9**).

Optic Nerve Sheath Meningioma

Although optic nerve sheath meningioma (ONSM) is rare, it nevertheless represents the second most common tumor to arise from the ONSC after optic glioma.[11] Like intracranial meningioma, ONSM is usually benign, but may cause progressive vision loss if left untreated. The vision loss is typically progressive over a prolonged course of months to years, and patients may come to medical attention with varying degrees of optic nerve atrophy. Radiation therapy is the most common treatment.

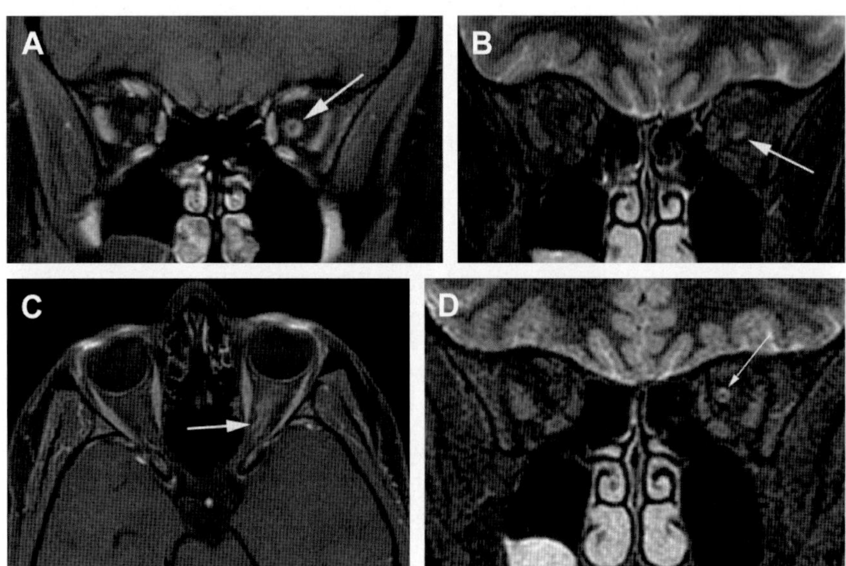

Fig. 7. IOI with perineuritis. A 31-year-old woman with acute left orbital pain and blurry vision. (*A*) Coronal postcontrast T1-weighted image shows abnormal enhancement of the left ONSC, predominantly involving the sheath (*arrow*). (*B*) Corresponding coronal STIR image shows abnormal signal hyperintensity of the left optic nerve sheath, relatively sparing the nerve (*arrow*). (*C*) Axial postcontrast T1-weighted image shows abnormal enhancement of the orbital segment of the left optic nerve sheath (*arrow*). (*D*) Follow-up coronal STIR image 14 months after treatment shows small caliber of the left optic nerve and relative prominence of the surrounding cerebrospinal fluid within its sheath, consistent with atrophy (*arrow*).

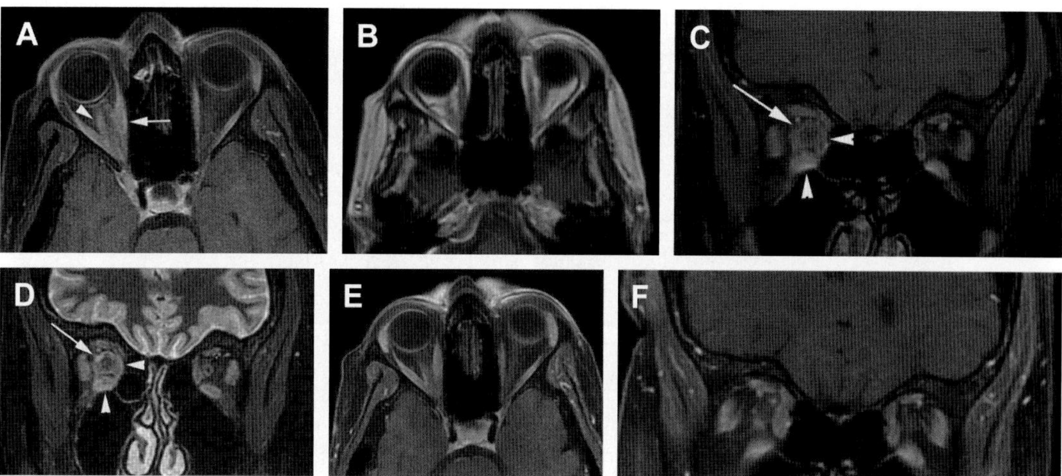

Fig. 8. IOI of ONSC and extraocular muscle (EOM). A 53-year-old woman with acute right orbital pain and diplopia. (*A*) Axial postcontrast fat-saturated T1-weighted image shows abnormal enhancement of the right ONSC (*arrowhead*). There is also enlargement and abnormal enhancement of the left medial rectus muscle (*arrow*). (*B*) These findings are not readily apparent on the routine postcontrast axial T1-weighted image of the head acquired at the end of the examination. (*C*) Coronal postcontrast T1-weighted image shows that the abnormal enhancement of the right ONSC is predominantly involving the nerve sheath (*arrow*). There is enlargement and abnormal enhancement of the medial and inferior rectus muscles (*arrowheads*). (*D*) Coronal STIR image shows corresponding signal abnormality in the nerve sheath (*arrow*) and extraocular muscles (*arrowheads*). (*E*) Follow-up axial and (*F*) coronal postcontrast fat-saturated T1-weighted images show near resolution of the abnormal findings after a course of steroid therapy.

ONSM may present with a variety of morphologic features and growth patterns at imaging, and these have been classified by investigators such as Schick and colleagues.[12] The shape of the perineural component may vary from bulblike (**Fig. 10**) to fusiform (**Fig. 11**), eccentric or concentric and diffuse or focal. The ONSM may or may not have an intracranial component, with contiguity through the superior or inferior orbital fissure into the cavernous sinus; extension into the optic canal is also a variable feature.

As with intracranial meningioma, the fibroblastic stromal elements of ONSM give it a characteristic T2 signal, which is hypointense compared with

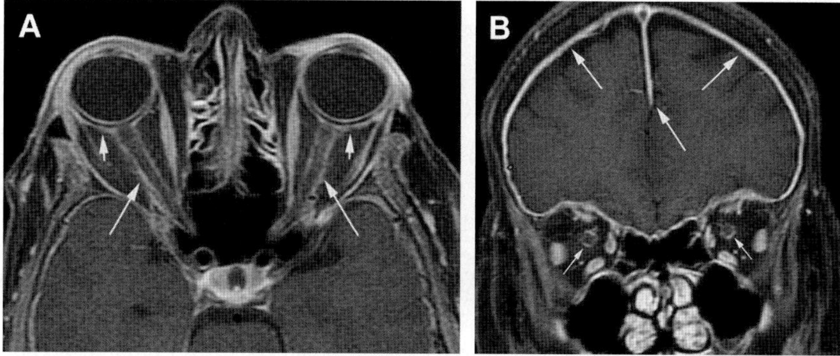

Fig. 9. Non-Hodgkin lymphoma of the ONSC. A 68-year-old woman with bilateral progressive vision loss. (*A*) Axial postcontrast fat-saturated T1-weighted image shows bilateral thin linear enhancement of the optic nerve sheaths (*long arrows*), continuous with similar abnormality along the bilateral posterior sclera (*short arrows*). (*B*) Coronal postcontrast fat-saturated T1-weighted image shows bilateral symmetric enhancement of the optic nerve sheaths (*small arrows*) and symmetric pachymeningeal enhancement (*large arrows*). The patient had a history of non-Hodgkin lymphoma.

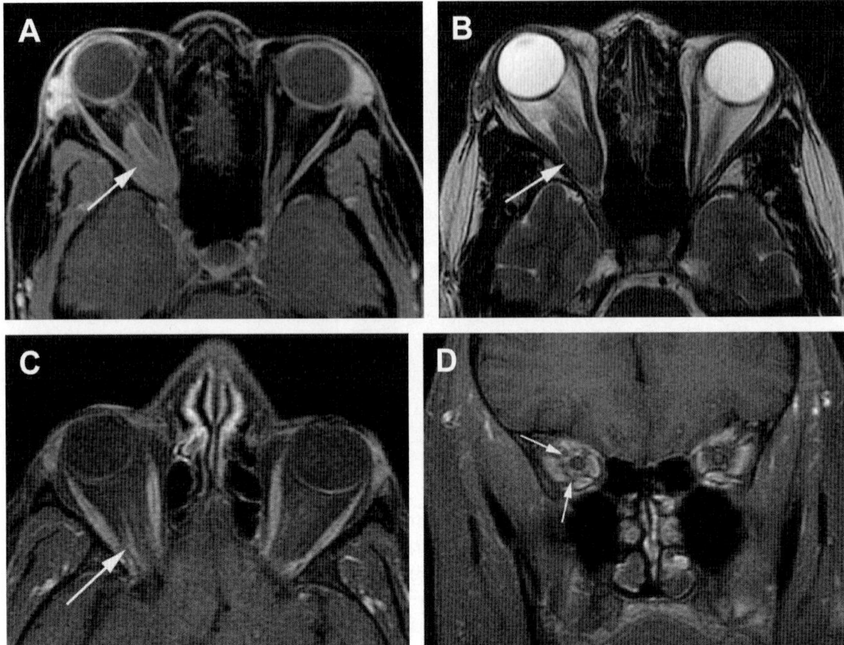

Fig. 10. Meningioma optic nerve sheath adult 1. A 41-year-old woman with slowly progressive right-sided vision loss. (*A*) Coronal postcontrast T1-weighted image shows an enhancing bulbous mass surrounding the posterior orbital segment of the right optic nerve (*arrow*). (*B*) Axial T2W image shows hypointense signal of the mass (*arrow*). (*C*) Follow-up axial and (*D*) coronal images several months after radiation shows marked decrease in size of the mass (*arrows*).

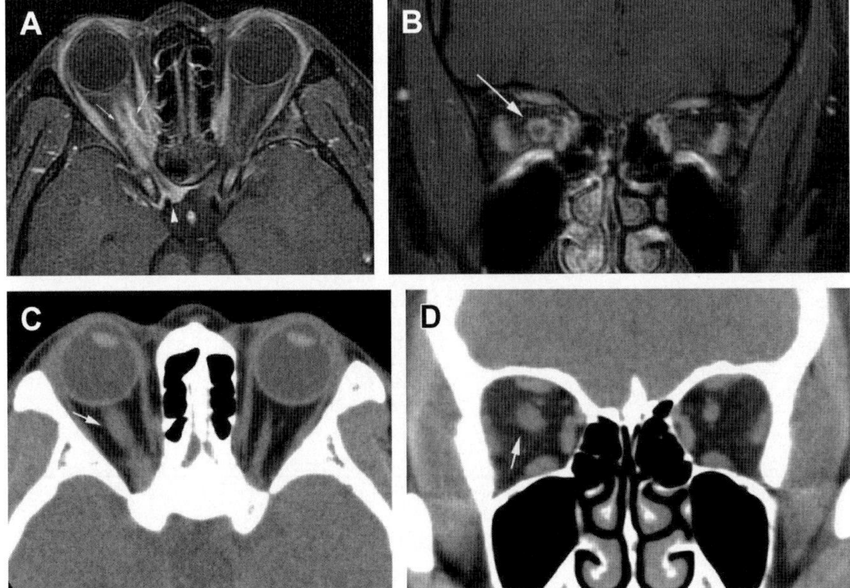

Fig. 11. Meningioma optic nerve sheath adult 2. A 40-year-old woman with slowly progressive right-sided vision loss. (*A*) Axial postcontrast T1-weighted image shows abnormal enhancement and thickening of the right optic nerve sheath, with a fairly uniform linear configuration (*arrows*). Note extension of nodular enhancement intracranially through the optic canal (*arrowhead*). (*B*) Corresponding coronal postcontrast T1-weighted image shows the concentric dural mass around the posterior orbital segment and anterior intracranial segments of the right optic nerve (*arrow*). (*C*) Axial and (*D*) coronal CT images show enlargement of the right ONSC, with density similar to muscle (*arrows*).

brain cortex.[13] ONSM may be dense on noncontrast CT, for similar reasons. There is typically brisk enhancement of the tumor on CT and MR imaging. If large enough, increased signal may be appreciable on diffusion-weighted imaging (DWI). ONSM is rare in children (**Fig. 12**) and must be distinguished from more common ONSC lesions, such as optic glioma. In children, ONSM tends to be more aggressive than in adults.[14] Neurofibromatosis type 2 is diagnosed in 28% of pediatric patients with ONSM.[15]

Optic Glioma

Most children with optic pathway glioma (OPG) have neurofibromatosis type I (NF-1).[16,17] About 20% of patients with NF-1 have OPG.[18,19] Most OPG in patients with NF-1 are diagnosed by age 6 years, and by age 8 years in cases of sporadic OPG.[20] Signs and symptoms at presentation include decreased visual acuity, visual field defect, proptosis, and afferent papillary defect.[20] These clinical findings may vary with the involved segments of the optic pathway. Any portion of the optic pathway may be involved. NF-1–associated OPG is more likely to involve the optic nerves, and sporadic OPG is more likely to involve the chiasm.[21] Bilateral OPG is virtually pathognomonic for NF-1. Histologically, OPG may be classified as a low-grade glioma, most commonly with features that resemble juvenile pilocytic astrocytoma.

In patients with NF-1, OPG tends to present either with tubular and tortuous enlargement of the nerve, with associated kinking (**Fig. 13**), or a spindle shape. The OPG of the orbital portions of the optic nerve, more commonly seen in NF-1, tend to show minimal or no enhancement on postcontrast T1-weighted (T1W) MR images. In patients with sporadic OPG, the tumor tends to resemble pilocytic astrocytoma, as seen in the brain, round with solid and cystic components (**Fig. 14**).[22]

Sarcoidosis

The incidence of sarcoidosis affecting the various structures of the orbit, including ocular and adnexal disease, varies according to different studies, possibly because of the populations or methods of diagnosis.[23] However, involvement of the ONSC in sarcoidosis occurs less frequently than uveitis or infiltration of the lacrimal gland.[24] Symptoms at presentation depend on the distribution of affected structures. Generally, a pattern of signs and symptoms consistent with inflammation is most common in orbital sarcoidosis, and involvement of the ONSC may affect visual acuity.[25] On MR imaging, the linear enhancement of the optic nerve sheath is similar to that seen in IOI or lymphoproliferative disease, hence, history of sarcoidosis is helpful (**Fig. 15**). However, orbital sarcoidosis has been well documented as the initial presentation of systemic disease (**Fig. 16**), although the incidence varies across studies.[25]

INTRACONAL LESION

Orbital Cavernous Malformation

Orbital cavernous malformation (OCM) (also known as cavernous hemangioma) has been cited as the most common orbital vascular lesion in adults.[26] However, the incidence is difficult to define, because these lesions have a typical imaging appearance, which frequently results in conservative management, especially if incidental, without histopathologic correlation. OCM has a predilection for middle-aged women, occurring in this demographic in approximately 60% to 70%

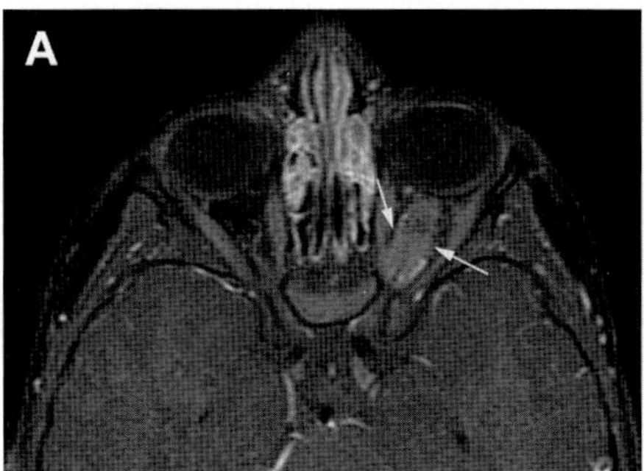

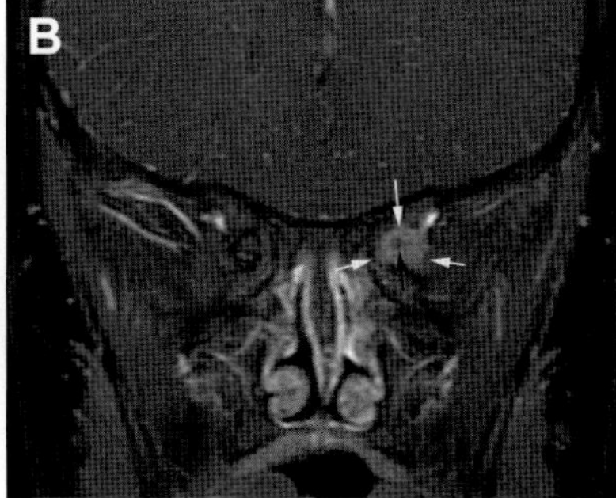

Fig. 12. Meningioma optic nerve sheath pediatric. A 4-year-old boy with loss of visual acuity in the left eye. (*A*) Axial postcontrast fat-saturated T1-weighted image shows a fusiform enhancing mass (*arrows*) along the left ONSC. (*B*) Coronal postcontrast fat-saturated T1-weighted image shows the mass (*white arrows*) surrounding the left optic nerve (*black arrow*).

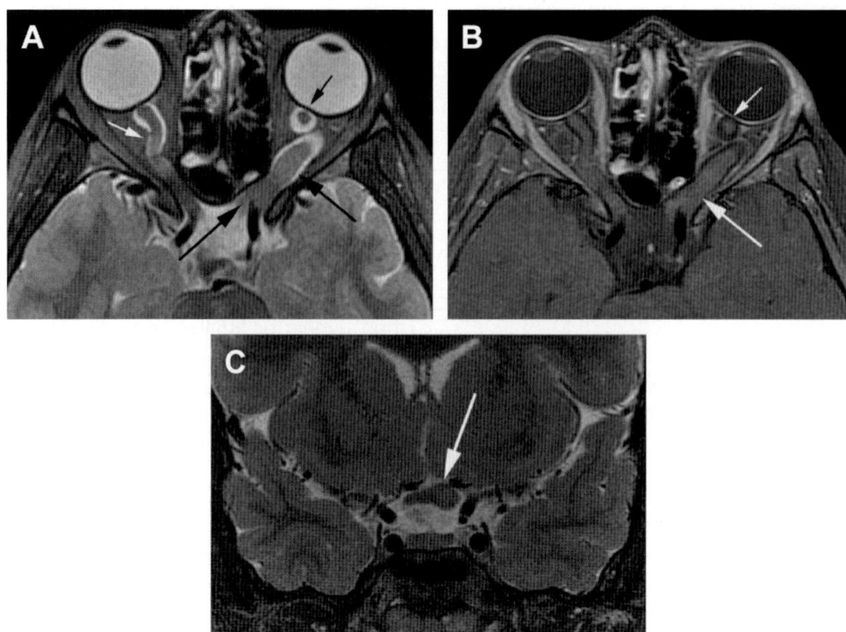

Fig. 13. Optic nerve glioma in NF-1. A 2-year-old girl with cutaneous findings suggestive of NF-1. (*A*) Axial T2W image shows abnormal thickening of the left optic nerve, with associated tortuosity of the ONSC (*black arrows*). There is mild tortuosity of the right ONSC (*white arrow*) without focal nodularity of the nerve, possibly caused by dural ectasia without a right-sided optic nerve glioma. (*B*) Axial postcontrast T1-weighted image shows a lack of enhancement of the optic nerve glioma (*arrows*). (*C*) Coronal T2W image shows involvement of the chiasmatic portion of the nerve (*arrow*).

of cases.[27] Painless, gradual proptosis is the most common presentation, with vision loss or pain being less frequent.

There has been controversy about the nature of OCM; however, some investigators now believe the entity to represent a low-flow arteriovenous malformation, with feeding and draining vessels that may be undetectable at imaging. On digital subtraction angiography, the only visible sign may be small areas of contrast pooling on delayed images.[28] Intralesional hemorrhage is uncommon, in contradistinction to cerebral cavernous malformations. This factor may be related to differences in their histologic features; for example, the orbital lesions do not have the irregular dysplastic vessel walls that are characteristic of cerebral cavernous malformations.[29] On imaging, OCM most commonly occurs in the lateral retrobulbar space, with involvement of the apex or extension into the superior orbital fissure being less common.[30] Bone remodeling may occur. OCM is typically well circumscribed, and has heterogeneous enhancement on MR imaging, which becomes more uniform on delayed images, frequently from central to peripheral (**Fig. 17**). Intralesional calcifications may be seen on CT imaging (**Fig. 18**).

Lymphatic Malformation

Lymphatic malformation (LM), also called venous lymphatic or venolymphatic malformation, is a vascular malformation that generally presents in childhood. LM is frequently multispatial, affecting several adjacent compartments of the face. The lymph-filled vascular channels are not in communication with the orbital vasculature and therefore not subject to postural changes such as those seen in venous varices.[31] Intralesional hemorrhage is likely related to the fragile vessels within the intralesional septations.[32]

Intralesional hemorrhage is a common cause of acute enlargement and associated exacerbation of symptoms in LM. MR is the optimal modality for showing the extent of the lesion and which structures are involved. Signal characteristics on MR imaging vary with the presence or absence of proteinaceous content or blood products in the fluid-filled components of the lesions.[33] There is typically minimal enhancement, within the walls

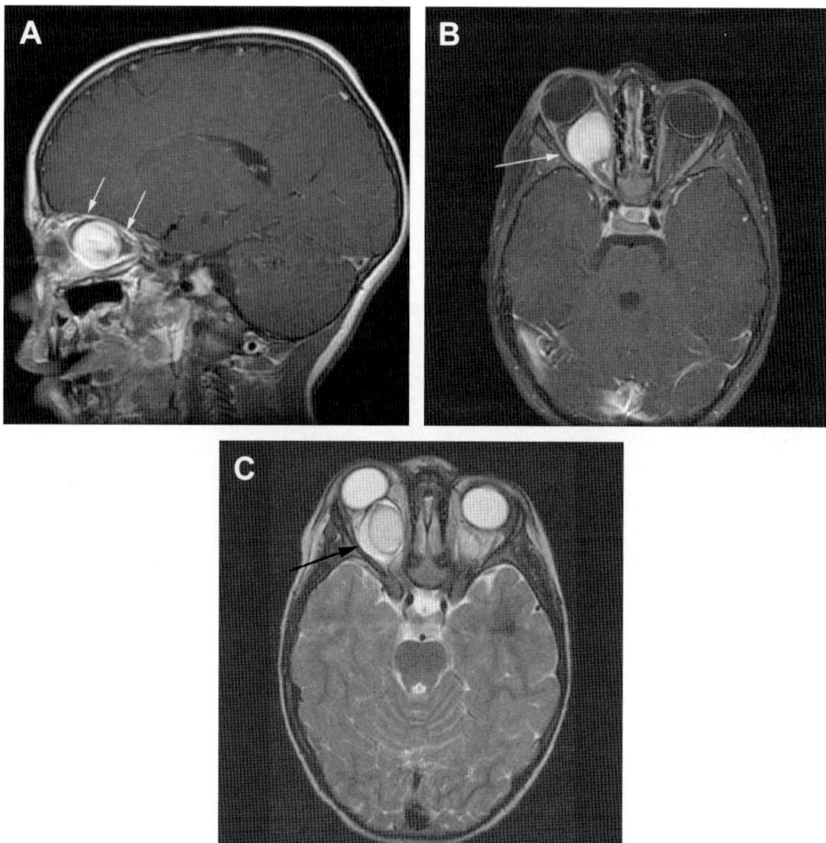

Fig. 14. Optic nerve glioma sporadic. A 4-year-old boy with slowly progressive right-sided proptosis. (*A*) Sagittal and (*B*) axial postcontrast T1-weighted images show an oblong enhancing mass within the right optic nerve (*arrows*). (*C*) Axial T2W image shows heterogeneous signal of the mass (*arrow*).

of the lesion or its internal septations, unless there is an associated venous component. Fluid-fluid levels are a characteristic finding in the setting of recent intralesional hemorrhage (**Fig. 19**).

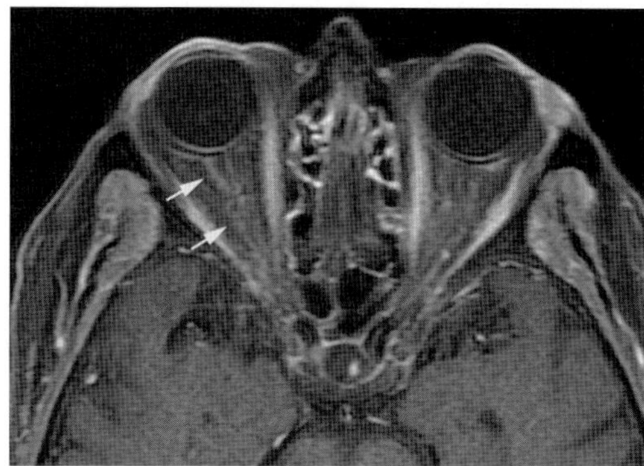

Fig. 15. Sarcoidosis ONSC 1. Axial postcontrast T1W image shows abnormal linear enhancement along the right optic nerve sheath (*arrows*) in this 78-year-old man with known sarcoidosis.

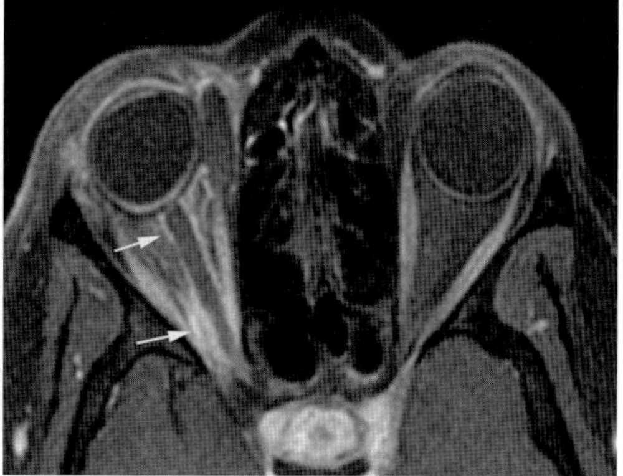

Fig. 16. Sarcoidosis ONSC 2. Axial postcontrast fat-saturated T1W image shows abnormal linear enhancement along the right optic nerve sheath, more infiltrative at the orbital apex (*arrows*) in this 56-year-old woman. Subsequent clinical evaluation led to a diagnosis of sarcoidosis.

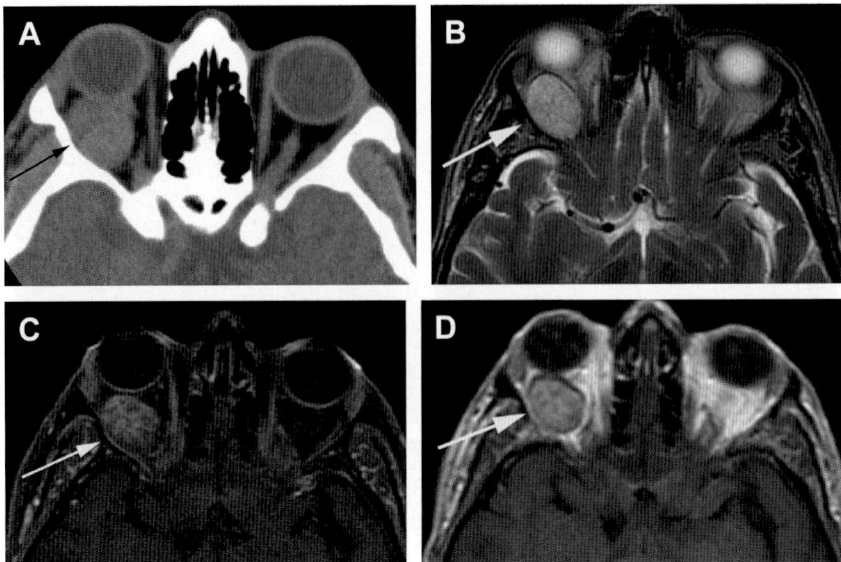

Fig. 17. OCM CT and MR with delay. A 43-year-old woman with slowly progressive right-sided proptosis. (*A*) Axial CT image shows a well-circumscribed ovoid intraconal mass (*arrow*). (*B*) Axial T2-weighted image shows homogeneous signal hyperintensity (*arrow*). (*C*) Thin-section axial fat-saturated postcontrast T1W image shows predominantly central enhancement (*arrow*), which becomes more homogeneous on the postcontrast T1 image of the brain obtained several minutes later (*arrow* in *D*).

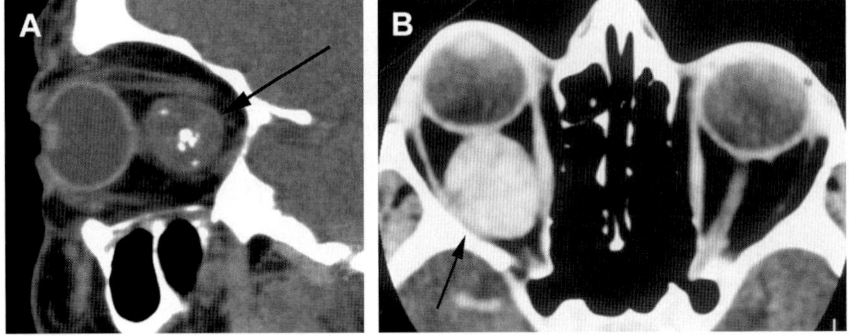

Fig. 18. OCM CT images. An 84-year-old woman with slowly progressive right-sided proptosis. (*A*) Noncontrast CT sagittal CT image shows intralesional calcifications in an ovoid intraconal mass, consistent with OCM (*arrow*). (*B*) Contrast-enhanced CT axial image shows brisk enhancement of an intraconal OCM (*arrow*).

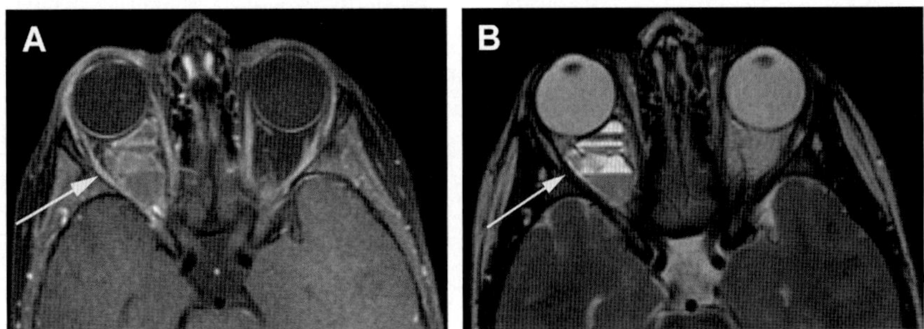

Fig. 19. LM. A 10-year-old girl with known orbital LM, presenting with rapid onset exacerbation of proptosis and orbital pain after recent upper respiratory infection. (*A*) Axial postcontrast fat-saturated T1W image shows faint enhancement of the walls and internal septations of an intraconal LM in the right orbit (*arrow*). Both on this image, and on the corresponding axial T2-weighted image (*B*), there are multiple fluid-debris levels (*arrow*) consistent with recent intralesional hemorrhage.

Venous Varix

Orbital varices represent a form of hamartoma, with thin-walled distensible venous channels that communicate with the normal orbital venous vasculature.[34,35] These lesions arise from a developmental weakness of the postcapillary venous wall, with ensuing proliferation and dilatation of valveless orbital veins.[30,35] Varices with a large communication with the venous system distend during maneuvers that increase venous pressure (**Figs. 20** and **21**), whereas those with small communications to the normal venous system are more likely to present with thrombosis and hemorrhage, resulting in persistent proptosis.[35,36]

Schwannoma

Orbital schwannomas may be intraconal or extraconal, or both, especially when large. Painless slowly progressive proptosis is the most common clinical presentation, and may be accompanied by diplopia, caused by mass effect on the extraocular muscles.[37] Any nerve in the orbit may be involved, commonly branches of the ophthalmic division of the trigeminal nerve.[38] Therefore, in keeping with the distribution of the orbital nerve branches, schwannomas tend to be extraconal about as often as they are intraconal.[39] Even the ONSC may rarely be involved, because the sheath receives innervation from the trigeminal distribution.[38] A large series of orbital schwannomas showed variable enhancement patterns on MR imaging, with homogeneous or ring enhancement being the most common.[40] Some schwannomas may have delayed homogenization of contrast enhancement, similar to cavernous malformations. Therefore, schwannoma may be difficult to distinguish from cavernous malformation, both clinically and at imaging. However, the progression from peripheral to central enhancement, a characteristic feature of OCM, tends not to occur so frequently in schwannomas (**Fig. 22**).[39]

Lymphoproliferative Disease and Intraconal Metastasis

When well circumscribed, intraconal metastases may be difficult to distinguish from other intraconal masses on imaging alone, unless there are additional findings to help lead to the correct diagnosis. For example, melanoma metastases may have intrinsic T1 signal hyperintensity, and there may be additional metastatic disease included in the imaged portion of the brain (**Fig. 23**). The progression of symptoms may be expected to be more rapid than with nonaggressive lesions such as cavernous malformations or schwannomas. Similar clinical considerations apply to lymphoproliferative disease, such as lymphoma (**Fig. 24**).

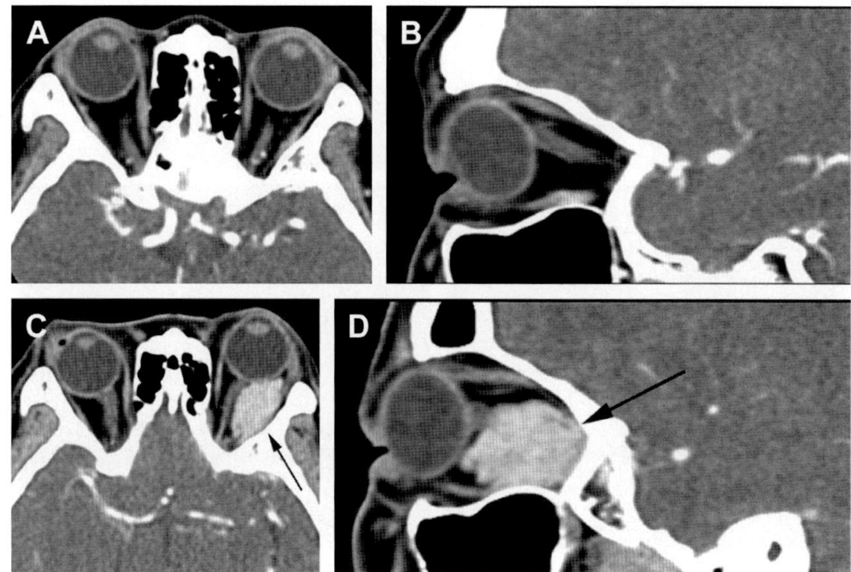

Fig. 20. Varix CT. A 58-year-old man with intermittent left-sided orbital pressure and proptosis. (*A*) Axial and (*B*) sagittal contrast-enhanced CT images obtained supine appear normal. Repeat imaging in the prone position, using a Valsalva maneuver, results in marked filling of clinically suspected venous varix in the lateral intraconal space on the repeat axial (*C*) and sagittal (*D*) images (*arrows*).

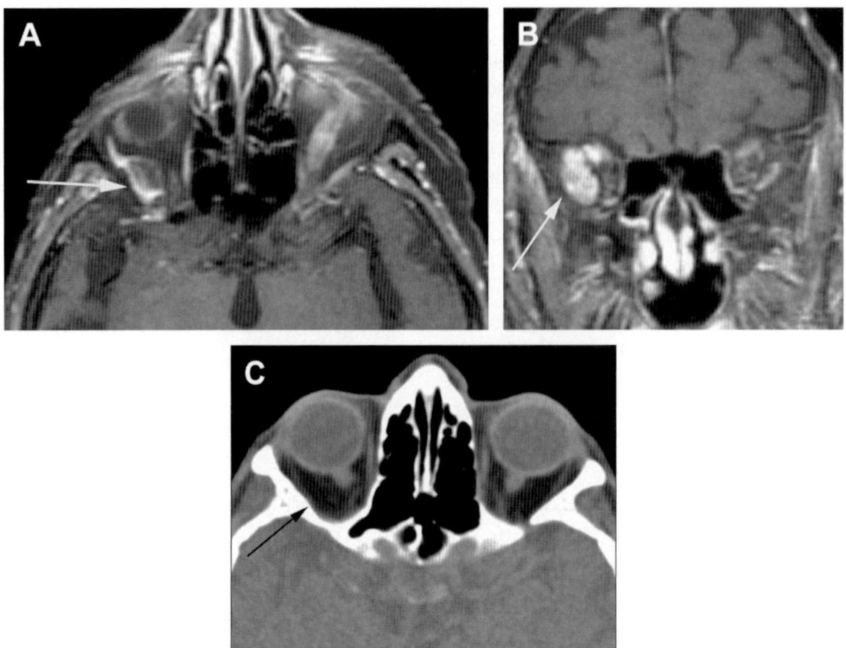

Fig. 21. Varix MR. (*A*) Axial postcontrast fat-saturated T1W image shows a heterogeneously enhancing intraconal mass in the right orbit (*arrow*), in a 52-year-old woman who presented with rapid onset of orbital pain. (*B*) Coronal postcontrast fat-saturated T1W image acquired after the axial image shows more homogeneous enhancement (*arrow*), consistent with venous filling with contrast. (*C*) Follow-up axial CT image 10 days later shows apparent resolution of the lesion (*arrow*).

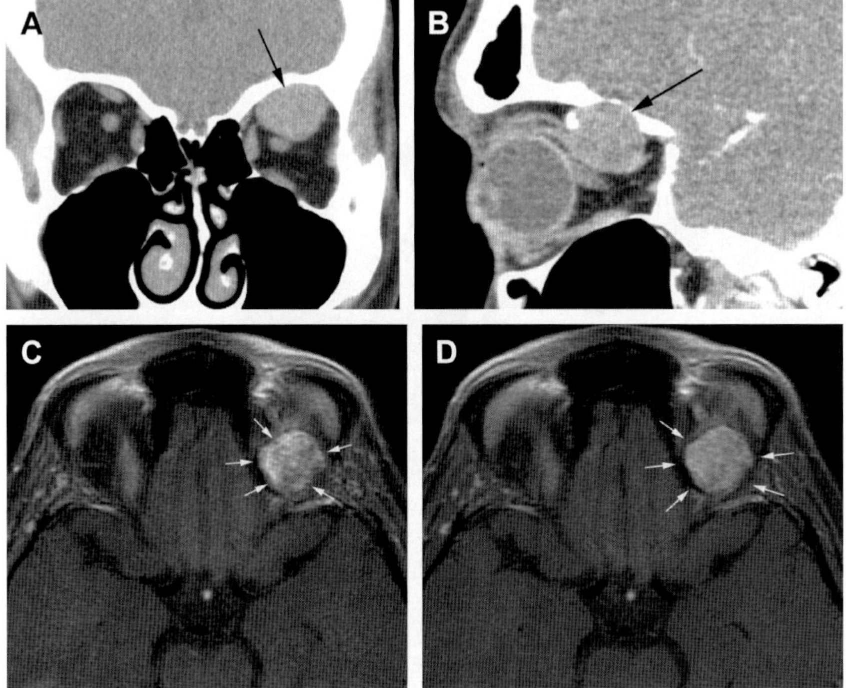

Fig. 22. Schwannoma. A 46-year-old woman with chronic left orbital pain and proptosis. (*A*) Coronal CT image shows a predominantly intraconal soft tissue mass in the left orbit (*arrow*). (*B*) Sagittal postcontrast CT image shows mild enhancement of the ovoid mass (*arrow*), visually inseparable from the superior muscle complex, and causing osseous remodeling. (*C*) Axial postcontrast fat-saturated T1W image shows enhancement that is slightly heterogeneous (*arrows*). (*D*) Delayed axial image 5 minutes later shows slight increase in the degree of enhancement (*arrows*).

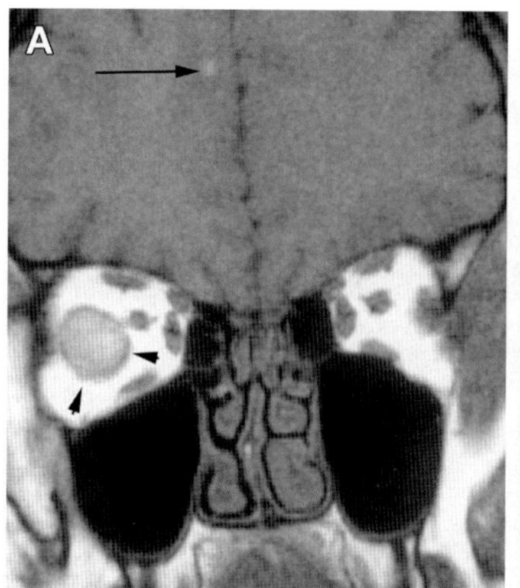

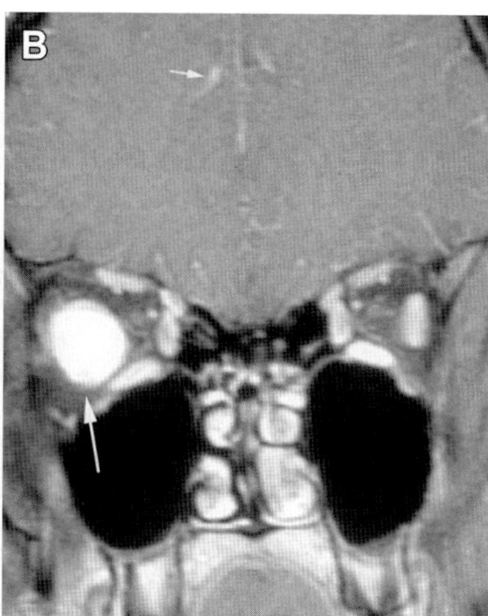

Fig. 23. Intraconal melanoma metastasis. A 66-year-old man with rapidly progressive right orbital pressure. (*A*) Coronal T1W image shows a well-circumscribed right intraconal ovoid mass, with some intrinsic signal hyperintensity before contrast administration (*arrowheads*). There is also a focus of abnormal T1 signal hyperintensity in the subcortical white matter of the right frontal lobe (*arrow*). (*B*) Coronal postcontrast fat-saturated T1W image shows marked enhancement of the orbital mass (*large arrow*), as well as the subcortical lesion (*small arrow*). The intrinsic T1 signal hyperintensity is consistent with melanoma.

EXTRACONAL LESION

DERMOID

Orbital dermoid cysts, usually seen in the pediatric population, most commonly occur near suture lines, the frontozygomatic suture being most common, in keeping with their classification as congenital choristomas. However, postseptal dermoid cysts may occur and are more likely to be discovered later in life.[41] The reported incidence of orbital dermoid cysts varies among different studies, ranging from 3% to 9% of orbital masses.[42] The lipid, proteinaceous, and hemorrhagic content of dermoid cysts result predominantly in fat density on CT (**Fig. 25**), and varying degrees of T1 signal hyperintensity on MR imaging. Signal dropout on fat-saturated images is helpful in imaging diagnosis (**Fig. 26**).

ORBITAL BONE LESIONS

The osseous boundaries of the orbit are subject to the same array of disease processes as any other bone in the body. Benign tumors and primary or secondary malignancy may affect the

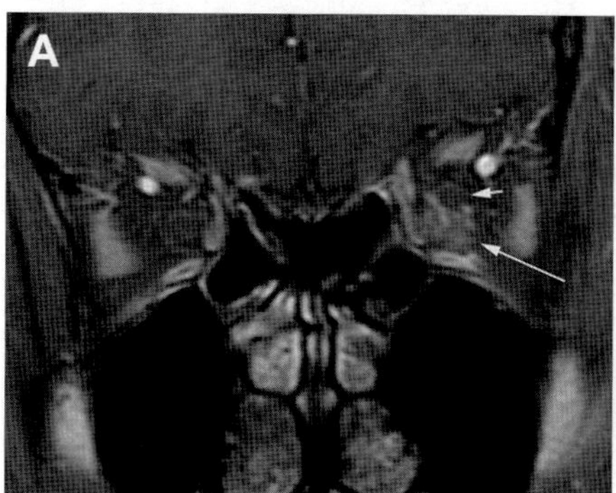

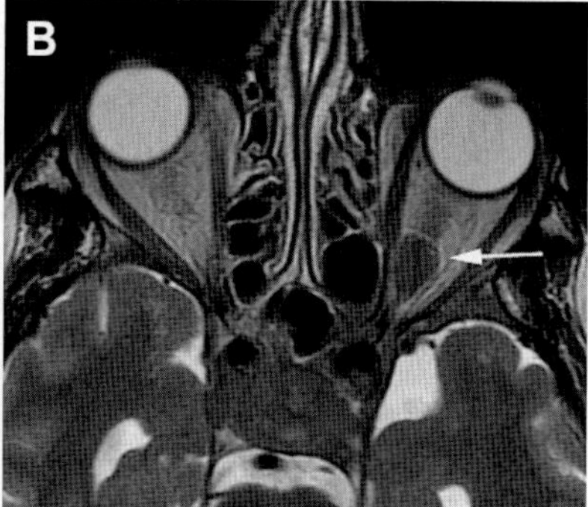

Fig. 24. Intraconal lymphoma. A 35-year-old woman with history of human immunodeficiency virus infection, presenting with pain and pressure in the left orbit progressing over several days. (*A*) Coronal postcontrast fat-saturated T1W image shows an ovoid intraconal enhancing mass (*large arrow*) just inferior to the ONSC (*small arrow*). (*B*) Axial T2-weighted image shows marked signal hypointensity of the mass (*arrow*), commonly seen in lesions that have high cellular nuclear/cytoplasmic ratio. Further evaluation led to a diagnosis of Burkitt lymphoma.

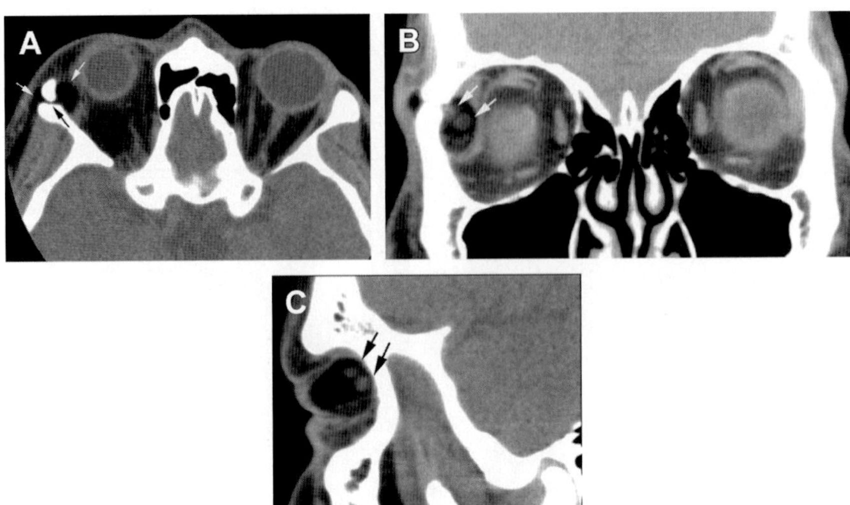

Fig. 25. Dermoid at suture CT. A 33-year-old man with long history of orbital mass. (*A*) Axial CT image shows a predominately fat density extraconal mass with components medial and lateral to the frontozygomatic suture (*white arrows*), with a visible connecting component in the suture (*black arrow*). (*B*) Coronal and (*C*) sagittal CT images show small components of the dermoid cyst with soft tissue density (*white arrows* in coronal image, *black arrows* in sagittal image), presumably representing proteinaceous debris or vestigial dermal appendage tissue.

orbital bones. In addition, various benign bone diseases may occur in this region. Of course, consideration of the patient's demographics and symptoms is paramount for generating a focused differential diagnosis, both clinically and at imaging.

The prevalence of primary sources of orbital metastases may vary from series to series;

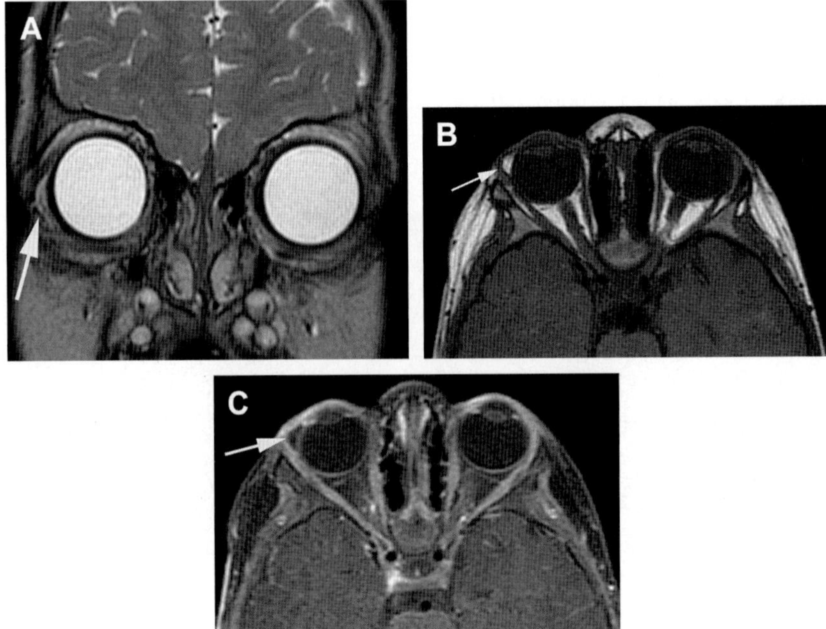

Fig. 26. Dermoid MR imaging. An 18-month-old boy with orbital mass. (*A*) Coronal T2W image, (*B*) axial T1W image, and (*C*) axial postcontrast fat-saturated T1W image show a subcentimeter mass along the anterolateral scleral surface (*arrows*), which follows fat signal on all sequences.

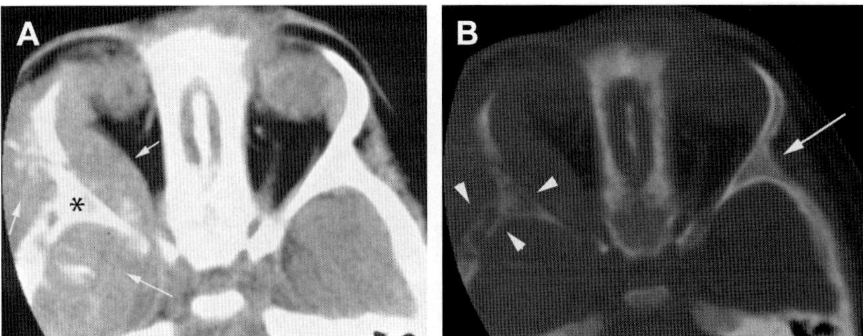

Fig. 27. Neuroblastoma metastasis orbital wall. An 11-month-old boy with neuroblastoma. (*A*) Axial CT image shows a large mass (*arrows*) centered at the right sphenotemporal buttress (*asterisk*). (*B*) Bone algorithm CT image at the same level shows irregular erosion of the involved bone (*arrowheads*). The normal contralateral sphenotemporal buttress is indicated for comparison (*arrow*).

however, it is not surprising that the more common primary malignancies, such as breast, lung, and prostate, are well represented.[43] Metastatic lesions of the orbital bones frequently manifest on imaging as a combination of osseous destruction and contiguous soft tissue mass (**Figs. 27** and **28**).[43]

Meningiomas of the greater sphenoid wing (also known as spheno-orbital meningioma, meningioma en plaque of the sphenoid wing, and so forth) originate from the dura along the intracranial surface of the sphenoid bone and commonly show intraosseous growth.[44] These tumors may have varying proportions of intraosseous, dural (intracranial), and orbital soft tissue components.[45] Local mass effect on structures such as the superior orbital fissure, optic canal, optic nerve sheath complex, or extraocular muscles determine the presenting signs and symptoms. The intraosseous component has strikingly hypointense signal on

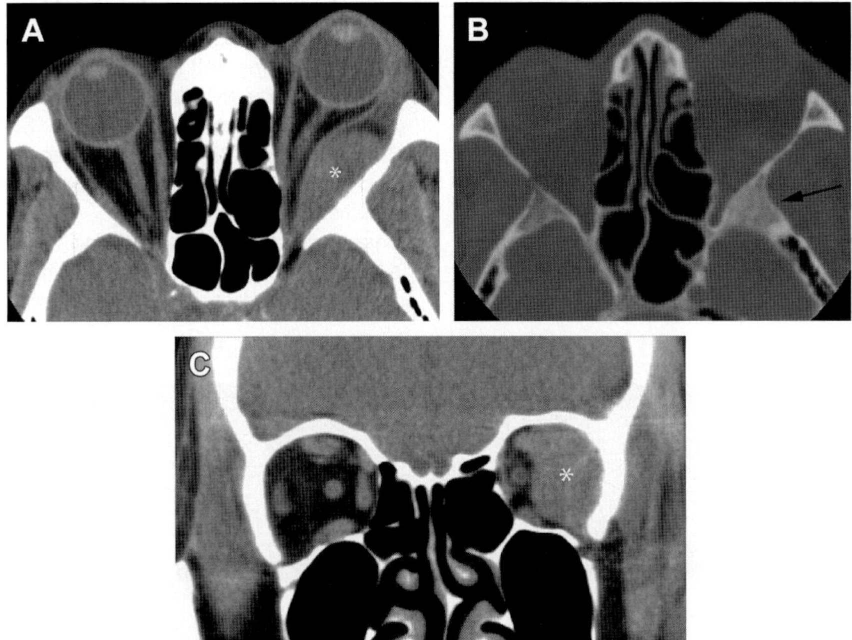

Fig. 28. Prostate metastasis orbital wall. A 67-year-old man with left lateral orbital pain. (*A*) Axial CT image shows a large extraconal mass (*asterisk*) associated with the left sphenotemporal buttress. (*B*) Bone algorithm CT image at the same level shows abnormal expansion and hyperdensity of the left sphenotemporal buttress. (*C*) Coronal CT image shows the soft tissue mass (*asterisk*) visually inseparable from the lateral rectus muscle. Further investigation showed metastatic prostate cancer.

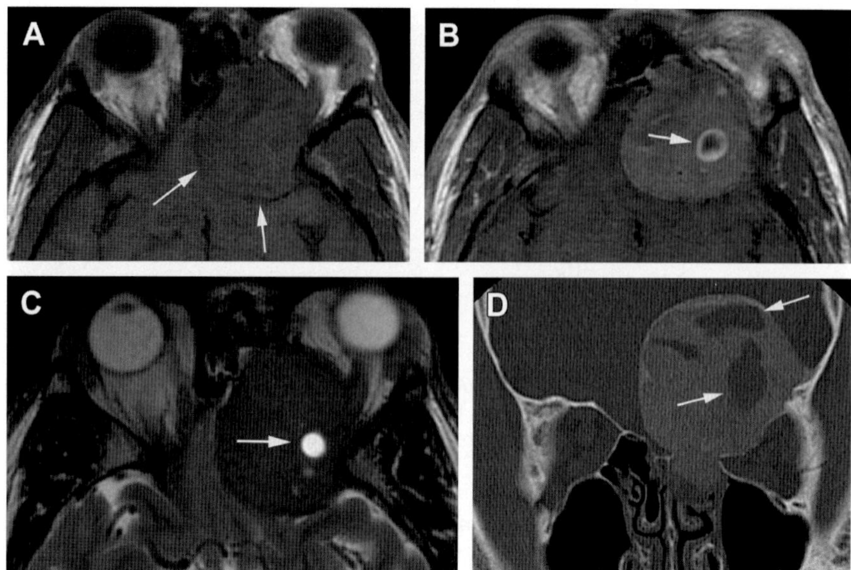

Fig. 29. FD orbital roof in a 22-year-old man. (*A*) Axial T1W image shows a large mass (*arrows*) at the left orbital roof and paracentral skull base. (*B*) Postcontrast axial T1W image shows faint enhancement of the mass, with a more robustly enhancing area laterally (*arrow*). This enhancing area corresponds to cystic change on the axial T2-weighted image (*arrow* in *C*). The remainder of the mass is otherwise hypointense on T2. (*D*) Coronal bone algorithm CT image shows the characteristic ground-glass density of FD, with areas of cystic change (*arrows*).

T2-weighted (T2W) MR images and appears on CT as abnormal expansion and sclerosis.

Nonneoplastic benign fibro-osseous entities, such as fibrous dysplasia (FD) and ossifying fibromas, may be detected at imaging. FD has a characteristic ground-glass density on CT and usually affects patients younger than 30 years.[46] On MR images, FD is typically hypointense on both T1W and T2W images, more strikingly so on T2. However, FD can have areas of T2 signal hyperintensity caused by cystic degeneration, as well as areas of enhancement on MR imaging, which may be misleading (**Fig. 29**). It is important to assess for narrowing of the optic canal or superior orbital at imaging (**Fig. 30**). Ossifying fibromas may have internal mineralization, which can mimic that of FD on CT imaging. However, ossifying fibroma usually has borders that are better defined (**Fig. 31**) than those of FD, which tends to have a poorly defined transition zone.[47,48]

Orbital subperiosteal hemorrhage (SpH) is a rare cause of rapid onset proptosis. SpH may be associated with trauma, or a variety of causes that increase central venous pressure, such as activities that require Valsalva, weight lifting, prolonged emesis, or scuba diving. The orbital roof is most commonly affected.[49] In most cases, orbital hematomas are resorbed without chronic

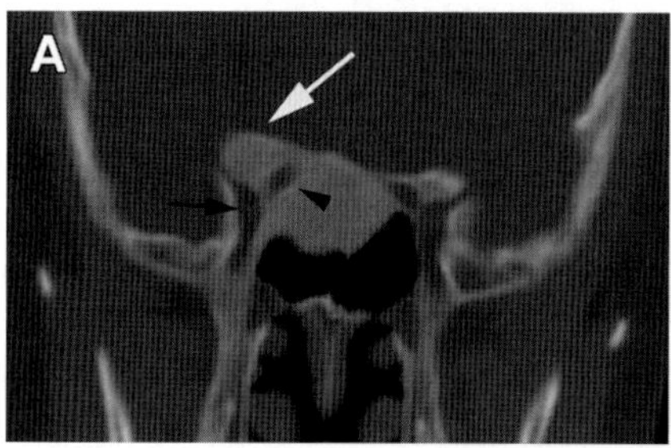

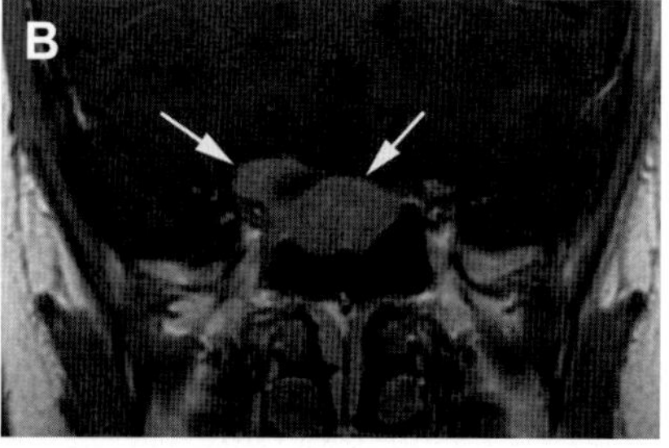

Fig. 30. FD orbital apex in a 24-year-old woman. (*A*) Coronal CT image shows abnormal hyperdensity and expansion of the right sphenoid body and lesser sphenoid wing, including the anterior clinoid process (*white arrow*). There is mild narrowing of the right superior orbital fissure (*black arrow*), but the optic canal maintains normal caliber (*arrowhead*). (*B*) Corresponding coronal T1W image shows moderate T1 signal hyperintensity of the lesion (*arrows*).

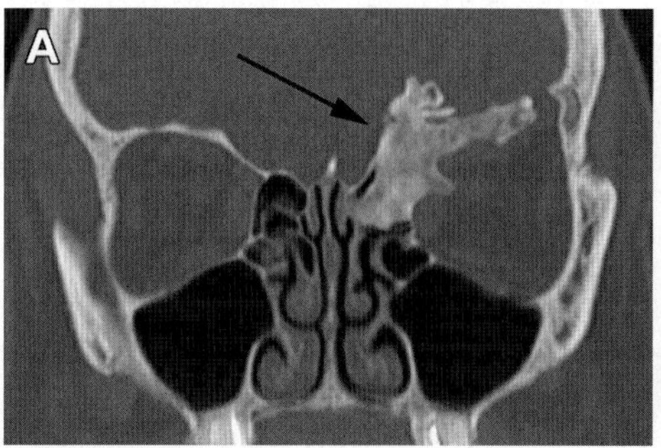

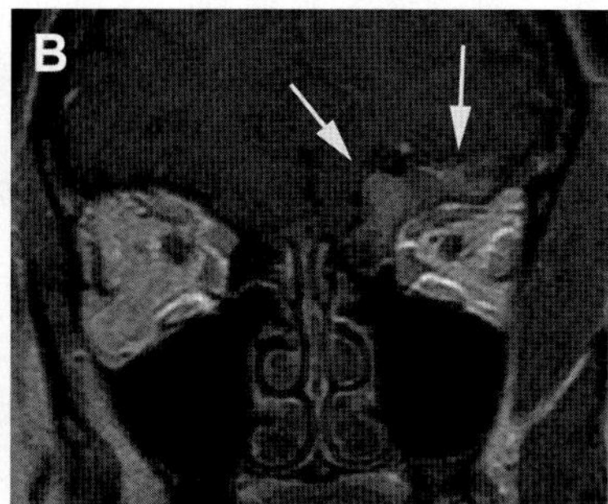

Fig. 31. Ossifying fibroma in a 49-year-old woman evaluated for seizures. (*A*) Coronal CT bone algorithm image shows a well-circumscribed mass with irregular morphology at the left orbital roof (*arrow*) and superior aspect of the medial orbital wall. (*B*) On the corresponding coronal T1W image, there is T1 signal hyperintensity (*arrows*), similar to that of normal marrow. The appearance is consistent with ossifying fibroma.

sequelae. However, the degrading blood products may provoke a granulomatous reaction, leading to the deposition of cholesterol and hemosiderin crystals, which are then phagocytized by histiocytes, leading to the formation of giant cells and calcification.[50] These subacute/chronic forms of SpH are known by several names, including hematocele, hematic cyst, and cholesterol granuloma. Depending on the chronicity of the findings at the time of presentation, and whether an inciting event can be reliably recalled, hematocysts may be difficult to distinguish from a metastatic lesion, both clinically and at imaging. However, on MR imaging, there is often a characteristic appearance with intrinsic T1 signal hyperintensity on noncontrast images, caused by the proteinaceous blood products (**Fig. 32**).

Intraosseous meningiomas frequently occur in the sphenotemporal buttress, and may be difficult to distinguish from metastasis, especially if there is no dural or orbital soft tissue component. Intraosseous meningioma manifests as expansile hyperostosis of the affected bone on CT (**Fig. 33**). They are characteristically hypointense on T2W images and result in varying degrees of mass effect on the neighboring orbital structures (**Fig. 34**).

SINONASAL LESIONS

Paranasal sinus disease, particularly infection and malignancy, may affect the adjacent soft tissues of the orbit. A well-known complication of pediatric ethmoid sinusitis is the development of orbital cellulitis (**Fig. 35**), caused by bacterial infiltration through small neurovascular channels; there need not be a visible osseous defect between the infected sinus and the adjacent orbital soft tissues. This sequence may occur in adults as well; for example, the frontal sinus is a potential source (**Fig. 36**).

Chronic obstruction of a paranasal sinus may lead to the formation of a mucocele, which may expand and deform the orbit. There may be dehiscence of the osseous boundaries of the mucocele. Hyperdense contents may signify proteinaceous debris and inspissated secretions, whether or not there is superimposed infection. If superinfected, these lesions are known as mucopyoceles (**Fig. 37**), and there is a risk of infection spreading to the orbital soft tissues.

Similarly, malignant lesions of the paranasal sinuses and nasal cavity can secondarily involve the orbit. CT and MR imaging are complementary in assessing the full extent of the tumor, for staging and therapeutic planning (**Fig. 38**).

LACRIMAL GLAND LESIONS

Disease of the lacrimal gland and fossa may be divided into epithelial and nonepithelial lesions. Epithelial lesions are mainly neoplastic, arising from the acini of the gland. Various inflammatory or infiltrative lesions comprise the nonepithelial lesions.[51]

Alternatively, diseases of the lacrimal gland may be subclassified by clinical presentation. With this approach, benign mixed tumor (pleomorphic adenoma) presents with slow painless enlargement of the gland over several months. By contrast, other conditions such as carcinoma, inflammatory disease, or lymphoproliferative disorders have a shorter time course and are often painful.[51,52]

As alluded to earlier, pleomorphic adenoma has an indolent course, with painless enlargement of the gland. Sudden onset of pain may indicate malignant transformation.[52] On MR imaging, pleomorphic adenoma is typically isointense to muscle and enhances vividly (**Fig. 39**). Adenoid cystic carcinoma is the most common malignancy of the lacrimal gland and usually presents with a rapidly

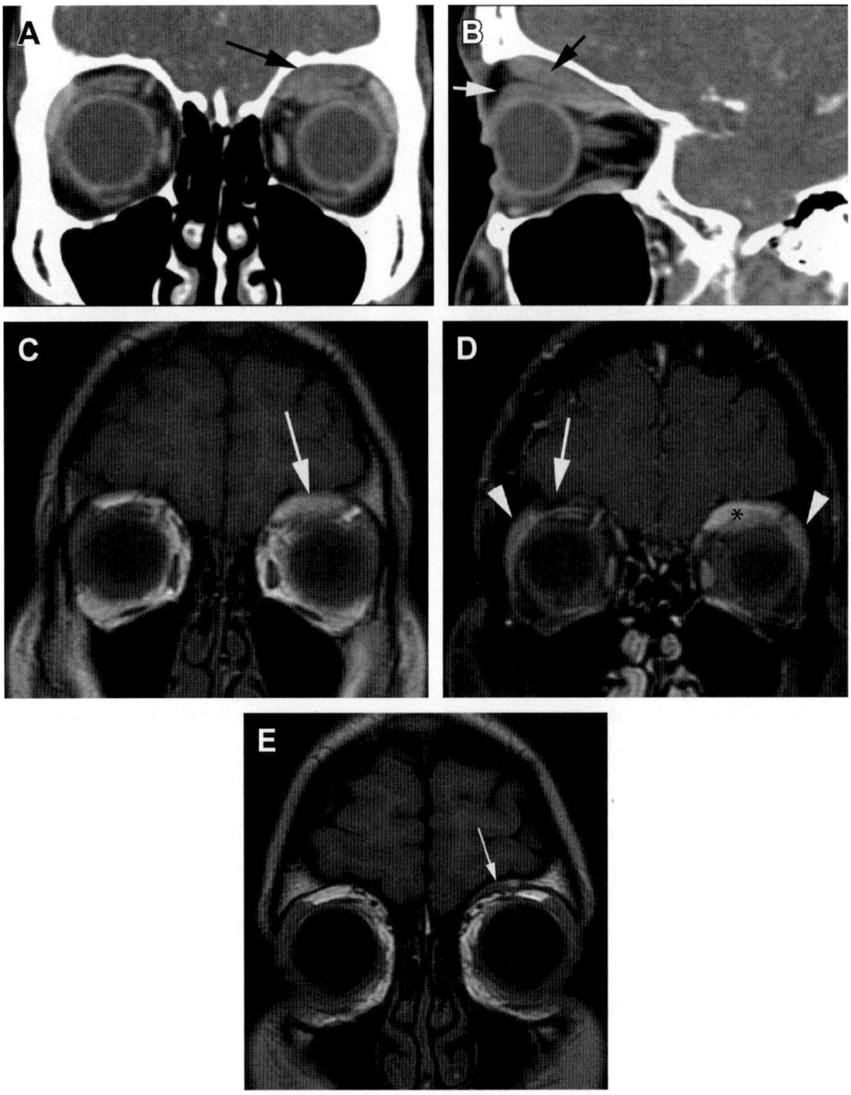

Fig. 32. Subperiosteal hematoma in a 29-year-old woman with rapid onset of painless left orbital mass. (*A*) Axial and (*B*) sagittal CT images show abnormal soft tissue density in the left superior extraconal orbit (*white arrows*). There is downward displacement of the left superior muscle complex (*white arrow* in *B*). (*C*) Coronal T1W image shows asymmetric signal hyperintensity in the superior extraconal space of the left orbit (*arrow*). (*D*) Coronal postcontrast fat-saturated T1W image shows no enhancement of this area (*asterisk*). Neither is there loss of signal as expected for normal fat, as seen on the normal contralateral side (*arrow*). There is normal enhancement of the lacrimal glands (*arrowheads*). Further history was significant for a recent episode of vomiting and retching, the night before the onset of symptoms. (*E*) Follow-up coronal T1W image 1 month later shows near resolution.

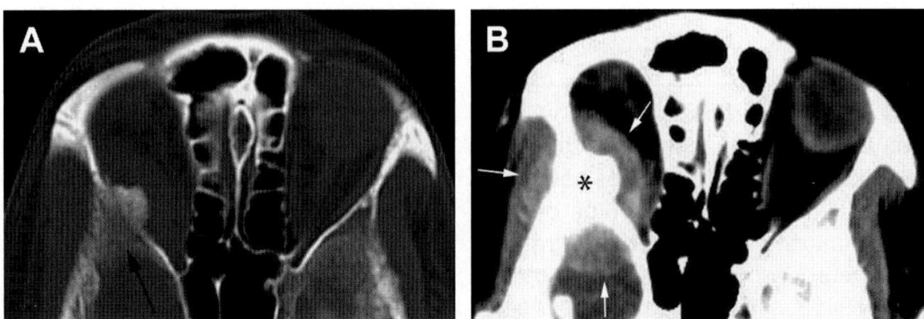

Fig. 33. Intraosseous meningioma CT in a 57-year-old woman with slowly progressive proptosis. (*A*) Axial CT image in bone algorithm shows expansile hyperostosis of the right sphenotemporal buttress (*arrow*). (*B*) Corresponding soft tissue image shows the expanded bone (*asterisk*), and associated soft tissue components in the extraconal orbit, suprazygomatic masticator space, and middle cranial fossa (*arrows*).

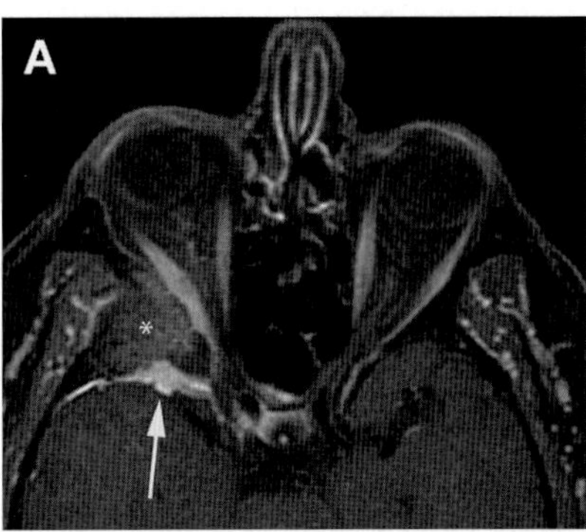

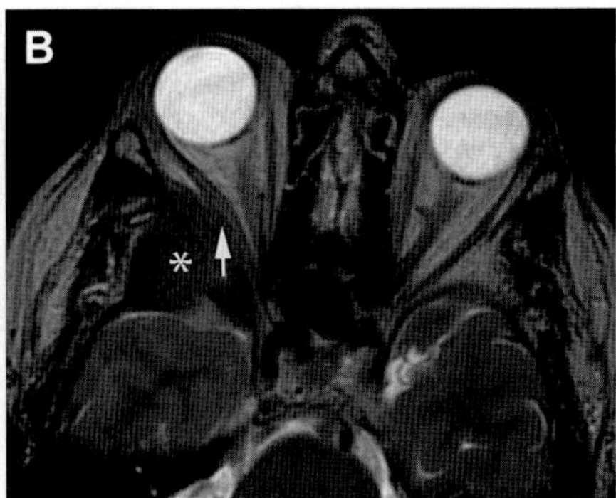

Fig. 34. Intraosseous meningioma MR imaging in a 64-year-old man with slowly progressive proptosis. (*A*) Axial postcontrast fat-saturated T1W image shows an intraosseous meningioma in the right sphenotemporal buttress (*asterisk*), with involvement of the adjacent dura in the middle cranial fossa (*arrow*). (*B*) Axial T2W image shows typical signal hypointensity of the osseous component (*asterisk*), and mass effect on the adjacent left lateral rectus muscle (*arrow*).

growing, painful, and firm mass in the lacrimal fossa (**Fig. 40**). As in the salivary glands, adenoid cystic carcinoma of the lacrimal gland has a propensity for perineural tumor spread. Nonepithelial disease of the lacrimal gland is chiefly inflammatory or lymphoproliferative, including dacryoadenitis, IOI, sarcoidosis, and lymphoma (**Figs. 41–43**). Primary lymphoma of the lacrimal gland is frequently of the MALT type, and secondary lymphoma has been found to be predominantly follicular.[53] As expected for lymphoproliferative disease, T2 signal of lymphoma is hypointense to muscle on MR imaging, and the mass may also show restricted diffusion (**Fig. 44**). The lacrimal gland is a common location for IOI, found to be second most common by Mafee and colleagues.[54,55] As described in the section on lesions of the ONSC, sarcoidosis has variable incidence in the orbit, and lacrimal gland involvement may be an initial presentation.

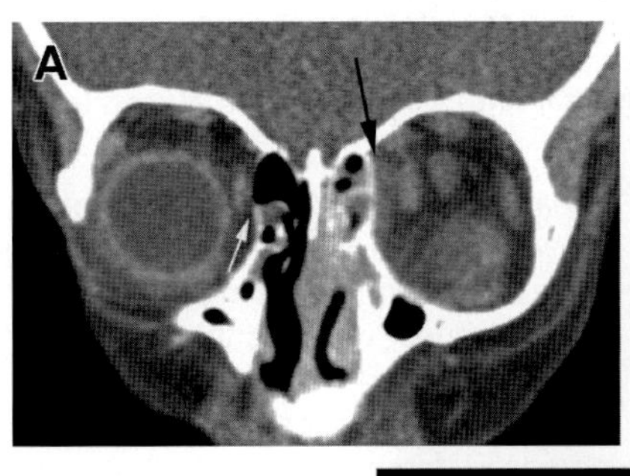

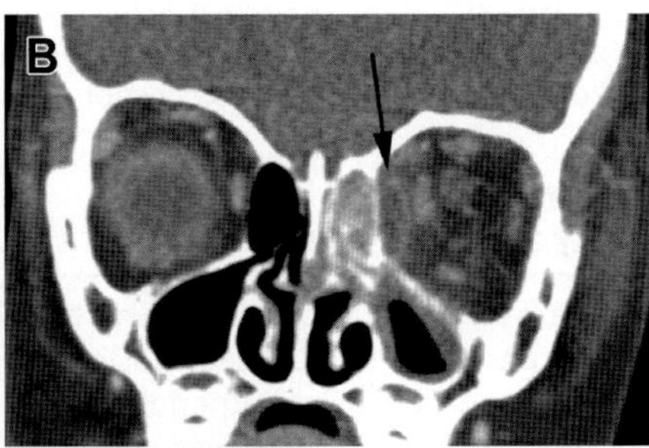

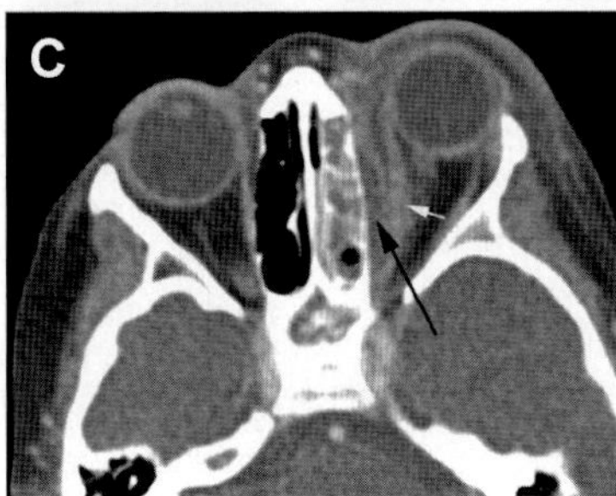

Fig. 35. Subperiosteal abscess from ethmoid sinusitis. A 5-year-old boy with rapid onset of left eye pain, fever, and limited ocular motion. (*A*) Coronal CT image shows abnormal density of the fat plane between the left medial rectus muscle and lamina papyracea (*black arrow*). The normal contralateral fat plane is indicated (*white arrow*). (*B*) Coronal contrast-enhanced CT (CECT) image shows peripheral enhancement of this area (*arrow*), consistent with a subperiostal abscess. (*C*) Axial CECT image shows the abscess (*black arrow*), displacing the medial rectus muscle (*white arrow*).

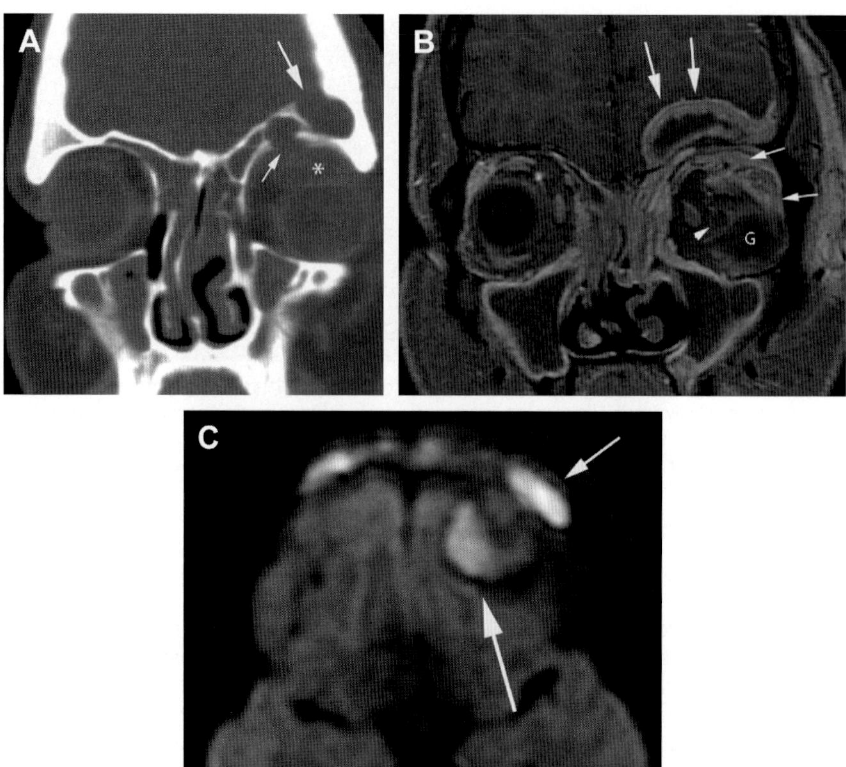

Fig. 36. Frontal sinusitis in a 45-year-old man with chronic pansinusitis who presented with acute left proptosis, headache, and fever. (*A*) Coronal CT image shows abnormal soft tissue in the superior left orbit (*asterisk*) depressing the ocular globe. There is associated opacification of the left frontal sinus with areas of dehiscence at the left orbital roof (*small arrow*) and at the interface with the cranial vault (*large arrow*). (*B*) Coronal postcontrast fat-saturated T1W image shows extraconal phlegmon in the left superior orbit (*small arrows*) inferiorly displacing the ONSC (*arrowhead*) and the globe (G). There is also an epidural abscess (*large arrows*). (*C*) Axial DWI shows restricted diffusion in the epidural collection and frontal sinus, consistent with abscess (*arrows*).

POSTSEPTAL INFECTION AND LYMPHOPROLIFERATIVE LESIONS

Infection may involve the periorbital soft tissues without underlying paranasal sinus disease. Minor trauma such as insect bites or superinfected dermal lesions may progress to cellulitis, which may then invade the postseptal soft tissues (**Fig. 45**). Lymphoma and other lymphoproliferative diseases may involve the periorbital soft tissues and may appear similar at imaging to an infectious process (**Fig. 46**). However, although some forms of lymphoma may have an unusually accelerated course, infection generally has a more rapid onset and progression of physical signs and symptoms than neoplasm.

EXTRAOCULAR MUSCLE ENLARGEMENT

Thyroid-Associated Orbitopathy

Thyroid-associated orbitopathy (TAO) is the most common extrathyroidal manifestation of Graves disease, affecting 23% to 50% of patients with Graves disease.[56,57] It has been suggested that there is a common antigen in the thyroid and orbital tissues, which is the target of this autoimmune process.[56,58] The accumulation of glycosaminoglycans in the orbital soft tissues, and increased fat volume, contribute to the clinical and radiographic findings.

The classic imaging findings of TAO (also known as Graves orbitopathy or Graves ophthalmopathy) are symmetric bilateral enlargement of the extraocular muscles (**Fig. 47**), with increased fat volume contributing to proptosis (**Fig. 48**). In contradistinction to IOI, the muscular enlargement typically spares the tendinous insertions, although tendinous involvement has been described.[56,59,60] Patients may less commonly present with unilateral disease (**Fig. 49**).

Approximately 4% to 8% of patients with TAO may develop dystrophic optic neuropathy (DON),[56,61] which presents with varying degrees of visual impairment. Mechanical compression of

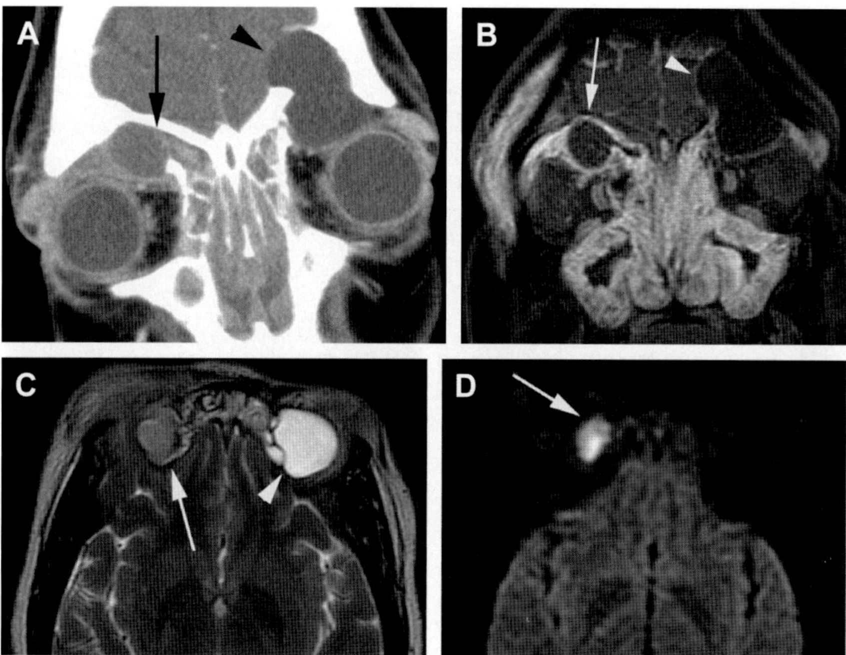

Fig. 37. Mucocele and mucopyocele in a 29-year-old woman with history of chronic sinusitis and recent onset of pain and fever. (*A*) Coronal contrast-enhanced CT image shows bilateral mucoceles. The left mucocele appears to be dehiscent with thin linear enhancement (*arrowhead*), but no brain edema. The right mucocele (*arrow*) is associated with thicker enhancing rim, and asymmetric enhancing tissue in the adjacent extraconal superior orbit. (*B*) Coronal T1W fat-saturated image shows thick peripheral enhancement of the right mucocele (*arrow*), with enhancing tissue in the more lateral aspect of the superior orbit, consistent with abscess (mucopyocele) and associated phlegmon. The left-sided mucocele again has T1 signal consistent with simple fluid, and thin linear dural enhancement at the area of dehiscence (*arrowhead*). (*C*) Axial T2W image shows simple fluid signal of the left mucocele (*arrowhead*). There is hypointense signal in the right mucocele (*arrow*). (*D*) Axial DWI shows restricted diffusion in the mucopyoceles (*arrow*), as would be seen in other forms of abscess.

the optic nerve by the enlarged extraocular muscles at the orbital apex is commonly held to be the cause of DON (**Fig. 50**). Several schemes have been proposed for quantifying and monitoring the degree of crowding of the optic nerve at the orbital apex, mainly by assessing the effacement of the perineural fat.

Idiopathic Orbital Inflammation

In a study of 65 patients, myositis was found to be the second most common orbital manifestation of IOI, after dacryoadenitis, with 5 patients presenting with concurrent involvement of the muscles and lacrimal gland.[7] In contradistinction to TAO, IOI of the extraocular muscles is typically unilateral, painful, and of rapid onset (hours to days). However, some patients may have an atypical presentation, with a relatively painless manifestation of IOI, or bilateral disease. Bilateral disease may occur in approximately 25% of patients and is more common in children.[8,62] On imaging, an additional distinguishing feature is that IOI often involves the tendinous insertions of the affected extraocular muscles,[5] and there may be concurrent inflammatory changes in the fat adjacent to the muscles (**Fig. 51**). The inflammatory changes of IOI are typically hypointense with respect to normal muscle on T2W MR images and enhance briskly with intravenous gadolinium.[63] IOI frequently responds dramatically to steroid treatment.

Carotid-Cavernous Fistula

Carotid-cavernous fistula (CCF) may be classified by their hemodynamics (high or low flow), cause (spontaneous or posttraumatic), or vascular anatomy (direct or indirect).[64] Direct CCF is frequently associated with trauma or, if spontaneous, with aneurysm rupture. Direct CCF typically progresses rapidly, in the days to weeks after the inciting event, and is caused by direct flow from the cavernous carotid artery to the venous space of the cavernous sinus. Because of venous engorgement of the extraocular muscles, exophthalmos

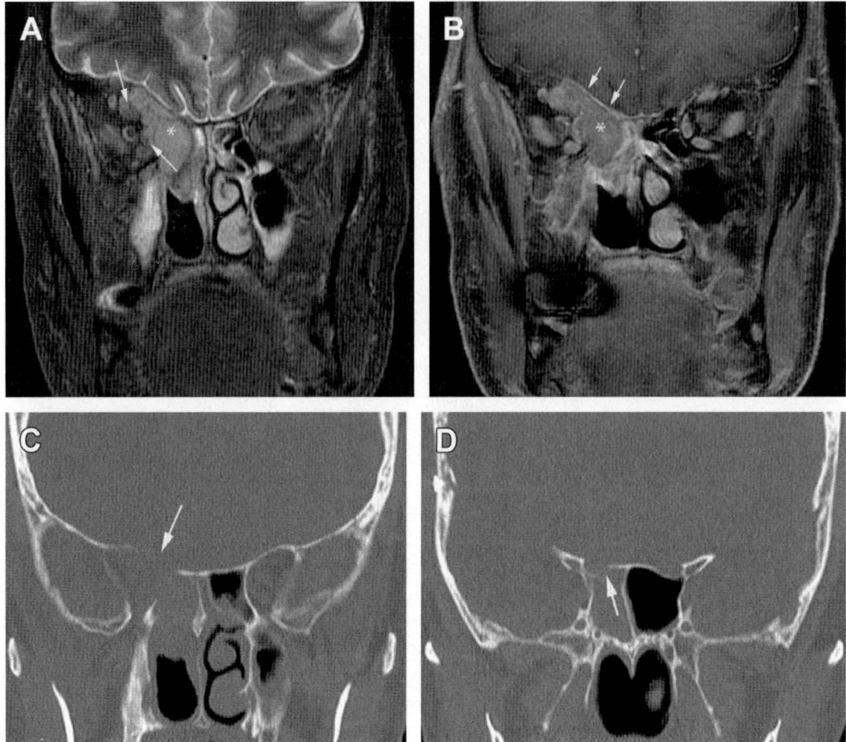

Fig. 38. Sinonasal melanoma invading orbit in a 72-year-old man with history of previously resected sinonasal melanoma. (*A*) Coronal STIR image shows extension of tumor from the posterior ethmoid operative bed into the right posterior orbit through the lamina papyracea (*asterisk*). The tumor is visually inseparable from the superior extraocular muscle complex and medial rectus muscles (*arrows*). (*B*) Coronal T1W fat-saturated image shows moderate enhancement of the mass (*asterisk*). There is abnormal enhancement of the overlying dura, raising concern for intracranial extension (*arrows*). (*C*) Corresponding coronal CT image shows erosion of the overlying bone (*arrow*). (*D*) Additional coronal CT image more posteriorly shows erosion of the floor of the right optic canal (*arrow*) from tumor that has extended into the right sphenoid sinus.

(possibly pulsatile) is one of the most common clinical signs, along with orbital bruit and chemosis.[64,65] Indirect or low-flow CCF has a similar constellation of presenting signs, but usually a more insidious onset, and less dramatic imaging findings. Indirect CCF is caused by dural shunting of arterial flow into the cavernous sinus from branches of the internal carotid artery, external carotid artery, or both.[66,67]

Engorgement of the extraocular muscles is one of the important cross-sectional imaging features of CCF. Engorgement of the superior ophthalmic vein may also be visible on CT, MR imaging, or MR angiography, with an appearance that is

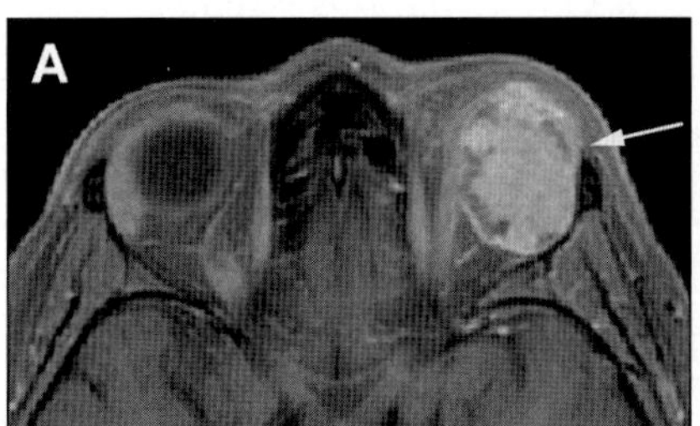

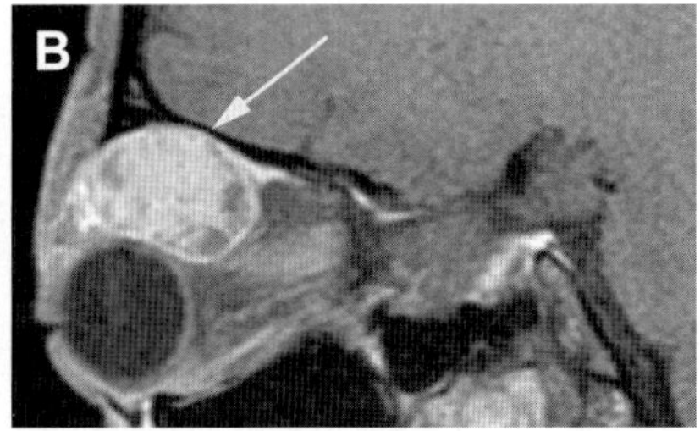

Fig. 39. Pleomorphic adenoma of the lacrimal gland in a 45-year-old man with slowly progressive painless orbital mass. (*A*) Axial and (*B*) sagittal postcontrast fat-saturated T1W images show a well-circumscribed ovoid enhancing mass in the left superior orbit (*arrows*), which was proved to be pleomorphic adenoma.

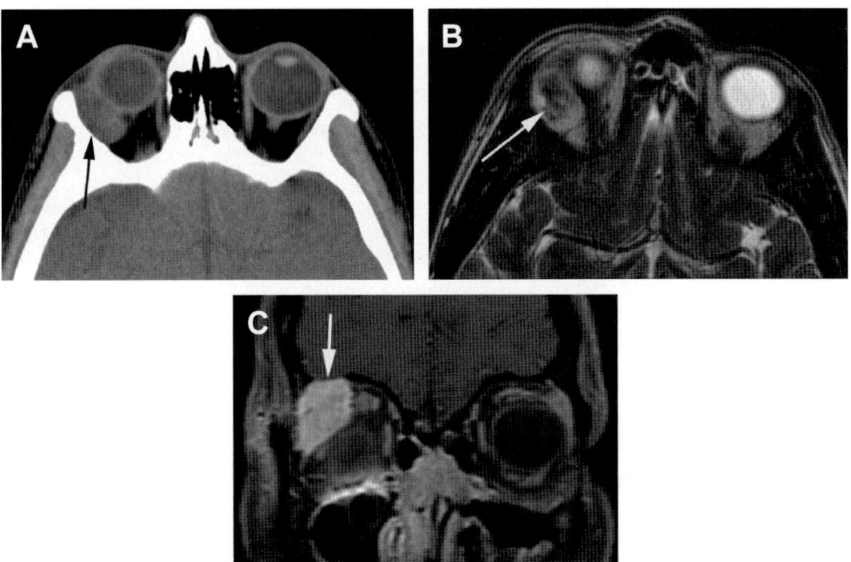

Fig. 40. Adenoid cystic carcinoma of the lacrimal gland in a 37-year-old woman with right orbital mass. (*A*) Axial CT image shows an ovoid mass in the right superolateral orbit (*arrow*). (*B*) Axial T2W image shows heterogeneous signal of the mass (*arrow*). (*C*) Coronal postcontrast T1W image shows avid enhancement of the mass (*arrow*), proved to be adenoid cystic carcinoma.

commensurate to findings on catheter angiography. The cavernous sinus may also show abnormal unilateral enlargement or the presence of abnormal flow voids (**Fig. 52**).

Sarcoidosis

Involvement of the extraocular muscles by sarcoidosis is unusual, but may be multiple or bilateral, painful or indolent, with or without

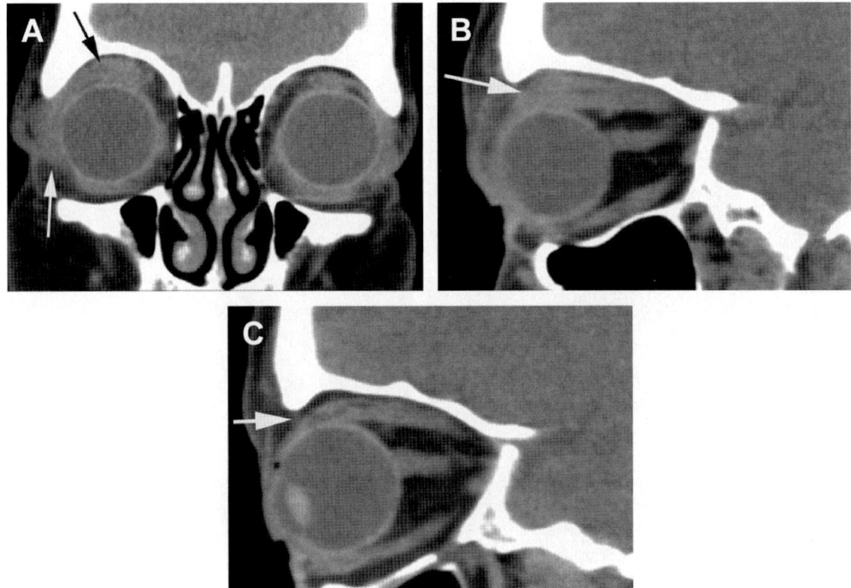

Fig. 41. IOI of the lacrimal gland. (*A*) Coronal CT image shows abnormal enlargement of the palpebral lobe (*white arrow*) and orbital lobe (*black arrow*) of the right lacrimal gland, in a 68-year-old woman who presented with acute onset of orbital pain and swelling. (*B*) Sagittal CT image shows accompanying enlargement of the right superior muscle complex (*arrow*), with an infiltrative appearance of the adjacent fat planes, consistent with inflammation. The normal contralateral superior muscle complex (*C*) is shown for comparison (*arrow*).

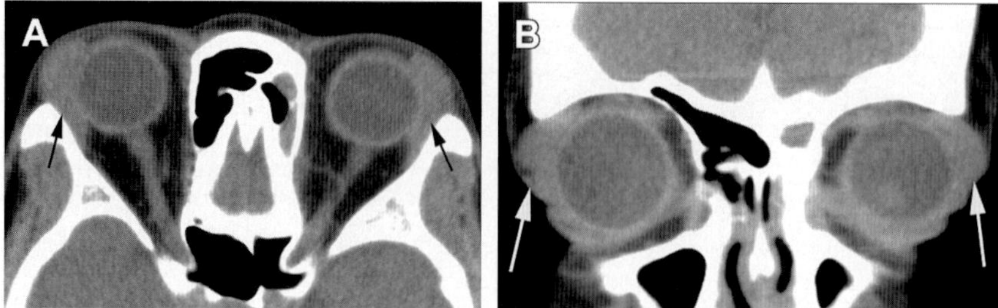

Fig. 42. Sarcoidosis of the lacrimal glands in a 35-year-old woman with painless slowly progressive bilateral orbital masses. (*A*) Axial and (*B*) coronal CT images show bilateral symmetric enlargement of the lacrimal glands (*arrows*) in this patient with sarcoidosis.

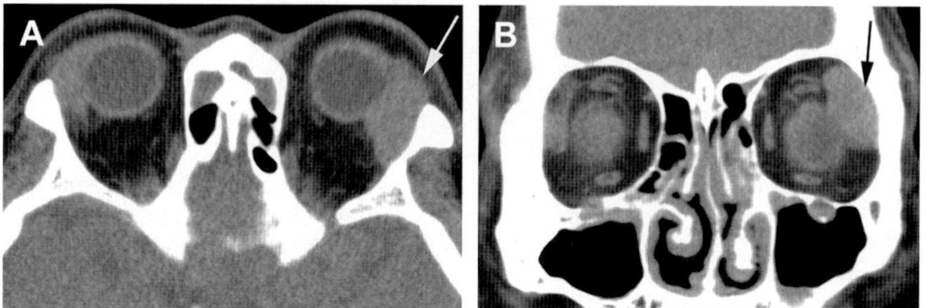

Fig. 43. Atypical lymphoid hyperplasia of the lacrimal gland in a 46-year-old man with a 10-year history of slowly enlarging left orbital mass. (*A*) Axial and (*B*) coronal CT images show abnormal enlargement of the left lacrimal gland (*arrows*). Biopsy confirmed atypical lymphoid hyperplasia.

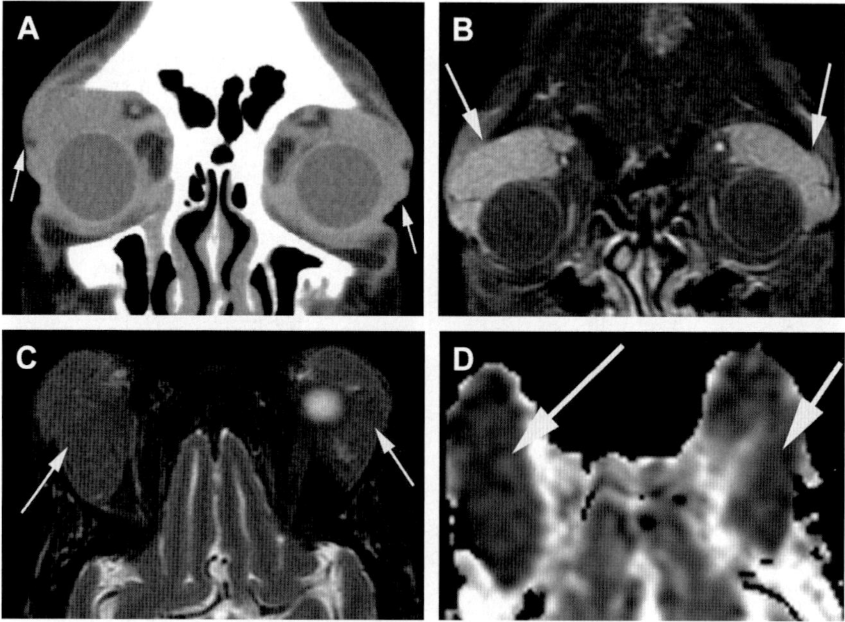

Fig. 44. Lymphoma of the lacrimal gland in a 58-year-old woman with bilateral painless orbital masses, progressive over several weeks. (*A*) Coronal CT image shows abnormal symmetric enlargement of the lacrimal glands (*arrows*). (*B*) Coronal postcontrast fat-saturated T1W image shows corresponding brisk enhancement of the enlarged lacrimal glands (*arrows*). (*C*) Axial fat-saturated T2W image shows hypointense signal of the lacrimal glands (*arrows*), and there is markedly restricted diffusion, corroborated on the apparent diffusion coefficient image (*D*), typical of lymphoma.

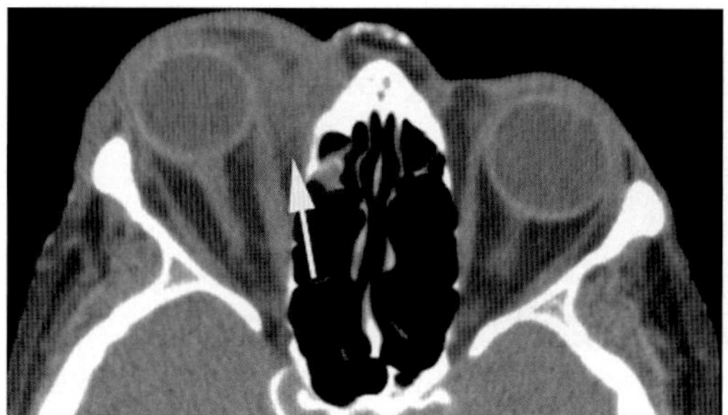

Fig. 45. Postseptal orbital cellulitis in an 85-year-old woman with rapidly progressive right orbital pain, redness and swelling, and impaired ocular movement. Axial CT image shows abnormal soft tissue density in the periorbital soft tissues, with postseptal extension (*arrow*), consistent with orbital cellulitis.

concomitant disease of other orbital soft tissues such as the lacrimal gland.[68] Both sparing[69] and involvement[70] of the tendinous insertions have been reported. With this range of presentation, it may be difficult to differentiate from TAO or IOI by physical examination and imaging, especially if there is no history of systemic sarcoidosis (**Fig. 53**).

Lymphoproliferative Disease and Metastases

Intramuscular metastases and lymphoma are rare, with most published reports describing extraorbital musculature.[71] Metastases and lymphoma or other lymphoproliferative diseases occurring in the extraocular muscles have been reported only sporadically in the literature. Carcinoma (predominantly breast) melanoma, non-Hodgkin lymphoma (**Fig. 54**), and neuroendocrine tumors such as carcinoid (**Fig. 55**) are prevalent.[71–73] As described in the section on intraconal metastases, signs and symptoms may vary according to the structures involved by the metastatic tumor. However, diplopia is a prevalent symptom when the extraocular muscles are involved. Patients may not necessarily have known metastatic disease at the time of discovery of the extraocular muscle metastases.[72] Breast carcinoma may involve the extraocular muscles in a bilateral symmetric pattern with sparing of the tendons, which may be difficult to distinguish from TAO at imaging (**Fig. 56**).[72]

Trauma

The extraocular muscles may appear enlarged because of traumatic edema and hyperemia. On imaging alone, there may be a close resemblance to infection or inflammatory disease, or even atypical TAO (**Fig. 57**). However, in most cases, the correct history makes the diagnosis clear.

INFILTRATIVE DISEASE

Metastasis

The most common primary malignancy to metastasize to the orbits is breast carcinoma.[74] Incidence of orbital metastases in patients with breast carcinoma has been reported between 8% and 10%.[75] Diffuse intraconal disease is one of many imaging patterns that may be seen in breast cancer, in addition to intramuscular or osseous masses.[43] Infiltrative schirrhous breast carcinoma may cause enophthalmos, because fibrous tissue replaces the normal orbital fat (**Fig. 58**).[26]

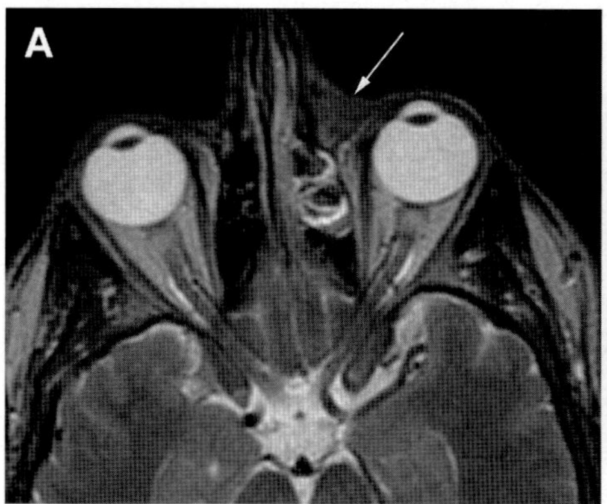

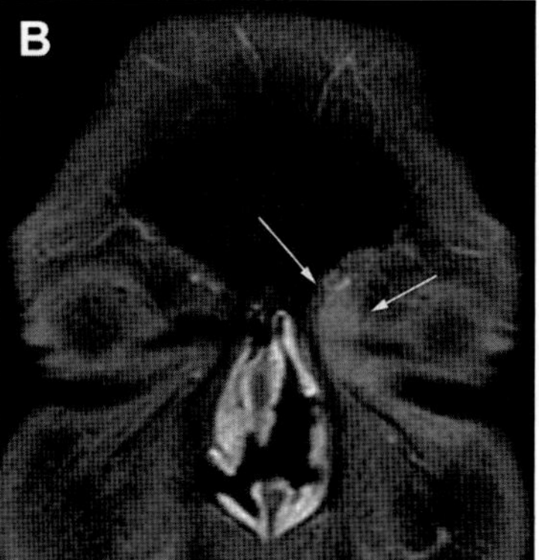

Fig. 46. Lymphoma of the lacrimal sac fossa in a 33-year-old man with painless left medial orbital mass progressing over several weeks. (*A*) Axial T2W image shows a hypointense mass in the left lacrimal sac fossa (*arrow*). (*B*) Coronal postcontrast fat-saturated T1W image shows enhancement of the mass (*arrows*), proved to be non-Hodgkin lymphoma.

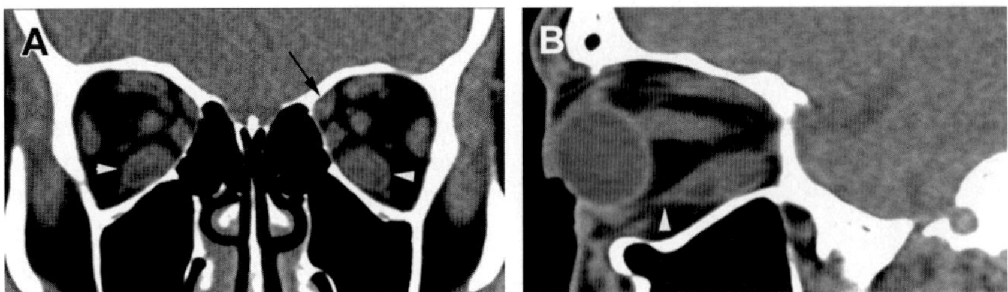

Fig. 47. Tendon-sparing TAO. (*A*) Coronal CT image shows symmetric enlargement of the inferior rectus muscles (*white arrowheads*). There is also asymmetric enlargement of the left superior oblique muscle (*black arrow*). (*B*) Sagittal CT image shows sparing of the inferior rectus tendon (*arrowhead*).

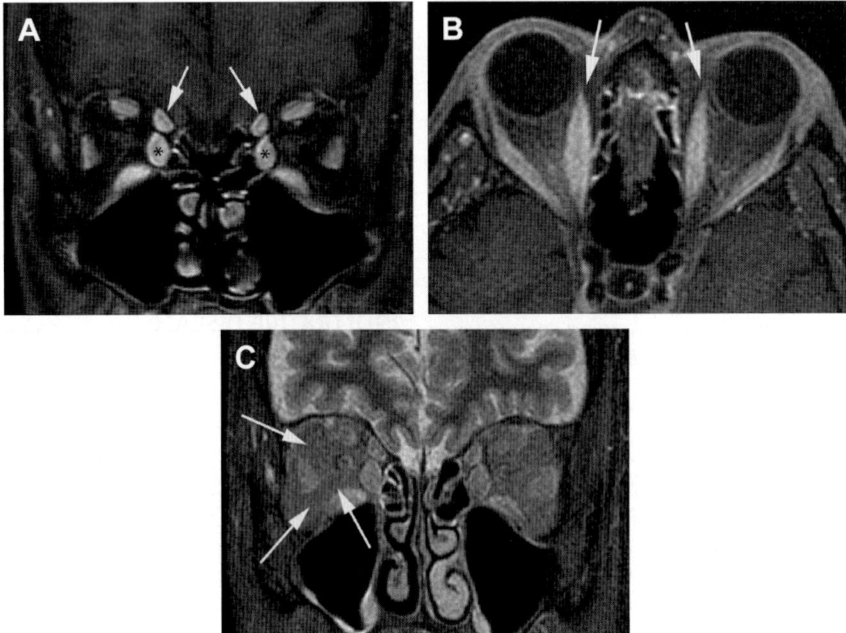

Fig. 48. Graves disease with fat proliferation in a 22-year-old man with proptosis and symptoms of hyperthyroidism. (*A*) Coronal postcontrast fat-saturated T1W image shows symmetric enlargement of the medial rectus muscles (*asterisks*) and superior oblique muscles (*arrows*) in this patient with TAO. (*B*) The axial postcontrast fat-saturated T1W image shows sparing of the tendinous insertions of the medial rectus muscles (*arrows*). (*C*) Coronal STIR image shows mildly hyperintense signal of the orbital fat (*arrows*), which may be secondary to deposition of glycosaminoglycans.

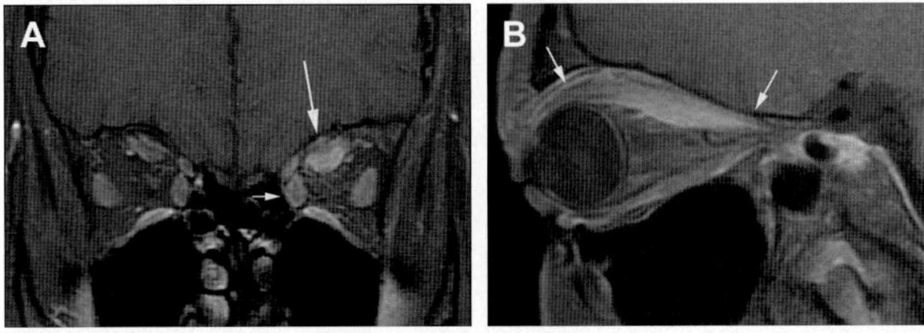

Fig. 49. Unilateral TAO in a 43-year-old woman with unilateral proptosis. (*A*) Coronal postcontrast fat-saturated T1W image shows abnormal enlargement of the left superior rectus muscle (*large arrow*). There is also subtle enlargement of the medial rectus muscle (*small arrow*). (*B*) Sagittal postcontrast fat-saturated T1W image shows sparing of the tendinous insertions of the superior rectus muscle (*arrows*). Subsequent clinical evaluation was diagnostic of TAO, with an atypical unilateral orbital presentation. (*Courtesy of* Ali Sepahdari, MD.)

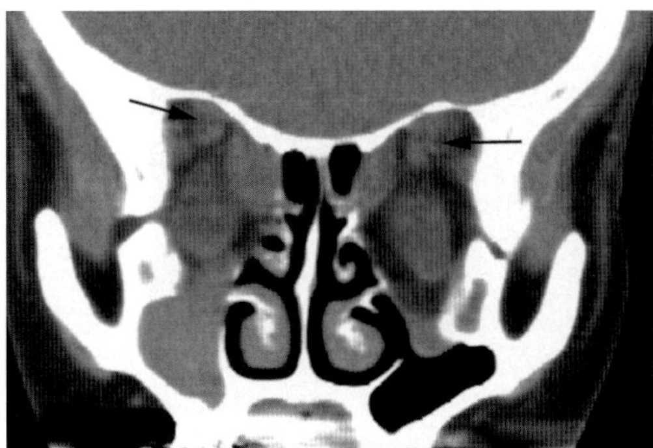

Fig. 50. DON in TAO. Coronal CT image shows early loss of the normal fat planes surrounding the bilateral ONSC at the orbital apices (*arrows*) in this 47-year-old woman with TAO, at risk for DON.

Idiopathic Orbital Inflammation

Diffuse involvement of the orbital fat is less common than involvement of other orbital structures such as the lacrimal gland or extraocular muscles.[7] As with IOI in general, unilateral pain of rapid onset is the classic presentation. There may be concurrent involvement of any of the other orbital structures; for example, there may be contiguous involvement of the sclera or ONSC (**Fig. 59**). The eponym Tolosa-Hunt syndrome applies when there is predominantly involvement of the orbital apex or cavernous sinus (**Fig. 60**).

Lymphoproliferative Disease

Similar to IOI, lymphoproliferative disease such as lymphoma may present with an infiltrative pattern, involving any orbital structure. However, in contrast to IOI, lymphoproliferative disease presents with minimal or no pain and with gradual progression.[76] In one large series, diffuse ill-defined orbital disease was slightly more common than a well-circumscribed round or oblong mass.[10] On MR imaging, T2W signal isointense or hypointense to muscle is typical of lymphoproliferative disease (**Figs. 61** and **62**), and restricted diffusion may also be seen.

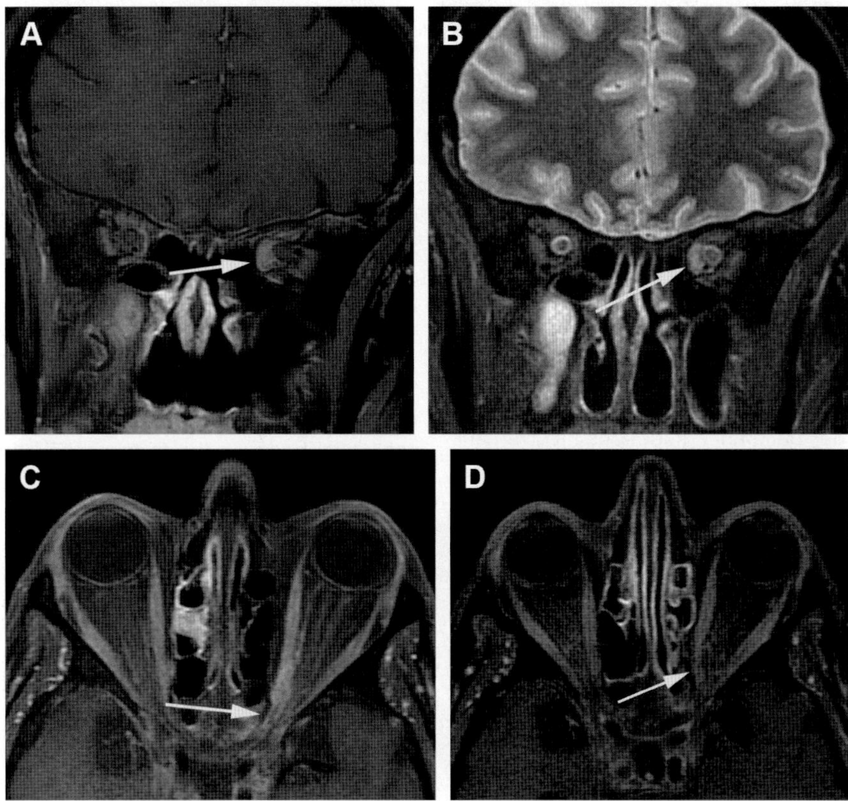

Fig. 51. IOI of the EOM. (*A*) Coronal postcontrast fat-saturated T1W image shows abnormal enlargement and enhancement of the left medial rectus muscle (*arrow*) in this 58-year-old man with rapid onset of orbital pain and diplopia. (*B*) Corresponding coronal STIR image shows abnormal signal in the muscle (*arrow*). (*C*) Axial postcontrast fat-saturated T1W image shows involvement of the posterior tendinous insertion (*arrow*). (*D*) Follow-up axial postcontrast fat-saturated T1W image shows near resolution of the previously seen findings (*arrow*) after steroid therapy.

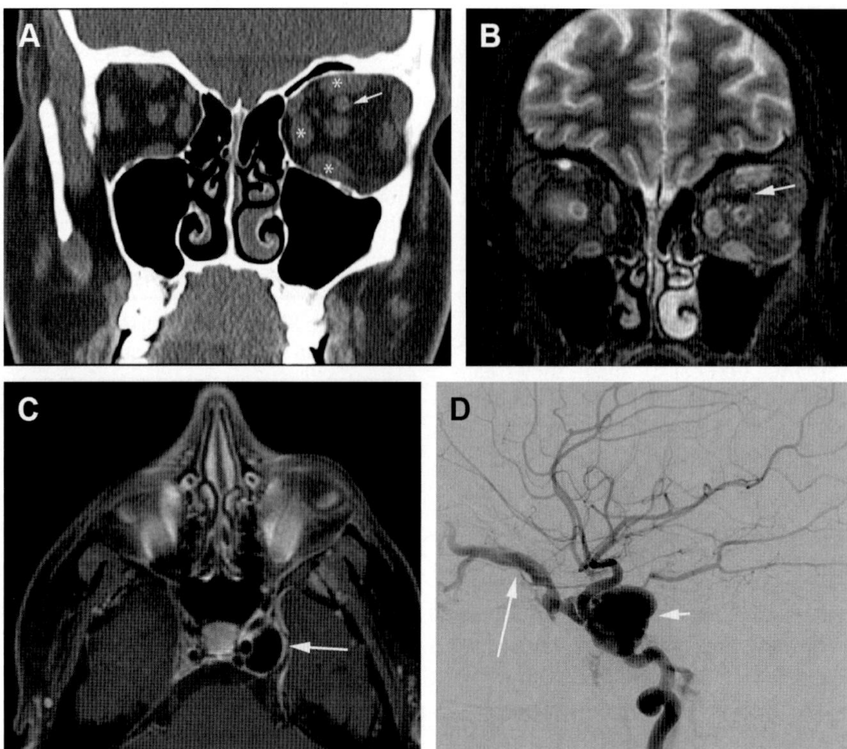

Fig. 52. CCF in a 29-year-old woman who presented with pulsatile exophthalmos approximately 3 weeks after falling off a horse. (*A*) Coronal CT image shows left-sided enlargement of the medial, lateral, and inferior rectus muscles (*asterisks*) and engorgement of the superior ophthalmic vein (*arrow*). (*B*) Coronal STIR image shows abnormal flow void in the left superior ophthalmic vein (*arrow*), consistent with arteriovenous shunting. (*C*) Axial postcontrast fat-saturated T1W image shows asymmetric enlargement of the left cavernous sinus, with prominent flow void (*arrow*). (*D*) Lateral catheter angiogram image shows abnormal contrast filling of the cavernous sinus venous space (*short arrow*) during the arterial phase of the internal carotid artery injection. Note the abnormal shunting into the enlarged ophthalmic venous system (*long arrow*).

Cellulitis

Orbital cellulitis predominantly affects children and adolescents and tends to have a more severe course in older patients.[77] Infectious involvement of the soft tissues posterior to the orbital septum is the imaging hallmark of orbital cellulitis, in contradistinction to preseptal cellulitis. It is important to distinguish orbital cellulitis from preseptal cellulitis, because the former may be associated

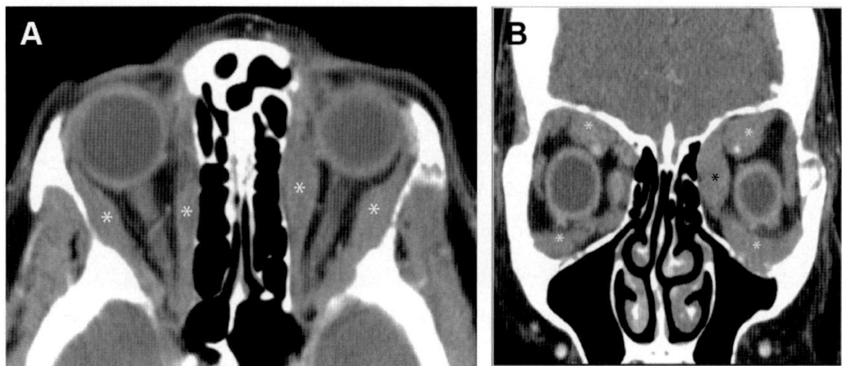

Fig. 53. Sarcoid of the EOM. (*A*) Axial and (*B*) coronal CT images show abnormal enlargement of the extraocular muscles (*asterisks*) in a patient with known sarcoidosis, who presented with bilateral proptosis. (*Courtesy of* C. Douglas Phillips, MD.)

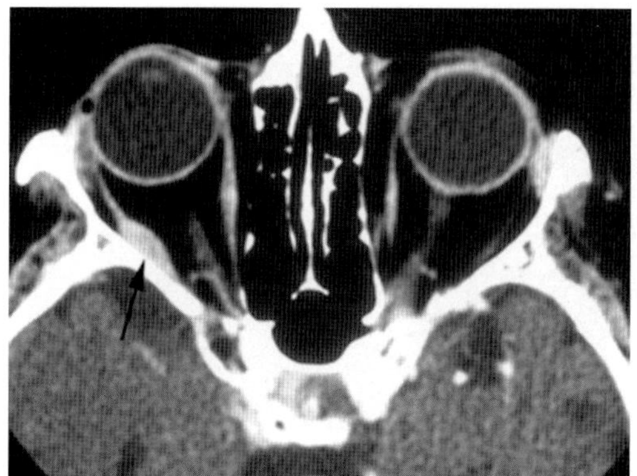

Fig. 54. Lymphoma of the EOM. Axial contrast-enhanced CT image shows abnormal enlargement and enhancement of the right lateral rectus muscle (*arrow*) in a patient with non-Hodgkin lymphoma.

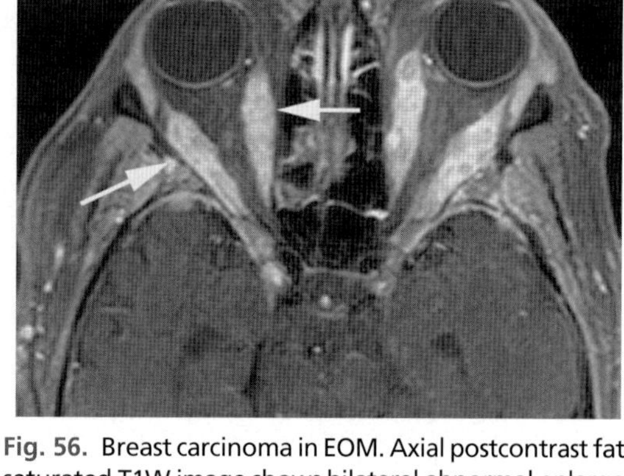

Fig. 56. Breast carcinoma in EOM. Axial postcontrast fat-saturated T1W image shows bilateral abnormal enlargement of the extraocular muscles (*arrows*), sparing the tendinous insertions, in a 59-year-old woman with metastatic breast carcinoma. (*Courtesy of* Yvonne Lui, MD.)

with complications including optic neuropathy, encephalomeningitis, cavernous sinus thrombosis, sepsis, and intracranial abscess.[78] The infiltrative appearance of orbital cellulitis may appear similar to neoplasm or lymphoproliferative processes (Fig. 63), and associated abscess formation may resemble tumor necrosis.

Sarcoidosis

Sarcoidosis may have an infiltrative appearance similar to malignancy in the orbit. The noncaseating granulomas contain many lymphocytes, which have a high nuclear/cytoplasmic ratio. This relatively low water content of the cells manifests as T2 hypointensity on MR imaging, which may mimic lymphoproliferative disorders, such as lymphoma, or metastatic disease (Fig. 64).

Plexiform Neurofibroma

Plexiform neurofibroma (PNF) occurs in about one-third of patients with NF-1.[79] When the head and neck are affected by PNF in the setting of NF-1, the trigeminal nerve may be involved, especially the ophthalmic and maxillary divisions.[80] Following the distribution of the nerves, PNF has a multispatial growth pattern, similar to some of the vasoformative anomalies, such as venous malformations and LMs, which follow vessels. However, the patient's age and relevant history should lead to the correct diagnosis. On imaging, PNF follows the distribution of the involved nerves through fascial boundaries into several contiguous anatomic compartments. When the enlarged nerves are caught in cross section, they have a characteristic targetoid appearance on T2W images (Fig. 65).

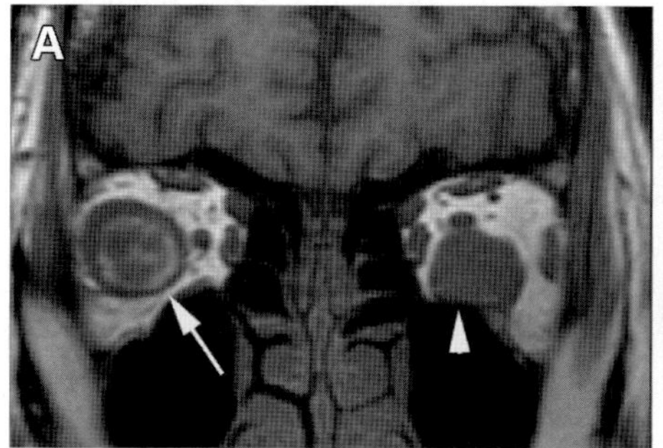

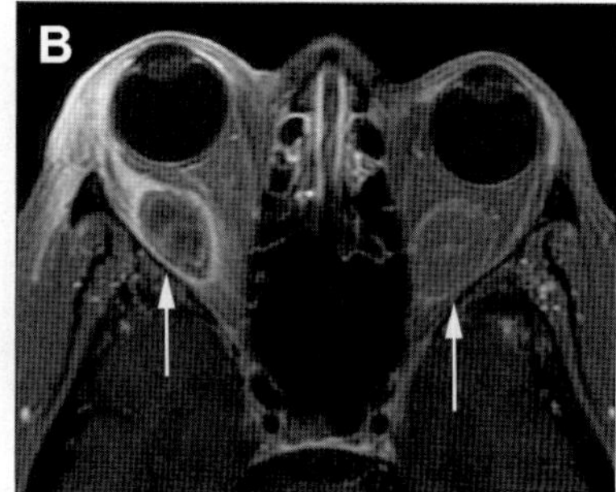

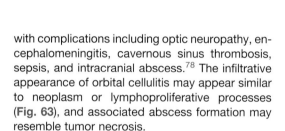

Fig. 55. Carcinoid to EOM. (*A*) Coronal T1W image shows abnormal enlargement of the right lateral rectus (*arrow*) and left inferior rectus (*arrowhead*) in a patient with metastatic carcinoid tumor. (*B*) On the axial postcontrast fat-saturated T1W image, there is minimal enhancement of the metastases (*arrows*). Asymmetric enhancement of the right lateral rectus muscle may be artifactual, judging by the ipsilateral preseptal soft tissues. (*Courtesy of* Deborah Shatzkes, MD.)

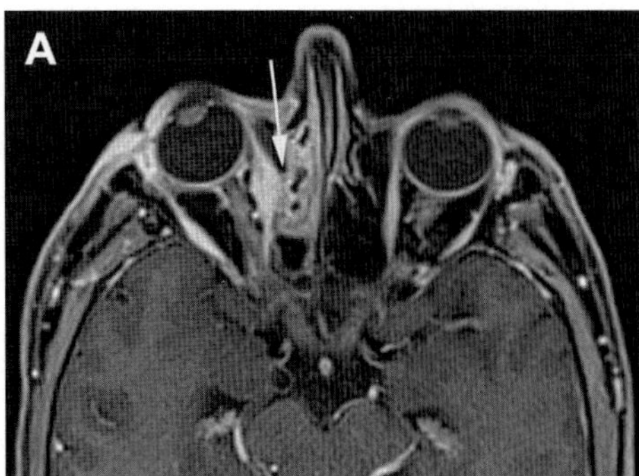

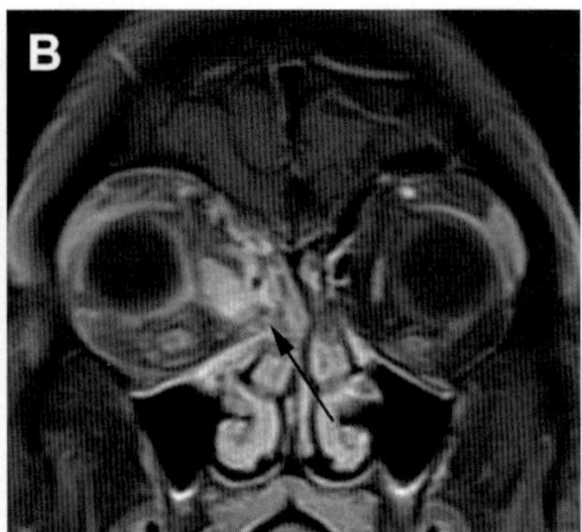

Fig. 57. Enlargement of the medial rectus muscle in a 47-year-old man with recent trauma to the right orbit. (*A*) Axial and (*B*) coronal postcontrast T1W images show abnormal enlargement of the right medial rectus muscle and abnormal enhancement of the fat plane between the muscle and the lamina papyracea (*arrows*). (*Courtesy of* Yvonne Lui, MD.)

Rhabdomyosarcoma

Rhabdomyosarcoma (RMS) is the most common soft tissue sarcoma of the head and neck in childhood, with 10% of all cases occurring in the orbit.[26,81] Although RMS may occur at any age, the mean is 8 years.[82] Proptosis and blepharoptosis are common presenting symptoms of orbital RMS. Pain is uncommon, and may indicate an advanced tumor. Rapidity of onset is variable.[82]

Although RMS is often a well-circumscribed mass without osseous destruction at presentation, more advanced cases tend to be more infiltrative and destroy bone (**Fig. 66**). Most RMS are extraconal in location at diagnosis, although many are both extraconal and intraconal.[81] RMS may involve any part of the orbit, including the extraocular muscles (**Fig. 67**). On noncontrast CT, the mass is isodense to muscle. With MR imaging, RMS is typically hyperintense to muscle and fat on T2, may have areas of high intrinsic T1 signal caused by hemorrhage, and enhances after gadolinium injection (**Fig. 68**).[81]

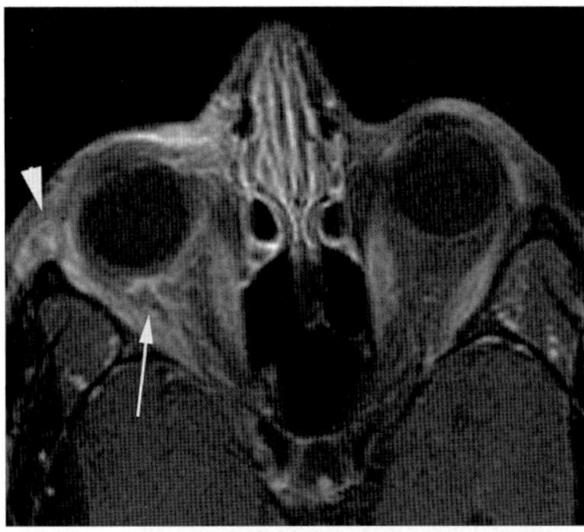

Fig. 58. Infiltrative metastatic disease. Axial postcontrast fat-saturated T1W image shows abnormal infiltrative enhancement of the retrobulbar fat (*arrow*) in this patient with metastatic breast carcinoma. There is also involvement of the lacrimal gland (*arrowhead*). There is mild enophthalmos.

INTRAOCULAR MASS

Metastasis

The reported incidence of orbital metastases ranges from 1% to 13%.[43,83,84] The prevalence of orbital metastases ranges from 2% to 4.7% in patients who have cancer.[85] Common signs and symptoms include proptosis, diplopia, pain, and decreased vision, with varying frequency across many studies.[43,83,86,87] However, progression over weeks to months is a unifying feature. Small orbital lesions are less likely to be detected than intraocular lesions of the same size,[88] presumably because of the presence of visual symptoms in the latter. Certain tumor types have been reported to have a propensity to metastasize to particular tissues (prostate to bone, melanoma to extraocular muscles, breast to fatty tissue and extraocular muscle); however, this is variable, and the overall distribution of orbital metastases is approximately in a 2:2:1 bone/fat/muscle ratio.[86]

Uveal metastases are the most common intraocular malignancy, most of which are localized to the choroid (**Fig. 69**).[89] The most common primary tumors are lung for men and breast for women.[90] In half of these cases, the intraocular metastases are asymptomatic, but in the other cases, they may present with vision loss or scotoma.[89] Choroidal metastases may rarely be the presenting manifestation of metastatic cancer.[91]

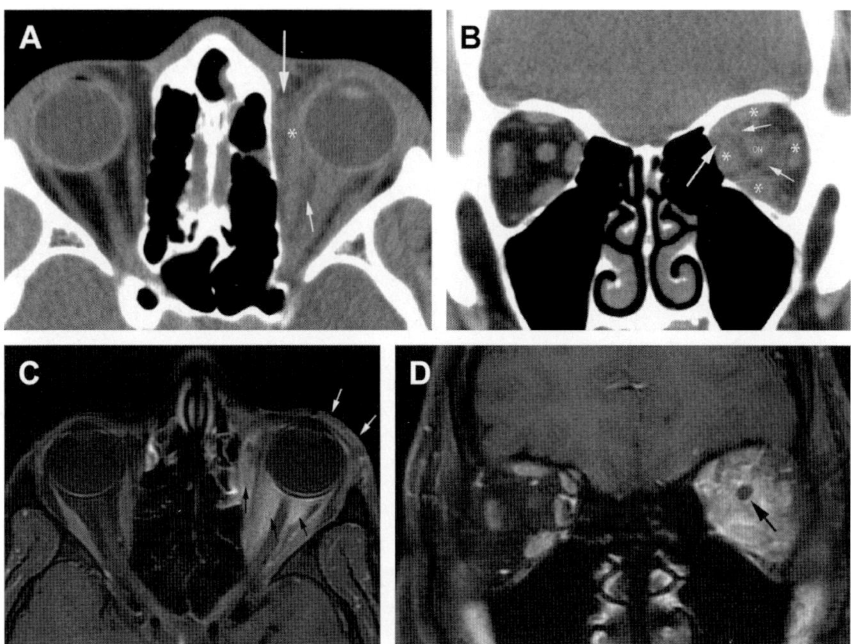

Fig. 59. IOI infiltrative in a 22-year-old man who presented with rapid onset of left orbital pain and diplopia, and mild left proptosis. (*A*) Axial CT image shows abnormal infiltrative soft tissue density in the extraconal (*large arrow*) and intraconal (*small arrow*) fat planes. There is abnormal enlargement of the medial rectus muscle, involving the tendinous insertion (*asterisk*). (*B*) Coronal CT image again shows infiltrative changes in the extraconal (*large arrow*) and intraconal (*small arrows*) fat planes, surrounding the ONSC (ON). There is involvement of the rectus muscles (*asterisks*). (*C*) Axial postcontrast fat-saturated T1W image shows abnormal infiltrative enhancement of the left retrobulbar and extraconal fat (*white arrows*). There is also involvement of the preseptal periorbital soft tissues (*white arrows*). (*D*) Corresponding coronal postcontrast fat-saturated T1W image shows relative sparing of the optic nerve (*arrow*).

Retinal Detachment

Retinal detachment (RD) typically begins with posterior vitreous detachment, and has a sudden onset of visual symptoms, such as floaters or flashes of light. This situation may progress to RD, with development of a visual field deficit or decreased vision. RD may be spontaneous or posttraumatic or occasionally caused by underlying tumors. Although RD is frequently diagnosed by the ophthalmologist, findings may be present on CT or MR imaging, commonly as an

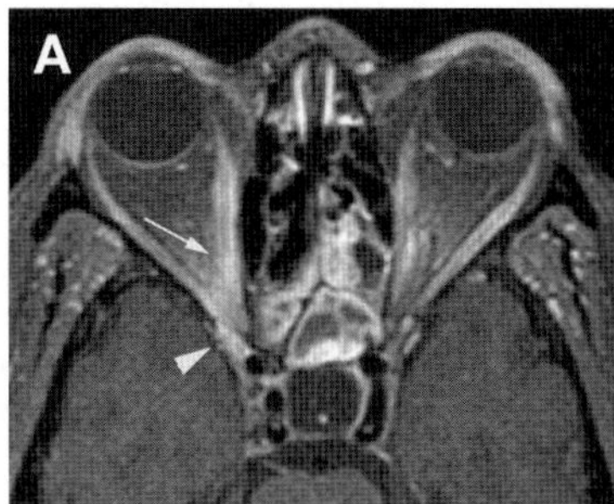

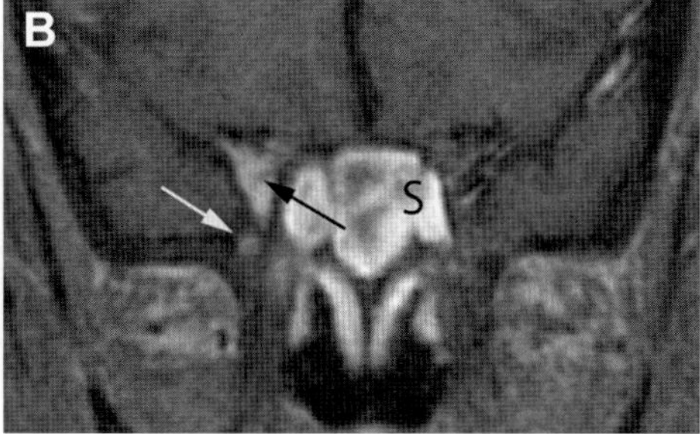

Fig. 60. IOI Tolosa-Hunt syndrome in a 48-year-old woman who presented with acute epiphora, pain, and blurry vision. (*A*) Axial postcontrast fat-saturated T1W image shows infiltrative enhancement at the orbital apex, involving the medial rectus muscle (*arrow*), and extending through the superior orbital fissure into the anterior cavernous sinus (*arrowhead*). (*B*) Coronal axial postcontrast fat-saturated T1W image shows abnormal enhancement in the right superior and inferior orbital fissure (*black arrow*), with involvement of the foramen rotundum (*white arrow*). Mucosal thickening in the sphenoid sinus is also noted (S).

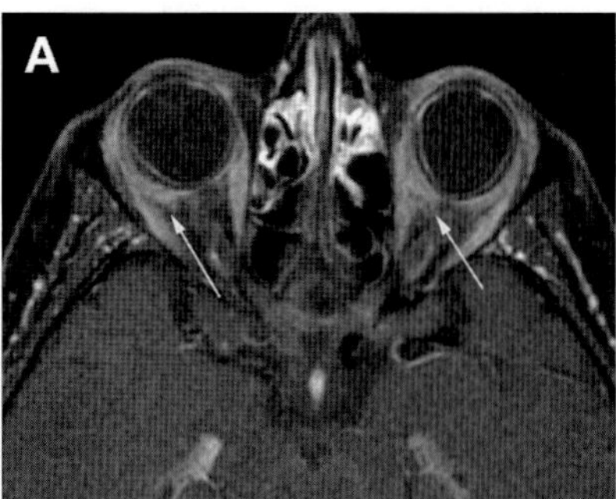

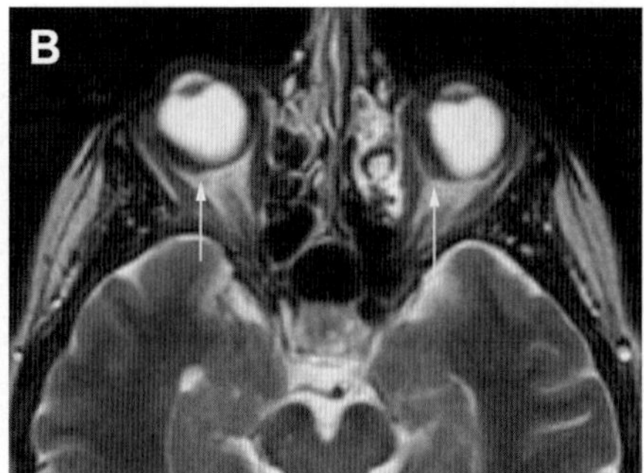

Fig. 61. Periscleral lymphoma in a 64-year-old woman with known non-Hodgkin lymphoma presented with blurry vision. (*A*) Axial postcontrast fat-saturated T1W image shows abnormal infiltrative enhancement predominantly in the bilateral periscleral areas (*arrows*). (*B*) Axial T2W image shows marked hypointense signal of the periscleral disease (*arrows*), in keeping with the diagnosis of lymphoma.

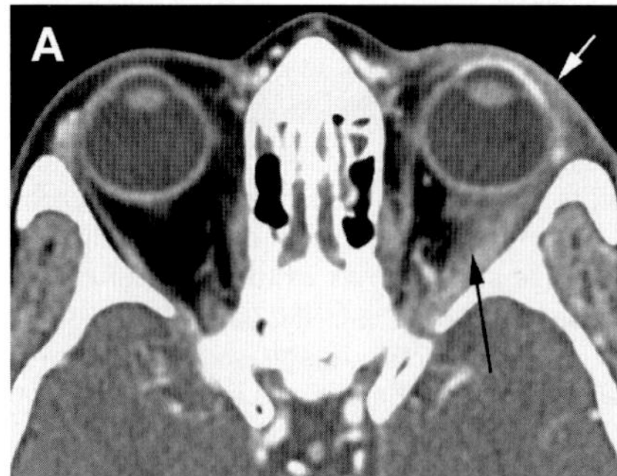

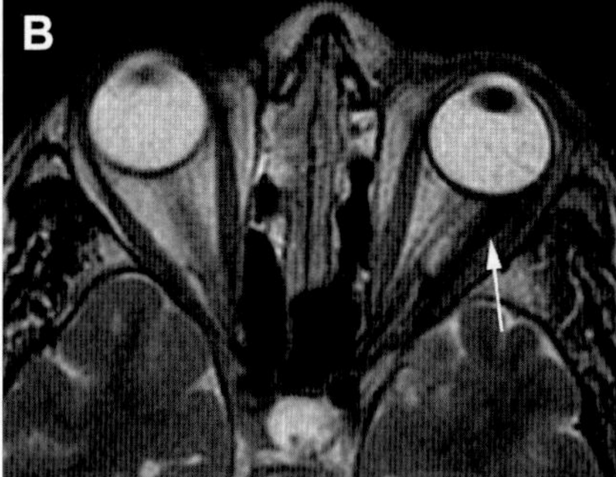

Fig. 62. Infiltrative lymphoma in a 55-year-old man with known non-Hodgkin lymphoma presented with left-sided orbital pressure and proptosis, and periorbital fullness. (*A*) Axial contrast-enhanced CT image shows infiltrative disease in the intraconal space (*black arrow*) as well as the preseptal soft tissues (*white arrow*). (*B*) Axial T2W image shows marked hypointense signal of the intraconal disease (*arrow*), consistent with lymphoma.

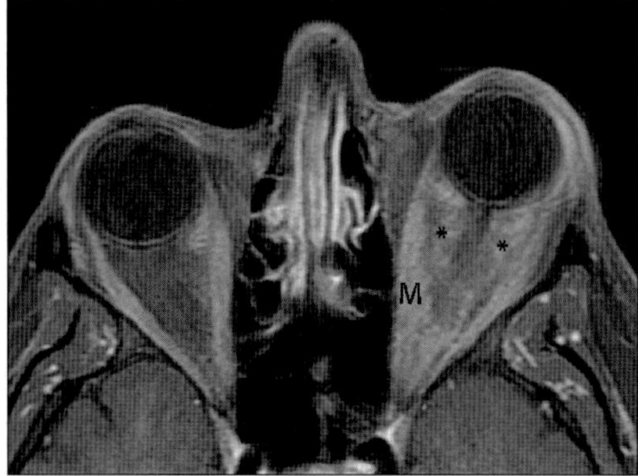

Fig. 63. Cellulitis in a 35-year-old man. Axial postcontrast fat-saturated T1W image shows abnormal infiltrative enhancement of the left retrobulbar fat (*asterisks*). There is also involvement of the left medial rectus muscle (M).

unexpected finding on head CT examinations performed for trauma (**Fig. 70**). There is a typical V-shaped area of abnormal density (CT) or signal (MR) in the posterior globe (**Fig. 71**). The anterior boundary of the subretinal collection is limited by the anterior attachment of the retina, in contradistinction to suprachoroidal collections, which may extend anteriorly to the level of the ciliary body. RD may be treated in a variety of ways, including scleral banding, which is frequently seen as an incidental finding on imaging. Postoperative infection of scleral bands can occur (**Fig. 72**). Silicone oil injection is another method of treatment (**Fig. 73**).

Uveal Melanoma

Uveal melanoma (UM) is the most common primary intraocular malignancy in adults, representing 5%

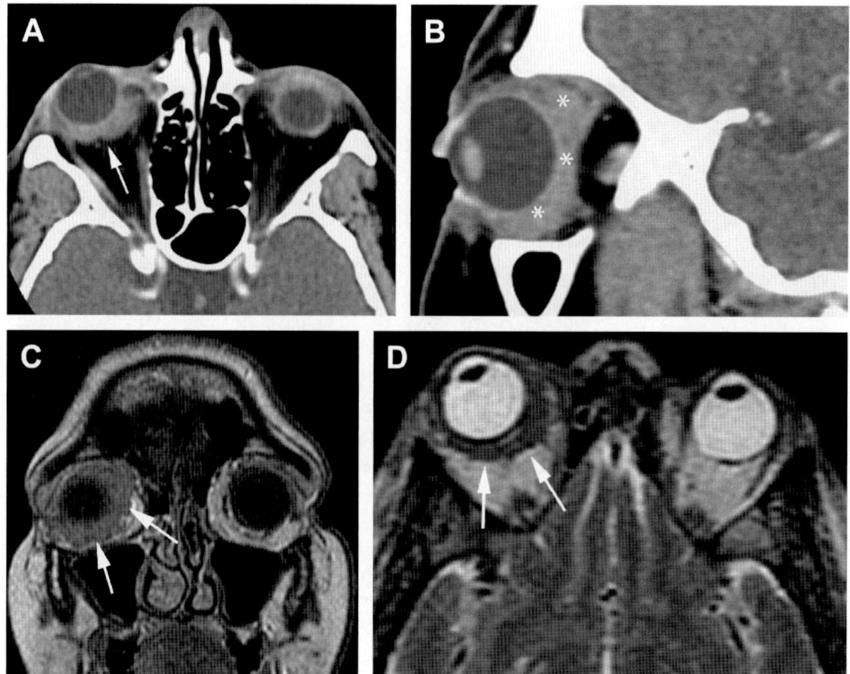

Fig. 64. Infiltrative sarcoidosis in a 57-year-old woman who presented with limitation of ocular mobility. (*A*) Axial contrast-enhanced CT image shows abnormal soft tissue along the posterior scleral surface of the right globe (*arrow*). (*B*) The sagittal contrast-enhanced CT image shows the same finding (*asterisks*). (*C*) Coronal postcontrast T1W image shows mildly enhancing ring of tissue around the posterior globe (*arrows*). (*D*) Axial T2W image shows hypointense signal of the abnormal tissue (*arrows*). Subsequent clinical evaluation led to a diagnosis of sarcoidosis.

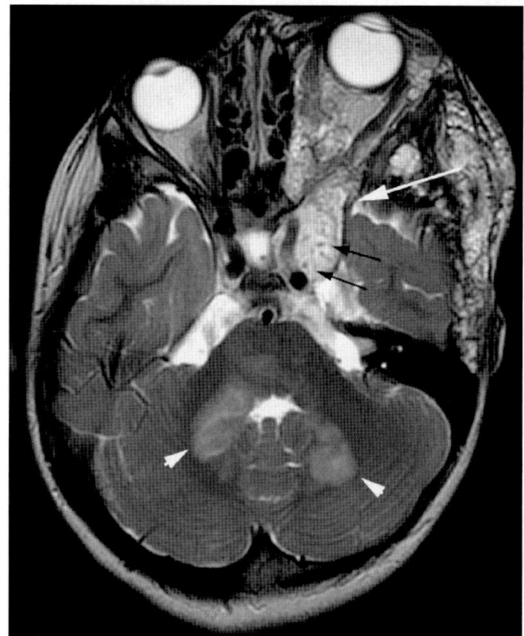

Fig. 65. PNF in an 8-year-old boy with known history of NF-1. Axial T2W image shows an infiltrative mass of the left orbit, extending intracranially thru the dysplastic left orbital apex region (*white arrow*). Targetoid appearance is shown in the cavernous sinus component of the mass (*black arrows*). There are bilateral signal changes in the medial cerebellum, typical of myelin vacuolization (*arrowheads*). (*Courtesy of* Yvonne Lui, MD.)

to 6% of melanoma diagnoses.[92] UM may arise in any of the divisions of the uvea, including the ciliary body, iris, or choroid. Choroidal UM is the most common subtype.[30] Up to 50% of patients develop distant metastases.[93]

UM is usually assessed by the ophthalmologist, possibly with the aid of ultrasonography or fluorescein angiography. However, ocular opacities may limit these modalities, in which case cross-sectional imaging may be of use.[94] UM moderately enhances on contrast-enhanced CT and has a characteristic signal pattern on MR imaging because of its melanin content; it is markedly hypointense on T2W images, and hyperintense on T1W images, which helps to distinguish it from other intraocular malignancies (**Fig. 74**).[30] MR is also excellent for distinguishing the borders of the tumor from associated hemorrhage caused by RD (**Fig. 75**).

Retinoblastoma

Retinoblastoma (RB) is the most common intraocular malignancy in pediatric patients.[95] Common presenting signs of RB include leukocoria and strabismus. Initial evaluation with ultrasonography may be useful to help distinguish RB from other diseases that present with leukocoria, such as Coat disease, persistent fetal vasculature (also known as persistent hyperplastic primary vitreous), and toxocariasis.[96] CT is superior to

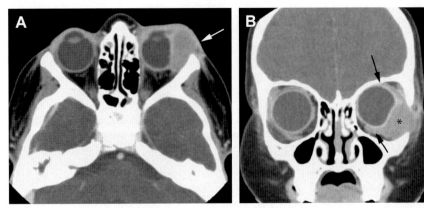

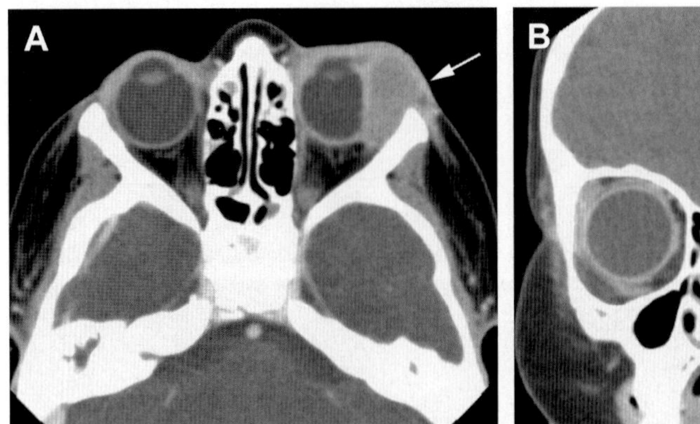

Fig. 66. RMS with bone defect in a 5-year-old boy with progressively enlarging painless orbital mass. (*A*) Axial contrast-enhanced CT image shows a moderately enhancing mass in the left lateral anterior orbit (*arrow*), deforming the globe. (*B*) Coronal contrast-enhanced CT image shows the mass (*asterisk*) eroding the bone of the lateral orbit, and infiltrating along the scleral surface of the globe (*arrows*). (*Courtesy of* Bernadette Koch.)

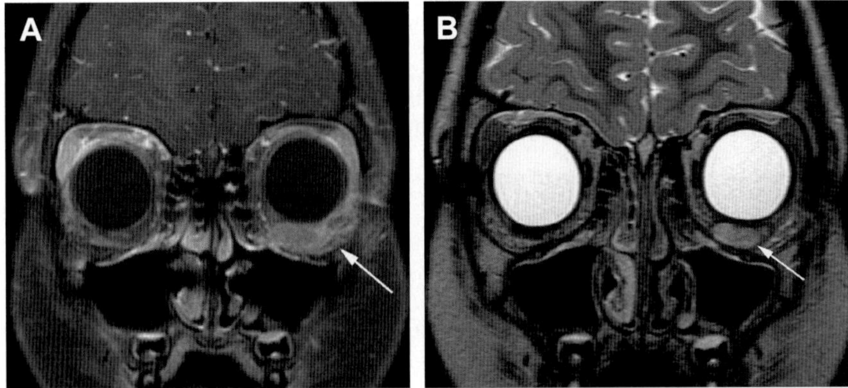

Fig. 67. RMS with EOM involvement in a 3-year-old boy with progressively enlarging painless orbital mass. (*A*) Coronal postcontrast fat-saturated T1W image shows an infiltrative enhancing mass in the left inferior orbit (*arrow*). (*B*) On the coronal STIR image, the mass is not visually separable from the left inferior rectus muscle (*arrow*). (*Courtesy of* Bernadette Koch.)

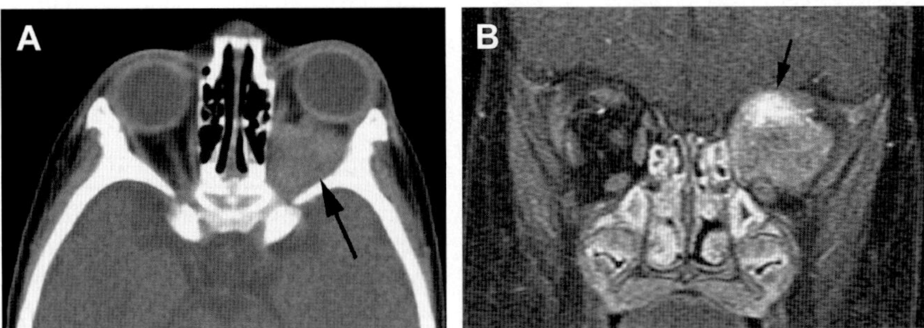

Fig. 68. RMS with hemorrhage in an 8-month-old boy with 2-week history of progressive unilateral proptosis. (*A*) Axial CT image shows a large mass in the left posterior orbit (*arrow*). (*B*) Coronal postcontrast fat-saturated T1W image shows the enhancing intraconal mass, with an area of more conspicuous signal hyperintensity (*arrow*), consistent with hemorrhage. (*Courtesy of* Caroline D. Robson, MBChB, Department of Radiology, Boston Children's Hospital.)

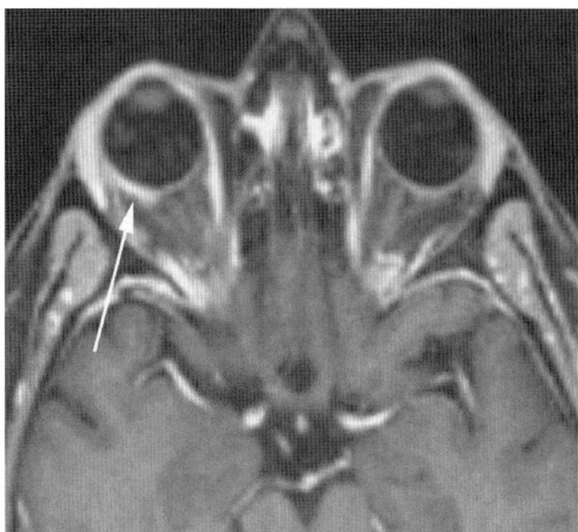

Fig. 69. Intraocular metastasis in a 57-year-old woman with history of breast carcinoma who presented with visual field defect. Axial postcontrast fat-saturated T1W image shows abnormal enhancement of the right choroid (*arrow*), consistent with a metastatic lesion.

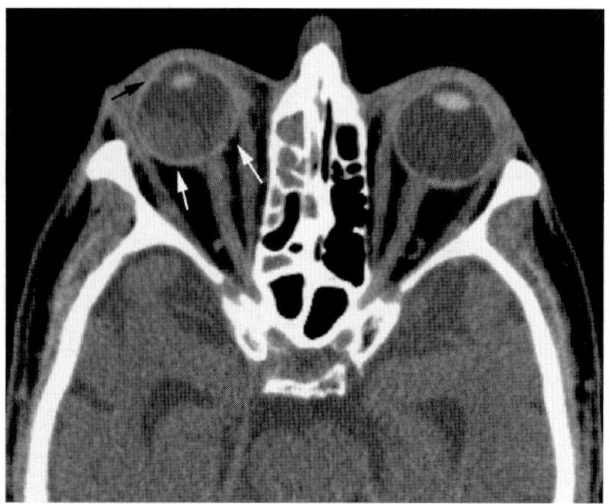

Fig. 70. RD CT in a 68-year-old woman who underwent a CT scan of the head for trauma. Axial CT image shows characteristic V-shaped posterior hyperdensity in the right globe (*white arrows*), consistent with RD and associated subretinal collections. Note that the collections do not reach the level of the ciliary body (*black arrow*), in keeping with subretinal location.

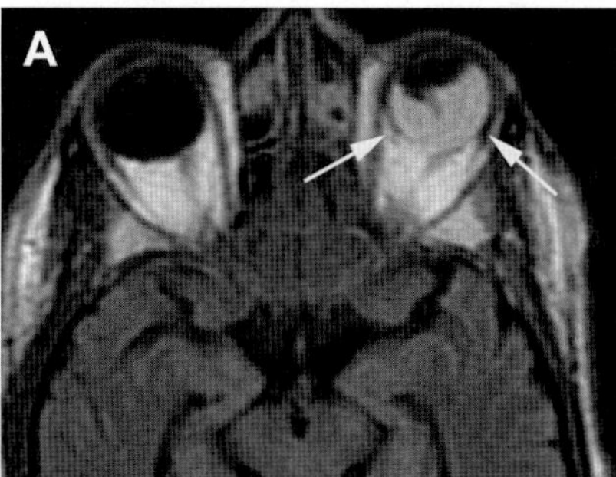

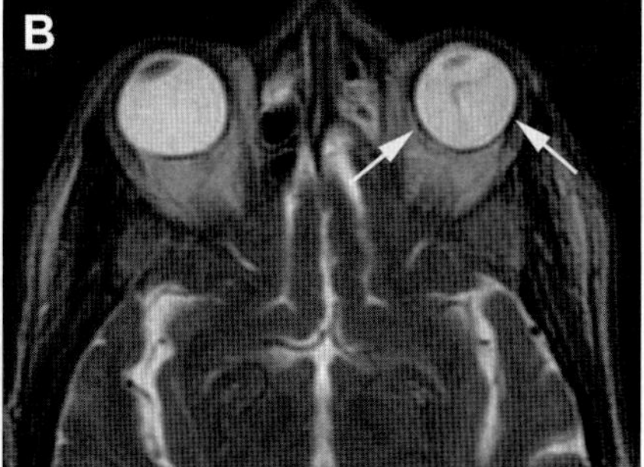

Fig. 71. RD MR imaging in a 39-year-old woman who had rapid onset of left-sided visual symptoms with no trauma. (*A*) Axial fluid-attenuated inversion recovery image shows large subretinal collections (*arrows*) consistent with RD. The findings are easier to see on the fluid-attenuated inversion recovery image than on the corresponding T2W image (*B*), in which the content of the collections more closely resembles vitreous (*arrows*).

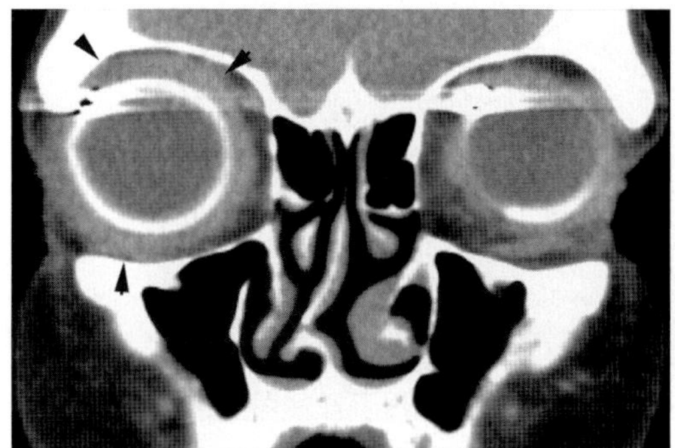

Fig. 72. RD banding. Coronal CT shows metallic bands for treatment of bilateral RDs. There is a band of asymmetric soft tissue density surrounding the right band (*arrowheads*), consistent with infection in the postoperative setting.

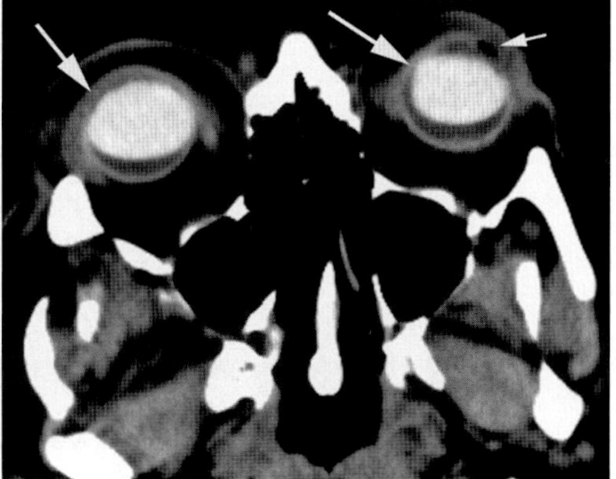

Fig. 73. RD injection. Axial CT image of the head performed for trauma in an 85-year-old man shows incidental finding of recent bilateral intraocular silicone oil injection for RD (*large arrows*). Small focus of gas consistent with recent procedure (*small arrow*).

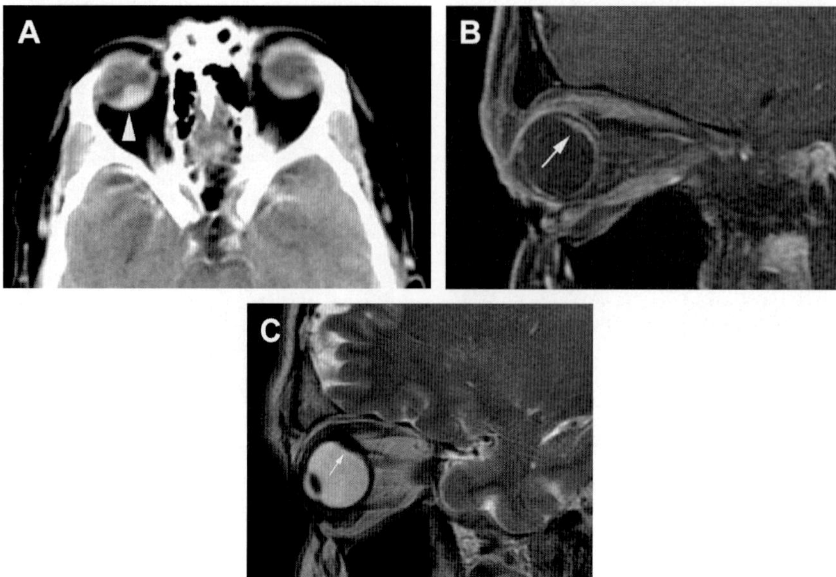

Fig. 74. Intraocular melanoma CT and MR in a 62-year-old man who presented with progressive vision loss in the right eye. (*A*) Axial CT image shows a hyperdense mass in the right globe (*arrowhead*). (*B*) On the sagittal postcontrast fat-saturated T1W image, there is a corresponding enhancing choroidal mass (*arrow*). (*C*) The mass is hypointense on the corresponding sagittal T2W image (*arrow*).

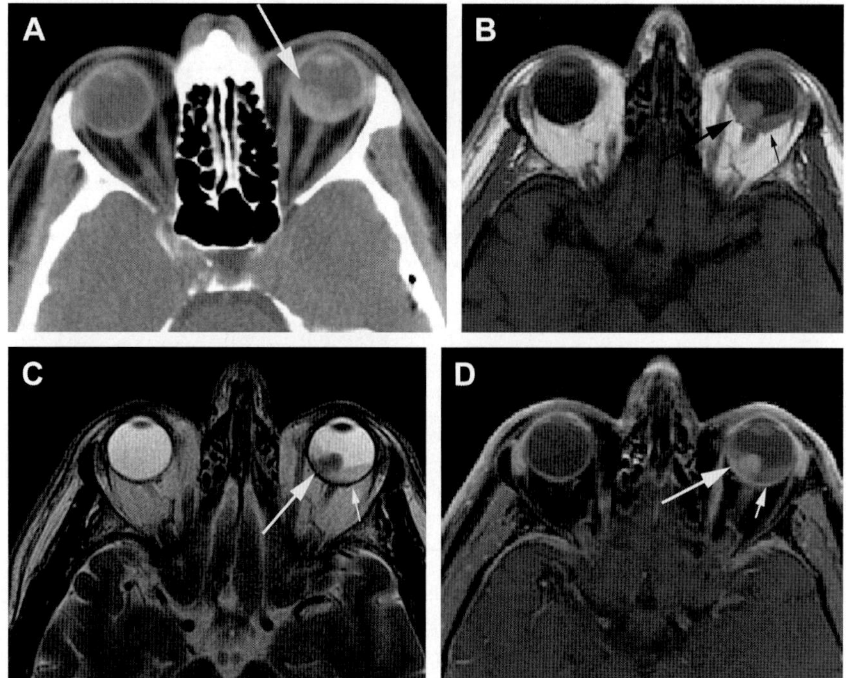

Fig. 75. Intraocular melanoma with RD in a 45-year-old man who presented with progressive vision loss in the left eye. (*A*) Axial CT image shows RD (*arrow*). (*B*) Corresponding axial T1W image shows relatively hyperintense signal of a nodular area in the posterior globe (*large arrow*), compared with the lower signal of the associated subretinal collection (*small arrow*). (*C*) On the axial T2W image, there is corresponding hypointense signal of the nodule (*large arrow*), compared with the subretinal collection (*small arrow*). (*D*) Axial postcontrast fat-saturated T1W image shows enhancement of the nodule (*large arrow*), but not the subretinal fluid (*small arrow*).

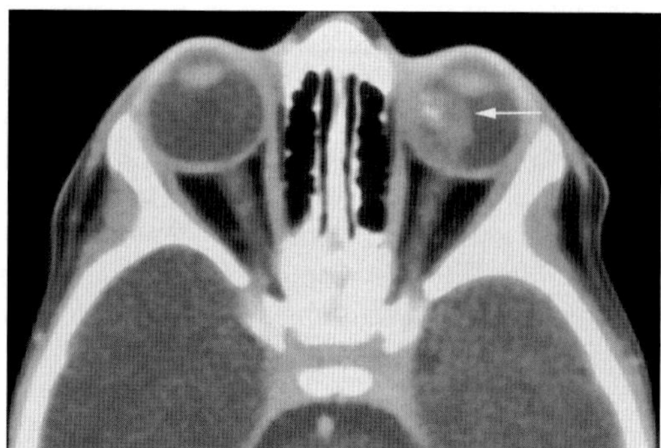

Fig. 76. RB on CT. Axial CT image of a 1-year-old boy with leukocoria shows a partially calcified mass in the left globe (*arrow*).

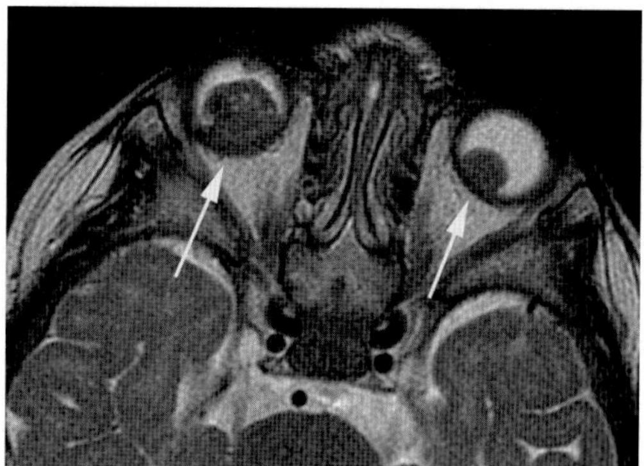

Fig. 78. RB bilateral in a 13-month-old girl with leukocoria. Axial T2W image shows bilateral hypointense ocular masses (*arrows*), consistent with RB.

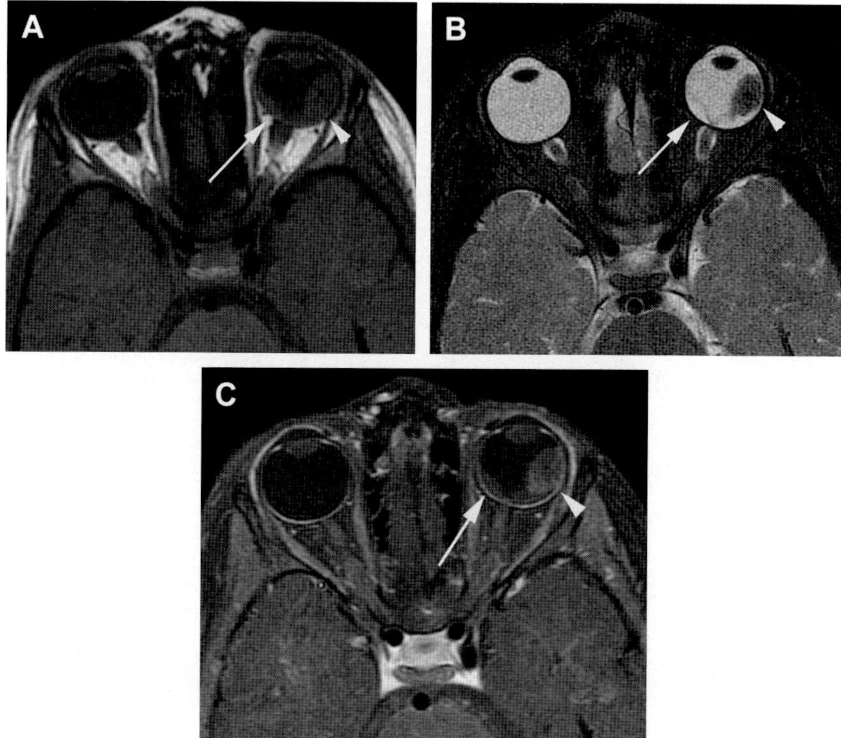

Fig. 77. RB with RD MR imaging in an 11-month-old boy with left leukocoria. (*A*) Axial T1W image shows abnormal signal in the bilateral posterior globe. The medial aspect has a relatively flat configuration (*arrow*), whereas the lateral aspect is more masslike (*arrowhead*). (*B*) Corresponding axial T2W image shows a markedly hypointense mass in the lateral globe (*arrowhead*), consistent with RB. The medial signal abnormality is consistent with secondary subretinal fluid collection (*arrow*). (*C*) On the axial postcontrast fat-saturated T1W image, there is abnormal enhancement of the mass (*arrowhead*), but not the medial subretinal fluid (*arrow*).

ultrasonography in detecting small calcifications, which are present in greater than 90% of RB cases, and ultrasonography is not reliable for detecting tumoral extension beyond the ocular globe into the optic nerve or retrobulbar space,[97] findings that portend a worse prognosis.

Although CT is the best for showing small calcifications (**Fig. 76**), MR is nevertheless the preferred imaging modality for delineating the morphology and extent of the tumor. RB is one of the small round blue cell tumors and has characteristic low T2 signal, because of its relatively high nuclear/cytoplasmic ratio (**Figs. 77** and **78**). Contrast-enhanced MR images increase sensitivity for leptomeningeal disease, the detection of which necessitates imaging of the entire neuroaxis (**Fig. 79**). When diagnosed early and treated with a combination of surgery, radiation, and chemotherapy, RB is curable in 95% of pediatric patients.[98]

Endophthalmitis

Endophthalmitis may occur after introduction of bacteria into the ocular globe after surgery or trauma, or hematogenously from a distant anatomic site. Clinical features include eye pain, decreased vision, and red eye.[99,100] Progression may be rapid. For example, certain pathogens such as *Bacillus cereus* may result in complete vision loss in the affected eye within 24 to 48 hours.[101] Although usually the province of the ophthalmologist, imaging findings of endophthalmitis may be present on cross-sectional imaging. Complications include the formation of intraocular abscess, RD, and development of phthisis bulbi (**Fig. 80**). Abscesses have been reported in both the suprachoroidal space[102,103] and the subretinal space.[104] On MR imaging, the intraocular infection may be difficult to distinguish from the normal T2 signal hyperintensity of the vitreous. However, the inflamed uveal tract stands out

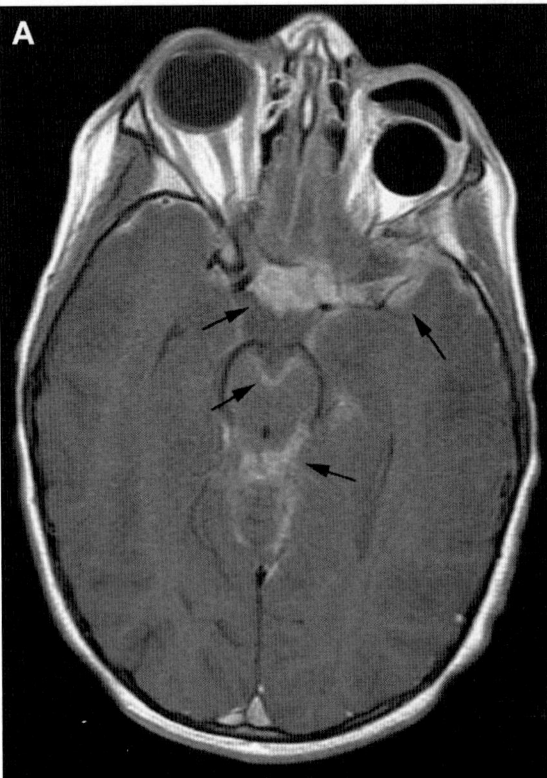

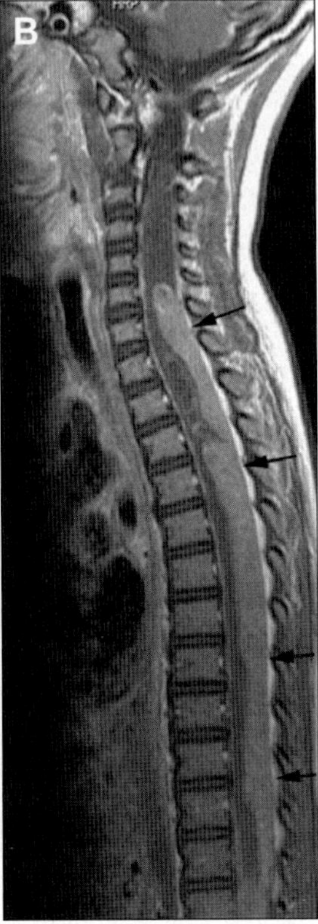

Fig. 79. RB with leptomeningeal disease in a 7-year-old patient with history of left ocular enucleation for RB. (*A*) Axial postcontrast T1W image of shows extensive leptomeningeal disease in the cisternal spaces (*black arrows*). (*B*) Sagittal postcontrast T1W image of the spine shows prominent nodular intradural enhancing tissue (*arrows*), consistent with intraspinal leptomeningeal disease.

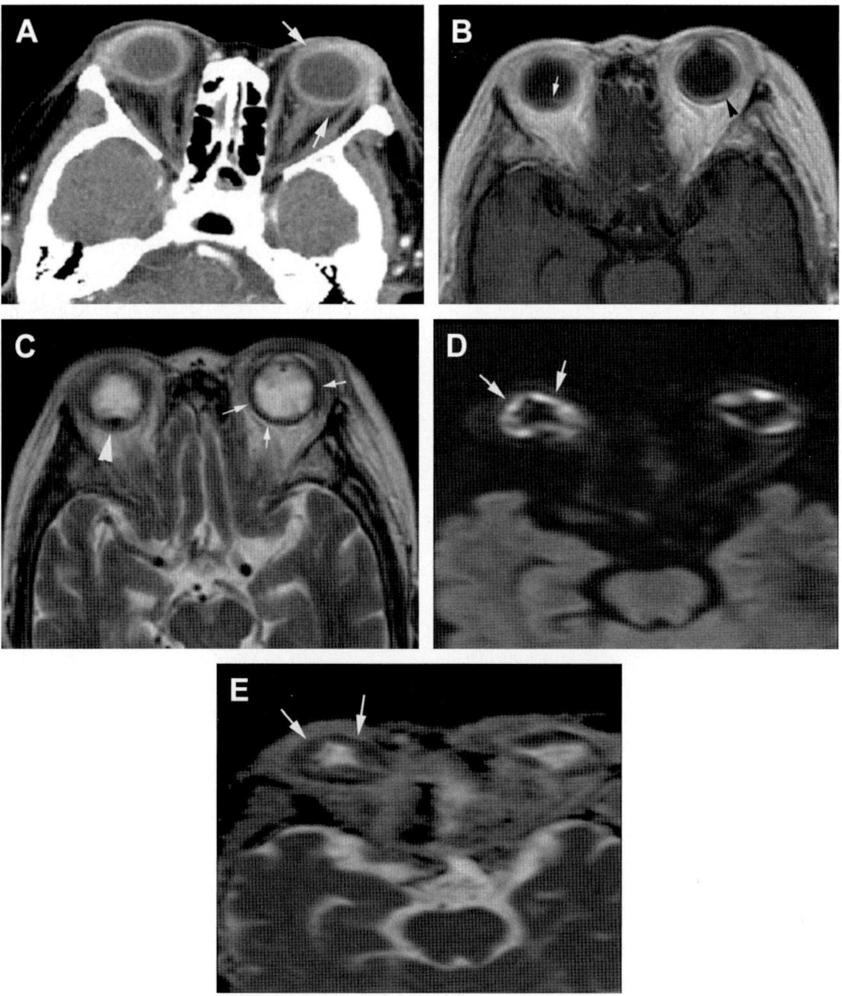

Fig. 80. Endophthalmitis in a 55-year-old man in hospital for treatment of endocarditis. (*A*) Axial CT image shows abnormal infiltrative changes of the retrobulbar fat and periscleral tissues (*arrows*), bilaterally but more pronounced on the left. (*B*) Axial postcontrast T1W image shows an abnormal degree of enhancement along the left uvea (*arrowhead*). There is peripheral enhancement of a small collection in the right globe (*arrow*). (*C*) Axial T2W image shows corresponding signal hypointensity of the left uveal tract (*arrows*). The small posterior collection in the right globe is markedly hypointense (*arrowhead*), which may be caused by blood products. (*D*) Axial DWI and (*E*) apparent diffusion coefficient images show markedly restricted diffusion in bilateral suprachoroidal collections (*arrows*).

from the vitreous on fluid-attenuated inversion recovery imaging. Also, DWI is useful to show the presence of infected intraocular fluid collections (abscesses).[100]

SUMMARY

There is a vast array of disease that involves the orbit. The possible causes span all the pathologic categories that are traditionally used to generate differential diagnoses, such as inflammatory, neoplastic, traumatic, infectious, and so forth, with considerable overlap. However, assignment of the cross-sectional imaging findings to specific patterns helps the radiologist focus on a few important, common differential considerations for each case of orbital disease.

Some diseases have a variety of possible imaging presentations or may involve several different orbital structures. IOI, lymphoproliferative disease, and sarcoidosis are particularly protean in their imaging characteristics and are therefore included in many of the pattern-based diagnostic categories. However, in conjunction with detailed clinical history and consideration of the patient's age, a pattern-based approach to interpretation of imaging studies should allow the radiologist to provide a concise and relevant differential diagnosis for the referring physician.

ACKNOWLEDGMENTS

Thanks to Deborah Shatzkes, MD, for the concept of pattern-based interpretation of orbital imaging.

REFERENCES

1. Rodriguez M, Siva, A, Cross SA, et al. Optic neuritis: a population-based study in Olmsted County, Minnesota. Neurology 1995;45(2):244–50.
2. Percy AK, Nobrega FT, Kurland LT. Optic neuritis and multiple sclerosis. An epidemiologic study. Arch Ophthalmol 1972;87(2):135–9.
3. Pau D, Al Zubidi N, Yalamanchili S, et al. Optic neuritis. Eye (Lond) 2011;25(7):833–42.
4. de la Cruz J, Kupersmith MJ. Clinical profile of simultaneous bilateral optic neuritis in adults. Br J Ophthalmol 2006;90(5):551–4.
5. Gordon LK. Orbital inflammatory disease: a diagnostic and therapeutic challenge. Eye (Lond) 2006;20(10):1196–206.
6. Lindfield D, Attfield K, McElvanney A. Systemic immunoglobulin G4 (IgG4) disease and idiopathic orbital inflammation: removing 'idiopathic' from the nomenclature? Eye (Lond) 2012;26(5):623–9.
7. Yuen SJ, Rubin PA. Idiopathic orbital inflammation: distribution, clinical features, and treatment outcome. Arch Ophthalmol 2003;121(4):491–9.
8. Espinoza GM. Orbital inflammatory pseudotumors: etiology, differential diagnosis, and management. Curr Rheumatol Rep 2010;12(6):443–7.
9. Demirchi H, Shields CL, Shields JA. Orbital tumors in the older adult population. Ophthalmology 2002; 109(2):243–8.
10. Demirci H, Shields CL, Karatza EC, et al. Orbital lymphoproliferative tumors: analysis of clinical features and systemic involvement in 160 cases. Ophthalmology 2008;115(9):1626–31, 1631.e1–3.
11. Shapey J, Sabin HI, Danesh-Meyer HV, et al. Diagnosis and management of optic nerve sheath meningiomas. J Clin Neurosci 2013;20(8):1045–56.
12. Schick U, Dott U, Hassler W. Surgical management of meningiomas involving the optic nerve sheath. J Neurosurg 2004;101(6):951–9.
13. Elster AD, Challa VR, Gilbert TH, et al. Meningiomas: MR and histopathologic features. Radiology 1989;170(3 Pt 1):857–62.
14. Monteiro ML, Goncalves ACP, Siqueira SA, et al. Optic nerve sheath meningioma in the first decade of life: case report and review of the literature. Case Rep Ophthalmol 2012;3(2):270–6.
15. Harold Lee HB, Garrity JA, Cameron JD, et al. Primary optic nerve sheath meningioma in children. Surv Ophthalmol 2008;53(6):543–58.
16. Kornreich L, Blaser S, Schwarz M, et al. Optic pathway glioma: correlation of imaging findings with the presence of neurofibromatosis. AJNR Am J Neuroradiol 2001;22(10):1963–9.
17. Nicolin G, Parkin P, Mabbott D, et al. Natural history and outcome of optic pathway gliomas in children. Pediatr Blood Cancer 2009;53(7):1231–7.
18. Listernick R, Charrow J, Greenwald M, et al. Natural history of optic pathway tumors in children with neurofibromatosis type 1: a longitudinal study. J Pediatr 1994;125(1):63–6.
19. Blazo MA, Lewis RA, Chintagumpala MM, et al. Outcomes of systematic screening for optic pathway tumors in children with neurofibromatosis type 1. Am J Med Genet A 2004;127A(3):224–9.
20. Avery RA, Fisher MJ, Liu GT. Optic pathway gliomas. J Neuroophthalmol 2011;31:269–78.
21. Chateil JF, Soussotte C, Pedespan J-M, et al. MRI and clinical differences between optic pathway tumours in children with and without neurofibromatosis. Br J Radiol 2001;74:24–31.
22. Lee YY, Van Tassel P, Bruner JM, et al. Juvenile pilocytic astrocytomas: CT and MR characteristics. AJR Am J Roentgenol 1989;152(6):1263–70.
23. Demirci H, Christianson MD. Orbital and adnexal involvement in sarcoidosis: analysis of clinical features and systemic disease in 30 cases. Am J Ophthalmol 2011;151(6):1074–80.e1.
24. Simon EM, Zoarski GH, Rothman MI, et al. Systemic sarcoidosis with bilateral orbital involvement: MR findings. AJNR Am J Neuroradiol 1998;19(2):336–7.
25. Mavrikakis I, Rootman J. Diverse clinical presentations of orbital sarcoid. Am J Ophthalmol 2007; 144(5):769–75.
26. Shields JA, Bakewell B, Augsburger JJ, et al. Classification and incidence of space-occupying lesions of the orbit. A survey of 645 biopsies. Arch Ophthalmol 1984;102(11):1606–11.
27. Ansari SA, Mafee MF. Orbital cavernous hemangioma: role of imaging. Neuroimaging Clin N Am 2005; 15(1):137–58.
28. Rootman J. Vascular malformations of the orbit: hemodynamic concepts. Orbit 2003;22(2):103–20.
29. Hejazi N, Classen R, Hassler W. Orbital and cerebral cavernomas: comparison of clinical, neuroimaging, and neuropathological features. Neurosurg Rev 1999;22(1):28–33.
30. Smoker WR, Gentry LR, Yee NK. Vascular lesions of the orbit: more than meets the eye. Radiographics 2008;28:185–204.
31. Harris GJ. Orbital vascular malformations: a consensus statement on terminology and its clinical implications. Orbital Society. Am J Ophthalmol 1999; 127(4):453–5.

32. Vu BL, Harris GJ. Orbital vascular lesions. Ophthalmol Clin North Am 2000;13(4):609.
33. Bilaniuk LT. Vascular lesions of the orbit in children. Neuroimaging Clin N Am 2005;15(1):107–20.
34. Islam N, Mireskandari K, Rose GE. Orbital varices and orbital wall defects. Br J Ophthalmol 2004; 88:833–4.
35. Rubin PA, Remulla HD. Orbital venous anomalies demonstrated by spiral computed tomography. Ophthalmology 1997;104(9):1463–70.
36. Shields JA, Dolinskas C, Augsburger JJ, et al. Demonstration of orbital varix with computed tomography and Valsalva maneuver. Am J Ophthalmol 1984;97(1):108–10.
37. Butt ZA, McNab AA. Orbital neurilemmoma: report of seven cases. J Clin Neurosci 1998;5(4):390–3.
38. Kapur R, Mafee MF, Lamba R, et al. Orbital schwannoma and neurofibroma: role of imaging. Neuroimaging Clin N Am 2005;15(1):159–74.
39. Xian J, Zhang Z, Wang Z, et al. Evaluation of MR imaging findings differentiating cavernous haemangiomas from schwannomas in the orbit. Eur Radiol 2010;20(9):2221–8.
40. Wang Y, Xiao LH. Orbital schwannomas: findings from magnetic resonance imaging in 62 cases. Eye (Lond) 2008;22(8):1034–9.
41. Cavazza S, Laffi GL, Lodi L, et al. Orbital dermoid cyst of childhood: clinical pathologic findings, classification and management. Int Ophthalmol 2011; 31(2):93–7.
42. Ahuja R, Azar NF. Orbital dermoids in children. Semin Ophthalmol 2006;21(3):207–11.
43. Char DH, Miller T, Kroll S. Orbital metastases: diagnosis and course. Br J Ophthalmol 1997;81(5): 386–90.
44. Saeed P, van Furth WR, Tanck M, et al. Natural history of spheno-orbital meningiomas. Acta Neurochir (Wien) 2011;153(2):395–402.
45. Oya S, Sade B, Lee JH. Sphenoorbital meningioma: surgical technique and outcome. J Neurosurg 2011; 114(5):1241–9.
46. Hanifi B, Samil KS, Yasar C, et al. Craniofacial fibrous dysplasia. Clin Imaging 2013;37(6):1109–15.
47. Wakefield MJ, Ross AH, Damato EM, et al. Review of lateral orbital wall ossifying fibroma. Orbit 2010; 29(6):317–20.
48. McCarthy EF. Fibro-osseous lesions of the maxillofacial bones. Head Neck Pathol 2013;7(1):5–10.
49. Crawford C, Mazzoli R. Subperiosteal hematoma in multiple settings. Digit J Ophthalmol 2013; 19(1):6–8.
50. Friedberg MH, David O, Woog J, et al. Orbital hematic cyst: case report and clarification of terms. Skull Base Surg 1997;7(2):95–9.
51. Vaidhyanath R, Kirke R, Brown L, et al. Lacrimal fossa lesions: pictorial review of CT and MRI features. Orbit 2008;27(6):410–8.
52. Wright JE, Stewart WB, Krohel GB. Clinical presentation and management of lacrimal gland tumours. Br J Ophthalmol 1979;63(9):600–6.
53. Farmer JP, Lamba M, Lamba WR, et al. Lymphoproliferative lesions of the lacrimal gland: clinicopathological, immunohistochemical and molecular genetic analysis. Can J Ophthalmol 2005;40(2): 151–60.
54. Mafee MF. Orbit: embryology, anatomy and pathology. In: Som PM, Curtin HD, editors. Head and neck imaging. St Louis (MO): Mosby; 2003. p. 543–7.
55. Mafee MF, Edward DP, Koeller KK, et al. Lacrimal gland tumors and simulating lesions. Clinicopathologic and MR imaging features. Radiol Clin North Am 1999;37(1):219–39, xii.
56. Gonçalves AC, Gebrim EM, Monteiro ML. Imaging studies for diagnosing Graves' orbitopathy and dysthyroid optic neuropathy. Clinics (Sao Paulo) 2012;67(11):1327–34.
57. Rabinowitz MP, Carrasco JR. Update on advanced imaging options for thyroid-associated orbitopathy. Saudi J Ophthalmol 2012;26(4):385–92.
58. Heufelder AE. Pathogenesis of ophthalmopathy in autoimmune thyroid disease. Rev Endocr Metab Disord 2000;1(1–2):87–95.
59. Trokel SL, Jakobiec FA. Correlation of CT scanning and pathologic features of ophthalmic Graves' disease. Ophthalmology 1981;88(6):553–64.
60. Ben Simon GJ, Syed HM, Douglas R, et al. Extraocular muscle enlargement with tendon involvement in thyroid-associated orbitopathy. Am J Ophthalmol 2004;137(6):1145–7.
61. Neigel JM, Rootman J, Belkin RI, et al. Dysthyroid optic neuropathy. The crowded orbital apex syndrome. Ophthalmology 1988;95(11):1515–21.
62. Jacobs D, Galetta S. Diagnosis and management of orbital pseudotumor. Curr Opin Ophthalmol 2002;13(6):347–51.
63. Lee EJ, Sung SL, Kim BS, et al. MR imaging of orbital inflammatory pseudotumors with extraorbital extension. Korean J Radiol 2005;6(2):82–8.
64. Ellis JA, Goldstein H, Connolly ES, et al. Carotid-cavernous fistulas. Neurosurg Focus 2012;32(5):E9.
65. de Kaiser RJ. Carotid-cavernous and orbital arteriovenous fistulas: ocular features, diagnostic and hemodynamic considerations in relation to visual impairment and morbidity. Orbit 2003;22(2):121–42.
66. Barrow DL, Spector RH, Braun IF, et al. Classification and treatment of spontaneous carotid-cavernous sinus fistulas. J Neurosurg 1985;62(2): 248–56.
67. Debrun GM, Vinuela F, Fox AJ, et al. Indications for treatment and classification of 132 carotid-cavernous fistulas. Neurosurgery 1988;22(2):285–9.
68. Lacey B, Chang W, Rootman J. Nonthyroid causes of extraocular muscle disease. Surv Ophthalmol 1999;44(3):187–213.

69. Brooks SE, Sangueza OP, Field RS. Extraocular muscle involvement in sarcoidosis: a clinicopathologic report. J AAPOS 1997;1(2):125–8.
70. Stannard K, Spalton DJ. Sarcoidosis with infiltration of the external ocular muscles. Br J Ophthalmol 1986;69:562–6.
71. Surov A, Behrmann C, Holzhausen H-J, et al. Lymphomas and metastases of the extra-ocular musculature. Neuroradiology 2011;53(11):909–16.
72. Wiggins RE Jr, Byrne SF. Metastatic tumor to the extraocular muscles: report of 5 cases. J AAPOS 2012;16(5):489–91.
73. Gupta A, Chazen JL, Phillips CD. Carcinoid tumor metastases to the extraocular muscles: MR imaging and CT findings and review of the literature. AJNR Am J Neuroradiol 2011;32(7):1208–11.
74. Reeves D, Levine MR, Lash R. Nonpalpable breast carcinoma presenting as orbital infiltration. Ophthal Plast Reconstr Surg 2002;18:84–8.
75. Buchanan CL, Morris EA, Dorn PL, et al. Utility of breast magnetic resonance imaging in patients with occult primary breast cancer. Ann Surg Oncol 2005;12(12):1045–53.
76. Bernardini FP, Bazzan M. Lymphoproliferative disease of the orbit. Curr Opin Ophthalmol 2007;18(5):398–401.
77. Harris GJ. Subperiosteal abscess of the orbit: older children and adults require aggressive treatment. Ophthal Plast Reconstr Surg 2001;17(6):395–7.
78. Lee S, Yen MT. Management of preseptal and orbital cellulitis. Saudi J Ophthalmol 2011;25(1):21–9.
79. Majoie CB, Hulsmans FJ, Castelijns JA, et al. Primary nerve-sheath tumours of the trigeminal nerve: clinical and MRI findings. Neuroradiology 1999;41(2):100–8.
80. Santaolalla F, Sanchez JM, Ereno C, et al. Severe exophthalmos in trigeminal plexiform neurofibroma involving the orbit and the infratemporal fossa. J Clin Neurosci 2009;16(7):970–2.
81. Jurdy L, Merks JHM, Pieters BR, et al. Orbital rhabdomyosarcomas: a review. Saudi J Ophthalmol 2013;27(3):167–75.
82. Jones IS, Reese AB, Krout J. Orbital rhabdomyosarcoma: an analysis of sixty-two cases. Trans Am Ophthalmol Soc 1965;63:223–55.
83. Font RL, Ferry AP. Carcinoma metastatic to the eye and orbit III. A clinicopathologic study of 28 cases metastatic to the orbit. Cancer 1976;38(3):1326–35.
84. Gunalp I, Gunduz K. Metastatic orbital tumors. Jpn J Ophthalmol 1995;39(1):65–70.
85. Ahmad SM, Esmaeli B. Metastatic tumors of the orbit and ocular adnexa. Curr Opin Ophthalmol 2007;18(5):405–13.
86. Goldberg RA, Rootman J. Clinical characteristics of metastatic orbital tumors. Ophthalmology 1990;97(5):620–4.
87. Shields JA, Shields CL, Brotman HK, et al. Cancer metastatic to the orbit: the 2000 Robert M. Curts Lecture. Ophthal Plast Reconstr Surg 2001;17(5):346–54.
88. Fenton S, Kemp EG, Harnett AN. Screening for ophthalmic involvement in asymptomatic patients with metastatic breast carcinoma. Eye (Lond) 2004;18(1):38–40.
89. Camarillo C, Ronco IS, Encinas JL. Choroidal metastases. An Sist Sanit Navar 2008;31:127–34 [in Spanish].
90. Shields CL, Shields JA, Gross NE, et al. Survey of 520 eyes with uveal metastases. Ophthalmology 1997;104(8):1265–76.
91. Singh N, Kulkarni P, Aggarwal AN, et al. Choroidal metastasis as a presenting manifestation of lung cancer. Medicine 2012;91:179–94.
92. Bedikian AY. Metastatic uveal melanoma therapy: current options. Int Ophthalmol Clin 2006;46(1):151–66.
93. Spagnolo F, Caltabiano G, Queirolo P. Uveal melanoma. Cancer Treat Rev 2012;38(5):549–53.
94. Mafee MF, Peyman GA, McKusick MA. Malignant uveal melanoma and similar lesions studied by computed tomography. Radiology 1985;156(2):403–8.
95. Mehta M, Sethi S, Pushker N, et al. Retinoblastoma. Singapore Med J 2012;53(2):128–35 [quiz: 136].
96. Houston SK, Murray TG, Wolfe SQ, et al. Current update on retinoblastoma. Int Ophthalmol Clin 2011;51(1):77–91.
97. Apushkin MA, Apushkin MA, Shapiro MJ, et al. Retinoblastoma and simulating lesions: role of imaging. Neuroimaging Clin N Am 2005;15(1):49–67.
98. Shields JA, Shields CL, Scartozzi R. Survey of 1264 patients with orbital tumors and simulating lesions: the 2002 Montgomery Lecture, part 1. Ophthalmology 2004;111(5):997–1008.
99. Durand ML. Endophthalmitis. Clin Microbiol Infect 2013;19(3):227–34.
100. Rumboldt Z, Moses C, Wieczerzynski U, et al. Diffusion-weighted imaging, apparent diffusion coefficients, and fluid-attenuated inversion recovery MR imaging in endophthalmitis. AJNR Am J Neuroradiol 2005;26(7):1869–72.
101. Callegan MC, Engelbert M, Parke DW, et al. Bacterial endophthalmitis: epidemiology, therapeutics, and bacterium-host interactions. Clin Microbiol Rev 2002;15(1):111–24.
102. Manka RH, Nozik RA, Stern WH. Intraocular *Staphylococcus aureus* abscess masquerading as chronic uveitis. Am J Ophthalmol 1988;105(5):555–6.
103. Bhuta S, Hsu CC, Kwan GN. *Scedosporium apiospermum* endophthalmitis: diffusion-weighted imaging in detecting subchoroidal abscess. Clin Ophthalmol 2012;6:1921–4.
104. Harris EW, D'Amico DJ, Bhisitkul R, et al. Bacterial subretinal abscess: a case report and review of the literature. Am J Ophthalmol 2000;129(6):778–85.

Squamous Cell Carcinoma of the Upper Aerodigestive Tract: A Review

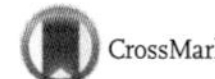

David Landry, MD, FRCPC, B.Eng,
Christine M. Glastonbury, MBBS*

KEYWORDS

• Pharynx • Squamous cell carcinoma • Staging • Human papilloma virus

KEY POINTS

- In nasopharyngeal carcinoma, extension to the skull base or paranasal sinuses indicates a T3 tumor, whereas intracranial extension, perineural spread, or involvement of the orbit, hypopharynx, infratemporal fossa, or masticator space denotes a T4 tumor.
- There is a rising incidence of human papilloma virus–related oropharyngeal squamous cell carcinomas, particularly in middle-aged white men, found over a much wider patient age range than tobacco-related oropharyngeal tumors. Cystic nodal metastases are more often found and should not be mistaken for branchial cleft cysts.
- Differentiation of T3 and T4 cancers in the larynx is important because larynx-sparing chemoradiation is not currently recommended for T4 tumors.

INTRODUCTION

Squamous cell carcinoma (SCCa) is the most common head and neck (HN) malignancy. There has been a steady decrease in the incidence of laryngeal, hypopharyngeal, and oral cavity malignancies since the late 1980s correlating with declining tobacco use, the primary risk factor for SCCa at these sites.[1] By contrast, the incidence of oropharyngeal squamous cell carcinoma has been increasing, owing to the rising incidence of human papilloma virus (HPV)-associated SCCa, particularly HPV-16–related SCCa.[1–3] The demographics of these patients are somewhat different to those of the traditional tobacco-related and alcohol-related oropharyngeal SCCa, in that there is a broader age demographic and a better overall tumor prognosis.[4,5]

The radiologist has several roles in the management of patients with SCCa, but initially imaging is performed to establish tumor staging. Specifically, the radiologist should determine the extent of local disease spread and determine whether there is evidence of nodal metastases. With advanced tumor presentation, distant metastasis should also be considered, and may necessitate whole-body positron emission tomography (PET) imaging. In the non-HPV–related SCCa patient group, consideration should always be given to the possibility of a synchronous or metachronous tobacco-related and/or alcohol-related second primary neoplasm. For initial tumor staging, knowledge of the involved anatomy and staging criteria is mandatory. The most widely used tumor staging system is the tumor node metastasis (TNM), created in a joint effort between the American Joint Committee on Cancer (AJCC) and the International Union for Cancer Control (UICC). This system is periodically updated, with the most recent (seventh) edition published in

Financial Disclosure: None.
Conflict of Interest: None.
Department of Radiology and Biomedical Imaging, University of California, San Francisco, Box 0628, Room L358, 505 Parnassus Avenue, San Francisco, CA 94143-0628, USA
* Corresponding author.
E-mail address: christine.glastonbury@ucsf.edu

Radiol Clin N Am 53 (2015) 81–97
http://dx.doi.org/10.1016/j.rcl.2014.09.013
0033-8389/15/$ – see front matter

2010.[6] Using the AJCC criteria as guidelines, the radiologist has much to contribute in the initial staging of SCCa patients.

In this article the relevant reportable findings of pharyngeal SCCa are explored, with particular attention to findings that change the T staging of the tumor and/or reorient therapy. Each subsite of the pharynx and larynx is addressed, from the nasopharynx to the hypopharynx.

NASOPHARYNGEAL CARCINOMA

Anatomic Considerations

The nasopharynx is the uppermost portion of the pharynx, extending from the skull base to the horizontal plane created by the soft palate. The nasopharynx is continuous with the nasal cavity anteriorly and the oropharynx inferiorly, and should always remain patent. There are 2 key anatomic landmarks to identify on imaging: the lateral pharyngeal recesses (fossae of Rosenmüller) and the midline lymphoid tissue known as the adenoids.

Epidemiologic and Demographic Factors

There have been many changes to the pathologic description of nasopharyngeal carcinoma (NPC). Keratinizing carcinoma, previously called SCCa or type I NPC, is rare; it is strongly associated with tobacco and alcohol use, and generally has a poor prognosis. Nonkeratinizing nasopharyngeal carcinoma (NK NPC) is much more common and is endemic in certain parts of the world, in particular southeastern China. NK NPC is strongly associated with the Epstein-Barr virus (EBV) and, as it is very radiosensitive, has a significantly better prognosis. NK NPC can be divided into differentiated (previously called type II NPC) and undifferentiated (previously called type III NPC) pathologic subtypes. Basaloid nasopharyngeal SCCa is very rare.

Imaging Manifestations

The nasopharynx is best imaged by magnetic resonance (MR) imaging to detect intracranial and bone invasion (particularly clival), in addition to perineural spread of malignancy. NPC, often arising in the fossa of Rosenmüller, invades or displaces the parapharyngeal fat laterally and can cause obstruction of the adjacent Eustachian tube ostium, leading to opacification of the ipsilateral middle ear and mastoid air cells. For this reason, close attention to the nasopharynx is mandatory in any adult presenting with otitis media. Close attention to this area, particularly in patients with middle ear or mastoid air cell opacification, can potentially detect early NPC and greatly affect the patient's outcome (**Fig. 1**). Because early NPC can be asymptomatic or may cause nonspecific symptoms, it may be an incidental imaging finding on a brain or cervical spine computed tomography (CT) scan.

Recent retrospective studies showed that NPC with extension to the nasal cavity and oropharynx has as favorable a prognosis as those confined to the nasopharynx. This finding led to modification of the T stage of NPC in the seventh edition of the AJCC, with such tumors now staged as T1.[6–10] Extension to the posterolaterally located parapharyngeal fat denotes a T2 tumor, whereas extension to the skull base or paranasal sinuses

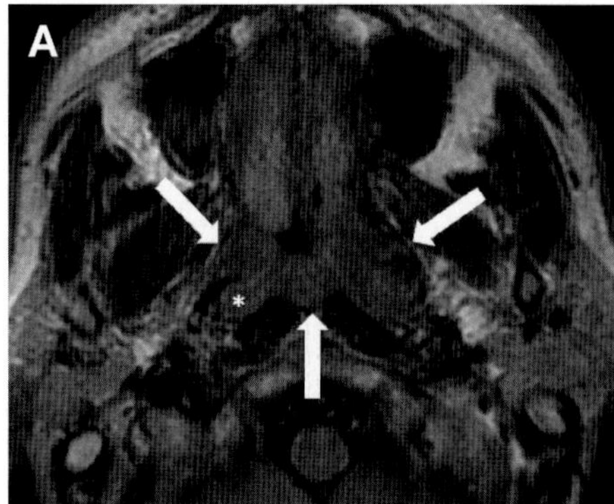

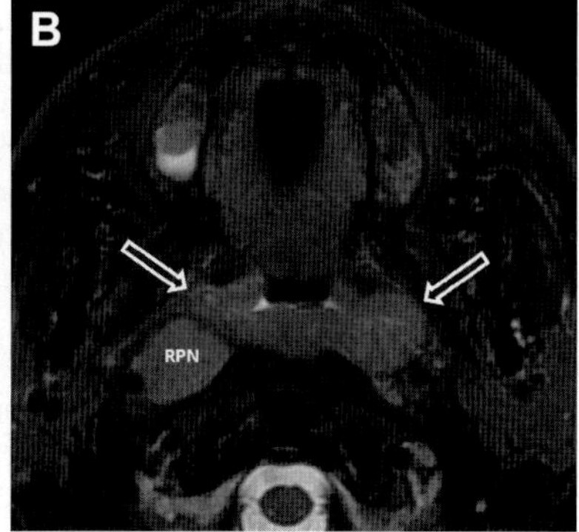

Fig. 1. (*A*) Brain magnetic resonance (MR) imaging of a 59-year-old man presenting with gradual decline in memory. Axial fluid-attenuated inversion recovery image of the nasopharynx shows incidental asymmetric thickening of the nasopharyngeal mucosa (*arrows*) with an enlarged right retropharyngeal node (*asterisk*). The patient refused further investigation. (*B*) Same patient, 15 months later, presents for imaging for left-sided humming tinnitus, poor left-side hearing, and left nasal congestion. Axial T2-weighted image centered on the nasopharynx shows progression in size of the asymmetric nasopharyngeal mass (*open arrows*) and further enlarged right retropharyngeal node (RPN). Tumor stage T3N2; this is incidentally detected nasopharyngeal carcinoma (NPC).

indicates a T3 tumor. Finally, intracranial extension, perineural spread, and involvement of the orbit, hypopharynx, infratemporal fossa, or masticator space denotes a T4 tumor. Of importance, involvement of the masticator space requires careful examination of the foramen ovale to exclude perineural spread along the mandibular division of the trigeminal nerve.[9]

As nodal metastases are much more common, larger, and more frequently bilateral in NPC, its nodal staging system is unique and different from all other HN SCCa subsites, which have a common nodal staging system (**Fig. 2**).

ORAL CAVITY SQUAMOUS CELL CARCINOMA

Anatomic Considerations

The oral cavity (OC) is the anterior most subdivision of the aerodigestive tract, separated from the oropharynx by a ring formed by the soft palate, the anterior tonsillar pillars, and the circumvallate papillae. The OC is bounded anteriorly by the lips, laterally by the cheeks, superiorly by the superior alveolar ridge and hard palate, and inferiorly by the inferior alveolar ridge and the mylohyoid muscle.

The OC is subdivided into 7 subsites: the lip, the floor of the mouth (FOM), the buccal mucosa, the oral tongue, the retromolar triangle, the upper and lower alveolar ridges, and the hard palate.

The FOM is a crescent-shaped space divided in 2 by the tongue frenulum, and contains the ostia of the submandibular and sublingual salivary glands. The most important landmark for delineating the anatomy of the FOM is the mylohyoid muscle, which is best visualized in the coronal plane. It forms the inferiormost limit of the FOM, thus dividing the sublingual from the submandibular spaces. This muscle originates from the mandible and inserts itself on the hyoid bone. It is innervated by a branch of the mandibular division (V3) of the trigeminal nerve. The lower gingiva forms the anterior border of the FOM, the alveolar ridge the lateral border, and the base of the anterior tonsillar pillar the posterior border. The buccal mucosa is contiguous with the retromolar trigone and covers the cheeks and the lips, extending anteroposteriorly from the lips to the pterygomandibular raphe, and craniocaudally from the upper to lower alveolar ridges. The oral tongue consists of the anterior two-thirds of the tongue and comprises both intrinsic and extrinsic muscles. The upper (maxilla) and lower (mandible) alveolar ridges consist of the gingiva-covered bones supporting the teeth. SCCa arising from the lower alveolar ridge is prone to bone invasion and then perineural spread along the inferior alveolar nerve (branch of V3). Panorex and bone CT can be used to detect bone erosion; however, MR imaging better defines perineural spread and extent of soft-tissue invasion and bone marrow infiltration, and is also less susceptible to dental amalgam artifacts. The retromolar trigone (RMT) is a small triangular mucosal space located behind the posteriormost inferior molar. It is an important location in the OC because of its proximity to many structures, permitting pathways for spread to the oral cavity, the oropharynx, the buccal space, the masticator space, and FOM (**Table 1**).[11] Hence when a primary lesion involves the RMT, close attention should be given to these subsites. The pterygomandibular raphe also deserves special attention. It consists of a fibrous band that anchors the buccinator and superior pharyngeal constrictor muscles and extends

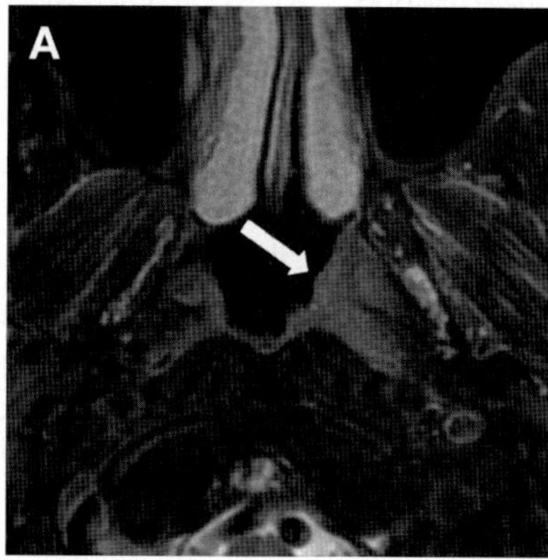

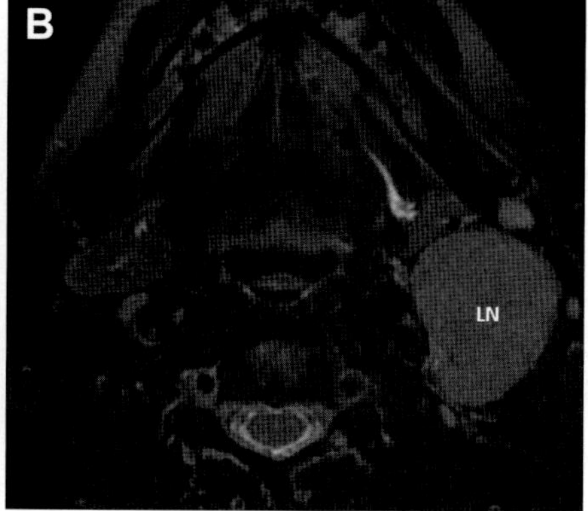

Fig. 2. (*A*) Axial T2-weighted image centered on the nasopharynx of a 61-year-old female patient with a history of slowly growing nontender left neck mass. The primary NPC is evident as a subtle well-defined mass filling the left lateral pharyngeal recess (fossa of Rosenmüller) (*arrow*). (*B*) Axial T2-weighted image in the same patient but centered at the level of the oropharynx shows an enlarged left lymph node (LN) at level 2A. Tumor stage T1N1, stage II.

Table 1
Typical spread of retromolar trigone squamous cell carcinoma (SCCa)

Direction of Spread	Structures Involved
Anterolaterally	Buccinator muscles Cheeks
Posterolaterally	Buccal fat Masticator space
Posteromedially	Tongue
Posteriorly	Anterior tonsillar pillar Oropharynx
Superiorly	Maxilla (by way of the pterygomandibular raphe)
Inferiorly	Mandible Inferior alveolar nerve

from the posterior mylohyoid line of the mandible to the hook of the medial pterygoid plate. The pterygomandibular raphe provides potential routes of spread for tumor to the posterior maxillary alveolus and pterygoid processes. The hard palate is an arch-like crescent-shaped mucosal surface extending from bilateral inner surfaces of upper alveolar ridges. It covers the maxillary bone and the horizontal plate of the palatine bone.

The OC mucosal surfaces are readily assessed by the clinician, and small mucosal lesions may not be visible on imaging. The role of the radiologist during the initial staging of tumors is to establish deep tissue involvement and assess for nodal metastases. The AJCC staging criteria are the same for all subsites of the OC, although there are several additional features for T4a staging of the lip and oral cavity.[6]

Lip

Although the lip is the most common site for SCCa in the OC, with approximately 40% of cases,[12] it is rarely imaged because tumors most often present as small T1 lesions. In addition to tobacco exposure, ultraviolet radiation is a risk factor for the development of lip carcinoma. SCCa of the lip has a tendency to spread superficially and laterally along the skin or deep to the orbicularis oris muscle. Imaging is usually obtained to evaluate large lesions with osseous involvement of the buccal surface of the maxillary bone or the mandibular alveolar ridge, or when metastatic nodal disease is clinically suspected. Both of these issues are adequately investigated by CT.

Floor of the mouth

The FOM is the second most frequent site for SCCa in the OC.[12] There is a strong association with alcohol and tobacco abuse and, as such, the incidence of FOM SCCa has been decreasing over the past 2 decades.[13] FOM SCCa has a tendency to occur within 2 cm of the anterior midline, and spreads laterally to the mandible or neurovascular bundle.[11] This bundle, which courses bilaterally in the sublingual space, is composed of the hypoglossal nerve and lingual artery. Special attention to involvement of contralateral neurovascular bundle is important, as this requires total glossectomy if a surgical approach is contemplated.[12] Attention to the midline of the FOM is also equally important, as involvement across midline precludes partial glossectomy.[14] Tumor may also directly invade the mylohyoid muscle.[12] FOM SCCa can be subtle, and may be revealed by secondary findings of muscle denervation or obstruction of salivary ducts (**Fig. 3**). Close attention to findings that increase the tumor stage to a T4 is required, such as invasion through the cortex of the mandible, the extrinsic muscles of the tongue, skin of the face, the masticator and pterygoid spaces, and the skull base.

Buccal mucosa

SCCa of the buccal mucosa is more common in southeast Asia, the south Pacific islands, and Taiwan than in the United States, because of its association with betel quid chewing and their substitutes, *gutkha* and *pan masala*.[15,16] Buccal mucosa SCCa can be subtle on imaging, even with clinical detailing of the primary site. To improve detection of the lesion, a technique may be used that consists in having the patient puff his or her cheeks during CT image acquisition, thus separating the opposing mucosal surfaces of the OC.[17,18] As acquisition times are longer with MR imaging, this technique is not feasible, but an alternative method is to pad the oral cavity at the site of the lesion with gauze.[19]

If a buccal mucosa lesion is found, care should be taken to evaluate its extent and establish if there is invasion of the masticator space, the pterygomandibular raphe, and the retromolar trigone. The goal of management is complete tumor and nodal resection, with or without adjuvant radiation therapy. Osseous invasion (T4) of the mandible or maxilla mandates bone resection. It is always important to carefully evaluate for involvement of the inferior alveolar nerve in the mandible (branch of V3) or the palatine nerves of the maxilla (V2 branches).

Oral tongue

Oral tongue SCCa is strongly associated with alcohol and tobacco use. Contrary to FOM SCCa, there is a rising incidence of SCCa arising

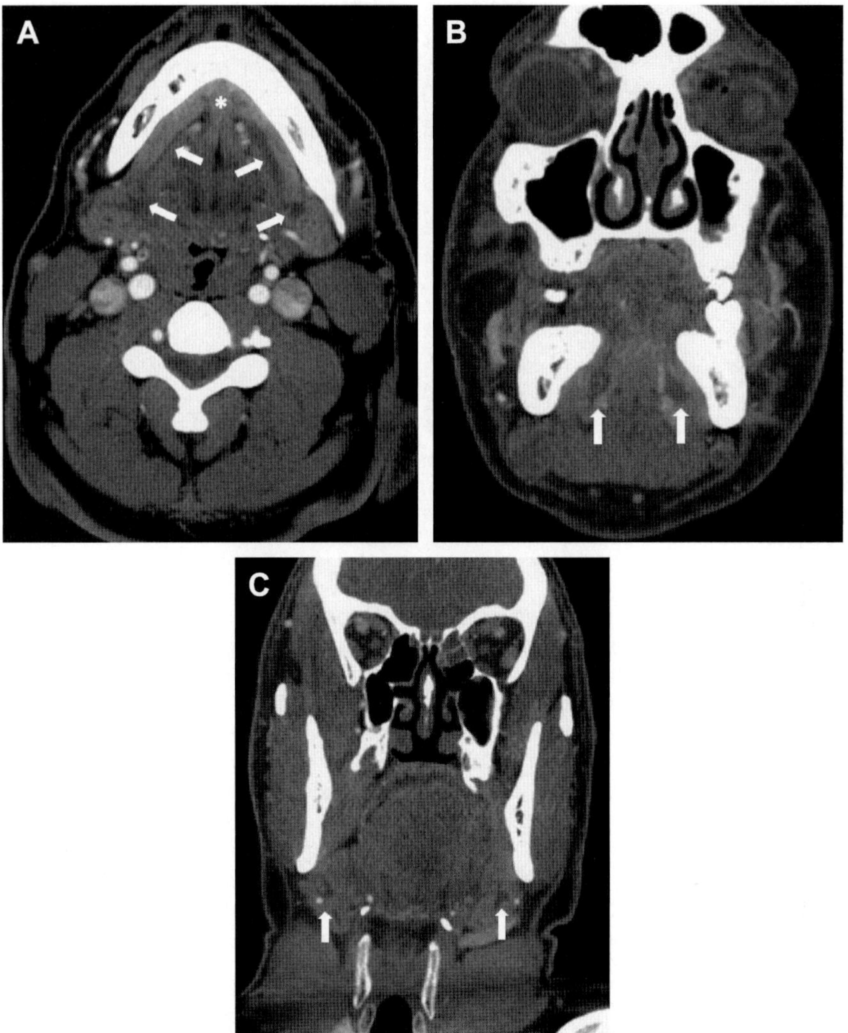

Fig. 3. (*A–C*) A 50-year-old male smoker and alcohol user who suffered a fall with subdural hematoma. During clinical examination an incidental floor-of-mouth tumor was found. Axial contrast-enhanced computed tomography (CECT) (*A*) and reformatted coronal images (*B, C*) shows dilated bilateral (left more than right) Wharton ducts and submandibular salivary glands (*arrows*). The obstructing floor-of-mouth midline lesion is very subtle (*asterisk*). Tumor stage T2N2c, stage IVA.

from the oral tongue, especially in young white females, and this increase does not seem to be related to tobacco or alcohol use, nor HPV infection.[20–25] Clinical examination or final pathologic evaluation better determine the mucosal size for tumor stages T1 to T3. Imaging is important for determining the deep extent and nodal involvement (most often levels IA/B and II).

Oral tongue SCCa most often arises from the lateral aspect of the tongue (**Fig. 4**), followed by the undersurface of the tongue. Involvement of the extrinsic muscles with SCCa determines at least T4a staging.[6] Knowledge of normal extrinsic musculature of the tongue greatly aids in staging, as loss of normal fat planes between these muscles is often the only imaging finding (**Fig. 5**). A potential pitfall, however, occurs in the presence of muscular atrophy such as from denervation. Care must be taken not to suggest disease when tongue asymmetry is the result of fatty atrophy, which is manifested by both high T1 and high T2 signal in the affected muscle.

Determining the extension of oral tongue SCCa is important, as margins of 1.5 to 2 cm are required to minimize recurrence. Attention to the contralateral side of the tongue is necessary because bilateral involvement prevents hemiglossectomy. As with staging of other SCCa subsites, special attention should be directed to any feature that upstages the tumor to T4,[6] such as invasion of the

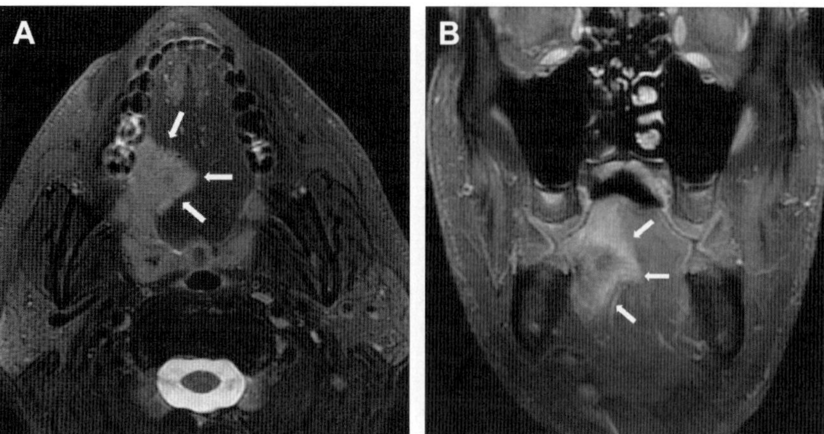

Fig. 4. (*A, B*) A 35-year-old nonsmoker and nondrinker presented with a history of several months of right tongue pain. Clinical examination revealed right tongue mass, pathologically proved to be squamous cell carcinoma (SCCa). Axial (*A*) and coronal (*B*) T2-weighted MR images show the well-circumscribed right tongue mass (*arrows*), which slightly crosses the tongue midline. Tumor stage T3N2c, stage IVA.

extrinsic muscles of the tongue. Further invasion to the mandible, skin of face, and masticator and pterygoid spaces can occur if the tumor transgresses through the FOM. Indeed, SCCa arising in the anterior third of the oral tongue has a tendency to invade the FOM. When arising from the middle third, there is a higher likelihood of involvement of the tongue musculature before the FOM. SCCa in the posterior third usually invades the anterior tonsillar pillars or the tongue base. Involvement of the tongue base often requires total laryngectomy to prevent aspiration.[14]

Alveolar ridge

SCCa of the upper alveolar ridge tends to spread medially to the palate, maxillary sinus, and nasal cavity. SCCa of the lower alveolar ridge tends to spread medially to the FOM and laterally to the buccal and masticator spaces. As the alveolar ridge and RMT are mucosal spaces overlying the mandible, bone involvement readily occurs and is associated with a poorer prognosis. Mandibular involvement also allows perineural tumor spread along the inferior alveolar nerve. MR imaging is more sensitive than CT in evaluating for such

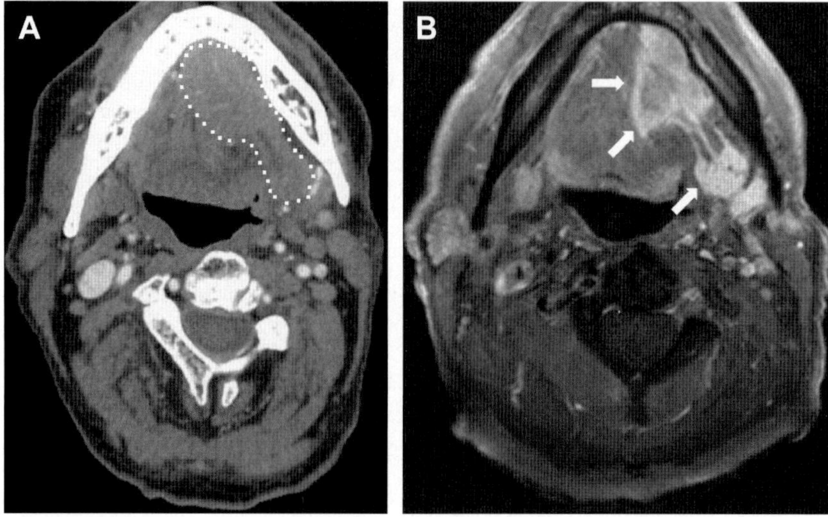

Fig. 5. (*A*) An 82-year-old smoker and active alcohol user presented with a palpable left tongue mass. Axial CECT shows the subtle mass (*dotted line*), which is revealed by noting the loss of normal fat plane between the intrinsic tongue muscles on the left. The tumor is also involving the left submandibular salivary gland. (*B*) Axial gadolinium-enhanced T1-weighted MR image better delineates the enhancing left tongue mass. Also better shown is the enhancement along the dilated left Wharton duct and abnormal enhancement of the left submandibular salivary gland (*arrows*). Tumor stage T4aN1, stage IVA.

invasion, especially on T1 sequences. On CT, tumoral invasion of the mandible can be seen as cortical disruption and sometimes marrow infiltration, whereas it is heralded by loss of normal bone marrow signal on MR imaging.

Hard palate

The hard palate is the least common location for SCCa in the OC. Most primary neoplastic lesions found in the hard palate consist of salivary gland tumors. Lesions of the hard palate are typically difficult to appreciate on imaging, sometimes even being occult. On MR imaging and CT, coronal plane imaging is most helpful for evaluating the primary tumor and the adjacent hard palate bone for invasion. SCCa can track along the greater palatine nerve, which runs in its canal, to reach the pterygopalatine fossa.

OROPHARYNGEAL SQUAMOUS CELL CARCINOMA

Anatomic Considerations

The oropharynx is posterior to the OC, between the nasopharynx and hypopharynx, the latter being separated from the oropharynx by the superior aspect of the hyoid bone. The oropharynx's anterior limit is defined by a plane formed by the circumvallate papillae, the anterior tonsillar pillars, and the soft palate. The posterior pharyngeal wall is its posterior limit. Laterally, the oropharynx is bounded by the palatine tonsils and the anterior and posterior tonsillar pillars. The retropharyngeal space is behind the oropharynx, and is a common nodal site for both oropharyngeal SCCa and NPC. The oropharynx is composed of 4 subsites: the base of tongue/lingual tonsils, the palatine tonsils, the posterior oropharyngeal wall, and the soft palate.

The lingual tonsils, also referred to as base of tongue, consist of the tonsillar tissue in the posterior third of the tongue. The palatine tonsils are lymphoid tissue nestled between the anterior and posterior tonsillar pillars, which are mucosal folds created by the palatoglossus and palatopharyngeus muscles, respectively. The posterior pharyngeal wall is between the soft palate superiorly and the hyoid bone inferiorly. The soft palate extends from the posterior aspect of the hard palate to the uvula (tip of soft palate).

Demographic and Epidemiologic Factors

There are more than 5000 new oropharyngeal malignancies diagnosed each year in the United States alone,[26,27] and SCCa represents 95% of all oropharyngeal cancers. There are well-established risk factors for oropharyngeal SCCa, the most important ones being tobacco and alcohol abuse (both separately and synergistically). Poor oral hygiene and radiation exposure are also known risk factors. Whereas the overall incidence of HN SCCa has been decreasing since the 1980s, mostly attributable to the decline in smoking, oropharyngeal SCCa incidence has been relatively stable, which is explained by the increasing incidence of HPV-related oropharyngeal SCCa. Indeed, HPV is found in up to 60% of oropharyngeal SCCa in the United States, most often in the palatine tonsils, followed by the lingual tonsils.[12,28] HPV-16, and less often HPV-18, are the most frequent oncogenic viral agents.

Risk factor profiles vary between HPV-positive and HPV-negative oropharyngeal SCCa. Indeed, studies have shown that patients with HPV-related oropharyngeal SCCa are less likely to be smokers than those with HPV-negative cancers.[2] HPV-related oropharyngeal SCCa patients tend to be younger, nonsmoking, nondrinking, white males of higher than average socioeconomic backgrounds.

HPV-positive oropharyngeal SCCa tends to be better circumscribed and more often presents with cystic nodal metastases than HPV-negative oropharyngeal SCCa, which has a tendency to have ill-defined contours and invade adjacent muscle.[29] However, there is an overlap of the imaging findings, and HPV-related tumors can be aggressive, invasive tumors with solid nodal metastases. HPV-related oropharyngeal SCCa is more likely than HPV-negative SCCa in a young male presenting with palatine or lingual tonsil mass and cervical lymph nodes.[11,27,30] It is important to always consider HPV-related oropharyngeal SCCa in any young adult presenting with a neck mass that might otherwise appear to represent a second branchial cleft cyst; HPV-related oropharyngeal SCCa metastatic lymph node should always be ruled out pathologically.

Nonsmoking patients with HPV-related oropharyngeal SCCa have significantly better outcomes than HPV-negative counterparts, with a 28% lower risk of death at 5 years.[31,32] Those with HPV-related oropharyngeal SCCa and a significant smoking history have an intermediate prognosis. Current AJCC staging does not differ for HPV-related oropharyngeal SCCa and non–HPV-related oropharyngeal SCCa, while there are ongoing trials to determine whether de-escalation of chemoradiation for HPV-related oropharyngeal SCCa in nonsmokers has equivalent outcomes. The AJCC staging criteria for all oropharyngeal SCCa are listed in Ref.[6]

Palatine tonsil

The palatine tonsils are the most common sites of involvement with SCCa in the oropharynx, representing 70% to 80% of oropharyngeal tumors.[11] Two subsets of patients exist: tobacco-related and alcohol-related SCCa and HPV-related SCCa. At presentation, more than three-quarters of patients will have adenopathy. Although asymmetry of the tonsils is almost invariably present in cases of palatine tonsil SCCa, this finding alone is insufficient to make the diagnosis, as asymmetry is often found in disease-free patients. However, in the setting of heterogeneous asymmetry accompanied by nodal disease, concern for SCCa should increase. Tumoral spread usually follows certain patterns, as are listed in **Table 2**.

Lingual tonsil

SCCa originating from this subsite have the highest rate of nodal disease,[12] so special attention should be given to retropharyngeal and cervical nodes. Lesions can be infiltrative and ulcerative or exophytic within the airway (**Fig. 6**). One should look for asymmetry on CT and MR imaging, with moderate to marked enhancement (**Fig. 7**). Because of the increasing incidence of HPV-related SCCa in this subsite, patients are often younger than for HPV-negative SCCa.

As most lingual tonsil tumors are treated with chemotherapy and radiation, important features to note on imaging are the tumoral dimensions, particularly the greatest diameter of the lesion, and tumor extent. Tumoral spread usually follows certain patterns, listed in **Table 3**. Extension to the preepiglottic fat (a triangular-shaped zone anterior to the epiglottis and below the hyoepiglottic ligament best visualized on sagittal images) is associated with higher probability of cervical node involvement.[12] Extension inferiorly to the lingual surface of the epiglottis indicates T3.[6] Because risk factors for non-HPV–associated lingual tonsil SCCa are tobacco and alcohol abuse, a synchronous or metachronous neoplasm should always be considered. Indeed, up to 15% of non-HPV patients have a synchronous or metachronous second primary SCCa of the HN.[11]

Table 2
Typical spread of palatine tonsil SCCa

Direction of Spread	Structures Involved
Anterior	Pharyngeal constrictor muscles Pterygomandibular raphe Oral cavity Retromolar trigone Buccinator muscle Thyroid cartilage
Posterior	Posterior pharyngeal wall
Lateral	Masticator space Pterygomandibular raphe Pharyngeal constrictor muscles
Superior	Soft palate Nasopharynx Base of skull
Inferior	Palatoglossus muscle to base of tongue Pharyngoepiglottic fold Superior aspect of pyriform sinus

Posterior pharyngeal wall

This site is a rare one for oropharyngeal SCCa. Risk factors are mostly tobacco and alcohol abuse. SCCa of the posterior pharyngeal wall are relatively rare entities and, when present, tumors are often large at presentation. A lobulated posterior oropharyngeal enhancing mass is the usual imaging finding (**Fig. 8**). Tumoral spread usually follows certain patterns, as listed in **Table 4**. The key nodal drainage site for these tumors is the retropharyngeal nodal group, and imaging must include the highest retropharyngeal nodes at the skull base.

Soft palate

SCCa at this location are very uncommon, and occur most often on the ventral aspect of the soft palate. Risk factors consist of tobacco and alcohol abuse. Although usually small at the time of diagnosis, patients commonly complain of odynophagia and present with T1 or T2 stage in approximately 75% of cases.[11] It is often difficult to appreciate the lesion and its soft-tissue extension on axial planes; SCCa of the soft palate is better evaluated with sagittal and coronal images. Lesions commonly extend across the midline and may involve the palatine tonsils. Tumoral spread usually follows certain patterns, as are listed in **Table 5**. Tumor can also spread submucosally and infiltrate the parapharyngeal fat. Close inspection of the pterygopalatine fossa and cavernous sinus for perineural spread is required, as extension along the palatine nerves can occur.

LARYNGEAL SQUAMOUS CELL CARCINOMA

Laryngeal SCCa, like other pharyngeal SCCa, is heavily associated with tobacco use, with this risk factor being present in up to 95% of patients.

Anatomic Considerations

The larynx is responsible for the production of the voice, and connects the oropharynx to the trachea. It therefore extends from the level of the

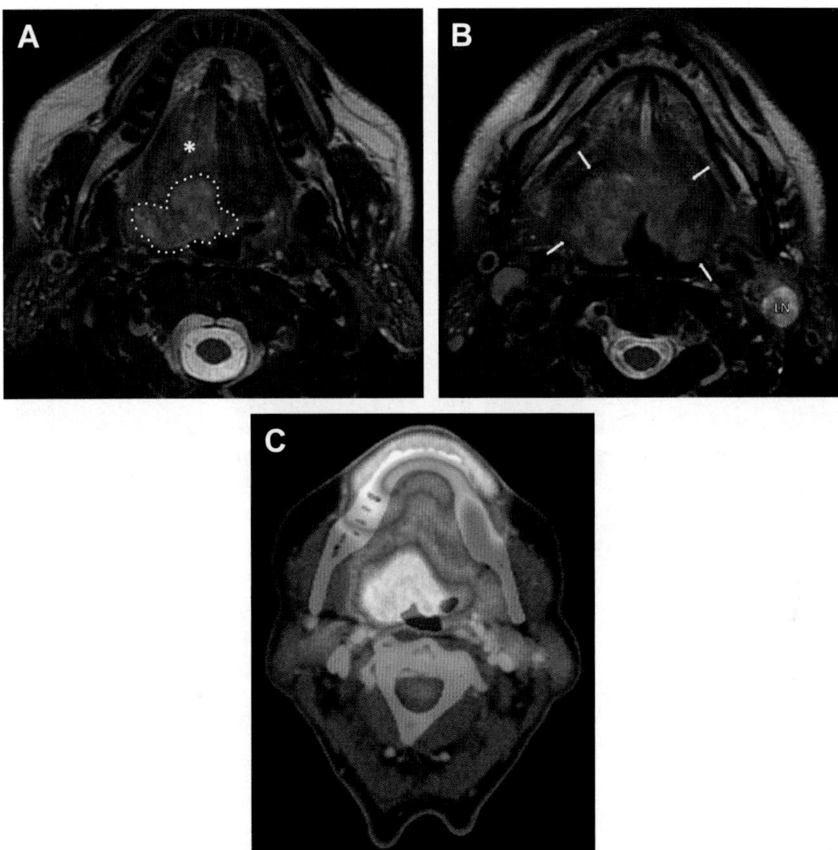

Fig. 6. (*A, B*) A 64-year-old former smoker presented with chronic cough and 50 lb (22.6 kg) weight loss over 6 months because of odynophagia and dysphagia. Axial T2-weighted MR image shows the well-circumscribed oropharyngeal mass (*arrows*) with spread to the bilateral base of tongue and right posterior intrinsic tongue muscles (*dotted line*). Note the slightly T2 hyperintensity of the right tongue (*asterisk*), related to denervation. Also present is a positive left level 2 cervical lymph node (LN in *B*). (*C*) Axial ^{18}F-fluorodeoxyglucose (FDG) positron emission tomography/computed tomography (PET/CT) in the same patient reveals hypermetabolism of the base of tongue mass, but no distant metastases were found. Tumor stage T3N2cM0, stage IVA.

hyoid bone to the inferior aspect of the cricoid cartilage. The larynx is subdivided into 3 subsites: supraglottis, glottis, and subglottis.

The supraglottic larynx extends from the tip of the epiglottis to the bottom of the laryngeal ventricles. This space encompasses the epiglottis, the aryepiglottic folds, the false vocal cords, the vestibule, the preepiglottic and paraglottic spaces, and the arytenoid cartilages. There are 3 sublocations where SCCa tends to occur: the epiglottis, the aryepiglottic folds, and the false vocal cords.

The glottic larynx contains the true vocal cords in addition to the anterior and posterior commissures. It is approximately 1 cm in height, extending down from the mid-plane of the laryngeal ventricles. The vocal cords attach to the thyroid cartilage at the anterior commissure by way of the Broyles ligaments. There is no perichondrium at this attachment site, which makes it vulnerable to early cartilaginous invasion.[33] As this is a fairly accessible area for the clinician to examine, the role of imaging lies in evaluating deep tissue extension. The true vocal cords can be located on axial imaging by finding the level where there is absence of submucosal fat and all 3 cartilages surrounding the cords are seen (which are the thyroid, cricoid, and vocal process of the arytenoid cartilages).[34]

The subglottic larynx extends from the inferior aspect of the true vocal cords to the inferior aspect of the cricoid cartilage.

In all cases of laryngeal SCCa, the most crucial imaging findings consist of those that differentiate a T3 from a T4 lesion, because larynx-sparing chemoradiation is not recommended for T4 lesions. Erosion of the inner lamina of the thyroid cartilage or paraglottic or preepiglottic fat involvement denotes T3. Involvement of the arytenoid cartilage does not change staging. T4 tumors present with

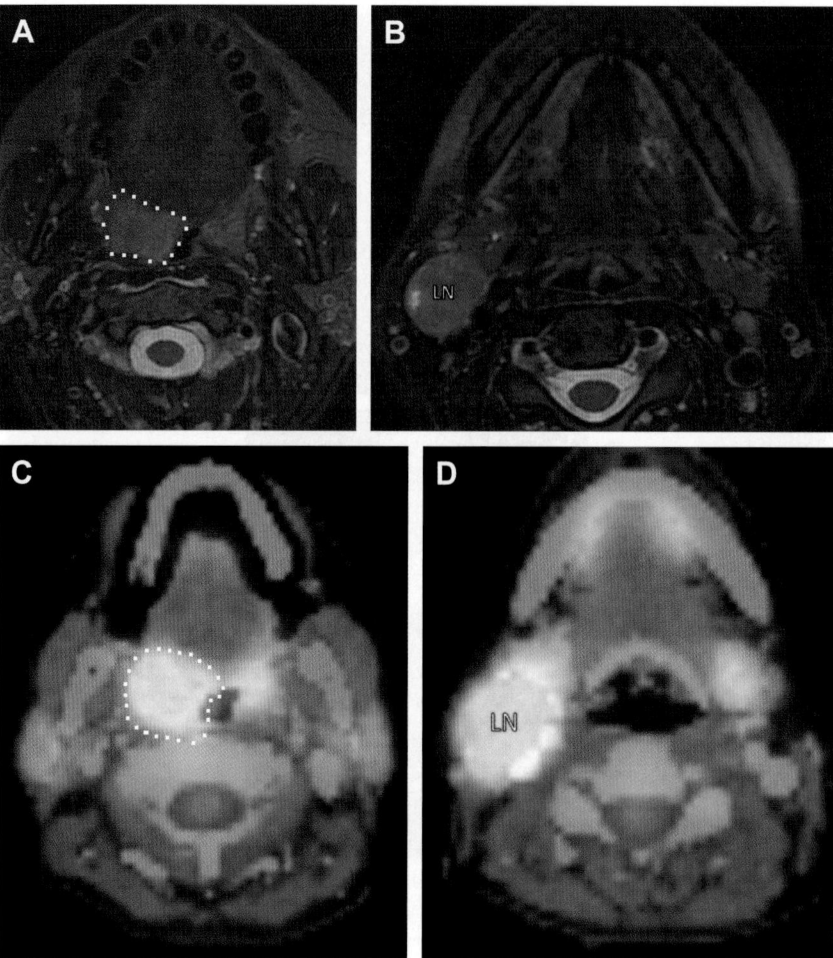

Fig. 7. (*A, B*) Axial T2-weighted MR image of a 45 year-old patient who presented with a right level 2 cervical node (LN) for which biopsy revealed SCCa. There is a well-circumscribed right tonsillar pillar mass (*dotted line*). (*C, D*) FDG-PET/CT scan of the same patient shows avid FDG uptake in both the right tonsillar pillar mass (*dotted line*) and right level 2 cervical node (LN). Tumor stage T2N1M0, stage III.

Table 3
Typical spread of lingual tonsil SCCa

Direction of Spread	Structures Involved
Anterior	Sublingual space Oral tongue Floor of mouth Neurovascular bundle of oral cavity
Posterior	Anterior tonsillar pillar Palatine tonsils
Lateral	Medial pterygoid Pterygomandibular raphe Mandible
Superior	Tonsillar pillars
Inferior	Valleculae Preepiglottic fat

extralaryngeal tumor spread and can also show penetration through the thyroid cartilage (T4a). Encasement of 270° or more of the carotid arteries by tumor denotes a T4b tumor. CT is usually adequate and sufficient for laryngeal SCCa staging. However, MR imaging can be a powerful tool to investigate equivocal thyroid cartilage penetration and distinguish a T3 from a T4 tumor.[35]

Supraglottis

Epiglottic SCCa may present as a midline, and therefore subtle and symmetric-appearing lesion. Because the supraglottic larynx is rich in lymphatics, patients presenting with enlarged cervical lymph nodes warrant high suspicion of disease, and epiglottic SCCa has a tendency for bilateral adenopathy at presentation. Aryepiglottic fold SCCa has a tendency to spread down to the pyriform sinus of the hypopharynx or anteriorly to the

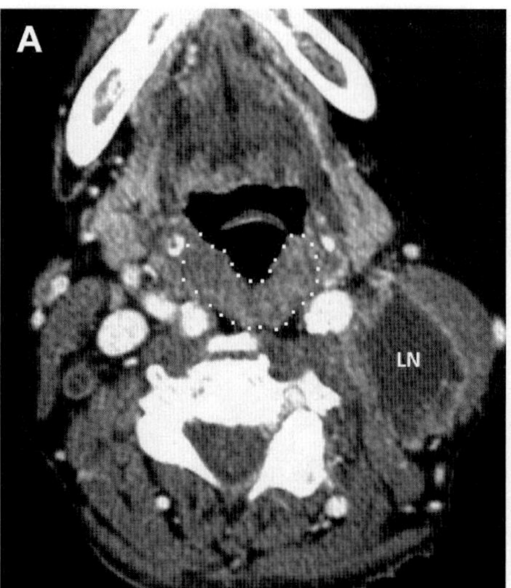

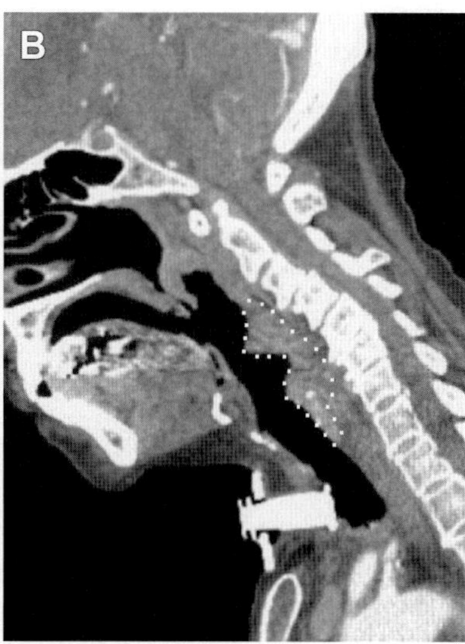

Fig. 8. Axial CECT (*A*) and sagittal reconstruction of the neck (*B*) in a 61-year-old female smoker with a 4-month history of left neck mass sensation. There is a posterior oropharynx mass (*dotted line*), extending from the nasopharynx to the junction of the oropharynx and hypopharynx. There is a large necrotic left level 2 cervical lymph node (LN) with extranodal spread, and a contralateral node was also found (not shown). Tumor stage T2N2c, stage IVA.

false cords. False cord SCCa has a propensity to invade the paraglottic space. Coronal images are helpful for evaluating craniocaudal extension, whereas sagittal and axial images best evaluate the preepiglottic space (Fig. 9).

Preepiglottic or paraglottic fat infiltration determines the tumor to be at least T3.[6] Preepiglottic spread may lead to invasion of the anterior commissure and the true vocal cords below. Whenever paraglottic space invasion is noted, close attention to both the true vocal cords and the thyroid cartilage is mandatory. Thyroid cartilage invasion can often be challenging to diagnose, and overstaging on pretreatment CT examination can result in unnecessary extensive surgery. If only erosion of the inner cortex is present, the tumor stage is T3. However, if there is cartilage penetration, with tumor extending through the cartilage, the tumor is staged as T4. Although sclerosis of the cartilage, as seen on CT, is often cited as indicating tumoral invasion, it is nonspecific and can result from inflammation rather than invasion.[35,36] True erosion or frank lysis of cartilage is more specific. MR imaging is more sensitive and specific than CT for detection of thyroid cartilage invasion (Fig. 10). Analysis of both enhancement and T2-weighted imaging characteristics have been reported to be sensitive and specific. If T2-weighted signal intensity and enhancement within the cartilage are equal to that of the tumor, cartilage invasion is likely present. However, if T2-weighted signal intensity and enhancement are more intense than that of the tumor, invasion is less likely, as this most likely

Table 4
Typical spread of posterior pharyngeal wall SCCa

Direction of Spread	Structures Involved
Anterior	Tonsillar pillars
Posterior	Prevertebral muscles (longus colli and capitis muscles)
Lateral	Parapharyngeal space
Superior	Nasopharynx
Inferior	Hypopharynx

Table 5
Typical spread of soft palate SCCa

Direction of Spread	Structures Involved
Anterior	Hard palate
Lateral	Palatine muscles Tonsillar pillars Parapharyngeal space
Superior	Nasopharynx Skull base
Inferior	Tonsillar pillars

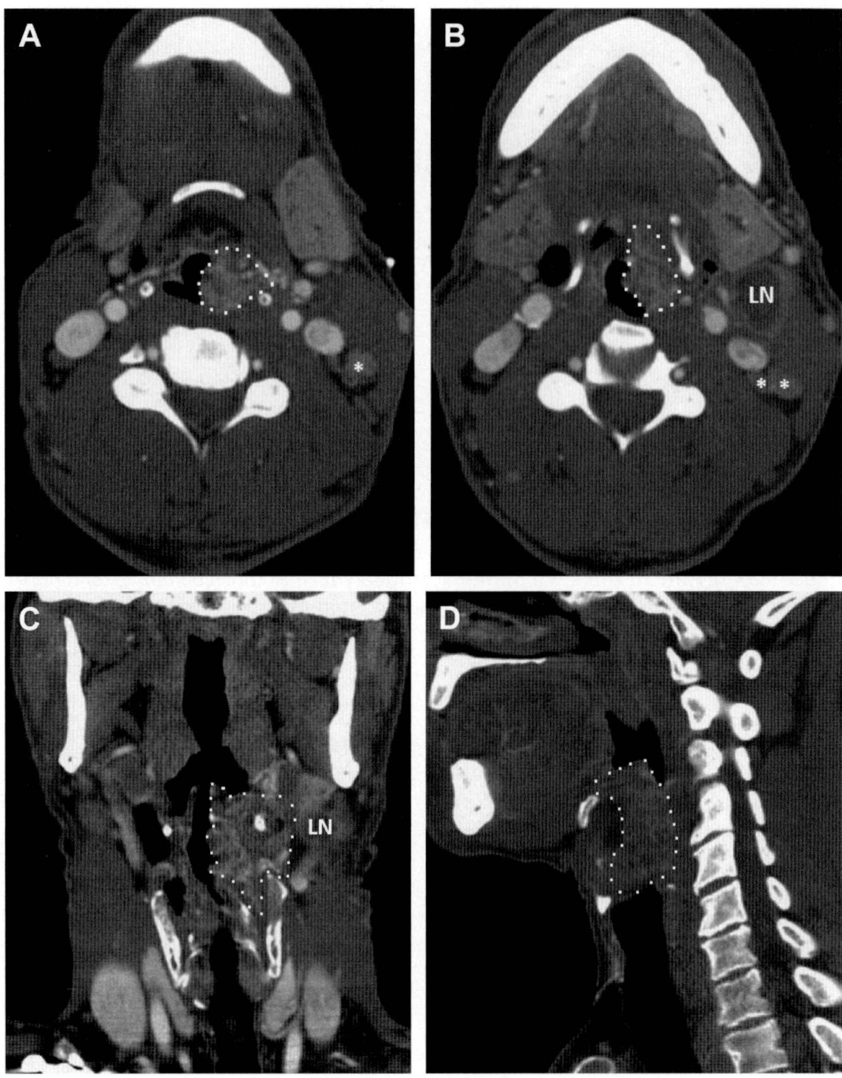

Fig. 9. Axial CECT (*A, B*) with coronal (*C*) and sagittal (*D*) reformatted images of a 57-year-old male smoker and heavy drinker, with 2-month history of increasing dysphagia and odynophagia. There is a large left supraglottic mass (*dotted line*), which extends inferiorly to the hypopharynx and superiorly to the oropharynx. There are also multiple left level 2 cervical lymph nodes (*asterisk*) with at least 1 being necrotic (LN). Tumor stage T3N2b, stage IVA.

represents inflammation. AJCC criteria for the staging of supraglottic SCCa are listed in Ref.[6]

Glottis

Most often, SCCa arises from the mucosa of the anterior third of the true vocal cords, and may extend to involve the anterior commissure. The tumor can be small and difficult to detect on imaging; often, patients will present at an early stage with voice hoarseness.

Coronal images are very helpful in evaluating extension of tumor and determining whether there is transglottic spread (cranial extension through the laryngeal ventricles) and/or subglottic extension. Such extensions denote T2 staging. Paraglottic and periglottic space invasion denote T3 staging. Tumors with hemilarynx fixation also denote T3 staging.[6]

Similar to thyroid cartilage in the case of supraglottic tumor, sclerosis of the arytenoid cartilages has often been reported as suggestive of tumoral invasion. However, it is also present in asymptomatic individuals, being often found as a normal variant on the left side in female patients.[37] Even in the presence of adjacent laryngeal tumor, sclerosis of the arytenoid cartilage is associated with only a 30% to 50% risk of tumoral invasion.[38,39] Arytenoid cartilage invasion does not change

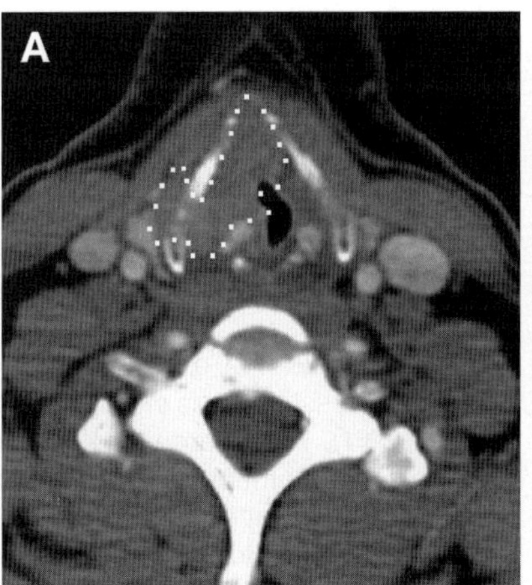

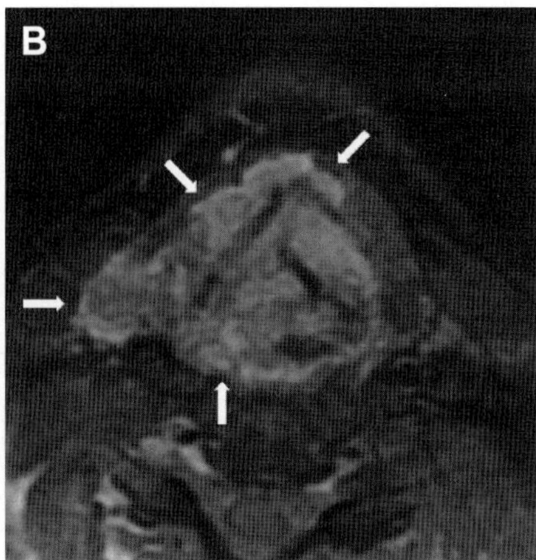

Fig. 10. (*A*) A 55-year-old male patient presenting with several-month history of progressive voice loss, increasing throat pain, and dysphagia. Axial CECT shows a right supraglottic mass (*dotted line*) extending anteriorly to the left and subtly eroding through the posterior aspect of the right thyroid cartilage. (*B*) Gadolinium-enhanced axial T1-weighted image of the same patient better demonstrates the well-circumscribed bilateral (right more than left) supraglottic mass (*arrows*), which clearly erodes through the right thyroid cartilage. Tumor stage T4aN2c, stage IVA.

staging or management. It is associated with increased risk of postradiation chondronecrosis. AJCC criteria for the staging of glottic SCCa are listed in Ref.[6]

Subglottis

Subglottic SCCa is rare, representing fewer than 5% of laryngeal tumors, and mostly affecting smokers and alcohol abusers. These SCCa commonly present at a late stage, with 50% of tumors being T4 at presentation, typically from invasion of the cricoid cartilage.

Imaging is very important, as clinical and endoscopic examinations are limited. Coronal images are helpful to evaluate craniocaudal extension and involvement of the true vocal cords. Because cricoid cartilage invasion upstages the primary tumor, close attention to its contour and density/signal is imperative. The mucosal layer is closely applied to the cricoid cartilage; any amount of tissue present in the subglottic larynx should be viewed with suspicion. The subglottic larynx is sparsely populated by lymphatics, and nodal metastases are infrequent. AJCC criteria for the staging of subglottic SCCa are listed in Ref.[6]

HYPOPHARYNGEAL SQUAMOUS CELL CARCINOMA

Anatomic Considerations

The hypopharynx is a difficult region for the clinician and endoscopist to adequately visualize. It is the lower portion of the pharynx located between the oropharynx and cervical esophagus. The hypopharynx is bounded superiorly by the hyoid bone, glossoepiglottic, and pharyngoepiglottic folds, and inferiorly by the inferior margin of the cricoid cartilage and cricopharyngeus muscle. The postcricoid mucosa and posterior cricoarytenoid muscle form the anterior margin, while the posterior mucosa with the middle and inferior constrictor muscles form the posterior margin. The hypopharynx is subdivided into 3 sites: the pyriform sinuses, the posterior wall, and the postcricoid region.

The pyriform sinuses are anterolateral recesses lateral to the aryepiglottic folds. The apices of the pyriform sinuses are at the same level as the true vocal cords. Craniocaudally, the pyriform sinuses extend from the thyrohyoid membrane to the thyroid cartilage. The aryepiglottic folds are not considered part of the pyriform sinuses; rather, they form part of the supraglottic larynx. The postcricoid region is the anterior wall of the hypopharynx, and divides the lumina of the hypopharynx and larynx. It runs down from the cricoarytenoids to the inferior portion of the cricoid cartilage. The posterior hypopharyngeal wall is the prolongation of the posterior wall of the oropharynx, extending from the soft palate to the cervical esophagus ostium.

Demographic and Epidemiologic Factors

Hypopharyngeal SCCa is relatively uncommon, and its main risk factors are tobacco and alcohol abuse. It has the worst prognosis of any SCCa of the pharynx, with a 5-year survival of only 40%

to 50%.[40] One of the proposed reasons for this poor prognosis is that patients frequently present with late-stage disease (stage III/IV). Other than presenting with metastatic nodal metastases as a new neck mass, patients may present with dysphagia, odynophagia, voice change, or otalgia.[41]

Imaging Manifestations

Imaging is often required to provide essential staging information. Patients with hypopharynx SCCa commonly have problems swallowing their secretions, which makes it difficult for them to do extensive breath-hold techniques. As a result, CT is often a better imaging technique than MR imaging, the latter often serving as an adjunct to better evaluate for involvement of prevertebral musculature. AJCC staging criteria are listed in Ref.[6]

Pyriform sinus

Approximately two-thirds of all hypopharyngeal SCCa arise from the mucosa lining the pyriform sinuses. As with other pharyngeal SCCa, there is a strong association with tobacco and alcohol abuse, in addition to prior radiation. Because these risk factors are also associated with other sites of SCCa, synchronous or metachronous primaries of the pharynx, lung, OC, or larynx are not uncommon. Most commonly, patients present with sore throat and sometimes referred pain to the ear.

Pyriform sinus SCCa can present as a small enhancing mass, which is often irregular and ulcerated (**Fig. 11**). When large, the tumor can fill the pyriform sinus. Sometimes the tumor spreads submucosally and involves the walls of the pyriform sinus circumferentially. Tumoral spread depends on primary tumor location within the sinus, and patterns of spread are listed in **Table 6**.

Although it may be difficult to detect, thyroid cartilage invasion is important to determine, as it denotes a T4a staging.[6] Encasement over 270° of the carotid arteries by tumor upstages the primary to a T4b.[6] When tumors arise from the

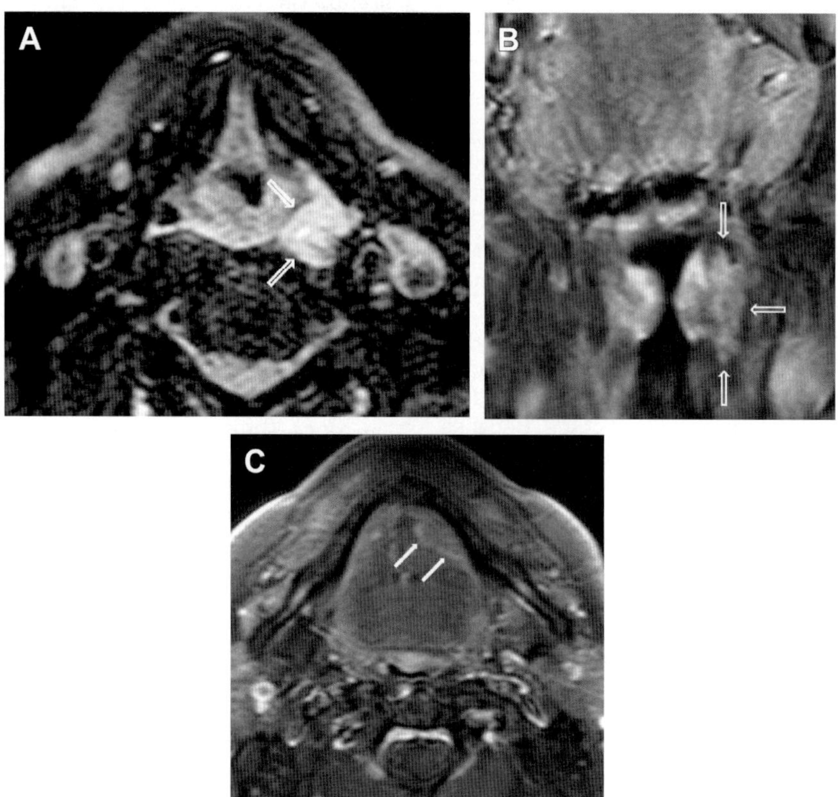

Fig. 11. (*A*) Axial T2-weighted image of a 75-year-old male drinker and smoker with a 2-month history of throat pain. There is a hyperintense mass in the left pyriform sinus apex (*open arrows*). (*B*) Coronal gadolinium-enhanced T1-weighted image with fat saturation in the same patient shows the enhancing mass involving the apex of the left pyriform sinus (*open arrows*). Tumor stage T2N0, stage II. (*C*) Axial gadolinium-enhanced T1-weighted image of the same patient at the level of the oral cavity shows an enhancing mass in the anterior left tongue (*arrows*), representing a synchronous second primary SCCa. Tumor stage by imaging also T2N0, stage II.

Table 6
Typical spread of pyriform sinus SCCa

Direction of Spread	Structures Involved
Apical	Inferiorly to postcricoid region
Anterior	Paraglottic fat
Lateral	Parapharyngeal soft tissues Through thyrohyoid membrane

posterior aspect of the pyriform sinus, they can extend into the prevertebral tissues, which may be better evaluated by MR imaging than with CT.

Postcricoid region

Though infrequent, postcricoid SCCa is the second most common hypopharyngeal location for SCCa, after pyriform sinus. Patients often present at a later stage with laryngeal, including cricoid cartilage invasion and nodal spread.

The lesion can extend cranially and/or laterally into the hypopharynx, inferiorly to the cervical esophagus, and anteriorly to the larynx. Postcricoid SCCa has a propensity to spread submucosally to the cervical esophagus, indicating a T3 tumor stage.

Posterior hypopharyngeal wall

Posterior hypopharyngeal wall is the least common hypopharyngeal location for SCCa, and has the poorest prognosis, with an overall 5-year survival estimated at approximately 30%. Patients usually present at a late stage, with referred otalgia, neck nodes, dysphagia, sore throat, or weight loss (**Fig. 12**). More than 75% will have positive cervical lymph node metastasis at presentation.

Lesions are usually irregular and mildly enhancing, with a tendency for submucosal spread to the oropharynx superiorly (T2) or cervical esophagus inferiorly (T3). Owing to its posterior

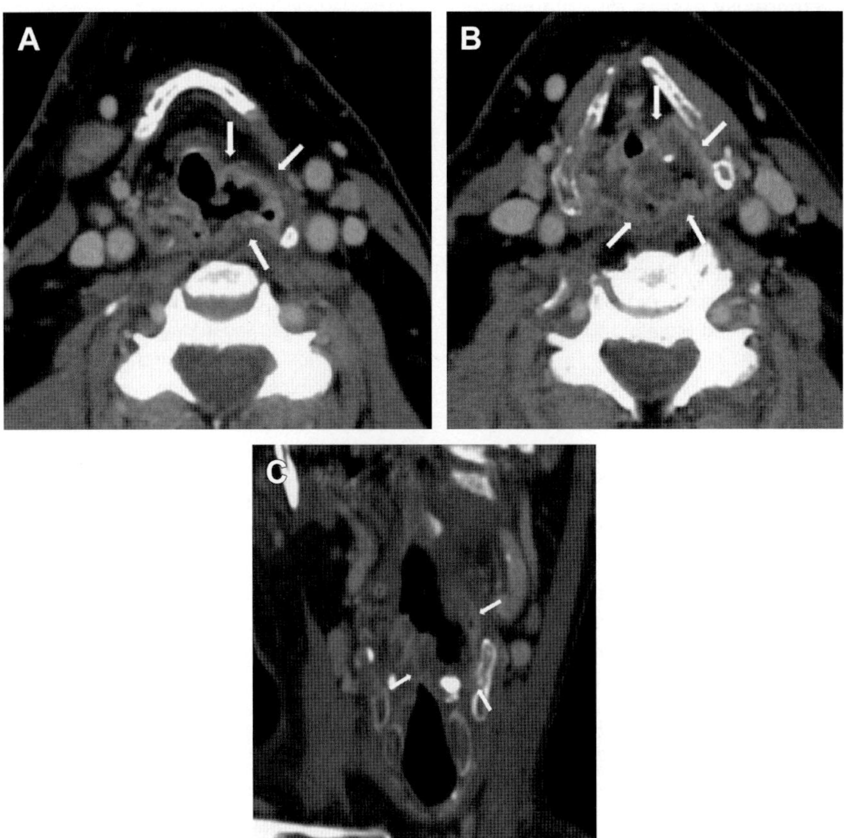

Fig. 12. Axial CECT (*A, B*) with coronal reformat (*C*) of a 62-year-old male smoker and drinker who presented with a several-week history of progressive odynophagia and dysphagia associated with left-sided otalgia and loss of 90 lb (40.8 kg) over the period of a year. There is an ulcerated posterior hypopharyngeal mass (*arrows*) extending into the pyriform sinus and anteriorly invading the paraglottic fat of the supraglottic larynx. Evident bilateral nodal disease also results in tumor stage T3N2c, stage IVA.

location, close attention to prevertebral muscle invasion is necessary, as invasion of these makes the tumor stage T4b. Although imaging is not very accurate in determining paravertebral muscle invasion, if there is preservation of the retropharyngeal fat, paravertebral muscle invasion is unlikely. Lateral spread to the carotid arteries with encasement of these can also occur, also denoting a T4b tumor.

SUMMARY

The epidemiology of pharyngeal SCCa is currently changing, with an increasing incidence of HPV-related oropharyngeal SCCa and a decrease in the traditional tobacco-related and alcohol-related SCCa. The radiologist plays a central role in tumor staging, posttreatment evaluation, and surveillance, and as such should be cognizant of the pertinent anatomy and staging criteria. Awareness of imaging findings pertinent to treatment planning is crucial. Finally, as most pharyngeal SCCa share identical risk factors, radiologists should always carefully assess for potential synchronous or metachronous tumors.

REFERENCES

1. Sturgis E, Ang K. The epidemic of HPV-associated oropharyngeal cancer is here: is it time to change our treatment paradigms? J Natl Compr Canc Netw 2011;9(6):9.
2. Chaturvedi A, Engels E, Pfeiffer R, et al. Human papillomavirus and rising oropharyngeal cancer incidence in the United States. J Clin Oncol 2011; 29(32):8.
3. Mehanna H, Beech T, Nicholson T, et al. Prevalence of human papillomavirus in oropharyngeal and non-oropharyngeal head and neck cancer—systematic review and meta-analysis of trends by time and region. Head Neck 2013;35(5):9.
4. D'Souza G, Kreimer AR, Viscidi R, et al. Case-control study of human papillomavirus and oropharyngeal cancer. N Engl J Med 2007;356:13.
5. Gillison M, D'Souza G, Westra W, et al. Distinct risk factor profiles for human papillomavirus type 16-positive and human papillomavirus type 16-negative head and neck cancers. J Natl Cancer Inst 2008; 100:14.
6. Edge S, Byrd D, Compton C, et al. AJCC cancer staging manual. 7th edition. New York: Springer; 2010. p. 649.
7. Lee A, Au J, Teo P, et al. Staging of nasopharyngeal carcinoma: suggestions for improving the current UICC/AJCC Staging System. Clin Oncol 2004;16:8.
8. Mao Y, Xie F, Liu L, et al. Evaluation of the sixth edition of AJCC staging system for nasopharyngeal carcinoma and proposed improvement. Int J Radiat Oncol Biol Phys 2008;70:9.
9. Glastonbury C, Salzman K. Pitfalls in the staging of cancer of nasopharyngeal carcinoma. Neuroimaging Clin N Am 2013;23:17.
10. Lee A, Ng W, Chan L, et al. The strength/weakness of the AJCC/UICC staging system (7th edition) for nasopharyngeal cancer and suggestions for future improvement. Oral Oncol 2012;48:7.
11. Glastonbury C. Specialty imaging head and neck cancer state of the art diagnosis, staging, and surveillance. Philadelphia: Lippincott Williams & Wilkins; 2013. p. 500.
12. Trotta B, Pease C, Rasamny J, et al. Oral cavity and oropharyngeal squamous cell cancer: key imaging findings for staging and treatment planning. Radiographics 2011;31(2):17.
13. Brown LM, Check DP, Devesa SS. Oral cavity and pharynx cancer incidence trends by subsite in the United States: changing gender patterns. J Oncol 2012;2012:10.
14. Aiken A. Pitfalls in the staging of cancer of oral cavity cancer. Neuroimaging Clin N Am 2013;23:18.
15. Nair U, Bartsch H, Nair J. Alert for an epidemic of oral cancer due to use of the betel quid substitutes gutkha and pan masala: a review of agents and causative mechanisms. Mutagenesis 2004;19(4):12.
16. Merchant A, Husain SSM, Hosain M, et al. Paan without tobacco: an independent risk factor for oral cancer. Int J Cancer 2000;86:4.
17. Weissman JL, Carrau RL. "Puffed-cheek" CT improves evaluation of the oral cavity. AJNR Am J Neuroradiol 2001;22:5.
18. Henrot P, Blum A, Toussaint B, et al. Dynamic maneuvers in local staging of head and neck malignancies with current imaging techniques: principles and clinical applications. Radiographics 2003;23:13.
19. Dillon JK, Glastonbury CM, Jabeen F, et al. Gauze padding: a simple technique to delineate small oral cavity tumors. AJNR Am J Neuroradiol 2011; 32:4.
20. Shemen L, Klotz J, Schottenfeld D, et al. Increase of tongue cancer in young men. JAMA 1984;252(14): 1857.
21. Depue R. Rising mortality from cancer of the tongue in young white males. N Engl J Med 1986;315:1.
22. Davis S, Severson R. Increasing incidence of cancer of the tongue in the United States among young adults. Lancet 1987;2:2.
23. Shiboski C, Shiboski S, Silverman S. Trends in oral cancer rates in the United States 1973-1996. Community Dent Oral Epidemiol 2000;28:8.
24. Myers J, Elkins T, Roberts D, et al. Squamous cell carcinoma of the tongue in young adults: increasing incidence and factors that predict treatment outcomes. Otolaryngol Head Neck Surg 2000;122:8.

25. Patel SC, Carpenter WR, Tyree S, et al. Increasing incidence of oral tongue squamous cell carcinoma in young white women, age 18 to 44 years. J Clin Oncol 2011;29(11):7.
26. Siegel R, Ward E, Brawley O, et al. Cancer statistics, 2011: the impact of eliminating socioeconomics and racial disparities on premature cancer deaths. CA Cancer J Clin 2011;61(4):25.
27. Corey A. Pitfalls in the staging of cancer of the oropharyngeal squamous cell carcinoma. Neuroimaging Clin N Am 2013;23:20.
28. Klussmann JP, Welssenborn SJ, Wieland U, et al. Prevalence, distribution, and viral load of human papillomavirus 16 DNA in tonsillar carcinomas. Cancer 2001;92(11):10.
29. Cantrell SC, Peck BW, Li G, et al. Differences in imaging characteristics of HPV-positive and HPV-negative oropharyngeal cancers: a blinded matched-pair analysis. AJNR Am J Neuroradiol 2013;34:5.
30. Goyal N, Zacharia TT, Goldenberg D. Differentiation of branchial cleft cysts and malignant cystic adenopathy of pharyngeal origin. AJR Am J Roentgenol 2012;199:6.
31. Fakhry C, Westr WH, Li S, et al. Improved survival of patients with human papillomavirus—positive head and neck squamous cell carcinoma in a prospective clinical trial. J Natl Cancer Inst 2008;100:9.
32. Ragin CC, Taioli E. Survival of squamous cell carcinoma of the head and neck in relation to human papillomavirus infection: review and meta-analysis. Int J Cancer 2007;121:8.
33. Chone CT, Yonehara E, Martins JEF, et al. Importance of anterior commissure in recurrence of early glottic cancer after laser endoscopic resection. Arch Otolaryngol Head Neck Surg 2007;133(9):6.
34. Baugnon KL, Beitler JJ. Pitfalls in the staging of cancer of the laryngeal squamous cell carcinoma. Neuroimaging Clin N Am 2013;23:26.
35. Becker M, Zbären P, Casselman JW, et al. Neoplastic invasion of laryngeal cartilage: reassessment of criteria for diagnosis at MR imaging. Radiology 2008;249(2):9.
36. Li B, Bobinski M, Gandour-Edwards R, et al. Overstaging of cartilage invasion by multidetector CT scan for laryngeal cancer and its potential effect on the use of organ preservation with chemoradiation. Br J Radiol 2011;84:6.
37. Schmalfuss I, Mancuso A, Tart R. Arytenoid cartilage sclerosis: normal variations and clinical significance. AJNR Am J Neuroradiol 1998;19:4.
38. Munoz A, Ramos A, Ferrando J, et al. Laryngeal carcinoma: sclerosis appearance of the cricoid and arytenoid cartilage- CT-pathologic correlation. Radiology 1993;189:5.
39. Becker M, Zbaren P, Laeng H, et al. Neoplastic invasion of the laryngeal cartilage: comparison of MR imaging and CT with histopathologic correlation. Radiology 1995;194:9.
40. Ozer E, Grecula J, Agrawal A, et al. Long-term results of a multimodal intensification regimen for previously untreated advanced resectable squamous cell cancer of the oral cavity, oropharynx, or hypopharynx. Laryngoscope 2006;116:6.
41. Uzcudun A, Bravo FP, Sanchez J. Clinical features of pharyngeal cancer: a retrospective study of 258 consecutive patients. J Laryngol Otol 2001;115(2):7.

Imaging of the Oral Cavity

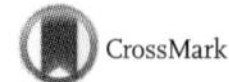

Indu Rekha Meesa, MD, MS[a,b], Ashok Srinivasan, MBBS, MD[a,*]

KEYWORDS

• Floor of mouth • Oral cavity carcinoma • Ludwig's angina • Ranula • Odontogenic lesions

KEY POINTS

- Mylohyoid muscle forms the floor of mouth and divides the sublingual and submandibular spaces.
- Oral mucosal space has bilateral drainage to submental and submandibular lymph nodes.
- Although a simple ranula is confined to the sublingual space, a diving ranula has extension into the submandibular space.

INTRODUCTION

The oral cavity is a challenging area in head and neck imaging because of its complex anatomy and the numerous pathophysiologies that involve its contents. This challenge is further compounded by the ubiquitous artifacts that arise from the dental amalgam, which compromise image quality. In this article, the anatomy of the oral cavity is discussed in brief, followed by a description of the imaging technique and some common pathologic abnormalities.

OVERVIEW OF ORAL CAVITY ANATOMY

The oral cavity comprises the lips anteriorly, the mylohyoid muscle, the alveolar mandibular ridge, and the teeth inferiorly, the gingivobuccal regions laterally, the circumvallate papillae, tonsillar pillars, and soft palate posteriorly, and the hard palate and maxillary alveolar ridge and teeth superiorly.[1]

The key muscles associated with the oral cavity include the anterior belly of the digastric, mylohyoid, genioglossus, geniohyoid, and hyoglossus. The anterior belly of the digastric is located in the submandibular space. The mylohyoid muscle divides the submandibular and sublingual spaces; the genioglossus and geniohyoid are at the root of the tongue, and the hyoglossus muscle is in the sublingual space (**Figs. 1** and **2**).

The Oral Tongue

The oral tongue consists of a supporting skeleton composed of the midline lingual septum and hyoglossus membrane (**Figs. 3** and **4**). There are both extrinsic and intrinsic muscles in the tongue: the 4 intrinsic muscles are the superior and inferior longitudinal, transverse, vertical/oblique muscles, and the major extrinsic muscles are the genioglossus, hyoglossus, palatoglossus, and styloglossus muscles. The extrinsic muscles allow attachment of the tongue to the hyoid bone, mandible, and styloid process of the skull base.[2,3] The tongue muscle fibers are arranged in various directions and their complex arrangement enables enunciation of various consonants.

Intrinsic and extrinsic tongue muscles receive motor innervation from the hypoglossal nerve, which courses between the mylohoid and hyoglossus muscles. The palatoglossus muscle is innervated by the pharyngeal plexus. The lingual nerve (a branch of the trigeminal nerve) courses adjacent to the hypoglossal nerve and carries sensory fibers from the anterior portion of the tongue. Special sensory taste fibers course with the lingual nerve before they coalesce to form the chorda tympani nerve, which joins the facial nerve after traversing the middle ear. The posterior one-third of the tongue is supplied by the glossopharyngeal nerve.

[a] Department of Radiology, University of Michigan Health system, 1500 E medical center, Ann Arbor, MI 48109, USA; [b] Summit Radiology, Fort Wayne, IN 46804, USA
* Corresponding author.
E-mail address: ashoks@med.umich.edu

Radiol Clin N Am 53 (2015) 99–114
http://dx.doi.org/10.1016/j.rcl.2014.09.003

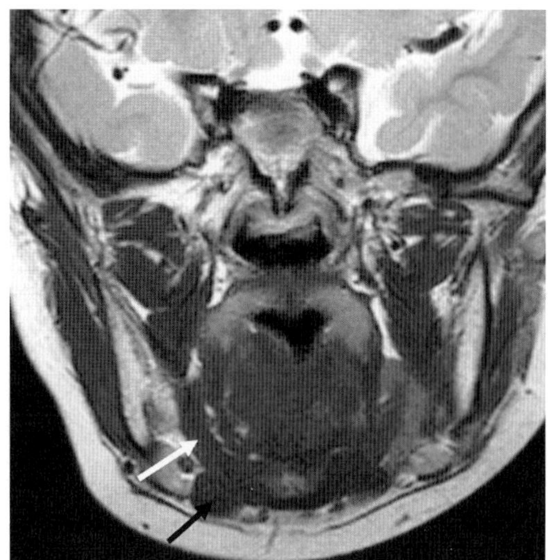

Fig. 1. Coronal T2-weighted image of the normal oral cavity. White arrow points to mylohyoid muscle; black arrow points to anterior belly of digastric muscle.

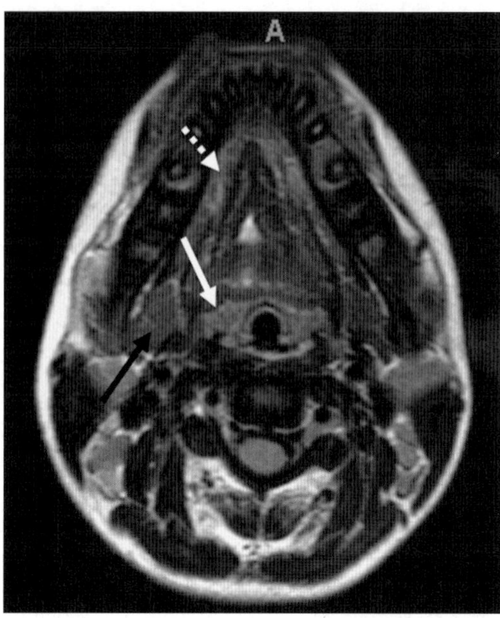

Fig. 3. Axial T2-weighted image of the normal oral tongue. Black arrow points to submandibular gland; white arrow points to palatine tonsils; dotted arrow points to sublingual gland.

Floor of Mouth

The floor of the mouth is U-shaped and covered by squamous mucosa. The primary muscles comprising the floor of the mouth are the mylohyoid muscles and a fibrous median raphe. Additional support is also provided by the paired anterior bellies of the digastric muscles and geniohyoid muscles. The mylohyoid muscle arises from the entire length of the mylohyoid ridge on the inner surface of the mandible and extends from the symphysis anteriorly to the last molar tooth posteriorly. Posterior fibers insert on the body of the hyoid bone and middle and anterior fibers insert into the fibrous medial raphe, which runs from the hyoid bone to the mandibular symphysis.[4] This forms

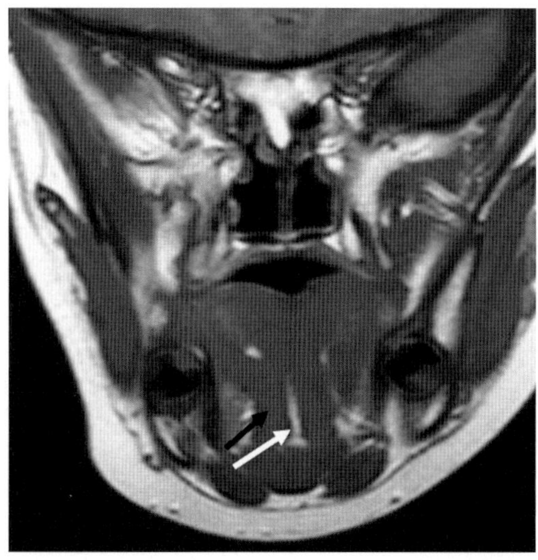

Fig. 2. Coronal postcontrast T1-weighted image of the normal oral cavity. White arrow points to fatty lingual septum; black arrow points to genioglossus muscle.

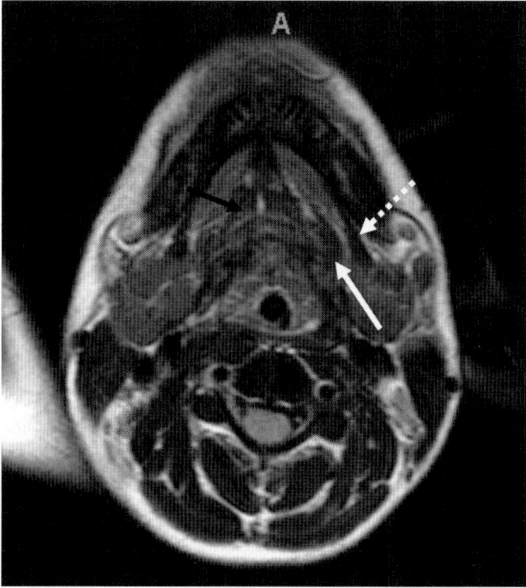

Fig. 4. Axial T1-weighted image of the normal oral tongue. White dotted arrow points to mylohyoid muscle; black arrow points to genioglossus muscle; white arrow points to hyoglossus muscle.

the U-shaped sling, best demonstrated on the coronal plane by CT or MR imaging.[5]

The mylohyoid branch of the inferior alveolar nerve (division of mandibular branch of trigeminal nerve) provides motor innervation to the mylohyoid muscle. There is a gap between the free edge of the posterior border of the mylohyoid muscle and between the hyoglossus muscle superiorly, through which the submandibular gland wraps around the mylohoid muscle, leading to the deep lobe of the gland lying cranial to the muscle fibers and the superficial lobe lying on the external surface.[5]

The digastric muscle consists of 2 bellies, the anterior belly and posterior belly. The anterior belly arises from the digastric fossa of the inner surface of the mandible and the posterior belly arises from the digastric fossa of the inner surface of the mastoid process of the temporal bone. The bellies terminate in a central tendon that pierces the stylohyoid muscle. The central tendon runs through a fibrous loop that is attached to the body and greater cornua of the hyoid bone. The anterior belly of the digastric muscle is innervated by the mylohyoid branch of the mandibular nerve and the posterior belly is innervated by the facial nerve.

Sublingual Space

The sublingual space contains the anterior aspect of the hyoglossus muscle, lingual nerve, artery, and vein, glossopharyngeal and hypoglossal nerves, sublingual glands and ducts, deep portion of the submandibular gland, and Wharton (submandibular) duct.[6] The hyoglossus, styloglossus, and palatoglossus muscles form the lateral muscular bundle in the sublingual space and form a surgical landmark because they separate the Wharton duct and the hypoglossal and lingual nerves, which lie laterally, from the lingual artery and vein, which lie medially.[5] The Wharton duct arises from the deep portion of the gland and runs anteriorly, in contact with the hypoglossal and lingual nerves, and drains into the floor of the mouth, just lateral to the frenulum of the tongue. The mylohoid muscle separates the submandibular space inferiorly from the sublingual space superomedially. These spaces are horseshoe-shaped and communicate across the midline. The submandibular, sublingual, and inferior parapharygneal spaces are also contiguous with one another.[6]

Submandibular Space

The submandibular space lies inferior to the mylohyoid muscle and is a fascially defined space expected at the posterior margin, where it is contiguous with the posterior aspect of the sublingual space and the parapharyngeal space anteriorly. The contents include fat, the anterior belly of the digastric, the superficial portion of the submandibular gland, the submandibular and submental lymph nodes, the facial vein and artery, and the inferior loop of the hypoglossal nerve.[6] The small fat-filled region between the 2 anterior digastric bellies is the submental portion of the submandibular space. Submental lymph nodes (level 1A) reside in this region, and level 1B lymph nodes and facial artery and vein lie lateral to the anterior digastric muscle in the fat surrounding the submandibular gland. The facial artery courses deep to the submandibular gland and the facial vein runs superficially.[5]

Lips and Gingivobuccal Region

The lips are composed of orbicularis oris muscle, primarily composed of muscle fibers from multiple facial muscles that insert into the lips. The motor innervation is from the facial nerve, and the lymphatic drainage is to the submental and submandibular lymph nodes.

The vestibule of the mouth separates the lips and cheeks from the teeth and gums. The mucosal covering over the medial (lingual) and buccal aspects of the alveolar processes of the mandible and maxilla is the gingiva.

Buccomasseteric Region

The buccomasseteric region includes the masseter and buccinator muscles, buccal space, and inferior body of the mandible. The buccal space is located lateral to the buccinator, deep to the zygomaticus major, and anterior to the mandibular ramus and masseter. The parotid gland duct (Stensen's duct) crosses the masseter, courses through the buccal fat pad and pierces the buccinator opposite the second maxillary molar, and drains into the vestibule of the mouth.

IMAGING OF THE ORAL CAVITY

CT and MR imaging are complementary in assessment of the oral cavity. The advantages of CT include better accessibility, faster acquisition time, and better cortical bone assessment.[7,8] The advantages of MR imaging include no ionizing radiation, better characterization of local tumor extent, better assessment of bone marrow involvement, and detection of perineural spread.[9,10]

Imaging of the oral cavity can be limited by artifacts from dental amalgam and opposed mucosal surfaces. Modified techniques, such as puffed cheek CT, have been shown to be useful in assessing mucosal-based tumors but require patient cooperation.[11] If there is significant dental amalgam artifact, limited repeat scan with imaging along the line of the mandible (parallel to the plane containing the metal) can provide a much improved imaging plane to visualize the oral cavity.[12]

Important Considerations in Oral Cavity Evaluation

- Oral mucosal space has bilateral drainage to submental and submandibular lymph nodes.
- Puffed cheek technique helps determine if the lesion is arising from the buccal surface or the gingival surface.
- Retromolar trigone (triangular region of mucosa posterior to the last mandibular molar) spread of cancers can occur from the tonsils or base of tongue.
- Pterygomandibular raphe, a fibrous band extending from the posterior mylohyoid line to the hook of the hamulus of the medial pterygoid plate, serves as the origin point for buccinator and superior constrictor muscles. Tumor invasion into this space therefore potentiates the spread in multiple directions into the buccal space and oropharynx.
- Involvement of root of the tongue upstages oral cavity tumors to T4, and involvement of the lingual septum makes the patient unsuitable for hemiglossectomy.[13]

PATHOLOGIES INVOLVING THE ORAL CAVITY

Major pathologic abnormalities involving the oral cavity are congenital, infectious/inflammatory, or neoplasms in cause. In the next section, some of the common lesions are discussed with pertinent imaging findings.

Congenital/Developmental Lesions

Second branchial cleft cysts

Clinical Features

- Bimodal distribution
- Child: mass seen at the angle of mandible, and, if a sinus tract or fistula, opening present anteriorly in neck just above the clavicle
- Young adult: trauma or viral infection provokes initial appearance, at the angle of mandible

Imaging Features

- CT or MR imaging scans: unilocular, "cystic" mass in the posterior submandibular space at the angle of the mandible (**Fig. 5**)
- Will displace the submandibular gland anteromedially, sternomastoid muscle posterolaterally, and carotid space contents posteromedially as the cyst grows[6]

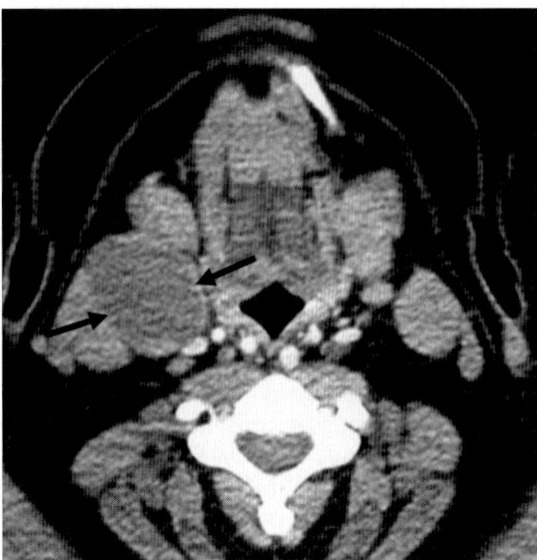

Fig. 5. Axial postcontrast CT image at the level of the floor of the mouth demonstrates a rounded cystic structure (*arrows*) anterolateral to the carotid vessels, causing anterior displacement of the right submandibular gland and posterolateral displacement of the right sternocleidomastoid muscle. This image was a pathology-proven second branchial cleft cyst.

Suprahyoid thyroglossal duct cysts

Clinical Features

- Suprahyoid thyroglossal duct cysts are most commonly nonodontogenic cysts and account for 70% of congenital neck abnormalities.[14,15]
- Suprahyoid thyroglossal duct cysts may occur anywhere along the course of thyroglossal duct or can involve the entire length of the duct from base of tongue (foramen cecum) to the thyroid gland.
- Secretions from epithelial lining into any persistent duct remnants can give rise to thyroglossal duct cyst.
- Suprahyoid thyroglossal duct cysts are about 65% infrahyoid, 15% level of hyoid bone, 20% suprahyoid.[16]
- Infrahyoid thyroglossal duct cysts tend to be paramedian; suprahyoid thyroglossal duct cysts often midline between bellies of anterior digastric muscles, embedded within or lying below the mylohyoid sling[15]
- Suprahyoid thyroglossal duct cysts may also present as masses in the floor of the mouth, and 1% to 2% of thyroglossal duct cysts are reported to be intralingual[17]

Imaging Features

- Imaging varies based on the protein content and with infection.

- Less than 1% of thyroglossal duct abnormalities are associated with coexisting carcinoma, papillary carcinoma.
- About 95% of thyroglossal duct carcinomas are thyrogenic and 5% are squamous.

Lingual thyroid

Clinical Features

- Thyroid gland normally descends from the foramen cecum area of the tongue base to the lower cervical neck.
- Failure to descend completely results in residual thyroid tissue along the thyroglossal duct tract.

Imaging Features

- CT or MR imaging: mass extends from midline mucosal surface of the tongue base into the medial sublingual space.
- Tongue is the most common location (90% of ectopic thyroid tissue).
- Most occur in the midline dorsum, with rare cases of involvement of the entire tongue.[18,19]
- CT: mass appears as a hyperdense mass on noncontrast and postcontrast studies with attenuation similar to that of the normal thyroid gland (**Fig. 6**).

Vascular lesions

There are 2 major types of vascular lesion in the neck: vascular tumor and vascular malformations (Mulliken and Glowacki classification). This classification is based on the natural history, cellular turnover, and histology of these lesions.[20]

Vascular tumors (hemangiomas)

Clinical Features

- Neoplastic lesions with increased proliferation and turnover of endothelial cells, mast cells fibroblasts, and macrophages[21]
- Most common tumors of the head and neck in infancy and childhood
- Account for 7% to 12% of all benign soft tissue tumors[22,23]
- Present in early infancy, enlarge rapidly, and involute by late childhood or early adolescence
- Often seen in the mucosal area and the deeper sublingual space[6]
- Often distinctive vascular hue to the skin overlying the lesion

Imaging Features

- CT: intense enhancement
- MR imaging: solid component demonstrates signal intensity isointense or slightly hyperintense to muscle on T1-weighted sequence and a higher signal on T2-weighted images[24]

Vascular malformations Vascular malformations are true congenital vascular anomalies that are almost always present at birth but may not manifest clinically until later in infancy or early childhood. These lesions demonstrate slow steady growth and do not regress or involute. There is sometimes rapid enlargement of these lesions in association with trauma, infection, or endocrine changes, such as during puberty or pregnancy.[25] Vascular malformations are classified based on the primary type of anomalous vessel involved: capillary, venous, arterial, and lymphatic malformations.[26,27]

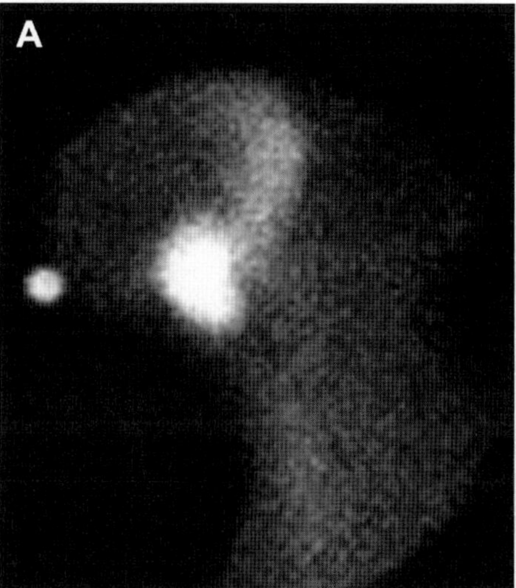

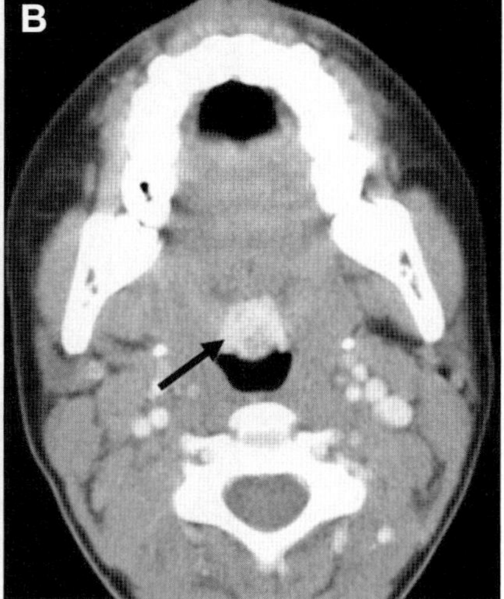

Fig. 6. (*A, B*) Lingual thyroid. Axial CT scan at the level of the foramen cecum/base of tongue in a 20-year-old woman demonstrates a large hyperdense structure (*black arrow*). Radioiodine scan demonstrates uptake at the level of foramen cecum consistent with a lingual thyroid. No thyroid tissue was seen in the rest of the neck.

Capillary malformations

Clinical Features

- Low-flow lesions, previously referred to as port-wine stains, are included, as well as capillary hemangiomas and nevus flammeus
- Underlying cheek, lip, and gingiva may be affected in the oral cavity and may be associated with gingival hypertrophy or chronic hemorrhage.[5,28]

Imaging Features

- Not commonly performed for evaluation of these lesions

Venous malformations

Clinical Features

- Most commonly affect the oral cavity and were earlier termed cavernous hemangiomas
- Unlike true hemangiomas, may involve bone and do not involute[24]
- Can infiltrate along the fascial planes and may also be entirely intramuscular[29,30]

Imaging Features (**Fig. 7**)

- CT: Imaging appears as isoattenuating to muscle and demonstrating various patterns of enhancement.[31]
- MR imaging: Imaging appears as iso-intense to hyperintense to muscle on T1-weighted images, hyperintense on T2-weighted images, and usually shows enhancement following contrast administration (often in a progressive delayed manner).
- Identifying areas of high signal, representing venous lakes, and the presence of phleboliths are helpful features in the diagnosis of venous malformation.[23,32,33]

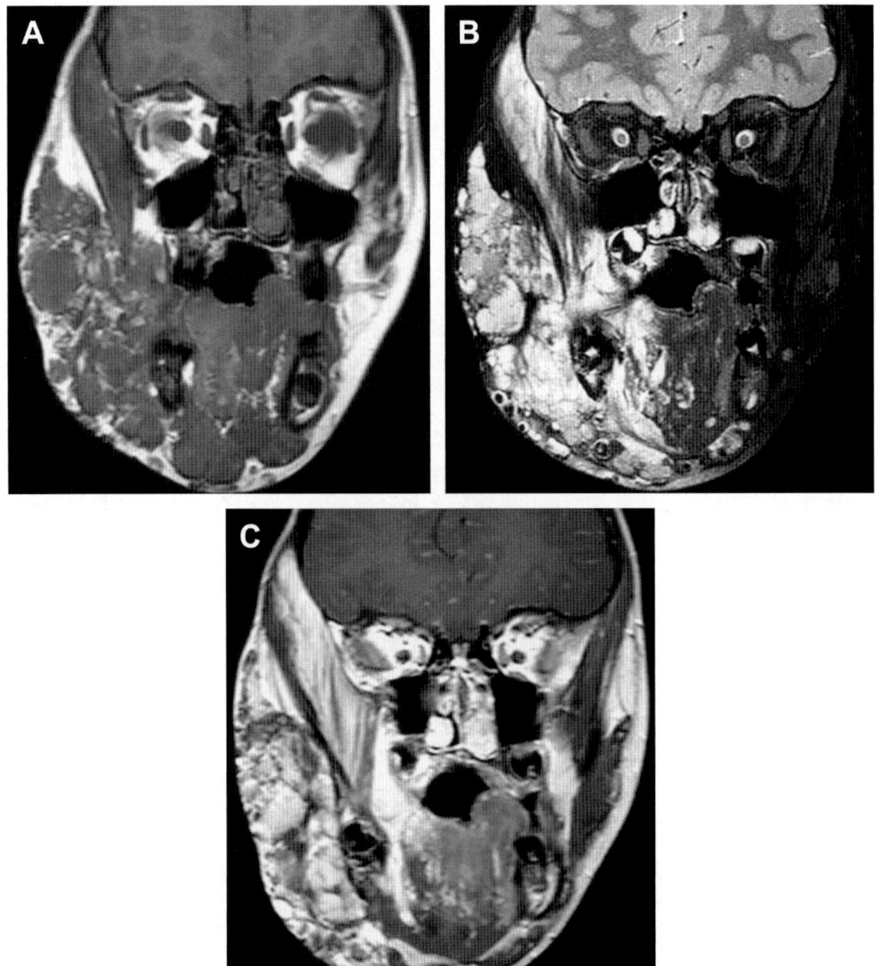

Fig. 7. (*A–C*) Venolymphatic malformation. Coronal T1, T2, and postcontrast T1 sequences demonstrate a large, partially enhancing multispatial, multiloculated cystic lesion consistent with a venolymphatic malformation.

Arteriovenous malformations

Clinical Features

- High-flow malformations and angiographically characterized by rapid flow and enlarged tortuous arteries and draining veins
- Result from abnormal blood vessel morphogenesis and are not very commonly encountered in the oral cavity

Imaging Features

- MR imaging: the enlarged vessels appear as flow voids on T1-weighted and T2-weighted images.

Lymphatic malformation (lymphangiomas)

Clinical Features

- Most are congenital in origin; some are acquired and present later in life[34,35]
- Most often extend through multiple spatial compartments.

Imaging Features

- CT: single-septated or multiseptated fluid-filled masses with low-density and variable enhancement depending on the presence of co-existing venous malformations[36]
- MR imaging: fluid signal on all imaging sequences unless there is superinfection, high-protein content, or hemorrhage[37,38]

Combined vascular malformations Combined vascular malformations that share features of both high-flow and low-flow lesions, including capillary-venous, veno-lymphatic, and arteriovenous malformations, have been described in a subgroup of patients.[39] For example, some lesions will demonstrate serpiginous flow voids characteristic of an arterial malformation and a soft tissue infiltrating component seen in a venous malformation.[27]

Epidermoid/dermoid cysts

Clinical Features

- Dermoid cysts can be classified into 3 forms: epidermoid, dermoid, and teratoid forms.
- The term dermoid cyst is often used to refer to all 3 types of lesions.[5]
- Epidermoid cysts are lined by simple squamous epithelium.
- Dermoid cysts contain various skin appendages, such as hair, sebaceous glands, and sweat glands.[6]
- It is important to distinguish them histologically because epidermoid cysts do not have malignant potential, but dermoid/teratoid cysts do have malignant potential.[40]
- In the oral cavity, epidermoid/dermoid cysts most commonly involve floor of the mouth (sublingual, submental, submandibular regions) with about 52% occurring in the sublingual region, 26% in the submental region, and 6% in the submandibular regions.[5]
- Dermoid cysts also occur in other areas, including the lips, tongue, buccal mucosa, but less frequently.

Imaging Features

- On imaging, in the absence of fat globules, epidermoids and dermoid cysts are indistinguishable.
- CT: epidermoids appear as low-density, well-circumscribed unilocular masses.
- MR imaging:
  a. Epidermoid cysts are of low signal on T1 images and high signal on T2 images.
  b. Compound dermoid cysts have a variable appearance, depending on their fat content (**Fig. 8**). Can present as multiple low-attenuation nodules due to coalescence of fat globules within the fluid matrix, giving it a sack-of-marbles appearance, which is pathognomonic for a dermoid cyst.[37]

Infection/Inflammation

Infections in the oral cavity can result from dental infections or stenosis or calculi within the salivary ductal systems. Dental manipulation, especially along the lower alveolar ridge, can also result in infection. Because the roots of the second and third molars lie below the mylohyoid ridge, infections involving these molars involve the submandibular space, whereas infections involving the first molar and premolars involve the sublingual spaces because they are above the mylohyoid ridge.[5]

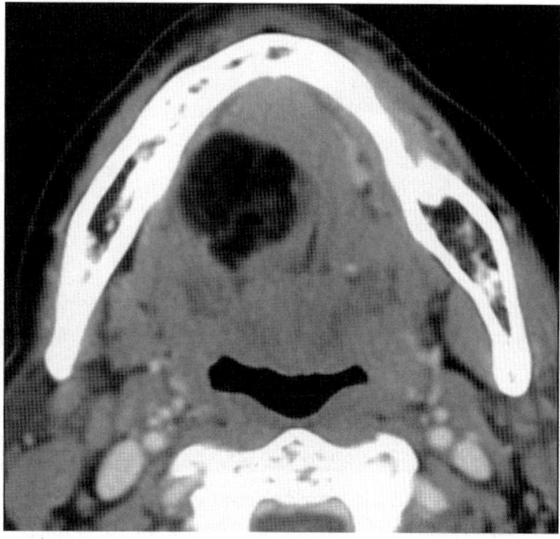

Fig. 8. Fat-containing lesion in the floor of the mouth in a 28-year-old man is consistent with dermoid.

Ludwig's angina

Clinical Features

- Extensive infection of the floor of the mouth with infections of the mandibular molars accounting for 90% of the reported cases
- Severe form of cellulitis that occurs 2 to 4 days after dental extraction from the lower alveolar ridge that involves both the sublingual and the submandibular spaces and is often bilateral[6]
- Spreads by contiguity and can result in gangrene, serosanguinous phlegmon, and abscesses in the sublingual and submandibular spaces

Imaging Features (**Fig. 9**)

- Can determine airway patency, document presence of dental infection and possible drainable neck abscesses[41]
- CT recommended over MR imaging in the evaluation of sublingual and submandibular infection due to better detection of

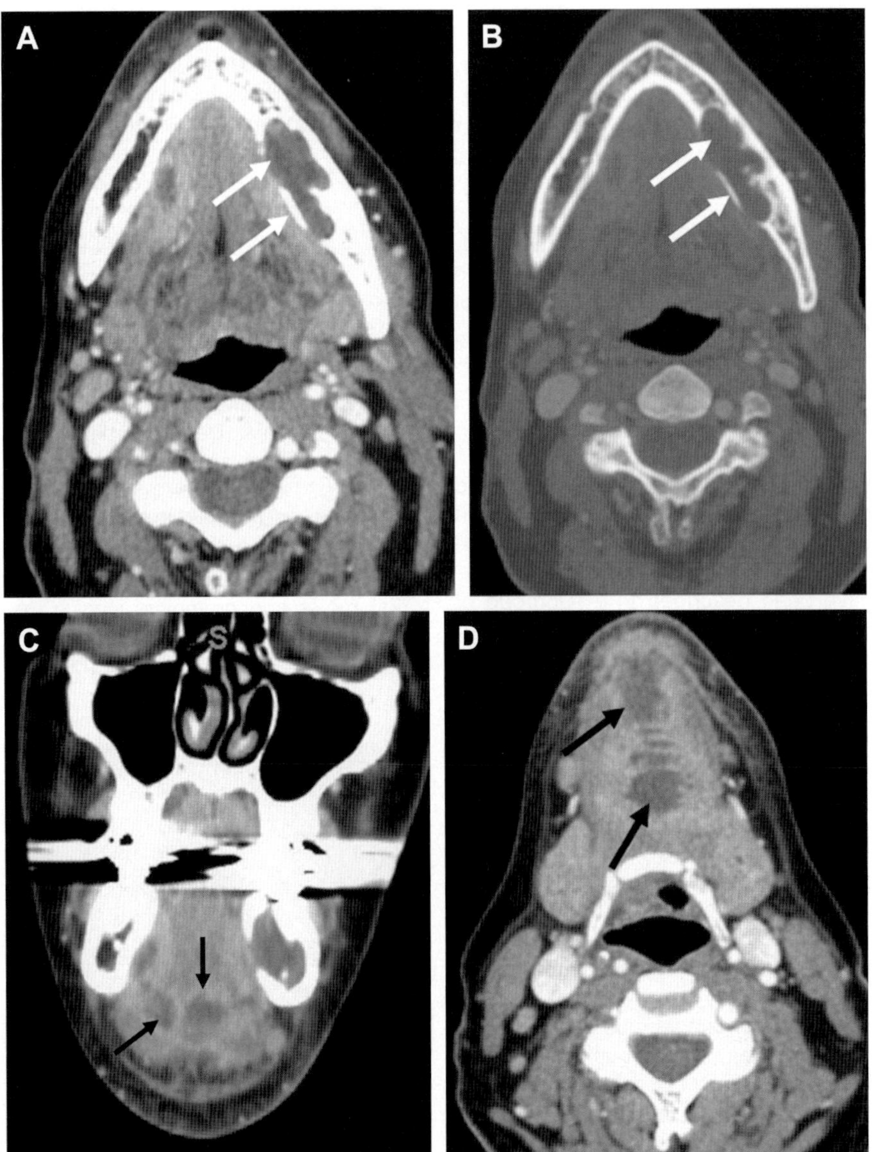

Fig. 9. (*A–D*) Ludwig angina from odontogenic infection. Axial and coronal postcontrast CT scans in a 38-year-old man with severe odynophagia demonstrate a large lytic area with irregular margins in the left mandible (*white arrows*) and associated extensive inflammatory changes (cellulitis) involving the floor of the mouth. Areas of central hypodensity with peripheral enhancement in the oral tongue and floor of mouth (*black arrows*).

precipitating factors, such as calculi and identification of areas of drainable pus[6]

Ranula

Clinical Features

- Also known as mucous retention cysts or mucoceles of the floor of the mouth
- Consists of 2 types: simple ranula and diving or plunging ranula
- Simple ranula:
  a. Postinflammatory retention cyst of the sublingual glands or the minor salivary glands of the sublingual space and has an epithelial lining
  b. Form usually caused by obstruction of the minor salivary gland or of the sublingual gland
- Diving or plunging ranula:
  a. Results if the ranula becomes large and ruptures from the sublingual space into the submandibular space
  b. Does not have an epithelial lining and is actually a pseudocyst lined by dense connective or granulation tissue
  c. Although most of the ruptured ranulas decompress posteriorly into the submandibular space, they can also extend into the adjacent upper cervical soft tissues

Imaging Features

- Simple ranula (**Fig. 10**) appears on imaging as a nonenhancing unilocular cystic mass in the sublingual space
- Diving ranula (**Fig. 11**) appears on imaging as a tail in the sublingual space (tail sign) with the bulk of the ruptured cyst (pseudocyst) seen in the submandibular space[6]
- Diving ranula versus second branchial cleft cysts: bulk of the diving ranula lies medial to the submandibular gland and displaces it laterally. Second branchial cleft cysts often located posterior to the gland and displace it anteriorly.[5]

Other inflammatory lesions in the sublingual and submandibular spaces

Occasionally, sialoliths (**Fig. 12**), trauma, or tumoral obstruction can lead to submandibular gland duct obstruction, leading to extravasation of the mucus in the surrounding tissues, eventually leading to cysts lined by granulation tissue and termed mucoceles of the extravasation type. A unilocular lymphatic malformation and epidermoid cyst can have similar imaging features and cannot be reliably differentiated on imaging alone. Other differential considerations of cystic-appearing masses in the sublingual and submandibular spaces include dermoids and thyroglossal duct cysts.[5]

Benign Tumors

Soft tissue tumors

Some of the common benign soft tissue tumors of the oral cavity include pleomorphic adenomas, aggressive fibromatosis, rhabdomyomas, lipomas, and nerve sheath tumors.

Pleomorphic adenomas

Clinical Features

- Most occur in the parotid gland; 8% arise in the submandibular gland, 0.5% in the sublingual gland, and 6.5% in the minor salivary glands

Imaging Features

- CT: pleomorphic adenomas are well-defined, homogenous, and slightly hyperdense to muscle on noncontrast images and do not demonstrate significant enhancement.
- MR imaging: pleomorphic adenomas are isointense to muscle on T1 images and become hyperintense on T2-weighted sequences.

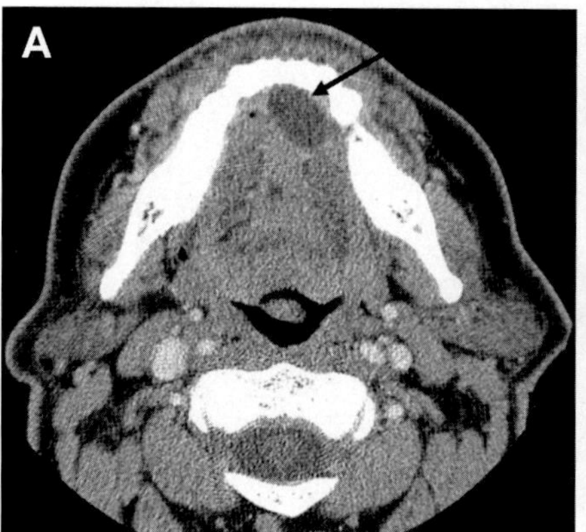

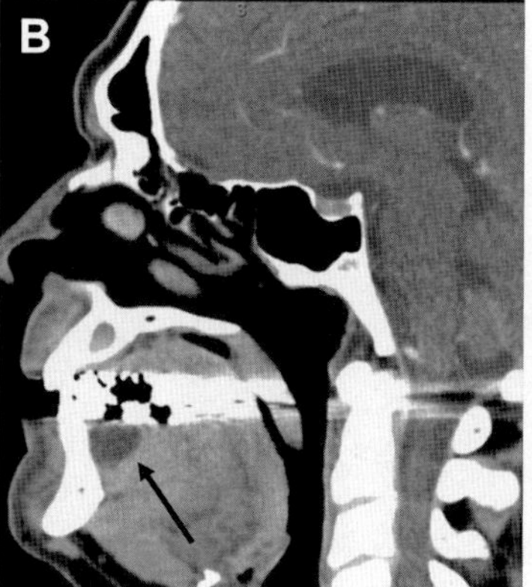

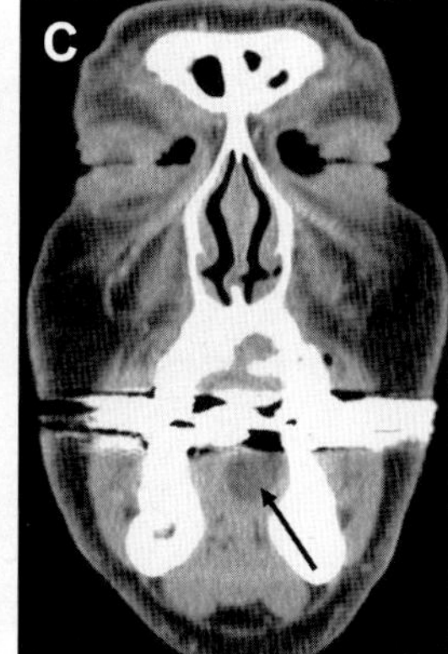

Fig. 10. (*A–C*) Simple ranula. Axial, sagittal, and coronal images at the floor of the mouth demonstrate a well-defined hypodense lesion (*black arrows*) in the left sublingual space consistent with a simple ranula.

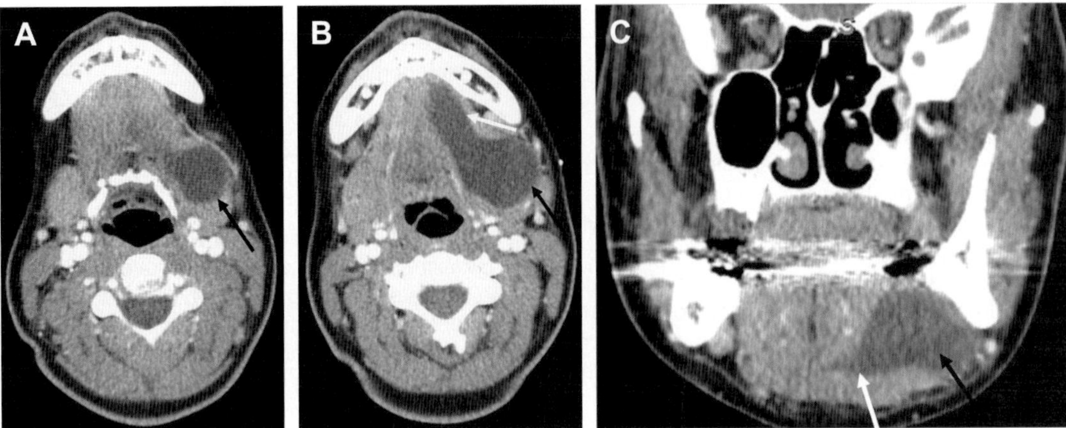

Fig. 11. (*A–C*) Diving ranula. Axial and coronal contrast-enhanced CT images reveal a cystic lesion in the submandibular region (*black arrows*) with a tail-like extension (*white arrow*) into the sublingual space.

Aggressive fibromatosis

Clinical Features

- About 11% of infantile fibromatosis occur in the extracranial head and neck, mainly in young children.
- Neck and supraclavicular regions are most commonly affected and the oral cavity is involved less frequently.
- Aggressive fibromatosis arise as solitary masses within the skeletal muscle or in the adjacent fascia, aponeurosis, or periosteum.

Imaging Features

- Variable signal intensity on MR imaging, demonstrates some degree of enhancement, sometimes making it inseparable from adjacent muscles[5]

Fibro-osseous lesions

Fibro-osseous lesions demonstrate replacement of bone with benign fibrous tissue containing various amounts of calcified or mineralized material. They are of 2 types: fibrous dysplasia, which results because of idiopathic arrest in the normal maturation of bone at the woven bone stage, and other lesions that are thought to originate from the periodontal ligament. Some of the common lesions belonging to the second group include central cementifying fibromas and periapical, focal, or florid cemento-osseous dysplasias.[42,43] Torus palatinus

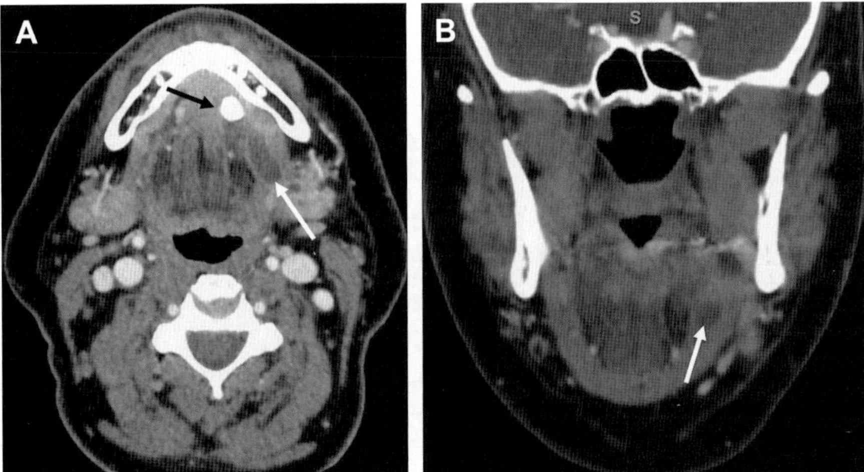

Fig. 12. (*A, B*) Sialolithiasis with sialectasia. Axial and coronal CT images in a 33-year-old woman with intermittent oral pain demonstrate a hyperdense calculus in the left sublingual space (*black arrow*) with proximal tubular dilatation of the Wharton duct (*white arrows*).

is a benign thickening of the cortical and medullary bone on the oral surface of the hard palate.

Fibrous dysplasia

Clinical Features

- Fibrous dysplasia can be monostotic or polyostotoic.
- Of the monostotic form, about 25% involve the head and neck, the maxilla and mandible being the common sites and about 40% to 60% of patients with polyostotic fibrous dysplasia have involvement of the skull and facial bones.[5]

Imaging Features (**Fig. 13**)

The plain radiographic features have been classified into 3 patterns: pagetoid (56%), sclerotic (23%), and radiolucent or cystic (21%).[26] CT reveals ground glass appearance and significant bone expansion.

Central cemento-ossifying fibromas

- Ossifying fibromas: primarily osteoid tissue (**Fig. 14**)
- Cementifying fibromas: primarily connective tissue
- Cement-ossifying fibromas: combination of osteoid formation and cementum-like tissue within the stroma.[5]

Benign odontogenic lesions

Clinical Features

- Radicular cyst (periodontal, periapical cyst): most common odontogenic cyst (**Fig. 15**)
    a. Arises from the apical end of an erupted, devitalized, infected tooth in a preexisting periapical granuloma[44]
- Follicular cysts
    a. 95% are dentigerous cysts and develop from the enamel organ of the unerupted tooth after the crown has developed.
    b. Remaining 5% represent primordial cysts and result from degeneration of enamel organ within the substance of the tooth crown.[5]

Odontogenic keratocysts and ameloblastomas are benign, locally aggressive lesions.

Odontogenic keratocysts

Clinical Features

- Contain keratin and occur 2 to 4 times more often in the mandible than in the maxilla
- Associated with basal cell nevus (Gorlin syndrome) and Marfan syndrome

Imaging Features

- MR imaging: variable signal intensity on T1-weighted images depending on the amounts of epithelial debris and blood degradation products, heterogeneous and intermediate signal intensity on T2-weighted sequences, and demonstrate weak enhancement with a thin wall[45]

Ameloblastomas

Clinical Features

- Occur in the mandible about 85% of the time
- Thought to arise from enamel organlike tissue composed of epithelial elements

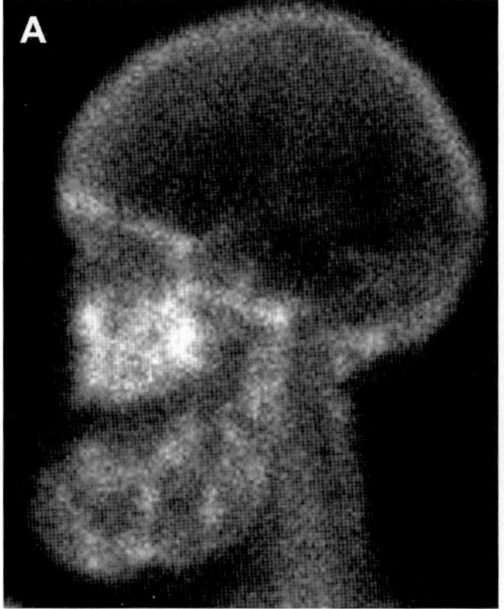

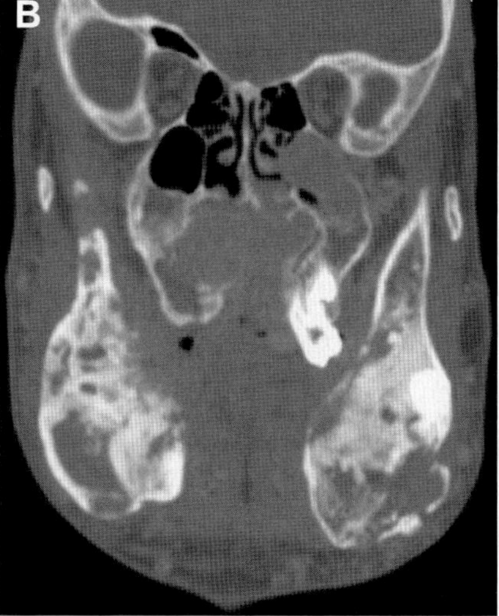

Fig. 13. (*A, B*) Polyostotic fibrous dysplasia, cherubism. Coronal CT scan at the level of the mandible demonstrates abnormal expansion of the mandibular condyles/rami/body with areas of sclerosis and cystic lucencies consistent with fibrous dysplasia. Bone scan demonstrates abnormal thickening, enlargement, and uptake in the mandible.

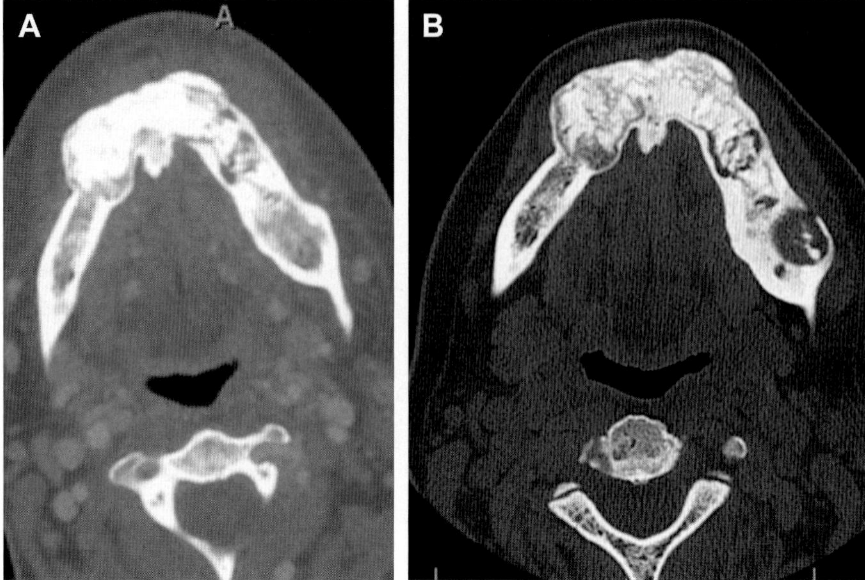

Fig. 14. (*A, B*) Cemento-osseous dysplasia. Axial images at the level of the mandible demonstrate irregular expansion of the mandible with areas of sclerosis and lucency in a patient with proven cement-osseous dysplasia.

Imaging Features (**Fig. 16**)

- CT: unilocular initially in younger individuals but become multiloculated (soap bubble), expansile neoplasms as the patient ages
- MR imaging: intermediate signal intensity on T1-weighted images, often isointense to muscle and higher signal on T2-weighted images. Postcontrast images demonstrate marked enhancement of the solid portions of the lesion.[45]

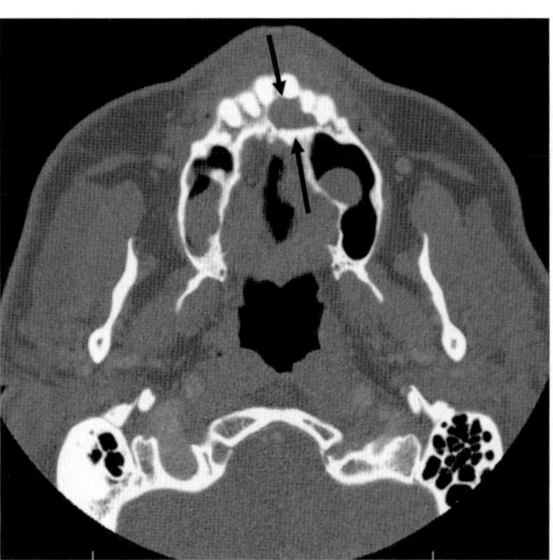

Fig. 15. Maxillary odontogenic cyst. Axial CT scan at the level of the maxilla in a 54-year-old woman demonstrates periapical lucencies (*black arrows*) involving the left central and lateral incisors consistent with periapical abscesses.

Malignant Tumors

Squamous cell carcinoma (SCC) accounts for 90% of all malignant oral cavity lesions and usually affects men aged 50 to 70 years with a long history of alcohol and tobacco abuse.[46,47] Other primary malignancies in this region include minor salivary gland tumors, such as adenoid cystic carcinoma, adenocarcinoma, mucoepidermoid carcinoma, lymphomas, and other rare sarcomas, including synovial sarcoma, liposarcoma, and rhabdomyosarcoma.[5]

Squamous cell carcinoma

Clinical Features

- Mucosa of the oropharynx, posterior to the circumvallate papillae, is derived from endoderm and the mucosa of the oral cavity is derived from ectoderm elements.
- SCC arising from the oral cavity tends to be affected by less aggressive lesions, whereas the SCC arising from the oropharynx tends to be affected by more aggressive, less well-differentiated carcinomas.[16,30]

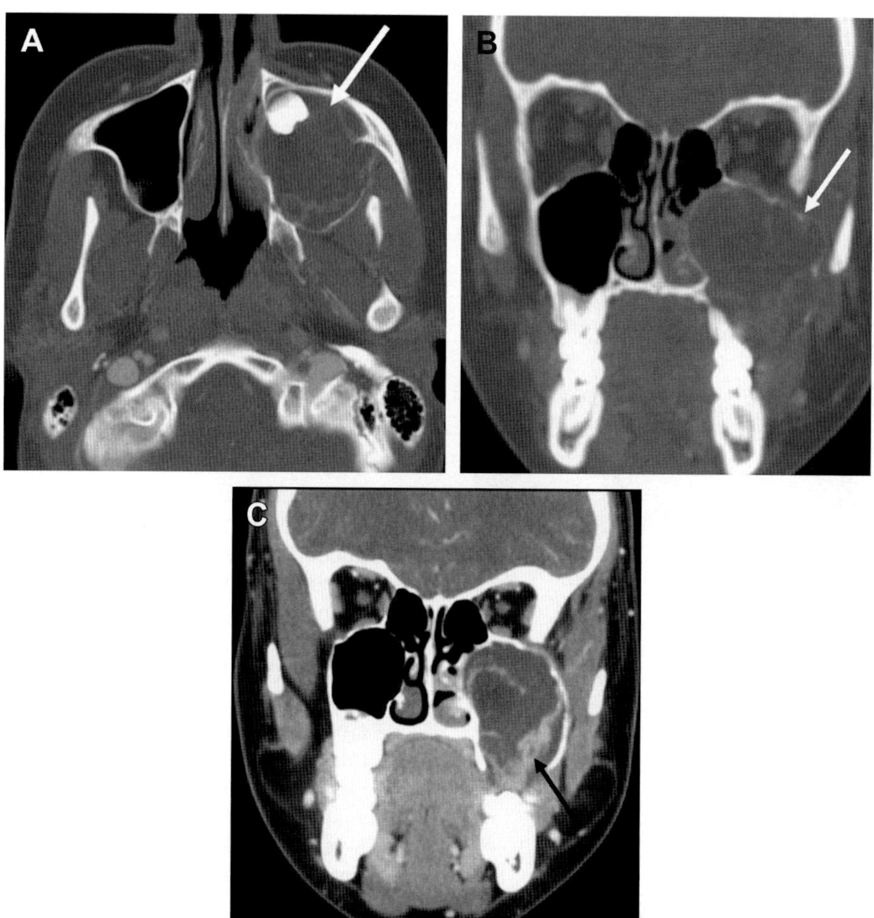

Fig. 16. (*A–C*) Ameloblastoma. Axial and coronal postcontrast images in a 64-year-old man with ameloblastoma demonstrate a large multiloculated expansile lucent lesion (*white arrows*) with thick enhancing septae and solid portions of enhancement (*black arrow*).

- Three of the most commonly affected intraoral areas include the floor of the mouth, ventrolateral tongue, and soft palate complex.[46,48]
- The soft palate complex comprises the soft palate proper, retromolar trigone, and anterior tonsillar pillar.[5]

Imaging Features

- Goal of imaging is to detect deep or submucosal extent.
- Staging of primary malignancies of the oral cavity is based on TNM system developed by the American Joint Commission on Cancer Staging.[49]
- With involvement of the floor of the mouth there is a potential for involvement of nerves and vessels within the neurovascular bundles, which would have adverse effects on overall patient survival because of distant spread of disease.[50,51]
- It is important to identify the presence of osseous involvement because this would classify the lesion as a stage T4 and a contraindication for treatment with wide local excision.[52]
- In oral tongue SCC (**Fig. 17**), it is very important to assess the extent of the tumor in relation to the midline and also involvement of the extrinsic musculature. Invasion across the midline would indicate that total glossectomy is necessary for curative resection or a nonsurgical organ preservation therapy is required.[5]

Other malignant tumors of the oral cavity

Other less common malignancies of the oral cavity include lymphoma, adenoid cystic carcinoma, and mucoepidermoid carcinoma. Liposarcoma and rhabdomyosarcoma are extremely rare.

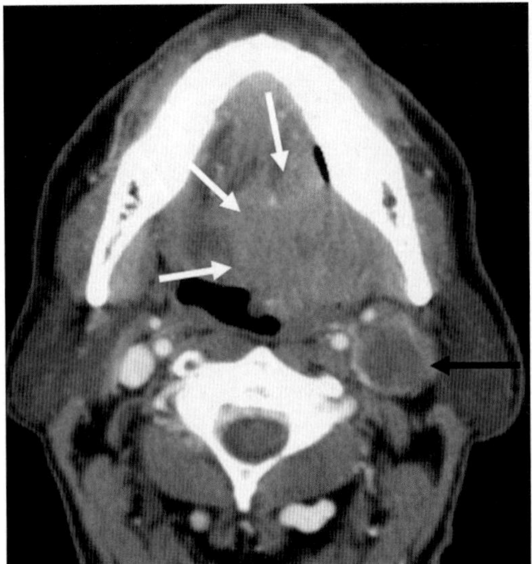

Fig. 17. Contrast-enhanced CT axial image in a 55-year-old male smoker with SCC of the tongue demonstrates an enhancing soft tissue mass involving the left oral tongue (*white arrows*) with extension to the midline. There is also a large necrotic-appearing left level 2 lymph node (*black arrow*) consistent with nodal metastasis.

Both Hodgkin and non-Hodgkin lymphomas occur in the head and neck region and the most common presenting symptom is lymph node enlargement.

Adenoid cystic carcinoma

- Accounts for only 5% of major salivary gland neoplasms but comprises about 25% of malignancies occurring in the minor salivary glands (**Fig. 18**)
- Shows a slow growth with a tendency toward extensive local invasion and a propensity for perineural spread
- Perineural extension occurs mainly along the maxillary and mandibular branches of the trigeminal nerve[5]

Mucoepidermoid carcinoma

Clinical Features

- Mucoepidermoid carcinoma arises from glandular ductal epithelium and about 30% arise from the minor salivary glands located in the buccal mucosa and palate.
- Mucoepidermoid carcinoma can be classified as low-grade, intermediate-grade, and high-grade lesions.
- Low-grade lesions tend to have a benign imaging appearance with fairly well-defined smooth margins and overall 5-year survival rate of about 90%.
- High-grade lesions are poorly circumscribed with indistinct infiltrating margins and overall 5-year survival rate of about 42%.[5]

Imaging Features

- On MR imaging, these tumors tend to be solid and demonstrate low-to-intermediate signal intensities on T1-weighted and T2-weighted images.

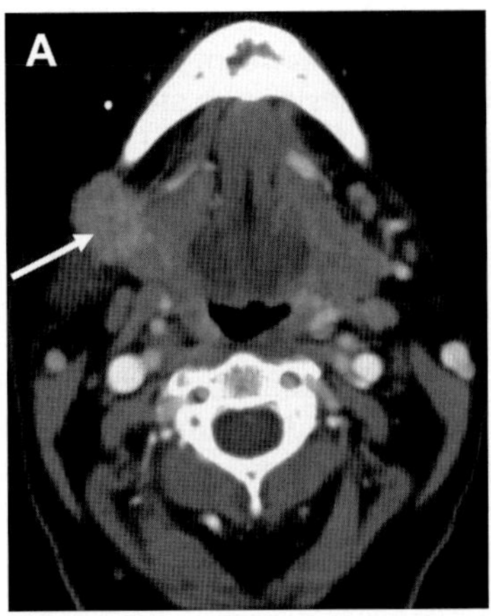

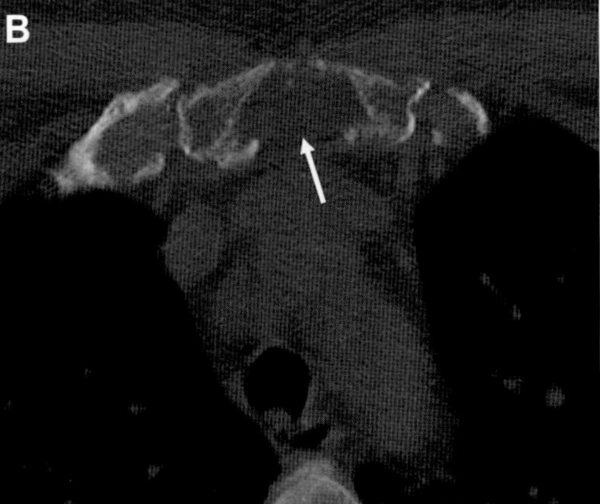

Fig. 18. (*A, B*) Contrast-enhanced CT axial image in a 60-year-old man with proven adenoid cystic carcinoma in the right submandibular gland demonstrates an irregular enhancing mass in the right submandibular gland (*arrow*). Axial bone window image at the level of the sternum shows a large lytic lesion in the manubrium (*arrow*) consistent with osseous metastatic disease.

SUMMARY

CT and MR imaging are important imaging tools for the comprehensive assessment of oral cavity pathologic abnormalities. Knowledge of the cross-sectional anatomy in multiple planes and the imaging appearances of common pathologies is crucial for providing an accurate diagnosis.

REFERENCES

1. MacDonald AJ, Harnsberger HR. Oral cavity anatomy and imaging issues. In: Harnsberger HR, Wiggins RH, Hudgins PA, et al, editors. Diagnostic imaging: head and neck. Salt Lake City (UT): Amirsys; 2004. p. 42–5, III.
2. Hollinshead W. 3rd edition. Anatomy for Surgeons. The head and neck, vol. 1. Hagerstown (NJ): Harper & Row; 1982.
3. Last RJ. Anatomy: regional and applied. 6th edition. Edinburgh (United Kingdom); London; and New York: Churchill Livingstone; 1978.
4. Gray H. Anatomy, descriptive and surgical. In: Pick TP, Howden R, editors. Philadelphia: Running Press; 1974. p. 33–1257.
5. Smoker WR. The oral cavity. In: Som PM, Curtin HD, editors. Head and neck imaging. vol. 2. St. Louis, Missouri: Mosby; 2003. p. 1055–2322.
6. Harnsberger HR. Handbook of head and neck imaging. 2nd edition. St Louis (MO): Mosby; 1995.
7. Stambuk HE, Karimi S, Lee N, et al. Oral cavity and oropharynx tumours. Radiol Clin North Am 2007; 45:1–20.
8. Mukherji SK, Isaacs DL, Creager A, et al. CT detection of mandibular invasion by squamous cell carcinoma of the oral cavity. AJR Am J Roentgenol 2001;177:237–43.
9. Beil CM, Kerberle M. Oral and oropharyngeal tumours. Eur J Radiol 2008;66:448–59.
10. Caldemeyer KS, Mathews VP, Righi PD, et al. Imaging features and clinical significance of perineural spread or extension of head and neck tumors. Radiographics 1998;18:97–110.
11. Weissman JL, Carrau RL. "Puffed-cheek" CT improves evaluation of the oral cavity. AJNR Am J Neuroradiol 2001;22:741–4.
12. Simon LL, Rubinstein D. Imaging of oral cancer. Otolaryngol Clin North Am 2006;39:307–17.
13. Law CP, Chandra RV, Hoang JK, et al. Imaging the oral cavity: key concepts for the radiologist. Br J Radiol 2011;84:944–57.
14. Thomas JR. Thyroglossal duct cysts. Ear Nose Throat J 1979;58:512–4.
15. Dolata J. Thyroglossal duct cyst in the mouth floor: an unusual location. Otolaryngol Head Neck Surg 1994;110:580–3.
16. Batsakis JG. Tumors of the head and neck: clinical and pathological considerations. 2nd edition. Baltimore (MD): Williams & Wilkins; 1979.
17. Allard RH. The thyroglossal cyst. Head Neck Surg 1982;5:134–46.
18. Douglas PS, Baker AW. Lingual thyroid. Br J Oral Maxillofac Surg 1994;32:123–4.
19. Wertz ML. Management of undescended lingual and subhyoid thyroid glands. Laryngoscope 1974;84:507–21.
20. Mulliken JB, Glowacki J. Hemangiomas and vascular malformation in infant and children: a classification based on endothelial characteristics. Plast Reconstr Surg 1982;69:412–20.
21. Mancuso AA, Harnsberger HR, Dillon WP. Workbook for MRI and CT of the head and neck. 2nd edition. Baltimore (MD): Williams & Wilkins; 1989. p. 163.
22. Watson WL, McCarthy WD. Blood and lymphatic vessel tumors: report of 1056 cases. Surg Gynecol Obstet 1940;71:569–88.
23. Bowers RE, Graham EA, Tomlinson KM. The natural history of the strawberry nevus. Arch Dermatol 1960;82:667–73.
24. Meyer JS, Hoffer FA, Barnes PD, et al. Biological classification of soft-tissue vascular anomalies: MR correlation. AJR Am J Roentgenol 1991;157: 559–64.
25. Mulliken JB. Vascular malformations of trhe head and neck. In: Mulliken JB, Young AE, editors. Vascular birthmarks, hemangiomas and malformations. Philadelphia: WB Saunders; 1988. p. 301–42.
26. Fries JW. The roentgen features of fibrous dysplasia of skull and facial bones. A critical analysis of 39 pathologically proved cases. AJR Am J Roentgenol 1957;77:71–80.
27. Baker LL, Dillion WP, Hieshima GB, et al. Hemangiomas and vascular malformations of the head and neck: MR characterization. AJNR Am J Neuroradiol 1993;14:307–14.
28. Mulliken JB. Classification of vascular birthmarks. In: Mulliken JB, Young AE, editors. Vascular birthmarks, hemangiomas and malformations. Philadelphia: WB Saunders; 1988. p. 24–37.
29. Elahi MM, Parnes L, Fox A. Hemangioma of the masseter muscle. J Otolaryngol 1992;21:177–9.
30. Paparella MM, Shumrick DA. Otolaryngology, vol. 3. Head and neck. Philadelphia: WB Saunders; 1980.
31. Braun IF, Hoffman JC Jr, Reede D, et al. Computed tomography of the buccomasseteric region. II. Pathology. AJNR Am J Neuroradiol 1984;5:611–6.
32. Itoh K, Nishimura K, Togashi K, et al. MR imaging of cavernous hemangiomas of the face and neck. J Comput Assist Tomogr 1986;10:831–5.
33. Gelbert F, Riche MC, Reizine D, et al. MR imaging of head and neck vascular malformations. J Magn Reson Imaging 1991;1:579–84.

34. Kennedy TL. Cystic hygroma-lymphangioma: a rare and still unclear entity. Laryngoscope 1989;99:1–10.
35. Yuh WT, Gleason TJ, Tali ET, et al. Traumatic cervical cystic lymphangioma in an adult. Ann Otol Rhinol Laryngol 1993;102:564–6.
36. Caro PA, Mahboubi S, Fearber EN. Computed tomography in the diagnosis of lymphangiomas in infants and children. Clin Imaging 1991;15:41–6.
37. Koeller KK, Alamo L, Adair CF, et al. Congenital cystic masses of the neck: radiologic-pathologic correlation. Radiographics 1999;19:121–46.
38. Yuh WT, Buehner LS, Kao SC, et al. Magnetic resonance imaging of pediatric head and neck cystic hygromas. Ann Otol Rhinol Laryngol 1991;100:737–42.
39. Kaban L, Mulliken JB. Vascular anomalies of the maxillofacial region. J Oral Maxillofac Surg 1986;44:201–13.
40. King RC, Smith BR, Burk JL. Dermoid cysts in the floor of the mouth. Oral Surg Oral Med Oral Pathol 1994;78:567–76.
41. Nguyen VD, Potter JL, Hersh-Schick MR. Ludwig angina: an uncommon and potentially lethal neck infection. AJNR Am J Neuroradiol 1992;13:215–9.
42. Mohammadi-Araghi H, Haery C. Fibro-osseous lesions of craniofacial bones. Radiol Clin North Am 1993;31:121–34.
43. Waldron CA. Fibro-osseous lesions of the jaws. J Oral Maxillofac Surg 1993;51:828–35.
44. DelBalso AM. Lesions of the jaws. Semin Ultrasound CT MR 1995;16:487–512.
45. Minami M, Kaneda T, Ozawa K, et al. Cystic lesions of the maxillomandibular region: MR imaging distinction of odontogenic keratocysts and ameloblastomas from other cysts. AJR Am J Roentgenol 1996;166:943–9.
46. Mashberg A, Samit A. Early diagnosis of asymptomatic oral and oropharyngeal squamous cancers. CA Cancer J Clin 1995;45:328–51.
47. American Joint Commission on Cancer, Beahrs OH, Henson DE, et al, editors. Manual for staging of cancer. 3rd edition. Philadelphia: JB Liippincott; 1988.
48. Crissman JD, Gluckman J, Whiteley J, et al. Squamous-cell carcinoma of the floor of the mouth. Head Neck Surg 1980;3:2–7.
49. Yarington CT. Pathology of the oral cavity. In: Paparella MM, Shumrick M, editors. Otolaryngology. Philadelphia: WB Saunders; 1980.
50. Close LG, Brown PM, Vuitch MF, et al. Microvascular invasion of the oral cavity and oropharynx. Arch Otolaryngol Head Neck Surg 1989;115:1304–9.
51. Close LG, Burns DK, Reisch J, et al. Microvascular invasion in cancer of the oral cavity and oropharynx. Arch Otolaryngol Head Neck Surg 1987;113:1191–5.
52. Mukherji SK, Pillsbury HR, Castillo M. Imaging squamous cell carcinomas of the upper aerodigestive tract: what clinicians need to know. Radiology 1997;205:629–46.

Imaging of Head and Neck Lymph Nodes

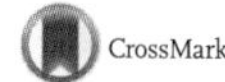

Laura B. Eisenmenger, MD[a,b], Richard H. Wiggins III, MD, CIIP, FSIIM[a,b,c,*]

KEYWORDS

• Cervical • Lymph nodes • CT • MR • PET • PET/CT • SCCa

KEY POINTS

- Knowledge of cervical lymph node anatomy, drainage pathways, and common pathology is key to cervical lymph node imaging interpretation.
- Correlation with clinical history and physical examination is vital to making the correct diagnosis or providing an appropriate differential.
- Contrast-enhanced computed tomography (CT) is considered the best modality for evaluating a neck mass of unknown cause; however, CT, MR, and PET/CT are complementary imaging modalities in the evaluation of the head and neck.

INTRODUCTION

Cervical lymph node evaluation and interpretation can be difficult for both the general radiologist and neuroradiologist alike. Lymph nodes facilitate lymph fluid transportation, filter foreign objects, and initiate an immune response, thereby making lymph nodes a location that can be affected by many different disease processes.[1] An understanding of cervical lymph node anatomy, lymph node drainage pathways, and common pathology (disease processes or abnormalities) is the foundation for interpretation of lymph node pathology. A location-specific approach to lymph node pathology as well as knowledge of various lymph node morphologies can further refine a differential diagnosis. Clinical information and physical examination can provide critical diagnostic information when combined with imaging.

This article reviews cervical lymph node anatomy as well as drainage pathways. Specific nodal morphologies with associated differential diagnoses and imaging findings are discussed. The article concludes with discussion of rare diseases affecting cervical lymph nodes as well as the importance of imaging in head and neck (HN) cancer.

NORMAL CERVICAL LYMPH NODE ANATOMY

Cervical lymph nodes can be classified based on basic anatomic location (such as groups and chains) or described with neoplastic processes using the formal American Joint Committee on Cancer's (AJCC) criteria.[1,2] The simple anatomic description of lymph node groups includes the submental group located inferior to the anterior mandible (**Fig. 1**A). The submandibular group of lymph nodes is located near the submandibular glands at the angles of the mandible (see **Fig. 1**B). The parotid lymph nodes include the intraglandular nodes (**Fig. 2**A) within the fascia circumscribing the parotid space (PS). Lymph nodes located within the subcutaneous tissues near the external auditory canal (EAC) can be referred to as *preauricular nodes* when found anterior to the EAC and *postauricular nodes* when found posterior to the EAC (see **Fig. 2**B).

The authors have no disclosures.

[a] Department of Radiology, University of Utah, 30 North 1900 East #1A071, Salt Lake City, UT 84132-2140, USA; [b] Department of Biomedical Informatics, University of Utah, 30 North 1900 East #1A071, Salt Lake City, UT 84132-2140, USA; [c] Division of Otolaryngology–Head and Neck Surgery, University of Utah, 30 North 1900 East #1A071, Salt Lake City, UT 84132-2140, USA

* Corresponding author. Department of Radiology, University of Utah, 30 North 1900 East #1A071, Salt Lake City, UT 84132-2140.

E-mail address: Richard.Wiggins@hsc.utah.edu

Radiol Clin N Am 53 (2015) 115–132

http://dx.doi.org/10.1016/j.rcl.2014.09.011

0033-8389/15/$ – see front matter

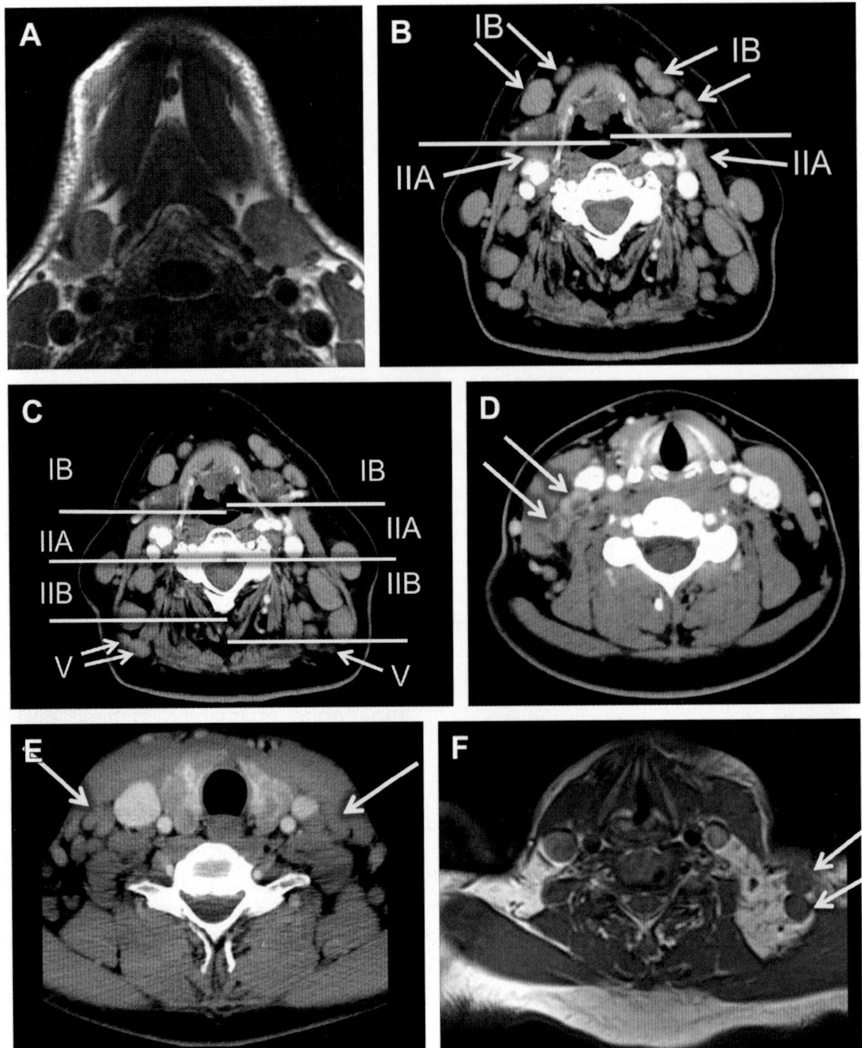

Fig. 1. (*A*) Axial T1-weighted (T1WI) MR of level IA or submental lymph node between the anterior bellies of the digastric muscles. (*B*) Axial contrast-enhanced computed tomography (CECT) of level IB and IIA lymph node enlargement in a confirmed case of non-Hodgkin lymphoma. (*C*) Axial CECT of enlarged bilateral level IB, IIA, IIB and V lymph nodes in a confirmed case of non-Hodgkin lymphoma. (*D*) Axial CECT of necrotic, right level III lymph nodes (*arrow*) in a confirmed case of squamous cell carcinoma. (*E*) Axial CECT of level IV lymph nodes (*arrow*). (*F*) Axial TIWI MR with prominent left supraclavicular (transverse cervical chain) lymph nodes (*arrow*).

A more general definition of periauricular nodes can be superficial lymph nodes near the EAC itself. The retropharyngeal space (RPS) lymph nodes include both the medial RPS nodes found in the paramedian RPS in the suprahyoid neck (SHN) and the lateral RPS nodes found lateral to the prevertebral muscles and medial to the internal jugular vein and internal carotid artery (CA) within the lateral RPS.

The facial lymph nodes include multiple nodes named for their anatomic location, such as the mandibular nodes superficial to the mandible, the buccinator nodes within the subcutaneous tissues of the cheek, the infraorbital nodes below the orbits, the malar nodes along the malar eminence, and the zygomatic nodes superficial to the zygomatic arch (see **Fig. 2**C). The occipital group of nodes is located within the subcutaneous tissues posterior and inferior to calvarium (see **Fig. 2**D). The retropharyngeal group is, as named, in the RPS (see **Fig. 2**E).

The major nodal chains within the cervical soft tissues can be thought of as 3 linear chains of lymph nodes, roughly forming a triangle on each side of the neck (**Fig. 3**A). Anteriorly, the internal jugular chain (IJC) surrounds the internal jugular

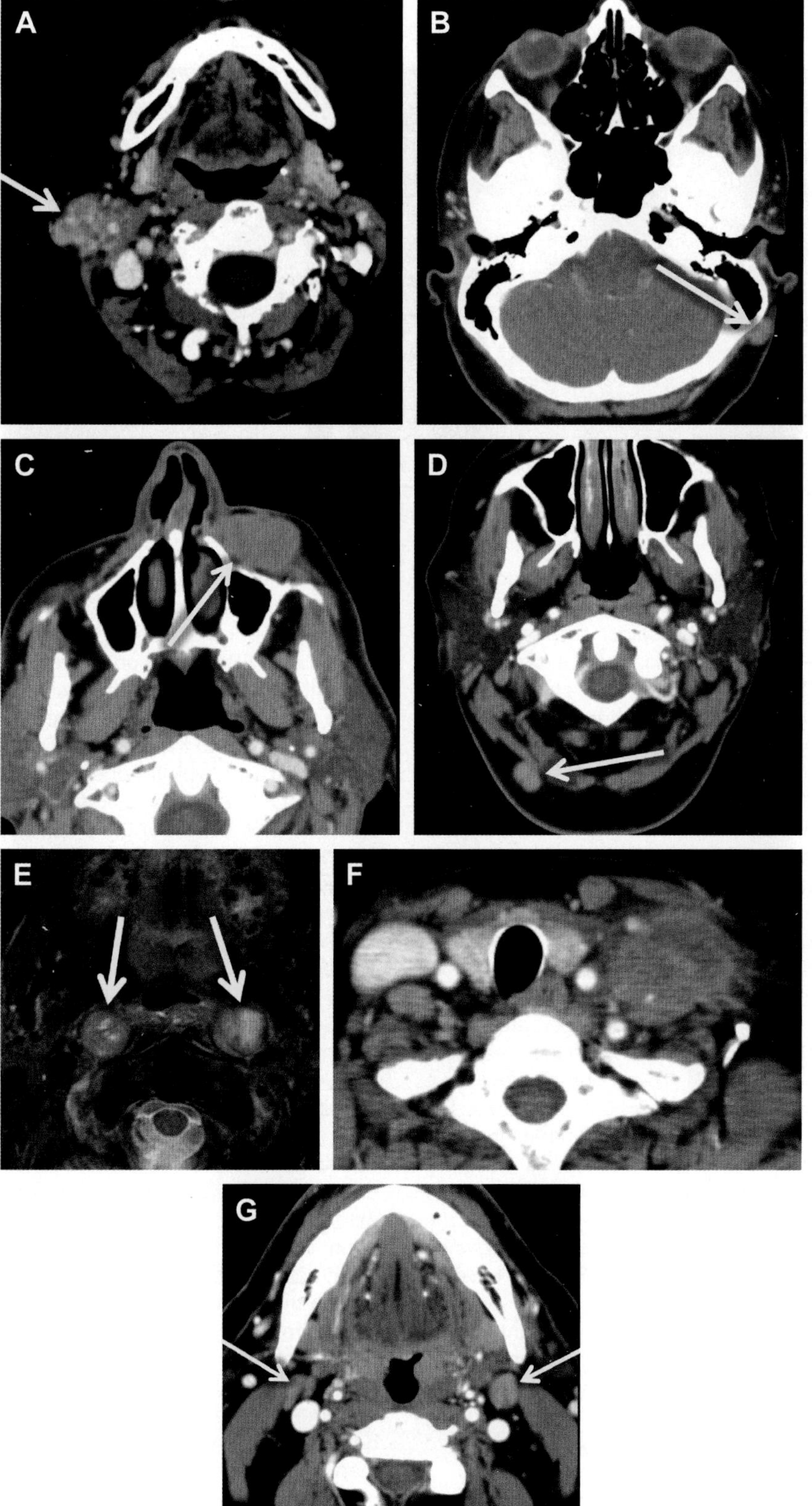

Fig. 2. (*A*) Axial contrast-enhanced computed tomography (CECT) of enlarged right parotid lymph nodes (*arrow*). (*B*) Axial CECT of an enlarged left posterior auricular lymph node (*arrow*). (*C*) Axial CECT of an enlarged left facial lymph node (*arrow*). (*D*) Axial CECT of an enlarged right occipital lymph node (*arrow*). (*E*) Axial T2-weighted MR of bilateral enlarged retropharyngeal lymph nodes (*arrow*). Specifically, these retropharyngeal nodes are also referred to as the nodes of Rouvière. (*F*) Axial CECT of an enlarged signal (Virchow) lymph node. (*G*) Axial CECT of sentinel (jugulodigastric) lymph nodes (*arrow*).

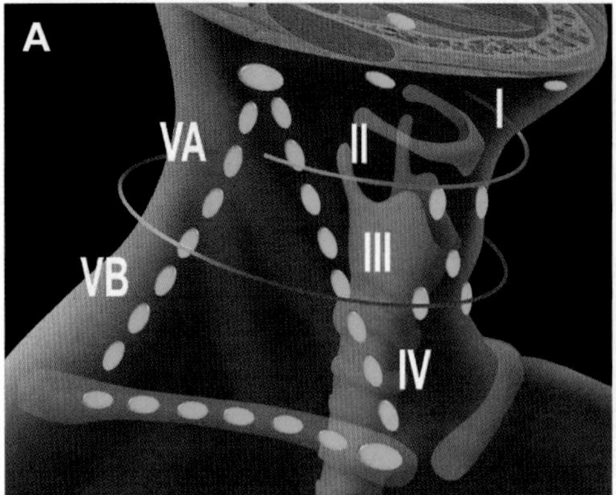

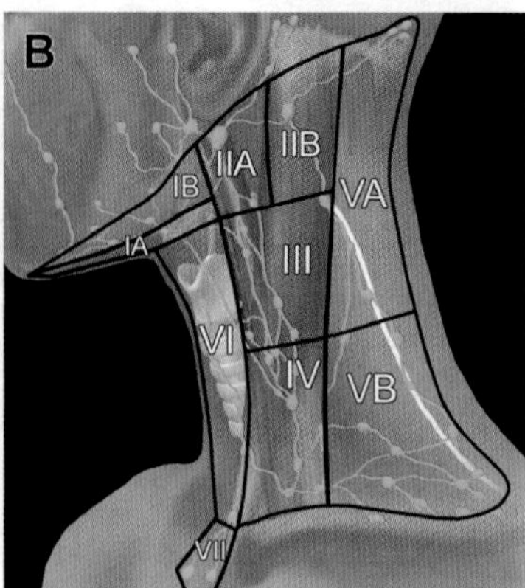

Fig. 3. (*A*) Cervical lymph node triangle made up of the internal jugular chain (anterior), the spinal accessory chain (posterior), and the transverse cervical chain (inferior). (*B*) Surgical lymph node levels.

vein (IJV) from the skull base to the thoracic inlet. Posteriorly, the spinal accessory chain (SAC) is along the course of the spinal accessory nerve across the posterior cervical space of the neck. Inferiorly, the transverse cervical chain (TCC) is along the transverse cervical artery in the supraclavicular fossa connecting the inferior aspects of internal jugular and SAC. The anterior cervical group (ACG) is divided into the prelaryngeal chain, pretracheal chain, and paratracheal chain. The prelaryngeal chain is the superficial midline chain in the cervical neck. The pretracheal chain follows the external jugular vein in the superficial fascia of the neck external to the strap muscles. The paratracheal chain follows the tracheoesophageal groove in the visceral space (VS) of the infrahyoid neck.

Cervical lymph nodes can also be categorized by surgical levels used for formal cancer treatment planning (see **Fig. 3**B). These surgical levels include 7 levels based on surgical landmarks. For imaging purposes, radiologic landmarks are used to approximate the surgical boundaries. Level I is divided into IA (the submental level) and IIA (the submandibular level). Level IA lymph nodes are found between the anterior bellies of the digastric muscles below the mandible (see **Fig. 1**A). Level IB lymph nodes are found lateral to the anterior bellies of the digastric muscles and anterior to the submandibular glands within the submandibular space (see **Fig. 1**B). Level II lymph nodes are the upper portions of the IJC and SAC, extending from the posterior belly of the digastric muscle to the hyoid.

The level II, III, and IV nodal groups extend along the IJC and are deep or anterior to the sternocleidomastoid muscle (SCM). Level IIA lymph nodes are found posterior to the posterior border of the submandibular gland (see **Fig. 1**B). These lymph nodes may be anterior, medial, lateral, or immediately posterior and adjacent to the IJV. If the lymph node is posterior to the IJV, it must be touching the IJV to be considered a level IIA node. Level IIB lymph nodes are posterior to the IJV with at least a fat plane visible between the node and the IJV, and the center of the node is located anterior to the posterior edge of the SCM (see **Fig. 1**C). Level III nodes correspond to the middle IJC nodes, extending from the hyoid bone to the inferior margin of the cricoid cartilage (see **Fig. 1**D). Level IV lymph nodes are the lower IJC nodes from the inferior margin of the cricoid cartilage to the supraclavicular fossa (see **Fig. 1**E).

The level V lymph nodes are the nodes of the posterior cervical space corresponding to the SAC, lying posterior to the posterior margin of the SCM in a coronal plane (see **Fig. 1**C). Level VA includes the upper SAC lymph nodes from the skull base to the inferior margin of the cricoid cartilage. Level VB lymph nodes are the lower SAC lymph nodes from the inferior margin of the cricoid to the supraclavicular fossa. Level VI lymph nodes are the nodes of the VS. These lymph nodes extend from the hyoid bone to the top of the manubrium including the prelaryngeal, pretracheal, and paratracheal subgroups. The level VI nodal group can be thought of as roughly all the nodal groups inferior to the hyoid bone and between the CAs; therefore, this group would also include the tracheoesophageal nodes. Level VII lymph nodes are the superior mediastinal nodes located between the CAs from the superior margin of the manubrium to the innominate vein.

It is important to note that several lymph nodes are not included in the AJCC's surgical classification but are important in patient care. These lymph nodes include the parotid, retropharyngeal, occipital, and facial node groups discussed in the group and chain anatomic classifications.

Although the term *supraclavicular lymph nodes* is common in radiology anatomic description reports, this is not a defined nodal group and incorporates portions of both levels IV and VB. From an imaging standpoint, the clavicle should be present on the imaging slice to use the term *supraclavicular node* (see **Fig. 1**F). The clinical definition of a supraclavicular fossa lymph node is one within the Ho triangle, which is outlined by 3 points: the sternal and lateral ends of the clavicle and the junction of the neck and shoulder. Although supraclavicular lymph nodes seem somewhat abstract from the imaging standpoint, supraclavicular nodes are important in cancer staging and should be accurately identified.

There are several specifically named lymph nodes present within the neck that have been associated with clinical significance. The signal (Virchow) node is a pathologic node within the left supraclavicular fossa (see **Fig. 2**F). This node is clinically significant in that if no primary tumor is evident in the neck, this left supraclavicular pathologic node may signal a primary chest or abdomen pathologic process and should be considered as a metastasis that may be carried via the thoracic duct to this nodal region. The high lateral retropharyngeal node (Rouvière node) lies within 2 cm of the skull base and is a common site of spread for nasopharyngeal carcinoma (see **Fig. 2**E). The jugulodigastric (sentinel) node is the high IJC node above the hyoid bone (see **Fig. 2**G). This node may normally be larger than surrounding nodes and will quickly enlarge with upper respiratory infectious conditions, which must be considered when deciding if this lymph node is pathologic.[1]

LYMPH NODE DRAINAGE

Lymphatic drainage patterns are important in many processes, as pathology at a certain location will usually drain to predictable nodal sites and chains. The opposite is also true, as nodal disease at certain locations can suggest a primary pathology site. Knowledge of expected lymph node spread can provide a road map leading to the source of disease. Because of the many lymphatic connections, the pattern of lymphatic spread is not definite; but certain pathways are more common. The cervical lymphatic drainage pathways are briefly discussed here.

Level I lymph nodes receive lymphatic drainage from the lips, floor of the mouth, and oral tongue. The level IA (submental) nodes normally drain into the level IB (submandibular) nodes, which usually then drain into level II. The intraparotid nodes receive lymphatic drainage from the EAC, the pinna of the ear, eustachian tube, skin of the lateral forehead and temporal region, posterior cheek, gums, and buccal mucous membrane. The parotid nodes commonly drain into the high IJC. The retropharyngeal nodes receive drainage from the sinonasal and pharyngeal mucosal surfaces and usually drain into the high IJC. Special attention should be paid to the retropharyngeal nodes as these nodes are often subclinical, with imaging being the first indicator of disease in this lymph node group.

The IJC (levels II, III, IV), as mentioned earlier, typically receive drainage from the PS, RPS, and level I nodes as well as the pharynx and facial nodes. The usual pattern of lymphatic drainage within the IJC progresses from level II to level III to level IV. The IJC then drains into the subclavian vein, the IJV, or the TCC. The SAC (level VA and level VB) receives drainage from the occipital nodes, mastoid nodes, parietal scalp, and lateral neck. The SAC nodes normally drain into the TCC. The TCC receives drainage from the IJS, SAC, subclavicular nodes, upper anterior chest wall, and skin of the anterolateral neck. The level VI (ACG) receives drainage from the VS including the larynx, thyroid, dermal lymphatics of the anterior neck, trachea, and esophagus. The ACG typically drains into the superior mediastinum and level IV nodes.

This summary is by no means the only lymphatic connections of the cervical lymph nodes, but it is a starting point to understand local nodal spread and help identify the origin of pathology. It is also important to remember, however, that some pathologies, such as thyroid carcinoma, may seem to completely ignore the normal expected lymphatic drainage, such as a thyroid carcinoma presenting with only retropharyngeal nodes.[1]

IMAGING TECHNIQUES

A common clinical presentation of abnormal cervical lymphadenopathy is a patient with a neck mass of uncertain cause. In this circumstance, contrast-enhanced computed tomography (CECT) is a recommended starting point, as it is a fast, high-quality imaging modality that is easily reproducible.[1,3,4] Size, shape, density, and location of the mass can all be determined with CECT in a matter of seconds; CECT is less affected by breathing and swallowing artifacts compared with MR. In addition, CECT can typically identify the primary site of origin and can accurately stage the nodes, search for recurrence or spread, and monitor treatment response.[1,3]

CECT of the cervical soft tissues is typically obtained helically from above the skull base through the carina. Slice thickness varies depending on the modality from 0.6 to 1.25 mm. The head should be positioned with the beam parallel to the inferior orbitomeatal line with no gantry tilt. Angled scans above and below dentition can help image around dental amalgam artifact, which may prove essential in evaluating the oral cavity and oropharynx. Images are reconstructed in soft tissue (standard) and bone algorithms (edge enhanced). Soft tissue window width (WW) near 400 and window center (WC) near 40 is preferable to allow easy differentiation of soft tissue from air, which is important in cervical pathology. Bone WW near 4000 and WC near 450 is preferable in order to differentiate osseous changes in density such as with the skull base and temporal bone. The typical kilovolt peak is near 100 kVp with a milliampere range of 100 to 800 mA depending on the body habitus and radiation minimizing techniques. Contrast administration should be delayed when evaluating the cervical soft tissues greater than that used for a CT angiography study, to allow contrast to leak into regions of pathology.[3] Please see **Box 1** for the CT protocol summary.

In the setting of a known malignancy, MR can also be used to stage the nodes, with CT and MR having approximately 80% sensitivity and specificity for detecting proven nodal metastases (**Fig. 4**).[3,5] In the SHN, MR imaging may be preferred for evaluation of the primary and to search for perineural tumor spread at the base of the skull.

When imaging the neck with MR, the skull base to at least the supraclavicular fossa should be imaged. A minimum of 3 sequences should be used with each in at least one plane. Recommended sequences include both coronal and axial T1-weighted images (T1WI), T2-weighted images (T2WI) with fat saturation (FS) (or other similar fluid bright sequence, such as short tau inversion recovery [*STIR*] in opposite planes), and postcontrasted T1WI with FS in both planes. The field of view is approximately 16 to 18 cm with a slice thickness of 3 to 4 mm and interslice gap of 0.5 to 1.0 mm. Matrix is typically 192 by 256. Surface coils should be used when possible to improve image quality, and saturation pulses will reduce vascular artifacts. Please see **Box 2** for the MR protocol summary.[3]

Whole-body PET and CT has also emerged as a useful modality for oncologic imaging, particularly for staging, monitoring, and surveillance of advanced HN squamous cell carcinoma (SCCa).[3,6,7] The combination of PET/CT is also very useful in detecting more than one primary neoplastic lesion and determining an unknown primary site; however, it is not always specific and frequently shows scintigraphic activity from other causes, with the most frequent being inflammation/infection. PET/CT is further limited by the metabolic activity of a lesion and can, therefore, miss some malignant lesions with low metabolic activity. Notably, the CT portion should be performed as a dedicated soft tissue neck CT with contrast and thin sections for nodal and primary evaluation, not solely for tissue attenuation correction. When imaging cervical SCCa of the HN, a dedicated high-resolution HN PET/CT protocol was found to be superior to a whole-body PET/CT in the detection of cervical nodal metastases and should be included in combination with whole-body PET/CT when evaluating HN SCCa (**Fig. 5**). This protocol is needed to increase the sensitivity and specificity of PET/CT because of the numerous false positives and false negatives of the technique when interpreted without vital knowledge of HN SCCa.[8]

Box 1
Imaging protocol for CECT when imaging unknown neck mass or evaluating an HN malignancy

CECT

Location: from the skull base through to carina

Slice thickness: ~0.6 to 1.25 mm

Head position: beam parallel to the inferior orbitomeatal line, no gantry tilt (angled scans above and below the mandibular dentition to reduce amalgam artifact)

Reconstructions: soft tissue (standard), bone algorithms (edge enhanced)

Soft tissue: WW 400, WC 40; 2.5 mm

Bone: WW 4000, WC 450; 0.65 to 1.25 mm

Kilovolt peak: 120 kVp

Milliampere range: 100 to 800 mA

Gantry rotation: ~0.7 seconds (should be increased for larger patients)

Beam collimation: 20 mm

Detector configuration: 32 × 0.625

Pitch: ~1

Table speed: ~20 mm per rotation

Contrast: 90 to 120 mL (safely given with a glomerular filtration rate >60)

Contrast rate: ~2 mL/s after an approximately 60-second delay

Split bolus technique: improves lesion/vascular enhancement

Saline chaser technique: clears intravenous injection of contrast, tighter contrast bolus

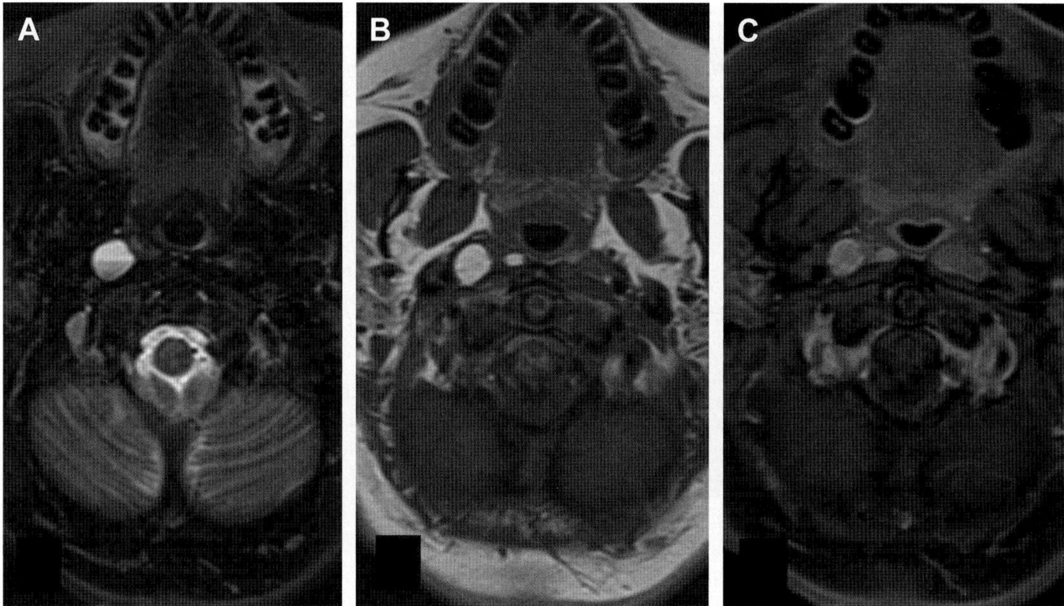

Fig. 4. Axial MR images of different morphology retropharyngeal (RP) lymph nodes in a single patient with undifferentiated thyroid carcinoma. (*A*) Axial short tau inversion recovery MR with a fluid-fluid level in an enlarged right RP lymph node. (*B*) Axial T1-weighted images (TIWI) precontrast with TI shortening of 2 right RP lymph nodes. No TI shortening of the left RP nodes. (*C*) Axial TIWI postcontrast with fat saturation showing variable RP lymph node enhancement.

If there is a low suspicion of malignancy, if patients are children or young adults, or if the mass appears to be thyroid based on examination, ultrasound (US) is a good initial imaging modality. US can characterize the internal structure of superficial lymph nodes and neck masses alike without radiation exposure, and vascularity can be assessed with Doppler.[9–11] Most importantly, US-guided fine-needle aspiration is an accurate method for detecting malignant cervical node metastasis.[12]

> **Box 2**
> **Imaging protocol for MR when imaging unknown neck mass or evaluating HN malignancy**
>
> *MR*
>
> Location: the skull base to at least the supraclavicular fossa
>
> Sequences: minimum of 3 sequences, each in at least one plane
>
> Recommend sequences: coronal & axial TIWI, T2WI FS or STIR, TIWI post-contrast FS (sagittal helpful but optional when imaging cervical nodes specifically)
>
> Field of view: ~16 to 18 cm
>
> Slice thickness: 4 mm
>
> Interslice gap: 0.5 to 1.0 mm
>
> Matrix: 192 × 256
>
> Surface coils: improve image quality
>
> Saturation pulses: reduce vascular artifact

Other promising techniques in the imaging of cervical lymph nodes include dynamic CT and MR; novel MR pulse sequences, such as T1-rho; quantitative diffusion imaging; and novel contrast agents, such as iron oxide particles. These modalities have demonstrated consistently high sensitivity or specificity[3,13–15] but have yet to become the standard of care for the imaging of cervical nodes.

To date, there is no consensus on which imaging modality should be used in monitoring malignancy and lymph nodes in the HN. The imaging used often depends highly on the ordering physician, the institution, and the personal preferences of the radiologist. One way the radiologist can help improve accuracy in follow-up imaging is to emphasize to the clinician the importance of using the same modality during surveillance to provide comparable studies.

IMAGING FINDINGS/PATHOLOGY

When evaluating an unknown neck mass, the distinction of a lesion as a lymph node or other pathology is often complicated. There are several

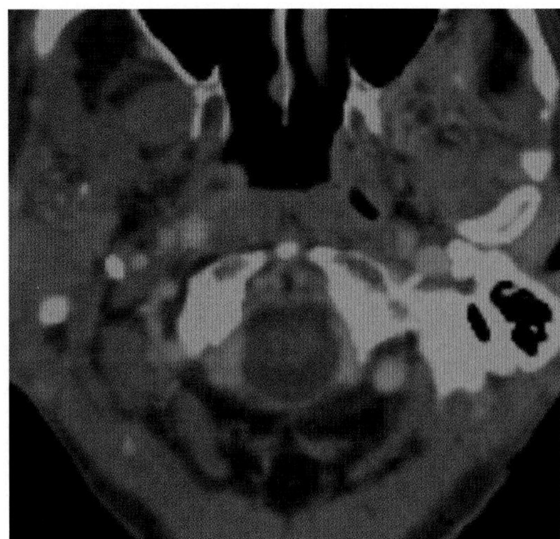

Fig. 5. Axial PET/CT with a small scintigraphically active right retropharyngeal lymph node. This lymph node does not meet size criteria for being pathologically enlarged but had avid fluorodeoxyglucose uptake and was found to have SCCa on pathology.

other pathologies that may mimic a node, including congenital cystic lesions, infectious and/or inflammatory processes, normal structures mimicking lymph nodes, or primary neoplastic processes. A strong knowledge of the neck spaces and normal structures and processes can improve accuracy in identifying lymph nodes and differentiating other processes.

Once a lymph node has been identified, the next step is the differentiation of a normal node from an abnormal node. Normal lymph nodes are typically reniform with a central fatty hilum that is contiguous with the surrounding cervical fat. A change in lymph node shape or a loss of the normal hilar fat may be a sign of nodal pathology.[9,10]

Lymph node size can also be a factor in deciding if a lymph node is normal or abnormal. Cervical lymph nodes have historically been considered abnormally enlarged if the longitudinal diameter of level I or level II nodes exceeded 15 mm, retropharyngeal nodes exceeded 8 mm, and other cervical nodes exceeded 10 mm. Other publications have described pathologic determinations of size when the axial diameter of level I or level II nodes exceeds 11 mm, retropharyngeal nodes exceed 5 mm, and other cervical nodes exceed 10 mm. Other publications have described a ratio of longitudinal to transverse measurements in order to determine normal from abnormal width of cervical lymph nodes. Although many publications have attempted to describe pathologic measurements, it is important to understand that approximately 50% of nodes harboring malignant cells measure less than 5 mm in size and 25% of nodes with ECS are less than 10 mm.[16] This point emphasizes the fact that size it not always the most important factor when evaluating for pathologies (see **Fig. 5**). Other findings, such as configuration, homogeneity, enhancement, loss of the normal fatty hilum, and the preservation of surrounding fat planes, are more important than any measurement techniques.

Once a lymph node is identified as abnormal, the next determination is whether the node harbors inflammation (reactive), infection (suppurative), or tumor (SCCa). This distinction is often quite difficult. It is important for radiologists to understand the typical appearances of normal and abnormal lymph nodes to provide a useful diagnosis or differential. The following section discusses the typical appearances of common lymph node pathologies.

REACTIVE LYMPHADENOPATHY

Reactive nodes are typically nodes that are enlarged in response to an antigen or infiltration and may be acute or chronic and localized or generalized.[11,17,18] Reactive lymph nodes can also be referred to as reactive adenopathy, reactive lymphoid hyperplasia, and nodal hyperplasia. Reactive lymph nodes by definition are benign.[19] Reactive lymph nodes are caused by a histologic reaction, which can be infectious or noninfectious. The cause can be a chemical, drug, foreign antigen, or an infectious agent, including viral, bacterial, parasitic, and fungal infectious agents.

Reactive nodes usually appear enlarged with a well-defined retained reniform shape.[20,21] On nonenhanced CT (NECT), reactive nodes are homogenous and isodense or hypodense to muscle. On CECT, the nodes have variable enhancement. Mildly enhancing linear markings are characteristic. On MR T1WI, reactive nodes typically show low to intermediate signal intensity, and T2WI shows intermediate to high signal intensity. Following contrast administration, these nodes typically show variable, mild enhancement with potential enhancing linear markings. On PET/CT, mild uptake of fluorine-18 fluorodeoxyglucose may be seen.[1] Children commonly get reactive nodes, especially with upper respiratory infections; these can reach several centimeters in size.[22] Although CECT is the study of choice for the evaluation of neck adenopathy, US can be considered in a child to reduce exposure to radiation.[11,20,21,23]

Clues to the specific cause can be found in the evaluation of the clinical presentation and in the careful evaluation of the surrounding tissues, such as stranding of adjacent fat in the case of a bacterial infection. Generalized adenopathy can also indicate a viral cause. On physical examination, reactive lymph nodes are typically firm, rubbery, mobile, and enlarged. Differential considerations for reactive nodes include other diffuse processes such as sarcoid, non-Hodgkin lymphoma (NHL), metastatic disease, and less commonly tuberculosis.[1] Please see **Box 3** for the reactive lymph node summary.

SUPPURATIVE LYMPHADENOPATHY

Suppurative lymph nodes are lymph nodes containing intranodal pus and are also known as adenitis, acute lymphadenitis, or intranodal abscess.[24] The most commonly involved nodes are the retropharyngeal, jugulodigastric, and submandibular nodes, although any node can be involved both unilaterally and/or bilaterally. Typically, the nodes are individually enlarged or a confluence of nodes forms before becoming an abscess. Surrounding inflammation is also an associated finding. The nodes are ovoid to round, cystic appearing, and frequently have poorly defined margins.[1,24,25]

> **Box 3**
> **Reactive lymph nodes**
>
> *Diagnostic criteria*
>
> Multiple, well-defined, oval nodes
>
> Nodes of normal size or mildly enlarged
>
> Location: Any of nodal groups of HN
>
> Size
>
> - Wide size range
> - Adult: often up to 1.5 cm
> - Child: reactive node may be 2 cm or more
>
> *Imaging recommendations*
>
> CECT is first-line tool for evaluation of adenopathy
>
> Differentiates reactive from suppurative nodes and cellulitis from abscess
>
> Allows determination of node extent and evaluation for potential malignant cause
>
> *Differential diagnoses*
>
> SCCa nodal metastases
>
> Systemic nodal metastases
>
> NHL nodes
>
> Tuberculous adenitis
>
> Sarcoid nodes

On CECT, stranding of the adjacent fat and subcutaneous tissues is seen with intranodal abscess formation with an irregular peripherally enhancing low-density fluid collection. On MR T1WI, low central signal intensity is often seen, and T2WI shows diffuse or central high signal intensity with surrounding high signal intensity in the subcutaneous tissues, best seen with FS sequences. US evaluation of suppurative nodal disease will show decreased central echogenicity with increased through transmission. Increased peripheral vascularity may be seen with Doppler. On PET/CT imaging, there is usually increased scintigraphic activity in the periphery of the node with low uptake centrally. CECT remains the study of choice and can best assist with the evaluation for an inciting process, such as dental infection and/or salivary gland calculus on bone windows.[1,3]

Suppurative lymph nodes are infectious in origin, and reactive nodes may transform into suppurative nodes. If left untreated, suppurative nodes may rupture with subsequent interstitial pus and may then become walled off resulting in adjacent soft tissue abscesses. Suppurative lymph nodes are most commonly seen in the pediatric and young adult population, and the most common organisms involved are staphylococcus and streptococcus.[24] Differential considerations for suppurative lymph nodes include fatty nodal metaplasia, second brachial cleft cyst, tuberculous adenitis, and nontuberculous mycobacterial adenitis. Please see **Box 4** for the suppurative lymph node summary.

CALCIFIED LYMPHADENOPATHY

The presence of calcifications within lymph nodes can indicate infection, granulomatous disease, or metastatic disease.[1,26–28] These densities are best seen with CT, either CECT or NECT, which can better characterize calcifications than MR. Bone windows can help evaluate the calcification extent and configuration. Although US can demonstrate calcifications, this modality is also limited, as calcifications will cause shadowing thereby limiting the evaluation of deeper structures. The most notable causes of calcified lymph nodes in the neck are tuberculous adenitis and thyroid cancer, specifically common in metastatic papillary thyroid carcinoma.[26,27,29] The configuration of the calcifications on CT can assist with the determination of their origin, as similar calcifications may be seen within the nodes and the primary lesion, such as with cases of differentiated thyroid carcinoma.[27] Lymph nodes may also have calcifications after treatment, such as radiation, again highlighting the importance of clinical

Box 4
Suppurative lymph nodes

Diagnostic criteria

Enlarged node with intranodal fluid and surrounding inflammation (cellulitis)

Ovoid to round, large node with cystic changes

Often poorly defined margins

Additional solid or suppurative nodes typically present

Location: any of nodal groups of HN

Size: typically enlarged node or confluence of nodes in the 1- to 4-cm range

Imaging recommendations

CECT usually first-line imaging modality with neck infections

Allows determination of focal absence of enhancement indicating pus

Carefully evaluate bone CT images

Differential diagnoses

SCCa nodes

Second branchial cleft anomaly

Non–*Mycobacterium tuberculosis* nodes

Tuberculosis nodes

Fatty nodal metaplasia

Pathology

Staphylococcus and streptococcus most frequent causative organisms

Pediatric infections show clustering of organisms by age range

Dental infections are typically polymicrobial and predominantly anaerobic

history whenever evaluating an HN imaging study. Please see **Box 5** for the calcified lymph node summary.

NECROTIC LYMPHADENOPATHY

Necrotic lymph nodes, as the name suggests, have central necrosis. This necrosis is highly suggestive of inadequate vascular supply in the presence of metastatic disease; however, necrotizing granulomatous disease, such as tuberculosis, should be considered in the correct clinical setting.[30] This sign is fairly specific for metastatic disease, and usually the frequency of nodal necrosis increases with metastatic nodal size.[1] Therefore, the detection of nodal necrosis in isolation is most useful if the necrotic nodes are less than 10 mm and there are no other abnormal nodes.[16]

Box 5
Calcified lymph nodes

Diagnostic criteria

Lymph nodes contain calcifications

Imaging

Best seen on NECT or CECT; less well characterized on MR

Bone windows best for assessing configuration of calcifications

Differential diagnoses

Tuberculous adenitis

Non–tuberculosis granulomatous adenitis

Differentiated thyroid carcinoma

Radiation-treated lymph nodes

Nodal necrosis on CECT will show low central density without the characteristic inflammatory changes seen with suppurative nodes (see **Fig. 1**D). Volume averaging through the normal fatty hilum and fat deposition may produce a low-attenuation focus in the suspected node on CT. Density measurements may, therefore, be of limited value in small lesions because of partial volume averaging. The location of the low-attenuation focus may be helpful, as necrosis may initially present at the pole of the reniform node, whereas fat is usually present in the central hilum. On MR, T1WI will generally show low central signal intensity, and T2WI typically shows central T2WI hyperintensity. Diffusion-weighted imaging can be used to show diffusion restriction, and low apparent diffusion coefficient (ADC) values ($<1.0 \times 10^{-3}$ mm^2/s) can be seen within malignant nodal disease, similar to primary site ADC values. Contrasted MR imaging evaluation will show low, nonenhancing signal intensity in the central necrotic region with surrounding enhancement of the portions of the lymph node that have increased vascular supply. US will show decreased central echogenicity with increased through transmission, similar to suppurative nodal disease.[1,31]

If a suspected necrotic lymph node is found, it must be a consideration that metastatic disease is present. Clinical history, such as age and smoking history, should be taken into account, although some cancers, such as human papillomavirus (HPV) positive (HPV+) SCCa, can occur in younger adults without a smoking history.[32–34] These HPV+ SCCa cases are most frequently found in the oropharynx and may be associated with necrotic nodal disease. If biopsy is indicated, tissue from the non-necrotic portion of the node

Box 6
Cystic and necrotic lymph nodes

Diagnostic criteria

Node with intranodal fluid

Ovoid to round, large node with cystic/necrotic changes

Often well-defined margins

Additional solid or cystic/necrotic nodes are often present

Location: any of nodal groups of HN

Size: typically enlarged but can be normal in size with fluid/necrotic material

Imaging recommendations

CECT usually first-line imaging modality

Allows determination of central fluid/necrotic changes

Carefully evaluate bone CT images

Differential diagnoses

Congenital cystic neck masses

- Brachial cleft cysts
- Thyroglossal duct cyst
- Lymphatic malformation
- Tornwaldt cyst

Inflammatory cystic masses

- Abscess
- Suppurative, granulomatous, necrotic adenopathy
- Ranula, retention cyst, sialocele

Vascular cystic masses

- Venous malformation, thrombosis, or thrombophlebitis
- Artery aneurysm or pseudoaneurysm

Visceral saccular cysts

- Laryngocele
- Zenker diverticulum

Parenchymal cysts

- Thyroid cyst
- Parathyroid cyst
- Thymic cyst

Cystic benign tumors

- Neural sheath tumors (schwannoma, neurofibroma)
- Lipoma
- Dermoid or epidermoid

Cystic malignant tumors

- Primary SCCa
- Nodal SCCa
- Primary or nodal thyroid carcinoma

must be taken. Please see **Box 6** for the necrotic and cystic lymph node summary.

CYSTIC LYMPHADENOPATHY

Many potentially cystic structures are located within the neck, including congenital cystic neck masses, such as brachial cleft cysts, thyroglossal duct cysts, lymphatic malformations, and retention cysts (**Fig. 6**A). Vascular malformations, parenchymal cysts, or benign cystic tumors may also present as cystic neck masses on imaging.[35] Malignant lymph nodes can be cystic in the case of nodal thyroid carcinoma or SCCa, especially with oropharyngeal HPV+ SCCa.[32–34,36]

If a cystic structure is found in the neck, a radiologist should try to identify if the structure is benign, congenital, or another structural abnormality, as the biopsy of a vascular malformation or aneurysm is to be avoided.[35] In the lower left neck, the signal node (of Virchow) and the distal thoracic duct have a similar location. A dilated distal thoracic duct may mimic an enlarged node; however, the duct is purely cystic and can be followed proximally into the superior mediastinum.[1]

When a cystic mass is found at the angle of the mandible, the radiologist should remember that second branchial cleft cyst (BCC) anomalies and lymph nodes can have a similar location, and metastatic disease from the oral cavity can often be purely cystic. In patients older than 50 years, SCCa should always be the preferred diagnosis (see **Fig. 6**B). In young children, BCC is more likely. Please see **Box 6** for the necrotic and cystic lymph node summary.

MATTED LYMPHADENOPATHY

Matted lymph nodes are a confluence of nodes that abut one another. These nodes can demonstrate individual nodal characteristics on imaging as described in the other nodal configurations mentioned earlier. Additional findings may be present around the matted nodal group, including fluid and/or inflammatory changes. Matted lymph nodes can also surround adjacent structures or cause mass effect with a differential, including infectious causes or metastatic disease.

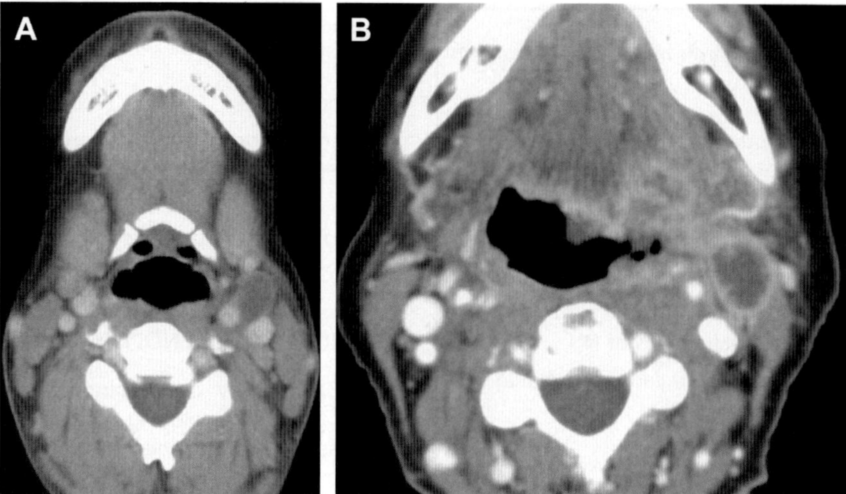

Fig. 6. (*A*) Axial CECT with a large left cystic lesion found to be an infected second brachial cleft cyst. (*B*) Axial CECT with cystic, left level IIB enlarged lymph node. Pathologically proven to be HPV+ SCCa.

In the case of SCCa, matted lymph nodes have been shown to be a novel marker for poor prognosis independent of T classification, HPV status, epidermal growth factor, and smoking status. Matted nodes have also been found to be distinct from extracapsular spread (ECS) and nodal status, conveying a worse prognosis independent of these conventional prognostic indicators. Matted nodes were found in one study to be more prevalent in the HPV− cohort when compared with HPV+ but were associated with distant metastasis in both groups. Mention of matted nodes in cases of HN SCCa may help to identify patients who are more likely to fail concomitant chemotherapy and radiation therapy.[37] Please see **Box 7** for the matted lymph node summary.

Box 7
Matted lymph nodes

Diagnostic criteria

Multiple lymph nodes without any space between

Lymph nodes often conform to the shape or push on adjacent nodes

Appear as a conglomerate mass

Imaging

CECT usually first-line imaging modality

Assess to the extent of the lymph node mass easily

Differential diagnoses

Cervical mass/malignancy

DIFFUSE LYMPHADENOPATHY

Diffuse involvement of the cervical lymph nodes or involvement of multiple levels has a wide differential, including local spread of infection, generalized systemic processes, or neoplasms (see **Fig. 1**B, C).

Systemic infection, such as a viral illness or bacterial sepsis, can cause diffuse nodal involvement. Human immunodeficiency virus adenopathy is a specific case of viral disease that should be considered in the appropriate clinical setting. Granulomatous disease, such as sarcoid, tuberculosis, or nontuberculous mycoplasma, can also present with diffuse nodal involvement.[1,38–42] Metastatic disease, however, is the most concerning cause of diffuse nodal disease and can indicate more advanced disease from the HN; superior spread from the lungs or mediastinum; or advanced, diffuse metastatic disease.[43–46] In the United States, lung, breast, kidney, and melanoma show a predilection for metastasizing to the HN.[44,47] In about 20% to 35% of cases, cervical metastasis may be the first manifestation of an otherwise occult malignancy.[44]

Primary malignancy, such as NHL or Hodgkin lymphoma (HL) is also a cause of diffuse cervical lymphadenopathy.[48–50] Lymphoma nodal disease, both HL and NHL, are typically both homogenous on CT with somewhat variable enhancement (see **Fig. 1**B, C). On MR, lymphoma is hypointense to isointense on T1WI and hyperintense on T2WI compared with muscle. Necrosis with or without extranodal spread implies more aggressive disease.[1] Please see **Box 8** for the diffuse lymph node summary.

Box 8
Diffuse lymph nodes

Diagnostic criteria

Multiple well-defined, oval nodes

Nodes of normal size or mildly enlarged

Location: any of nodal groups of HN

Imaging

CECT is first-line tool for evaluation of adenopathy

Differentiates types of lymph nodes

Allows determination of node extent and evaluation for potential malignant cause

Differential diagnoses

Infection/reactive: viral or bacteria

Sarcoid

Tuberculosis

Non–tuberculous mycoplasma

Lymphoma: HL and NHL

Metastatic disease

RARE LYMPHADENOPATHY DISEASES

There are a few diseases not previously mentioned that affect the cervical lymph nodes specifically. Castleman disease is a benign lymphoproliferative disorder of unknown cause characterized with lymph node enlargement and is divided into 2 types: hyaline vascular type and plasma cell type (**Box 9**). One nodal group or multiple nodal groups can be involved with greater than 90% of neck lesions being unifocal.[51–55] CECT typically demonstrates moderate to marked homogenous nodal contrast enhancement. Nodes are typically hypointense or isointense on T1WI and hyperintense on T2WI. Branching T2 hypointense striations are suggestive of Castleman disease, although this finding is not often present.[1]

Kimura disease is another disease of lymph node enlargement also known as eosinophilic lymphogranuloma or eosinophilic hyperplastic lymphogranuloma (**Box 10**). Painless unilateral cervical adenopathy or subcutaneous nodules is characteristic. Kimura disease is a chronic inflammatory disorder of the HN seen primarily in young Asian men with blood and tissue eosinophilia as well as elevated serum allergen-specific immunoglobulin E. Involvement of the parotid or submandibular gland must be present, although the lacrimal gland is rarely involved.[56–58]

Kikuchi disease, or Kikuchi-Fujimoto disease, is a rare, benign, self-limited disorder characterized by tender, regional cervical lymphadenopathy and is usually accompanied by mild fever and night sweats (**Box 11**). The prevalence is higher among Japanese and other Asian individuals. This disease is typically diagnosed by excisional biopsy of the affected lymph nodes showing irregular cortical areas of coagulation necrosis, abundant karyorrhectic debris, and several different histiocyte types.[57,59–63]

Rosai-Dorfman disease, or sinus histiocytosis with massive lymphadenopathy, is another extremely rare, benign process with proliferation of hematopoietic cells and fibrous tissue often presenting in the HN region. This disease usually manifests with symmetric, painless, bilateral cervical adenopathy. This disease is also diagnosed on

Box 9
Castleman disease

Synonyms

Angiofollicular lymphoid hyperplasia

Follicular lymphoreticular

Angiomatous lymphoid hamartoma

Lymph nodal hamartoma

Diagnostic criteria

Most often mediastinum (60%), then HN (15%)

Greater than 90% HN lesions are unifocal disease

Moderate to markedly enhancing nodal mass

CECT: central nonenhancing scar may be evident

T2 MR hypointense striations described, uncommon

Hypoechoic on US with intense peripheral vascular flow

Top differential diagnoses

Reactive lymph nodes

NHL lymph nodes

Differentiated thyroid carcinoma

Carotid body paraganglioma

Pathology

Probably reactive process, although cause unclear

Most often unifocal, hyaline vascular type, asymptomatic, and cured by excision

Multifocal form rare, plasma cell histology, often symptomatic, and aggressive disease course

Diagnosis requires core biopsy or node excision

Box 10
Kimura disease

Synonyms

Eosinophilic hyperplastic lymphogranuloma

Eosinophilic lymphogranuloma

Diagnostic criteria

Painless subcutaneous HN masses with regional adenopathy

Blood and tissue eosinophilia

Markedly elevated serum immunoglobulin E

Differential diagnoses

Nodal NHL

Nodal sarcoidosis

Parotid metastatic nodal disease

Parotid mucoepidermoid carcinoma

Pathology

Unknown cause; allergic and autoimmune theories favored

15% to 60% have renal dysfunction

pathologic examination and is frequently self-limited.[1,64,65]

Although these diagnoses are less common, one should be aware of these processes when forming a differential diagnosis of cervical node enlargement.

IMAGING ROLE IN SQUAMOUS CELL CARCINOMA

Imaging is integral to the evaluation of HN neoplastic disease. The involvement of the cervical lymph nodes remains the most important prognostic indicator in HN SCCa, decreasing the overall survival by approximately half.[7] ECS worsens the prognosis by yet another 50%.[16,66]

Imaging is frequently obtained to confirm N0 disease. Even with no evident nodal involvement, occult metastasis is common in some primary HN lesions, including 41% in the oral cavity, 36% in the oral pharynx, 36% in the hypopharynx, and 29% in supraglottic carcinomas. Many surgeons will perform neck dissections in the case of these high-risk lesions. Parotid gland, maxillary sinus, and glottic carcinomas have less than a 5% chance of occult metastatic disease and, therefore, can be spared surgical removal if the lymph nodes appear normal on imaging.[16,67] Despite these statistics, the decision to perform surgery often depends on the surgeon, institution, and individual patients.

Box 11
Kikuchi disease

Terminology

Histiocytic necrotizing lymphadenitis

Synonym: Kikuchi-Fujimoto disease

Benign idiopathic necrotizing cervical adenitis of young Asian adults

Diagnostic criteria

Unilateral, homogeneous, mildly enlarged nodes with inflammatory stranding

Posterior cervical and jugular chain

Nodes appear solid or rim enhancing but not necessarily necrotic

Most commonly in female Asians in third decade

High fever with 30% to 50% having other systemic symptoms

Diagnosis requires excisional biopsy

Top differential diagnoses

NHL lymph nodes

Systemic nodal metastases

Cat scratch disease

Tuberculosis lymph nodes

Pathology

Cortical and paracortical coagulative necrosis

Cellular infiltrate of histiocytes and immunoblasts

Possibly exuberant T cell–mediated immune response to variety of nonspecific stimuli

Associated with increased incidence of systemic lupus erythematosus

If malignant lymph nodes are present, the location and involvement can decide the type of surgery performed. Variations include the radical neck dissection, modified radical neck dissection, selective neck dissection, and extended neck dissection. Imaging may also identify disease that is nonsurgical. ECS can invade the carotid sheath thereby rendering patients as nonsurgical candidates. Variations of the use of radiation and chemotherapy can also be decided depending on lymphatic spread.[67]

ECS is relativity common on histology. ECS is classically diagnosed on imaging when the nodes appear matted or the nodal outline appeared streaky; however, imaging is not always accurate for identifying extracapsular spread.[16,66,68,69] Given the impact on prognosis and highly variable appearance of lymph nodes without extracapsular spread, many experts are now moving away from trying to identify extracapsular extension on imaging without blatant destruction of the lymph node capsule or evident adjacent spread into the surrounding tissues.

The modality of imaging used to monitor HN SCCa is highly variable.[13–15,31,70–73] The appearance of posttreatment necks is also highly variable with postsurgical and postradiation changes distorting and altering the surrounding structures. As mentioned in the imaging section, emphasis on consistent use of the same imaging modality can help to make comparison and more accurate assessment of disease evolution possible.

CARCINOMA OF UNKNOWN PRIMARY

The presence of definite pathologic adenopathy on imaging without an obvious primary site is often described as carcinoma of unknown primary (CUP). As almost half of patients with a HN carcinoma will have nodal disease at the time of presentation, it is crucial for the radiologist to search for pathologic nodes with each HN cancer case.[74]

The understanding of the importance of normal lymphatic drainage is most important in cases of CUP. When SCCa is present at a certain location along the upper aerodigestive tract, the radiologist should consider normal lymphatic drainage from that site and inspect those nodes at that location more closely. If a definite pathologic node is found within the cervical soft tissues, the radiologist should consider what regions should drain to that location and inspect those regions of the upper aerodigestive tract more closely.

Because SCCa of the HN usually follows predictable lymphatic drainage patterns, borderline suspicious nodes at unusual drainage locations may be considered less suspicious than nodes within the expected drainage patterns. It is also true that definite pathologic nodes in a location not considered within the expected lymphatic drainage site of a known primary can prompt the search for a second primary of HN carcinoma.

Box 12
Pearls, pitfalls, variants

Pearls

Lymph node appearance on imaging can lead to a diagnosis

Lymph node location can lead to both diagnosis/identification of primary pathology

Correct identification of pathologic lymph node can affect prognosis

Pitfalls

Misidentification of lymph nodes versus other structures

Incorrect identification of normal versus abnormal lymph nodes

Incorrect interpretation caused by posttreatment appearances

Variants

CECT can help distinguish different types of lymph nodes

Additional imaging modalities can compliment CECT to diagnose pathologic nodes

Box 13
What the referring physician needs to know

CECT is the first line for evaluation of lymph nodes.

Other imaging modalities can be used to compliment CT.

Consistent modality in follow-up scans makes for more accurate comparison.

Provide relevant clinical history to guide the diagnosis or follow-up treatment response.

SUMMARY

Cervical lymph node evaluation and interpretation can be difficult for not only the general radiologist but also the experienced neuroradiologist. An understanding of cervical lymph node anatomy, lymph node drainage pathways, and common pathology is essential for accurate interpretation. A location-specific approach to lymph node pathology as well as knowledge of various lymph node morphologies can further refine a differential diagnosis. Clinical information and examination can provide critical diagnostic information when combined with imaging (**Boxes 12** and **13**).

REFERENCES

1. Harnsberger HR, Glastonbury CM, Michael MA, et al. Diagnositc imaging. Head and neck. Salt Lake City (UT): Amirsys Publishing, Inc; 2011. Part 1 section 12. p. 1–39 and part 2 section 1. p. 1–48.
2. Edge SB, Byrd DR, Compton CC, et al. Lymphoid neoplasms. AJCC cancer staging manual. 7th edition. Salt Lake City (UT): Springer; 2010. p. 599–615.
3. Glastonbury CM, Harnsberger HR, Michael MA, et al. Specialty imaging. Head and neck cancer.

section 1. Canada: Amirsys Publishing, Inc; 2013. p. 1–47.
4. Yousem DM, Som PM, Hackney DB, et al. Central nodal necrosis and extracapsular neoplastic spread in cervical lymph nodes: MR imaging versus CT. Radiology 1992;182(3):753–9.
5. Ishikawa M, Anzai Y. MR imaging of lymph nodes in the head and neck. Magn Reson Imaging Clin N Am 2002;10(3):527–42.
6. Haerle SK, Strobel K, Ahmad N, et al. Contrast-enhanced ^{18}F-FDG-PET/CT for the assessment of necrotic lymph node metastases. Head Neck 2011;33(3):324–9. http://dx.doi.org/10.1002/hed.21447.
7. Mevio E, Gorini E, Sbrocca M, et al. The role of positron emission tomography (PET) in the management of cervical lymph nodes metastases from an unknown primary tumour. Acta Otorhinolaryngol Ital 2004;24(6):342–7.
8. Rodrigues RS, Bozza FA, Christian PE, et al. Comparison of whole-body PET/CT, dedicated high-resolution head and neck PET/CT, and contrast-enhanced CT in preoperative staging of clinically M0 squamous cell carcinoma of the head and neck. J Nucl Med 2009;50(8):1205–13. http://dx.doi.org/10.2967/jnumed.109.062075.
9. Ahuja AT, Ying M, Ho SY, et al. Ultrasound of malignant cervical lymph nodes. Cancer Imaging 2008;8:48–56. http://dx.doi.org/10.1102/1470-7330.2008.0006.
10. Esen G. Ultrasound of superficial lymph nodes. Eur J Radiol 2006;58(3):345–59.
11. Chan JM, Shin LK, Jeffrey RB. Ultrasonography of abnormal neck lymph nodes. Ultrasound Q 2007;23(1):47–54.
12. Lo CP, Chen CY, Chin SC, et al. Detection of suspicious malignant cervical lymph nodes of unknown origin: diagnostic accuracy of ultrasound-guided fine-needle aspiration biopsy with nodal size and central necrosis correlate. Can Assoc Radiol J 2007;58(5):286–91.
13. Vandecaveye V, De Keyzer F, Dirix P, et al. Applications of diffusion-weighted magnetic resonance imaging in head and neck squamous cell carcinoma. Neuroradiology 2010;52(9):773–84.
14. Holzapfel K, Duetsch S, Fauser C, et al. Value of diffusion-weighted MR imaging in the differentiation between benign and malignant cervical lymph nodes. Eur J Radiol 2009;72(3):381–7.
15. Kawai Y, Sumi M, Nakamura T. Turbo short tau inversion recovery imaging for metastatic node screening in patients with head and neck cancer. AJNR Am J Neuroradiol 2006;27(6):1283–7.
16. Chong V. Cervical lymphadenopathy: what radiologists need to know. Cancer Imaging 2004;4(2):116–20. http://dx.doi.org/10.1102/1470-7330.2004.0020.
17. Annam V, Kulkarni MH, Puranik RB. Clinicopathologic profile of significant cervical lymphadenopathy in children aged 1-12 years. Acta Cytol 2009;53(2):174–8.
18. Leung AK, Robson WL. Childhood cervical lymphadenopathy. J Pediatr Health Care 2004;18(1):3–7.
19. Ahuja AT, Ying M, Ho SS, et al. Distribution of intranodal vessels in differentiating benign from metastatic neck nodes. Clin Radiol 2001;56(3):197–201.
20. Papakonstantinou O, Bakantaki A, Paspalaki P, et al. High-resolution and color Doppler ultrasonography of cervical lymphadenopathy in children. Acta Radiol 2001;42(5):470–6.
21. Ahuja A, Ying M. Grey-scale sonography in assessment of cervical lymphadenopathy: review of sonographic appearances and features that may help a beginner. Br J Oral Maxillofac Surg 2000;38(5):451–9.
22. Hudgins PA. Nodal and nonnodal inflammatory processes of the pediatric neck. Neuroimaging Clin N Am 2000;10(1):181–92, ix.
23. Robson CD, Hazra R, Barnes PD, et al. Nontuberculous mycobacterial infection of the head and neck in immunocompetent children: CT and MR findings. AJNR Am J Neuroradiol 1999;20(10):1829–35.
24. Luu TM, Chevalier I, Gauthier M, et al. Acute adenitis in children: clinical course and factors predictive of surgical drainage. J Paediatr Child Health 2005;41(5–6):273–7.
25. Ide C, De Coene B, Trigaux JP. Internal carotid artery narrowing in children with retropharyngeal lymphadenitis and abscess. AJNR Am J Neuroradiol 2000;21(1):233–4.
26. Liu GC, Gao S, Cai L, et al. Characteristics of extrapulmonary tuberculosis in (18)F-2-fluoro-2-deoxy-D-glucose positron emission tomography-computed tomography: experience from 39 cases. Zhonghua Jie He He Hu Xi Za Zhi 2012;35(3):184–8.
27. Erdem T, Miman MC, Oncel S, et al. Metastatic spread of occult papillary carcinoma of the thyroid to the parapharyngeal space: a case report. Kulak Burun Bogaz Ihtis Derg 2003;10(6):244–7.
28. Eisenkraft BL, Som PM. The spectrum of benign and malignant etiologies of cervical node calcification. AJR Am J Roentgenol 1999;172(5):1433–7.
29. Choi EC, Moon WJ, Lim YC. Case report. Tuberculous cervical lymphadenitis mimicking metastatic lymph nodes from papillary thyroid carcinoma. Br J Radiol 2009;82(982):e208–11.
30. Jiang XS, West DS, Lagoo AS. Lymph node infarction: role of underlying malignancy, tumour proliferation fraction and vascular compromise–a study of 35 cases and a comprehensive review of the literature. Histopathology 2013;62(2):315–25. http://dx.doi.org/10.1111/j.1365-2559.2012.04361.x.

31. King AD, Tse GM, Ahuja AT, et al. Necrosis in metastatic neck nodes: diagnostic accuracy of CT, MR imaging, and US. Radiology 2004;230(3): 720–6.
32. Goldenberg D, Sciubba J, Koch WM. Cystic metastasis from head and neck squamous cell cancer: a distinct disease variant? Head Neck 2006;28(7):633–8.
33. Cantrell SC, Peck BW, Li G, et al. Differences in imaging characteristics of HPV-positive and HPV-Negative oropharyngeal cancers: a blinded matched-pair analysis. AJNR Am J Neuroradiol 2013;34(10):2005–9. http://dx.doi.org/10.3174/ajnr.A3524.
34. Goldenberg D, Begum S, Westra WH, et al. Cystic lymph node metastasis in patients with head and neck cancer: an HPV-associated phenomenon. Head Neck 2008;30(7):898–903. http://dx.doi.org/10.1002/hed.20796.
35. Harnsberger HR. Handbook of head and neck radiology. Philadelphia: Mosby; 1995. p. 199–223.
36. Morani AC, Eisbruch A, Carey TE, et al. Intranodal cystic changes: a potential radiologic signature/biomarker to assess the human papillomavirus status of cases with oropharyngeal malignancies. J Comput Assist Tomogr 2013;37(3):343–5. http://dx.doi.org/10.1097/RCT.0b013e318282d7c3.
37. Spector ME, Gallagher KK, Light E, et al. Matted nodes: poor prognostic marker in oropharyngeal squamous cell carcinoma independent of HPV and EGFR status. Head Neck 2012;34(12):1727–33. http://dx.doi.org/10.1002/hed.21997.
38. Esparcia O, Navarro F, Quer M, et al. Lymphadenopathy caused by Mycobacterium colombiense. J Clin Microbiol 2008;46(5):1885–7.
39. Wang WC, Chen JY, Chen YK, et al. Tuberculosis of the head and neck: a review of 20 cases. Oral Surg Oral Med Oral Pathol Oral Radiol Endod 2009; 107(3):381–6.
40. Menon K, Bem C, Gouldesbrough D, et al. A clinical review of 128 cases of head and neck tuberculosis presenting over a 10-year period in Bradford, UK. J Laryngol Otol 2007; 121(4):362–8.
41. Baskota DK, Prasad R, Kumar Sinha B, et al. Distribution of lymph nodes in the neck in cases of tuberculous cervical lymphadenitis. Acta Otolaryngol 2004;124(9):1095–8.
42. Moon WK, Han MH, Chang KH, et al. CT and MR imaging of head and neck tuberculosis. Radiographics 1997;17(2):391–402.
43. Gani C, Eckert F, Müller AC, et al. Cervical squamous cell lymph node metastases from an unknown primary site: survival and patterns of recurrence after radiotherapy. Clin Med Insights Oncol 2013;7:173–80. http://dx.doi.org/10.4137/CMO.S12169. eCollection 2013.
44. Barnes L. Metastases to the head and neck: an overview. Head Neck Pathol 2009;3(3):217–24. http://dx.doi.org/10.1007/s12105-009-0123-4.
45. Giridharan W, Hughes J, Fenton JE, et al. Lymph node metastases in the lower neck. Clin Otolaryngol 2003;28(3):221–6.
46. Weissman JL. Building a better mousetrap: the diagnosis of metastatic cervical adenopathy. AJNR Am J Neuroradiol 2003;24(3):297.
47. Zuur CL, van Velthuysen ML, Schornagel JH, et al. Diagnosis and treatment of isolated neck metastases of adenocarcinomas. Eur J Surg Oncol 2002; 28(2):147–52.
48. Gaini RM, Romagnoli M, Sala A, et al. Lymphomas of head and neck in pediatric patients. Int J Pediatr Otorhinolaryngol 2009;73(Suppl 1):S65–70.
49. Abramson SJ, Price AP. Imaging of pediatric lymphomas. Radiol Clin North Am 2008;46(2): 313–38, ix.
50. Matasar MJ, Zelenetz AD. Overview of lymphoma diagnosis and management. Radiol Clin North Am 2008;46(2):175–98, vii.
51. Liang J, Newman JG, Frank DM, et al. Cervical unicentric Castleman disease presenting as a neck mass: case report and review of the literature. Ear Nose Throat J 2009;88(5):E8.
52. Barker R, Kazmi F, Bower M. Imaging in multicentric Castleman's disease. J HIV Ther 2008;13(3): 72–4.
53. Souza KC, Silva SJ, Salomão E, et al. Cervical Castleman's disease in childhood. J Oral Maxillofac Surg 2008;66(5):1067–72.
54. Newlon JL, Couch M, Brennan J. Castleman's disease: three case reports and a review of the literature. Ear Nose Throat J 2007;86(7):414–8.
55. Puram SV, Hasserjian RP, Faquin WC, et al. Castleman disease presenting in the neck: report of a case and review of the literature. Am J Otol 2013; 34(3):239–44. http://dx.doi.org/10.1016/j.amjoto.2012.11.007.
56. Gopinathan A, Tan TY. Kimura's disease: imaging patterns on computed tomography. Clin Radiol 2009;64(10):994–9.
57. Mrówka-Kata K, Kata D, Kyrcz-Krzemień S, et al. Kikuchi-Fujimoto and Kimura diseases: the selected, rare causes of neck lymphadenopathy. Eur Arch Otorhinolaryngol 2010;267(1):5–11.
58. Sun QF, Xu DZ, Pan SH, et al. Kimura disease: review of the literature. Intern Med J 2008;38(8):668–72.
59. Ito K, Morooka M, Kubota K. F-18 FDG PET/CT findings showing lymph node uptake in patients with Kikuchi disease. Clin Nucl Med 2009;34(11): 821–2.
60. Lee DH, Lee JH, Shim EJ, et al. Disseminated Kikuchi-Fujimoto disease mimicking malignant lymphoma on positron emission tomography in a child. J Pediatr Hematol Oncol 2009;31(9):687–9.

61. Nomura Y, Takeuchi M, Yoshida S, et al. Phenotype for activated tissue macrophages in histiocytic necrotizing lymphadenitis. Pathol Int 2009;59(9):631–5.
62. Pilichowska ME, Pinkus JL, Pinkus GS. Histiocytic necrotizing lymphadenitis (Kikuchi-Fujimoto disease): lesional cells exhibit an immature dendritic cell phenotype. Am J Clin Pathol 2009;131(2): 174–82.
63. Chase SP, Templer JW, Miick R, et al. Cervical lymphadenopathy secondary to Kikuchi-Fujimoto disease in a child: case report. Ear Nose Throat J 2008;87(6):350–3.
64. La Barge DV 3rd, Salzman KL, Harnsberger HR, et al. Sinus histiocytosis with massive lymphadenopathy (Rosai-Dorfman disease): imaging manifestations in the head and neck. AJR Am J Roentgenol 2008;191(6):W299–306.
65. Otta Ottaviano G, Doro D, Marioni G, et al. Extranodal Rosai-Dorfman disease: involvement of eye, nose and trachea. Acta Otolaryngol 2006;126(6):657–60.
66. Kann BH, Buckstein M, Carpenter TJ, et al. Radiographic extracapsular extension and treatment outcomes in locally advanced oropharyngeal carcinoma. Head Neck 2013. http://dx.doi.org/10.1002/hed.23512.
67. Seethala RR. Current state of neck dissection in the United States. Head Neck Pathol 2009;3(3):238–45. http://dx.doi.org/10.1007/s12105-009-0129-y.
68. Ghadjar P, Simcock M, Schreiber-Facklam H, et al. Incidence of small lymph node metastases with evidence of extracapsular extension: clinical implications in patients with head and neck squamous cell carcinoma. Int J Radiat Oncol Biol Phys 2010;78(5):1366–72.
69. Kimura Y, Sumi M, Sakihama N, et al. MR imaging criteria for the prediction of extranodal spread of metastatic cancer in the neck. AJNR Am J Neuroradiol 2008;29(7):1355–9.
70. Subramaniam RM, Alluri KC, Tahari AK, et al. PET/CT imaging and human papilloma virus-positive oropharyngeal squamous cell cancer: evolving clinical imaging paradigm. J Nucl Med 2014; 55(3):431–8.
71. Mack MG, Rieger J, Baghi M, et al. Cervical lymph nodes. Eur J Radiol 2008;66(3):493–500.
72. Nakamura T, Sumi M. Nodal imaging in the neck: recent advances in US, CT and MR imaging of metastatic nodes. Eur Radiol 2007;17(5):1235–41.
73. Gor DM, Langer JE, Loevner LA. Imaging of cervical lymph nodes in head and neck cancer: the basics. Radiol Clin North Am 2006;44(1):101–10, viii.
74. Layland MK, Sessions DG, Lenox J. The influence of lymph node metastasis in the treatment of squamous cell carcinoma of the oral cavity, oropharynx, larynx, and hypopharynx: N0 versus N+. Laryngoscope 2005;115(4):629–39.

Imaging Evaluation of the Suprahyoid Neck

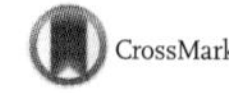

Caryn Gamss, MD, Ajay Gupta, MD, J. Levi Chazen, MD, C. Douglas Phillips, MD*

KEYWORDS

• Suprahyoid neck • Parapharyngeal space • Masticator space • Parotid space • Carotid space • Pharyngeal mucosal space • Magnetic resonance imaging • Computed tomography

KEY POINTS

- The suprahyoid neck is anatomically complex but can be organized into specific spaces based on the fascial planes and the individual space contents. The ability to place a pathologic process within a specific suprahyoid neck space is the first step in generating a differential diagnosis.
- The parapharyngeal space (PPS) deserves close attention in all cases of suprahyoid neck masses because the mass effect on the parapharyngeal fat follows a particular pattern and can help localize the pathology to a specific neck space.
- The masticator space (MS) demonstrates a variety of pathologic processes. It can serve as a conduit to other areas, including intracranial extension through foramen ovale, and, therefore, imaging along the entire course of the V3 should be performed.
- The purpose of parotid imaging is not necessarily to provide an exact diagnosis. Rather, it should aid in planning the next step. If a lesion is discrete, fine-needle aspiration (FNA) or core biopsy may be appropriate but an aggressive-appearing lesion may warrant total resection with margins and neck dissection.
- The carotid space (CS) should be evaluated carefully in a work-up for hoarseness. This space originates at the skull base and includes pathologic processes of the jugular foramen (JF).
- Squamous cell carcinoma (SCC) is by far the most common malignancy of the pharyngeal mucosal space (PMS). The role of imaging is to characterize the extent of the mass deep to the mucosal surface.

INTRODUCTION

The suprahyoid neck extends from the hyoid bone inferiorly to the skull base. The anatomic spaces created by fascial planes in the suprahyoid neck are the PMS, PPS, MS, parotid space (PS), CS, retropharyngeal space, and prevertebral space. This article emphasizes imaging considerations for the PMS, PPS, MS, PS, and CS. The retropharyngeal and prevertebral spaces are covered in greater depth elsewhere (**Fig. 1**).

A systematic approach is crucial in approaching neck masses on imaging studies. Establishing the location of a mass and identifying the space of origin are invaluable initial steps in developing a differential diagnosis. Utilization of the 3 layers of the deep cervical fascia to delineate multiple compartments of the suprahyoid and infrahyoid neck is the current paradigm and allows segmentation of pathology into well-defined fascially enclosed spaces. Next, the relationship to the surrounding spaces and structures, including the skull base, oral cavity, and infrahyoid neck, must be evaluated. A differential diagnosis can be generated based upon the unique anatomic contents of each space.

Department of Radiology, Weill Cornell Medical College, New York-Presbyterian Hospital, 525 East 68th Street, New York, NY 10065, USA
* Corresponding author.
E-mail address: cdp2001@med.cornell.edu

Radiol Clin N Am 53 (2015) 133–144
http://dx.doi.org/10.1016/j.rcl.2014.09.009
0033-8389/15/$ – see front matter

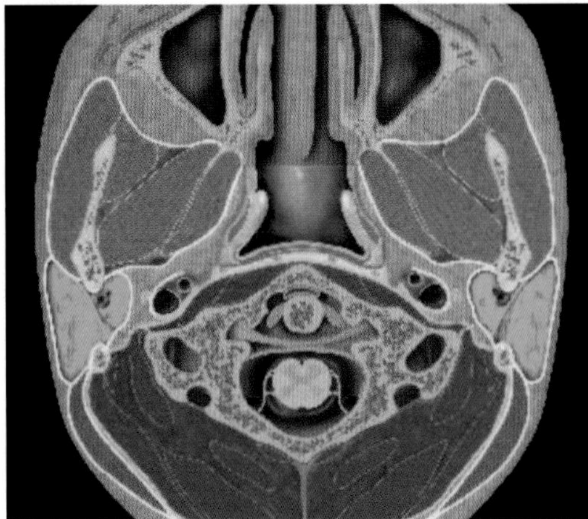

Fig. 1. The axial graphic depicts the suprahyoid neck spaces. Each space is separated and contained within the investing fascial layers. The paired MS (*purple*) surrounds the PMS. Posterior to the MS are the paired PS (*green*) and, medially, the CS (*orange*). Nestled between the MS, PMS, and CS lies the triangular-shaped PPS.

PARAPHARYNGEAL SPACE

Anatomy

The PPS is a symmetric crescent-shaped space in the suprahyoid neck lateral to the pharynx. It is an anatomic recess that was historically separated into the prestyloid and retrostyloid spaces by the tensor veli palatini,[1] styloid process, and associated musculature and ligaments. The anteriorly located prestyloid compartment is deep to the MS and lateral to the pharyngeal mucosa and borders the deep lobe of the parotid gland laterally.[2] The more posterior retrostyloid compartment contains the carotid sheath and its contents. For the purpose of an imaging differential diagnosis, it is convenient to consider the retrostyloid space as part of the carotid sheath or more contemporarily as the CS, because they are as one.[3] Thus, the focus in this section, the PPS, is on the contemporary PPS, previously known as the prestyloid space.

The PPS extends from the skull base down to the angle of the mandible. It is enclosed by layers of investing fascia laterally, separating it from the MS and PS and by the buccopharyngeal and prevertebral fascia, medially and posteriorly. The PPS is continuous with the submandibular and sublingual spaces, lacking a fascial barrier anteriorly. The lack of ventral border allows for spread of disease from the PPS along the pterygomandibular raphe, which connects the medial pterygoid plate to the lingual surface of the mandible along the posterior margin of the mylohyoid muscle. In addition, it is the superior attachment site of the superior pharyngeal constrictor muscle and the buccinators muscle.

Contents

1. Fat (the predominant component)
2. Vascular structures, including the maxillary and ascending pharyngeal artery and the pterygoid venous plexus

Pathology

1. Infections, such as cellulitis and abscess
2. Benign masses, specifically benign mixed tumor (BMT); rare venous, lymphatic, or mixed venolymphatic malformations; rare branchial cleft cyst
3. Disease from contiguous spaces extending into the PPS (such as deep lobe parotid tumors)

The PPS is largely fat. Fat is conspicuous on MR imaging and CT and readily distinguished from other tissue types on imaging. As a result, the PPS is easily identified by head and neck radiologists on normal neck imaging. Displacement and distortion of the PPS secondary to mass effect from lesions arising along the PPS border is an informative finding (Fig. 2). The importance of the PPS is, therefore, not only to identify pathology arising from this location (because it is rare) but also to provide confirmation as to the origin of adjacent pathology. Surrounding mass lesions shift the PPS in specific directions, serving as a signature for the source of origin (Fig. 3). As a result, the PPS can be used to help determine

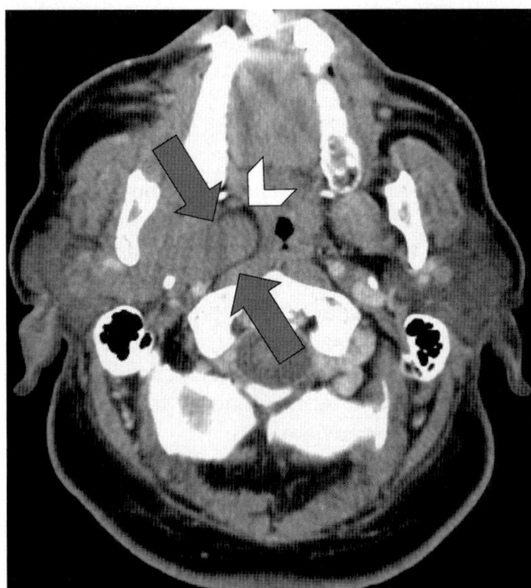

Fig. 2. Axial contrast-enhanced CT demonstrates a soft tissue mass (*arrows*) deforming the PPS and displacing it anteromedially (*arrowhead*). Based on the displacement pattern, the mass is arising from the deep lobe of the right parotid gland. PS origin was confirmed pathologically with a diagnosis of a BMT.

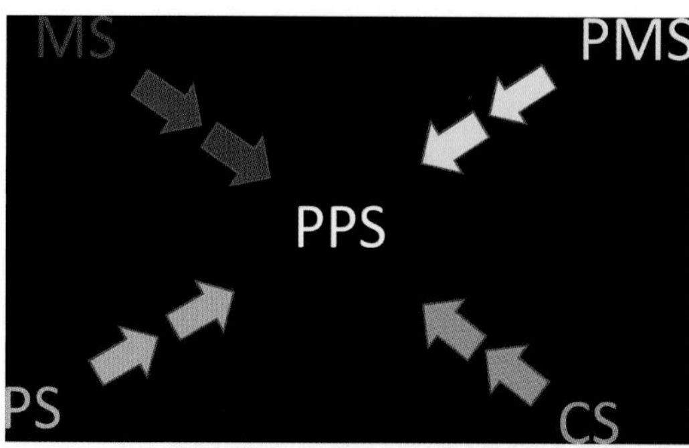

Fig. 3. Diagram demonstrating the relationship between the suprahyoid neck spaces and the parapharyngeal fat. A mass or pathologic process displaces the fat in a predictable pattern, allowing the radiologist to correctly identify the space of origin. As diagrammed, a mass in the MS pushes the PPS posteriorly, whereas a mass in the CS pushes it anteriorly. PMS deviates the PPS laterally and anterolaterally. (*Courtesy of* Kevan Shifteh.)

the originating space of a simple or complicated-appearing pathologic process. Primary PPS masses are rare, but if no clear contributor from the surrounding spaces is identified, the source is likely minor salivary gland ectopic rests.[4] The most common tumor arising from these rests is a BMT (**Fig. 4**).

MASTICATOR SPACE

Anatomy

The MS is located lateral to the PPS and divided into the suprazygomatic and infrazygomatic portions. It is the largest suprahyoid neck space, extending superiorly to the skull base, contacting foramen ovale, and foramen spinosum and inferiorly terminating along the margin of the posterior body of the mandible.

Contents

1. Muscles of mastication: masseter, medial, and lateral pterygoids and temporalis muscle
2. Posterior body and ramus of mandible (including temporomandibular joint)
3. Mandibular branch of the trigeminal nerve (cranial nerve [CN] V3)

The MS is delineated by the superficial layer of the deep cervical fascia (SLDCF). The SLDCF is made up of inner and outer layers, which encase the medial and lateral pterygoids, the masseter, and the temporalis muscles. These two layers fuse along the anterior and posterior borders of the mandibular ramus, enclosing the MS. In addition to these muscles, the mandibular ramus is included in the MS. The mandibular branch of the trigeminal nerve (cranial nerve [CN] V3) enters the MS through foramen ovale, providing motor supply to the aforementioned muscles of mastication plus the mylohyoid, anterior belly of the digastric, tensor veli palati, and tensor tympani. It also provides sensory innervation to the lower face. Benign masses and malignant lesions involving the MS have the potential to spread into other locations, including intracranial extension through foramen ovale, via perineural tumor spread along the course of this nerve (**Fig. 5**). Because the nerve spans from the bottom of the mandible to the skull vertex, all cross-sectional imaging should include the entire course of V3, including the lateral

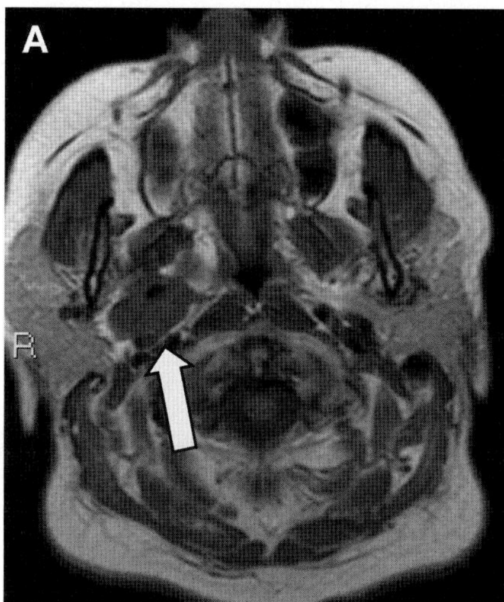

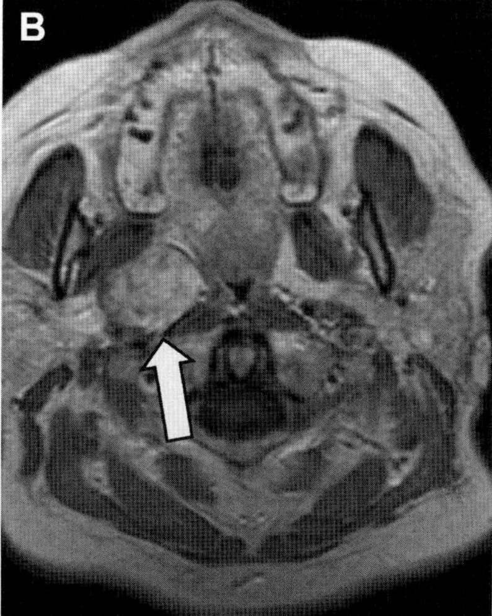

Fig. 4. Axial T1WI (*A*) without contrast and (*B*) after contrast demonstrates a mass within the PPS (*arrow*). There are clear fat planes surrounding the lesion precluding its origin from surrounding spaces. The mass is a BMT arising from ectopic parotid rests within the PPS.

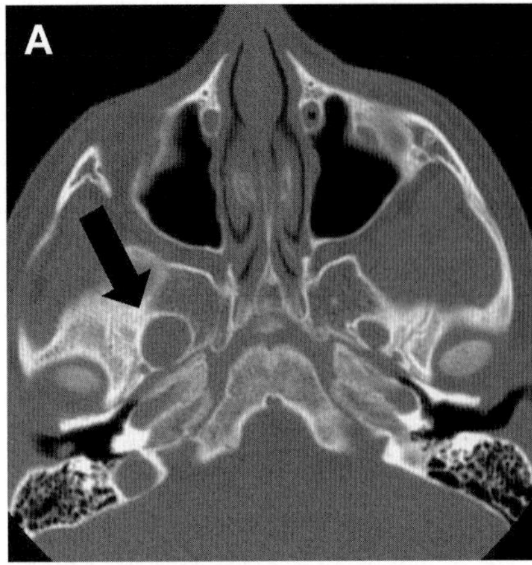

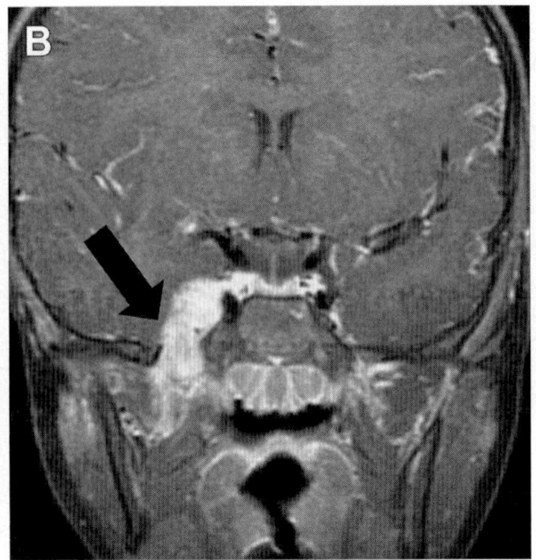

Fig. 5. (*A*) Axial CT, bone window, demonstrates asymmetric enlargement of the right foramen ovale (*arrow*). (*B*) Coronal contrast-enhanced T1WI demonstrates an enhancing schwannoma (*arrow*) extending through foramen ovale along the course of the V3.

pons, Meckel cave, foramen ovale, mandibular foramen, inferior alveolar canal, and mental foramen (**Fig. 6**).

Pathology

1. Inflammatory/infectious conditions (most commonly of dental origin)
2. Vascular lesions
3. Sarcomas arising from muscle, bone, and other soft tissues

Imaging plays an important role because clinical evaluation of the MS space is limited. Patients may complain only of trismus, which is a nonspecific finding. If other signs and symptoms are present, however, including fever, high white blood cell count, or a tender swollen cheek, an infection is the likely culprit. Because odontogenic infections stemming from dental caries and tooth extractions are by far the most common entity, CT is often the preferred imaging modality. Dental caries or recent dental manipulation may be evident. These infections can manifest as cellulitis, myositis, and/or abscess (**Fig. 7**).[5] Contrast administration is important in evaluating the extent of infection and to differentiate cellulitis/phlegmon from abscess.

The second most common MS masses are vascular lesions. The pterygoid venous plexus is a normal structure in the MS but commonly this plexus is asymmetric and can be mistaken for a mass. It is often described as a pseudolesion of

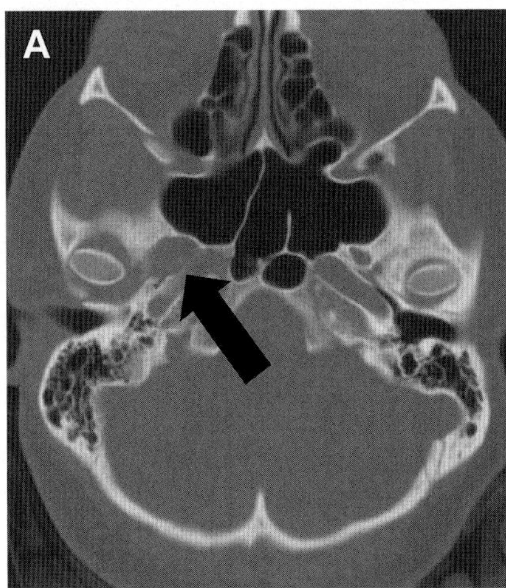

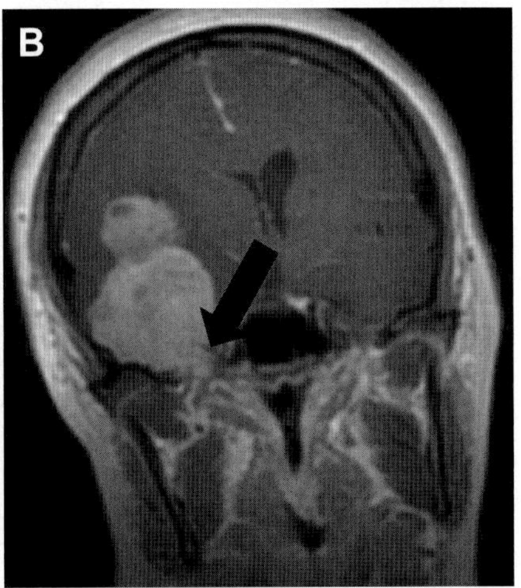

Fig. 6. (*A*) Axial CT, bone window, demonstrates asymmetric enlargement of the right foramen ovale (*arrow*). (*B*) Coronal contrast-enhanced T1WI depicting an enhancing extra-axial intracranial mass (hemangiopericytoma) extending through the skull base at foramen ovale (*arrow*).

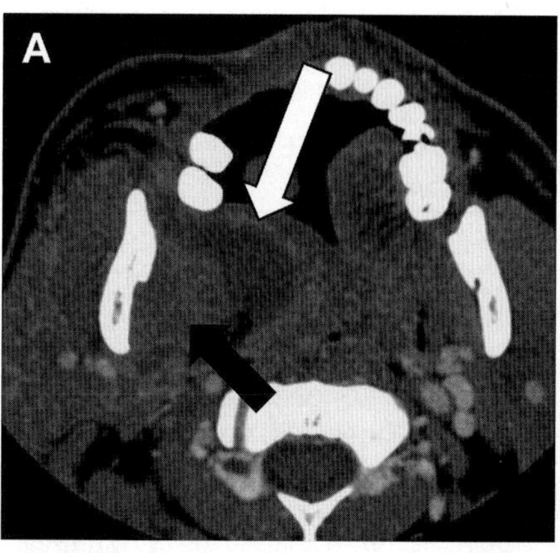

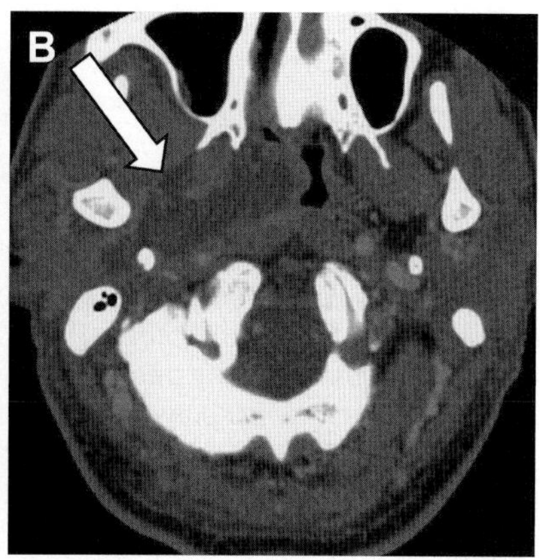

Fig. 7. Axial contrast-enhanced CT images (*A, B*) demonstrate low-density collection (*white arrows*) with peripheral enhancement in the right MS stemming from a dental infection. Important findings to evaluate include dental caries, missing teeth, and a fistulous connection between the infected tooth and the MS abscess (not seen). Inflammatory changes are seen in the MS with edema and enlargement of the pterygoids (*black arrow*).

the MS. True vascular lesions generally fall into 2 categories: (1) hemangiomas and (2) vascular malformations.[6]

Hemangiomas are true neoplasms and the most common pediatric tumor of the MS.[7] They are present at birth, grow rapidly during the first year of life, and undergo fatty replacement and involution by adolescence.[8] On MR imaging, the mass is well defined and demonstrates intermediate T1 signal and high T2 signal, depending on size. Prominent contrast enhancement is seen, particularly during the proliferative phase.[9]

Vascular malformations are present at birth but are often not clinically apparent until infancy or later. As opposed to hemangiomas, these lesions increase in size with age. They are the result of abnormal vessel morphogenesis and are labeled by their predominant tissue. They are divided into high-flow lesions and low-flow lesions. Low-flow lesions are venous, lymphatic, or mixed malformations (**Fig. 8**).[10] The lesions have low signal on CT, and the MR imaging characteristics are intermediate T1 and high T2, with prominent enhancement. Venous and lymphatic malformations can be confined to a muscle, most often the masseter, or can cross fascial planes within the deep spaces of the head and neck.[9]

High-flow vascular malformations contain arterial components and include both arterial venous malformations and arterial venous fistulas.[8] Large flow voids can be seen on T1-weighted image (T1WI) and T2-weighted image (T2WI) and often bone involvement is noted. When the bone is involved, it may be expanded and the lesion's margin can be eroded.[11]

Primary MS muscular lesions have a nonspecific imaging appearance. Clinical information, including patient age, can help limit the differential diagnosis. Primary neoplasms of the MS are rare and, therefore, systemic malignancy, head and neck malignancy, and infection should all be excluded before a primary MS sarcoma is considered. The mass often presents as an aggressive, poorly marginated lesion with bone destruction and violation of adjacent fascial planes. The most

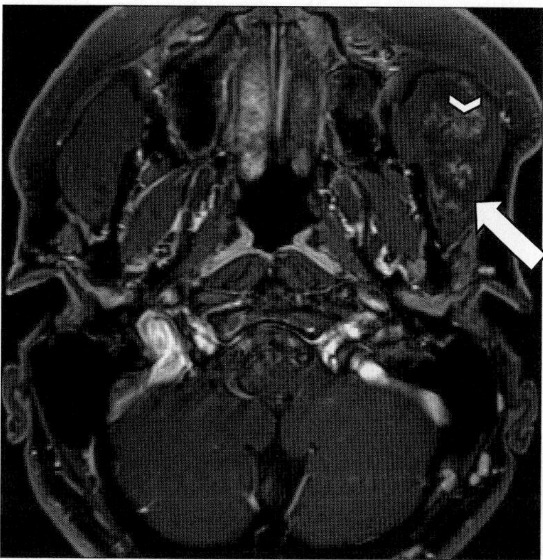

Fig. 8. Contrast-enhanced axial T1WI demonstrates a heterogeneously enhancing mass in the left MS (*white arrow*) causing enlargement of the masseter muscle. The enhancement (*arrowhead*) is due to abnormal venous structures in the setting of a venous malformation.

common neoplastic lesion in an adult is a leiomyosarcoma or malignant fibrous histiocytoma, whereas rhabdomyosarcoma is the most prevalent MS neoplasm in a child.

Neurogenic masses of the MS are tumors associated with the mandibular division of CN V or its branches, most commonly schwannomas. These lesions classically splay the medial and lateral pterygoid muscles away from each other. Proximally, a trigeminal schwannoma may demonstrate a "dumbbell" if it spans the porous trigeminus (**Fig. 9**).

Bony lesions of the MS include lesions of the mandible that are more likely odontogenic in origin.[1] These lesions include odontogenic cysts, such as dentigerous cysts or keratocystic odontogenic tumors (KOTs). Dentigerous cysts often form around the crown of an unerupted molar (**Fig. 10**). KOT often extend toward the ramus of the mandible and may be locally aggressive. Ameloblastoma is a locally aggressive odontogenic tumor that can be associated with a dentigerous cyst or an impacted tooth and in rare cases ameloblastoma can undergo malignant degeneration.

Malignant bone/cartilage lesions include osteogenic sarcoma, chondrosarcoma, Ewing sarcoma, and metastatic disease.[12] Metastases most commonly occur within the posterior body and angle of the mandible.

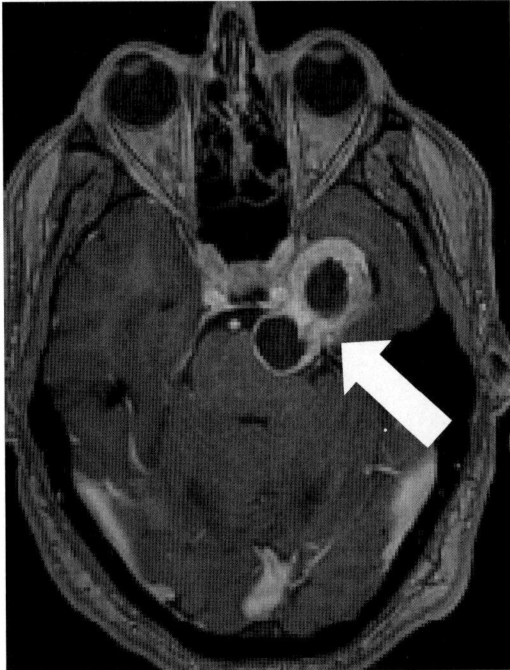

Fig. 9. Axial contrast-enhanced T1WI demonstrates a nerve sheath tumor (schwannoma) (*arrow*) with peripheral enhancement and central cystic change in a figure 8 formation as it passes through the porus trigeminus.

PAROTID SPACE

Anatomy

As its name indicates, the PS contains the parotid gland. The fascia about the PS is inseparable from the gland itself, such that an attempt to dissect out the gland leaves no "space" behind.[13] The parotid gland is traditionally divided into the deep and superficial lobes, separated by the plane of the facial nerve. Identifying the facial nerve, however, is difficult on imaging, and the adjacent retromandibular vein is often used as a landmark on cross-sectional imaging. In 20% of the population, there is an accessory third lobe, superficial to the masseter muscle. The parotid duct travels along the surface of the masseter muscle, then pierces the buccinator muscle at the level of the second maxillary molar. The normal duct should be small in size and often is not identifiable on imaging. The gland density decreases with increasing age due to normal fatty involution. At times, one gland may undergo premature fatty degeneration, which should not be mistaken for pathology. The PS also includes numerous intraparotid lymph nodes, because the parotid is encapsulated later in development.

Contents

1. Parotid gland
2. Facial nerve
3. External carotid artery (ECA) branches and retromandibular vein
4. Lymph nodes (a normal finding due to embryologically late encapsulation of the gland)

When approaching a PS mass, key imaging considerations include benign versus aggressive margins, unifocal versus multifocal location, and homogeneous versus heterogeneous appearance. Often the purpose of parotid imaging is not necessarily to provide an exact diagnosis. If a lesion is discrete, FNA or core biopsy may be the next step but an aggressive-appearing lesion may warrant total resection with margins and even potentially a neck dissection. Malignant pathology may appear well defined and benign on cross-sectional imaging. On the other hand, an ill-defined appearance more likely suggests malignancy. Multiplicity may also be helpful in the differential diagnosis of parotid pathology. CT and MR imaging can both aid in the diagnosis, however, there are particular circumstances where one modality is preferred. For example, in the setting of suspected inflammatory disease,

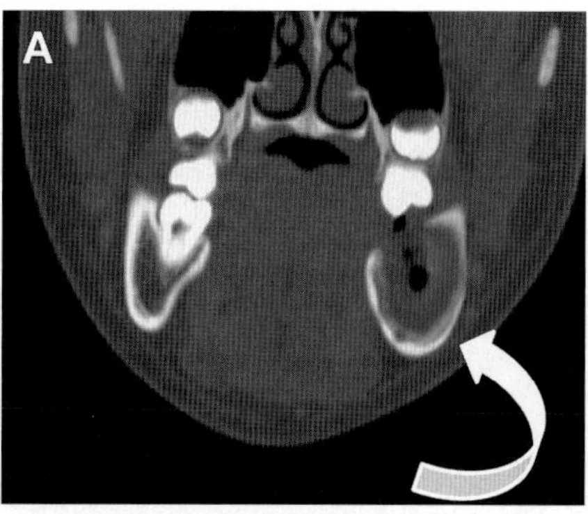

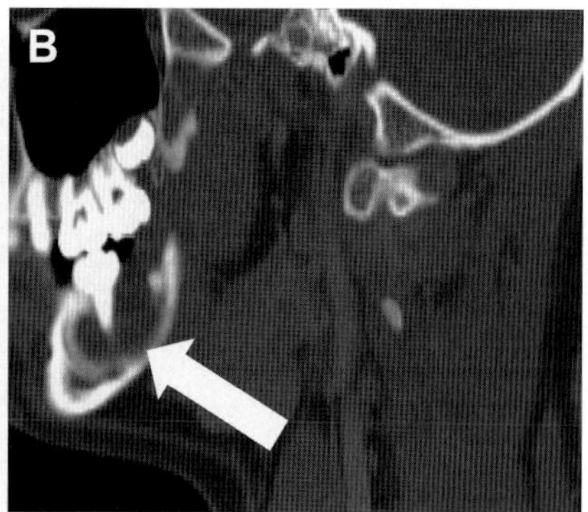

Fig. 10. (*A*) Coronal and (*B*) sagittal CTs, bone window, demonstrate a well-circumscribed (*curved arrow*), expansile radiolucent lesion surrounding the crown of an unerupted or impacted tooth (*arrow*).

CT is often the first imaging study. A calculus is more conspicuous on CT imaging. The presence of iodinated contrast media does not limit the detection of a potential calculus. Ductal dilatation and the presence of bilateral or unilateral processes should always be addressed. Important clinical information to have at the time of interpretation is the status of the facial nerve (CN VII). Benign neoplasms should not result in a facial nerve palsy. On the other hand, a patient with a significant ipsilateral CN VII paresis may harbor a malignant lesion. If facial palsy is the clinical indication, MR imaging is indicated to evaluate potential perineural spread of tumor. Perineural tumor can render the lesion unresectable or more difficult to resect, for example with extension into the temporal bone, internal auditory canal, or brainstem. Tumors may extend across the auriculotemporal branch of the trigeminal nerve (CN V) to reach CN VII, serving as an additional route of perineural spread of tumor to the parotid gland.

Pathology

1. Benign and malignant masses
2. Inflammatory/infectious processes

Approximately 80% of parotid tumors are benign.[14] The most common benign mass is a pleomorphic adenoma also known as a BMT (**Fig. 11**). The classic MR imaging appearance is a well-defined mass with uniform hyperintense T2 signal and homogeneous enhancement. When characteristic MR imaging findings are present along with concordant FNA results, a greater than 95% positive predictive value has been shown for pleomorphic adenoma diagnosis.[15] No additional features are 100% specific however, and tissue sampling or resection is almost invariably performed. Although these lesions are benign, they are often surgically removed for cosmetic reasons and because they carry a potential risk of malignant degeneration. A complete resection at the time of initial surgery is critical because residual tumor can create multiple daughter lesions that are difficult to resect. Schwannomas of the facial nerve, when small, can present as solidly enhancing masses and may develop central cystic degeneration when large. Benign parotid masses do not cause CN VII palsy; therefore as mentioned previously, malignant causes should be considered in that clinical scenario.

When multiple lesions are present, a differential diagnosis, including non-Hodgkin lymphoma, HIV with lymphoepithelial lesions, Sjögren's disease, and Warthin tumor, should be considered. Warthin tumors are usually well-defined cystic masses, with varying enhancement seen well on both MR imaging and CT (**Fig. 12**).

An oncocytoma is a rare benign parotid gland mass. There are no reliable distinguishing features on CT and ultrasound but oncocytomas demonstrate well-demarcated contours on T1WI and appear isointense to parotid tissue of postcontrast T1WI with fat saturation, categorizing it as a vanishing lesion. Preoperative identification of correct histology may help in surgical planning.[16]

Malignant parotid lesions include mucoepidermoid carcinoma (MEC) and adenoid cystic carcinoma (ACC). MEC is the most common primary malignancy of the parotid, arising from the ductal epithelium. The lesion characteristically contains areas of low T2 signal and can often be inconspicuous on postcontrast imaging because it demonstrates similar enhancement to normal parotid tissue. High-grade lesions are commonly associated with nodal spread.

ACC is the second most common parotid malignancy, arising from the peripheral parotid ducts. It demonstrates moderate T2 signal intensity and its aggressive appearance increases with tumor grade. ACC has the greatest propensity for perineural spread among the head and neck cancers

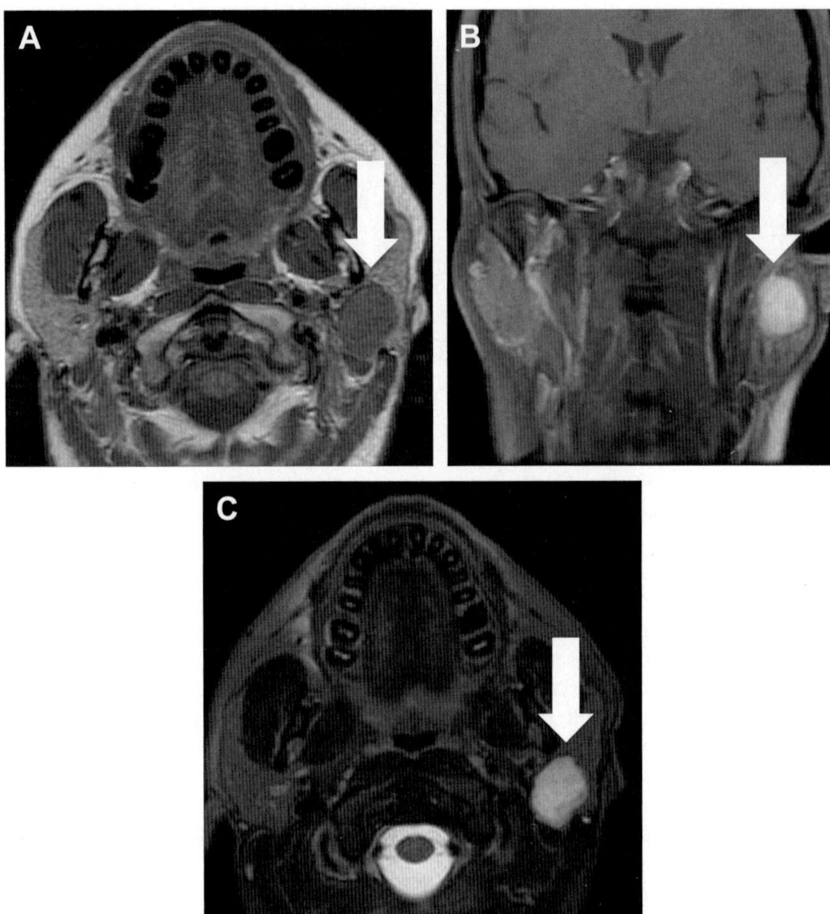

Fig. 11. (*A*) Axial T1 demonstrates a well-circumscribed hypointense mass (*white arrow*) in left parotid gland, which demonstrated homogeneous enhancement on the T1 post-contrast image (*B*). (*C*) The mass is T2 hyperintense and lobulated, typical findings of a BMT.

and local recurrence can occur 20 years after diagnosis, creating a favorable short-term but poor long-term prognosis.[17]

CAROTID SHEATH

Anatomy

The carotid sheath is a space that traverses both the suprahyoid and infrahyoid neck. It is located posterior to the styloid process, lateral to the retropharyngeal space, anterior to the prevertebral space, and medial to the parotid glands. The wall is made up of 3 layers with contributions from the superficial, middle, and deep cervical fascial layers. Caudal to the level of the bifurcation, the carotid sheath is a well-defined structure with circumferential borders. This space has been referred to using different terminology, such as the CS and the retrostyloid PPS (discussed previously). The CS has nasopharyngeal, oropharyngeal, cervical, and mediastinal segments.

Contents

1. Carotid artery
2. Internal jugular vein (IJV)
3. CNs IX, X, and XI and sympathetic chain
4. Lymph nodes are located lateral to the CS. Disease can spread into the space because the sheath is inconstant.

Pathology

1. Vascular pathology related to the carotid artery, include aneurysm, dissection, and arteritis. Jugular vein thrombosis and thrombophlebitis may also affect in this space.
2. Mass lesions, including neurogenic tumors and paragangliomas. They often arise in similar locations; imaging characteristics, including

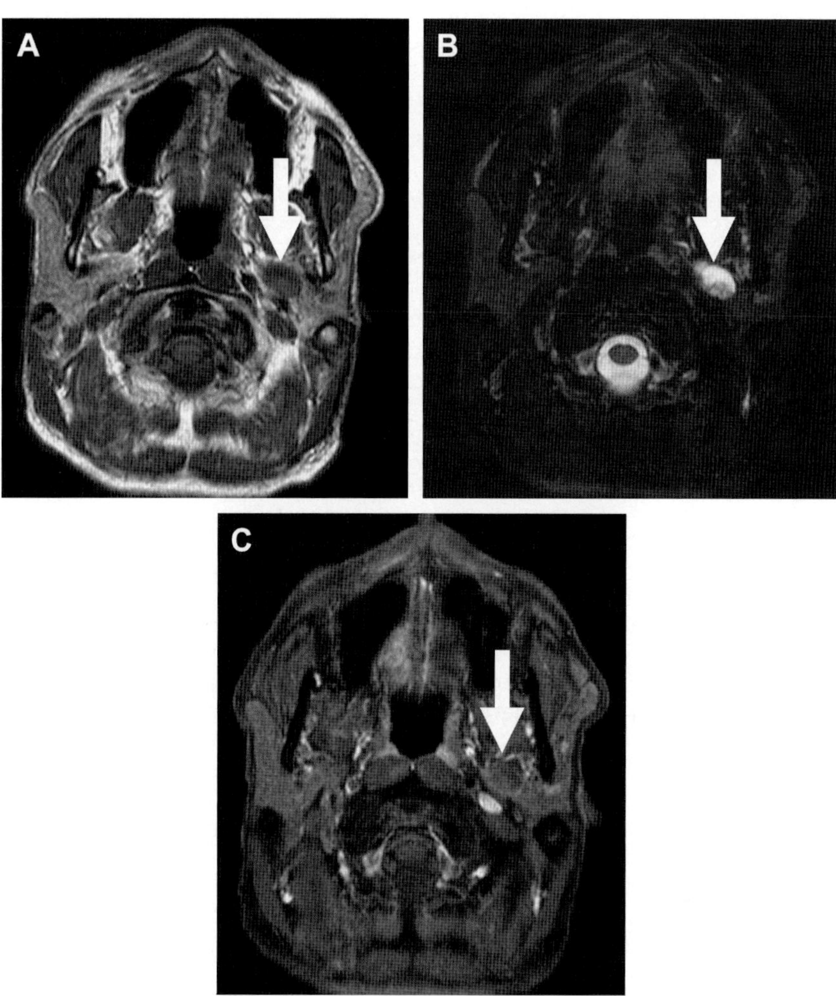

Fig. 12. Axial T1 (*A*), axial fat-suppressed T2 (*B*), and axial fat-suppressed postcontrast T1 (*C*) demonstrates a T1 hypointense, T2 hyperintense but heterogeneous, hypoenhancing mass (*arrow*) in the left deep lobe of the parotid gland. Surgical excision revealed a Warthin tumor.

prominent flow voids (salt-and-pepper appearance) within a paraganglioma, can reliably distinguish the two.

3. Lymph nodes either from neoplastic or inflammatory causes, located lateral to but closely approximating the CS.
4. Neoplastic causes, either contiguous or from perineural spread of tumor, most commonly SCC.

Vascular pathology can either be intrinsic to the internal carotid artery (ICA) or intrinsic to the IJV. Imaging options include CT and CT angiography as well as MR imaging and magnetic resonance angiography (MRA). Disease, including vessel tortuosity, thrombosis/phlebitis, pseudoaneurysm, dissection, and stenosis, is readily diagnosed using either technique. Acute IJV thrombophlebitis can mimic cellulitis/abscess whereas more chronic thrombosis can have the appearance of a mass. It is important to identify the IJV as the epicenter of these pathologic processes (**Fig. 13**).

CS lesions may come to a clinicians' attention during a work-up for hoarseness. Masses within the CS may arise from or compress CNs IX, X, and XII within the space, most commonly detected if CN X is involved. The skull base must be reviewed with special attention to the JF. Masses at the JF include glomus jugulare paraganglioma, schwannoma, and meningioma. Masses within the nasopharyngeal segment of the CS may actually represent lesions projecting downward from the skull base. CT may be helpful based on adjacent bony changes. A glomus jugulare paraganglioma typically results in permeative destructive osseous changes whereas a schwannoma incites smooth, expansile remodeled margins of the JF.

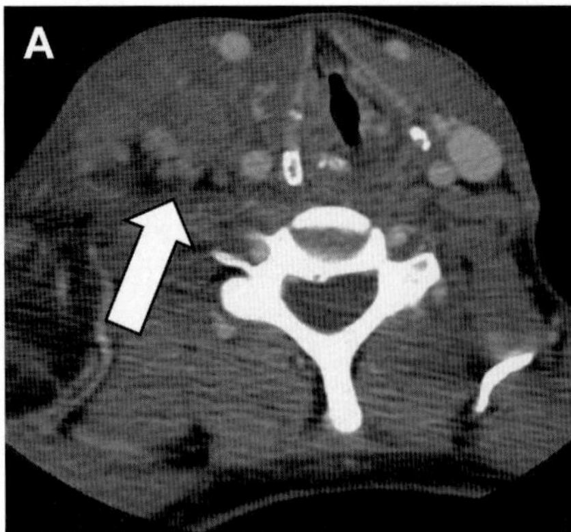

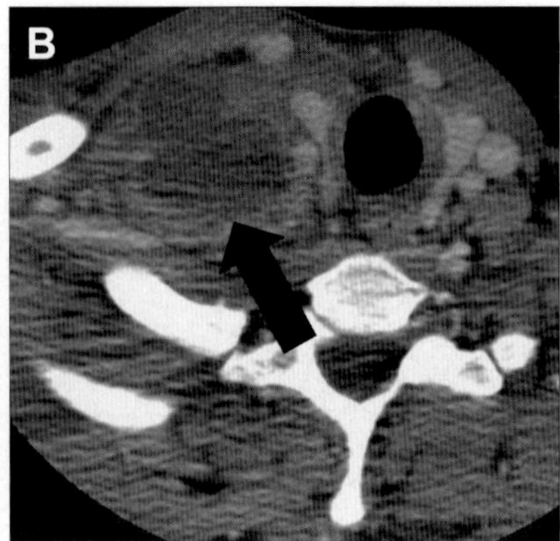

Fig. 13. Contrast-enhanced CT images showing (*A*) thrombosis of the right IJ (*white arrow*) with surrounding inflammatory change and (*B*) a fluid collection (*black arrow*). This patient was found to have pharyngitis with resulting septic IJ thrombophlebitis caused by *Fusobacterium necrophorum* seen in Lemierre syndrome.

Hyperostotic or permeative-sclerotic changes can be seen from a meningioma.

Glomus carotid paraganglioma is a slow-growing, painless vascular mass located at the carotid bifurcation, splaying the ICA and ECA. Contrast-enhanced CT and MR imaging demonstrate avid enhancement (**Fig. 14**). Larger lesions have a salt-and-pepper appearance on T2WIs, namely foci of subacute hemorrhage and punctuate vascular flow voids, respectively.

Masses within the CS space push adjacent structures in different directions depending on the level. If the mass is located within the nasopharyngeal segment of the CS, it displaces the PPS anteriorly, whereas at the oropharyngeal level, in addition to pushing the PPS forward, the posterior belly of the digastric muscle is displaced laterally. In addition, the structures within the CS are displaced depending on the pathology and can serve as a differentiating characteristic. For example, a vagal schwannoma and a sympathetic schwannoma share the same imaging appearance but a vagal schwannoma more likely divides the ICA and IJV whereas a sympathetic schwannoma displaces both structures anteriorly.[18]

The distinction between a glomus vagale tumor and a vagus schwannoma can be made based on location, because the glomus tumor is within 2 cm of the skull base and contains flow voids; these features are not characteristic of vagal schwannomas.[19] Differentiating a schwannoma from a neurofibroma can be difficult. CT may be helpful; a neurofibroma is typically lower in density relative to a schwannoma.

PHARYNGEAL MUCOSAL SPACE

Anatomy

The PMS extends the length of the pharyngeal mucosal surface and is divided into nasopharyngeal, oropharyngeal, and hypopharyngeal segments. Superiorly, it abuts the skull base along the superior/posterior aspect of the nasopharyngeal roof and extends inferiorly to the level of the hypopharynx. The PMS is bordered by the middle layer of the deep cervical fascia at its lateral and posterior deep margins but is not a truly enclosed fascial space because there is no fascia along the surface. A PMS mass can disrupt the mucosal/submucosal surfaces or can displace surrounding spaces, in particular the PPS laterally.

Contents

1. Mucosal surface of the pharynx
2. Pharyngeal lymphatic ring (includes adenoids, palatine, and lingual tonsils)
3. Minor salivary glands contained in the submucosa in highest concentration within the hard and soft palate

Pathology

1. Malignant tumors
   a. Nasopharyngeal carcinoma (NPC)
   b. Oropharyngeal carcinoma (palatine and lingual tonsil)
   c. Non-Hodgkin lymphoma
   d. Minor salivary gland carcinoma
2. Inflammatory lesions
   a. Tonsillar lymphoid hyperplasia
   b. Pharyngitis or postradiation change
3. Infectious causes
   a. Tonsillar or peritonsillar abscess
4. Musculoskeletal tumors
   a. Rhabdomyosarcoma
   b. Chordoma
5. Miscellaneous
   a. Tornwaldt cyst

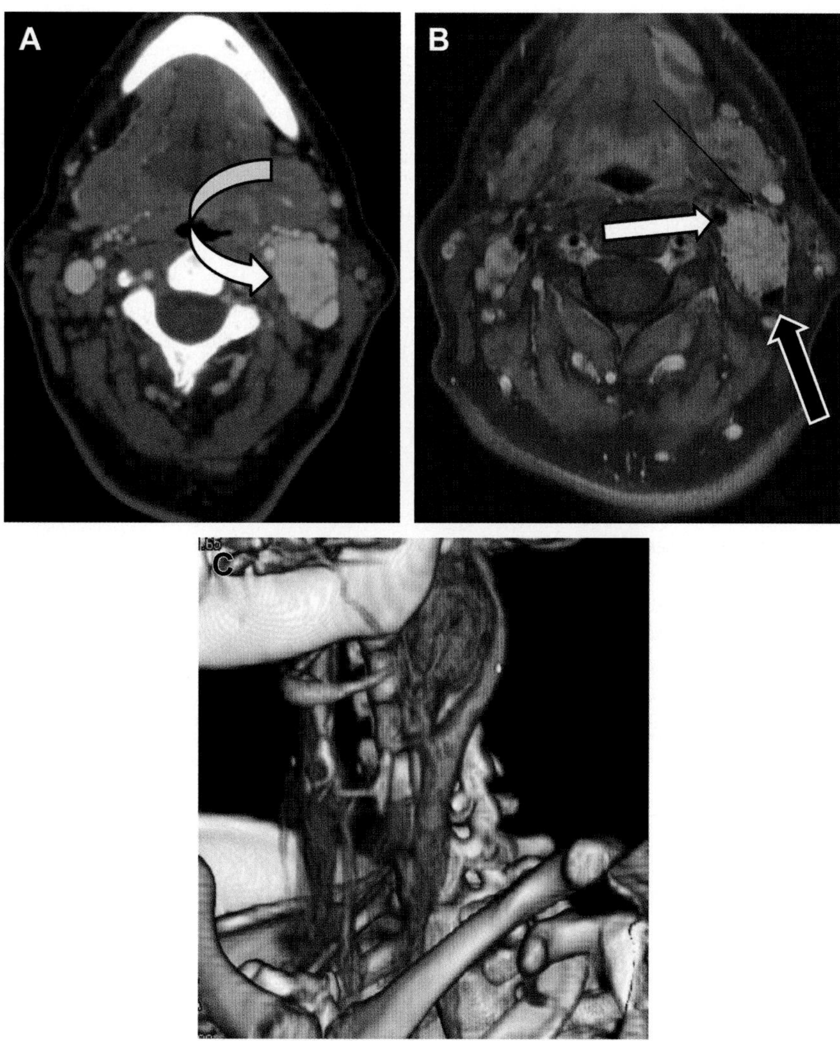

Fig. 14. (*A*) Axial contrast-enhanced CT shows a classic glomus carotid paraganglioma with avid uniform enhancement (*curved arrow*). (*B*) The contrast-enhanced T1WI depicts the mass located between splayed branches of the carotid artery. ECA anteriorly (*white arrow*) and the ICA posterolaterally (*black arrow*). (*C*) 3-D reformatted image clearly shows the mass sitting within the carotid notch.

Understanding and correctly identifying the pathology within the PMS is largely related to the imaging appearance, location of origin, and its effect on the PMS airway. Clinical input is often helpful in this regard as well. A clinical note indicating the site of primary lesion evident on endoscopy may be very helpful at the time of image review. Patient demographic information and age are also important. For example, in the setting of a tonsillar mass in a young patient, considerations include tonsillar lymphoid hyperplasia, especially if recurrent bouts of tonsillitis are reported. Although tonsillar inflammation has a characteristic striated appearance of mixed attenuation on CT, if rim enhancement is identified surrounding a fluid density collection, an abscess should be considered. Extension of abscess beyond the tonsillar tissue gives rise to a peritonsillar abscess.

SCC is by far the most common malignancy in this location. The site of origin is important to describe although the surface lesion itself can be directly visualized with greater accuracy by a referring endoscopist. Therefore, the role of imaging in guiding treatment decisions in SCC is to characterize the extent of the mass deep to the mucosal surface, including the presence of invasion into the surrounding spaces and whether nodal spread is present. Review of current American Joint Committee on Cancer staging criteria allows radiologists to note the important sites of disease spread to aid clinical staging.

The relationship between the PMS and the skull base is important in the setting of NPC. This tumor has a propensity for early intracranial spread largely because of its proximity to the foramen lacerum. Tumors can invade through the foramen's cartilaginous floor and travel along the ICA to invade the cavernous sinus. NPC may also spread via perineural tumor spread into the skull base and cavernous sinus. Although this is almost invariably non-operable disease, careful localization of tumor to determine radiation portals can be critical.

SUMMARY

Evaluating the complex anatomy of the suprahyoid neck on imaging studies can be a daunting task without a sound understanding of anatomy and a systematic approach. In this article, the suprahyoid neck is divided into characteristic anatomic spaces, which allow for accurate localization of both normal structures and abnormal pathology in the neck. Once a lesion is localized to a specific suprahyoid space, imaging characteristics and clinical data can be used in a logical fashion to provide a clinically useful imaging differential diagnosis.

REFERENCES

1. Mukherji SK, Castillo M. A simplified approach to spaces of the suprahyoid neck. Radiol Clin North Am 1998;36(5):761–80.
2. Gupta A, Chazen JL, Phillips D. Imaging evaluation of the parapharyngeal space. Otolaryngol Clin North Am 2012;45:1223–32.
3. Chong VF, Mukherji SK, Goh CH. The suprahyoid neck: normal and pathological anatomy. J Laryngol Otol 1999;113(6):501–8.
4. Shahab R, Heliwell T, Jones AS. How we do it: a series of 114 primary pharyngeal space neoplasms. Clin Otolaryngol 2005;30(4):364–7.
5. Schuknecht B. Masticator space abscess derived from odontogenic infection: imaging manifestation and pathways of extension depicted by CT and MR in 30 patients. Eur Radiol 2008;18(9):1972–9.
6. Fernandes T, Lobo JC, Castro R. Anatomy and pathology of the masticator space. Insights Imaging 2013;4:605–16.
7. Yousem DM, Grossman RI. Neuroradiology; the requisites. 3rd edition. Philadelphia: Mosby; 2010.
8. Finn MC, Glowaki J, Mulliken JB. Congenital vascular lesions: clinical application of a new classification. J Pediatr Surg 1983;18:894–9.
9. Nour SG, Lewin JS. Parapharyngeal and masticator spaces. In: Mafee MF, Valvassori GE, Becker M, editors. Imaging of the head and neck. 2nd edition. New York: Thieme; 2005. p. 580–624.
10. Som PM, Smoker WRK, Curtin HD, et al. Congenital lesions. In: Som PM, Curtin HD, editors. Head and neck imaging. 4th edition. St Louis (MO): Mosby; 2003. p. 1828–64.
11. Scholl RJ, Kellett HM, Neumann DP, et al. Cysts and cystic lesions of the mandible: clinical and radiologic-histopathologic review. Radiographics 2005;19(5):1107–24.
12. Atanosov DT. Sarcomas of the mandible: literature review and case reports. Folia Med (Plovdiv) 2004; 46(2):31–5.
13. Som PM, Curtin HD. Fascia and Spaces of the Neck. In: Som PM, Curtin HD, editors. Head and neck imaging. 5th edition. St Louis (MO): Mosby; 2011. p. 2203–34.
14. Freling NJ. Malignant parotid tumors: clinical use of MR imaging and histologic correlation. Radiolology 1992;185(3):691–6.
15. Heaton CM, Chazen JL, van Zante A, et al. Pleomorphic adenoma of the major salivary glands: diagnostic utility of FNAB and MRI. Laryngoscope 2013;123(12):3056–60.
16. Patel ND, Zante A, Eisele DW, et al. Oncocytoma. The vanishing parotid mass. AJNR Am J Neuroradiol 2011;32:1703–6.
17. Maroldi R. Perineural tumor spread. Neuroimaging Clin N Am 2008;18(2):413–29.
18. Anil G, Tan TY. Imaging Characteristics of Schwannoma of the cervical sympathetic chain: a review of 12 cases. AJNR Am J Neuroradiol 2013;34:628–33.
19. Yousem MD, Zimmerman MD, Grossman MD. Neuroradiology: the requisites. 3rd edition. Philadelphia: Mosby; 2010. p. 498.

Imaging Thyroid Disease

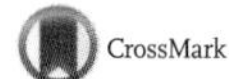

Updates, Imaging Approach, and Management Pearls

Jenny K. Hoang, MBBS[a,b,*], Julie A. Sosa, MD, MA[c], Xuan V. Nguyen, MD, PhD[d], P. Leo Galvin, MD[a], Jorge D. Oldan, MD[a]

KEYWORDS

• Thyroid cancer • Incidental thyroid nodule • Ultrasonography • Radioactive iodine scan • CT • MR imaging • Hyperthyroidism

KEY POINTS

- Thyroid cancer is the fastest increasing cancer in the United States. An exponential increase in incidence of thyroid cancer has been partly attributed to an increased work-up of incidentally detected thyroid nodules on imaging, especially ultrasonography and computed tomography (CT).
- A categorization method has been proposed for guiding the evaluation of incidental thyroid nodules detected on CT, MR imaging, or PET/CT. The method is a 3-tiered system and is based on the patient's age, nodule size, and suspicious imaging findings.
- The most common cause of hyperthyroidism is Graves disease, followed by toxic adenoma, toxic multinodular goiter, and subacute thyroiditis.
- Most patients do not have preoperative imaging with CT or MR imaging because ultrasonography adequately evaluates the primary tumor and nodal disease. CT or MR imaging is only performed in some cases of advanced local invasion to guide operative approach or decide whether surgery is possible.
- Ultrasonography of the neck is the first imaging investigation for suspected thyroid cancer recurrence. If the ultrasonography is negative and the histology is differentiated thyroid cancer, the next investigation should be radioiodine whole-body scintigraphy.

INTRODUCTION

There are many disorders that can occur in the thyroid gland, ranging from benign to malignant entities. Diseases in the thyroid can be subclinical or present with symptoms from structural or functional abnormalities. Imaging of the thyroid gland can also be complex because it includes different modalities such as ultrasonography, computed tomography (CT), MR imaging, and nuclear scintigraphy. Hence, expertise in the thyroid spans the subspecialties of neuroradiology, nuclear medicine, and body imaging. It is important for general radiologists and subspecialty radiologists to

Funding: No grant support or funding was received for this project.
Disclosure: The authors have nothing to disclose.

[a] Department of Radiology, Duke University Medical Center, Box 3808, Erwin Road, Durham, NC 27710, USA; [b] Department of Radiation Oncology, Duke University Medical Center, Durham, NC 27710, USA; [c] Division of Surgical Oncology, Department of Surgery, Duke University Medical Center, Box 2945, Durham, NC 27710, USA; [d] Department of Radiology, The Ohio State University Wexner Medical Center, 395 West 12th Avenue, Columbus, OH 43210, USA
* Corresponding author.
E-mail address: jennykh@gmail.com

Radiol Clin N Am 53 (2015) 145–161
http://dx.doi.org/10.1016/j.rcl.2014.09.002

understand key aims of imaging and treatment in order to provide helpful information to help guide management.

This article focuses on 5 common problems of the thyroid that require special consideration with regard to optimizing imaging strategies in a multidisciplinary and collaborative platform. These problems are the incidental thyroid nodule (ITN), preoperative evaluation of goiter, hyperthyroidism, invasive thyroid cancer, and recurrent thyroid cancer. For each problem, essential facts, interesting updates, optimal imaging approach, and management pearls are reviewed.

PROBLEM 1. THE INCIDENTAL THYROID NODULE DETECTED ON COMPUTED TOMOGRAPHY

A 51-year-old woman has an incidental 10-mm thyroid nodule on CT of the cervical spine performed for trauma. She has no personal or family history of thyroid disease. Should this nodule receive further work-up?

Essential Facts and Updates

ITNs on imaging are common, seen in 16% to 18% of CT scans that cover the neck.[1–4] Although ultrasonography has greater resolution than CT, several recent studies show that CT is the most common modality responsible for detection of asymptomatic thyroid nodules because CT is performed more commonly than ultrasonography.[5–7] The rate of incidental thyroid findings on CT increases with age with a prevalence of ITN in one-third of patients more than 65 years of age.[1] ITNs are also twice as common in women.[1]

The decision to work up an ITN is driven by the possibility that the nodule may be malignant, but the malignancy rate is as low as 1.2% according to a large population-based case-control study.[8] In addition, most thyroid cancers are indolent in behavior.[4,9,10] Most patients with small thyroid cancers die with rather than from the thyroid cancer.[4,9] In addition, the work-up of ITN detected on imaging has been partly attributed to an exponential increase in thyroid cancer incidence with little change in mortality.[10,11] Since 1975, the incidence of thyroid cancer has nearly tripled, from 4.9 to 14.3 per 100,000 individuals.[11]

Imaging Recommendations and Findings

Components of work-up

If work-up is necessary after an ITN is detected on CT or MR imaging, the next investigation is ultrasonography. Ultrasonography has higher spatial resolution and allows better characterization of nodules. Many sonographic signs of thyroid cancer have been evaluated in the literature.[12] In the largest retrospective study to date, the only useful sonographic signs of malignancy were microcalcifications, solid composition, and size greater than 2 cm (odds ratios of 8.1, 4.0, and 3.6, respectively).[8]

Which incidental thyroid nodule to select for work-up?

Most ITNs on CT and MR imaging do not have reliable signs of malignancy, which has resulted in highly variable reporting practices.[13] A categorization method has recently been proposed for guiding the evaluation of ITN detected on CT, MR imaging, or PET/CT.[1,5,14] The method is a 3-tiered system and is based on patient's age, nodule size, and suspicious imaging findings (**Table 1**). Two retrospective studies found that the 3-tiered system had the potential to reduce radiographic and endocrinologic work-up without missing malignancies in the respective cohorts. Compared with an academic institution's clinical practice without specific guidelines, there was a 35% reduction in ITN work-up with the 3-tiered system.[5] Compared with a 1 cm size cut-off, there was a 46% reduction in ITN work-up with the 3-tiered system.[1]

Tip

Signs of focal fluorodeoxyglucose (FDG) activity and corresponding thyroid nodule on CT is worrisome for thyroid cancer (**Fig. 1**). The rate of malignancy in ITNs with focal FDG uptake in a euthyroid patient ranges between 26% and 50%, with an overall incidence of 33% in one systematic review.[15–19]

Management Pearls

The decision to perform subsequent evaluation of ITN with ultrasonography can lead to fine-needle aspiration (FNA) in a large number of patients with asymptomatic, benign disease. Ultrasonography criteria for FNA are different for various societies, resulting in highly variable practices among radiologists and clinicians.[13,20–23] Smith-Bindman and colleagues[8] recently found that an approach to FNA of thyroid nodules with 2 or more of 3 ultrasonography findings (size>2 cm, entirely solid composition, and microcalcifications) reduced unnecessary biopsies while maintaining a low risk of missed cancers (0.5%).

It is also valuable to appreciate that evaluation does not end with an FNA in one-third of

Table 1
The 3-tiered system of risk categories for thyroid nodules detected using CT, MR imaging, or PET

Category	Criteria for Categories	Recommendations
Risk category 1: highly suspicious for malignancy	PET avid thyroid nodule Suspicious lymphadenopathy[a] Extrathyroid spread with or without signs of vocal cord palsy on side of nodule Lung metastases	Strongly consider work-up with ultrasonography for nodules of any size
Risk category 2: indeterminate with risk factor of young age	Age<35 y	Consider work-up with ultrasonography if ≥1 cm in adults Consider work-up with ultrasonography for any size in pediatric patients
Risk category 3: indeterminate without risk factors	Age ≥35 y	Consider work-up with ultrasonography if ≥1.5 cm

Note: intended for management of ITN in low-risk patients.
[a] Suspicious lymph nodes are defined as nodes greater than 10 mm in short axis (with the exception of jugulodigastric lymph nodes, which were permitted to be up to 15 mm in short axis), or nodes that contained calcifications, cystic components, or irregular margins.

patients; cytology results can lead to repeat biopsies and even diagnostic lobectomy.[24] A recent study found that imaging-detected ITN contributed to nearly one-quarter of surgeries for thyroid nodules, and, despite indeterminate or suspicious cytology results that led to surgery, more than half were benign on final pathology.[7]

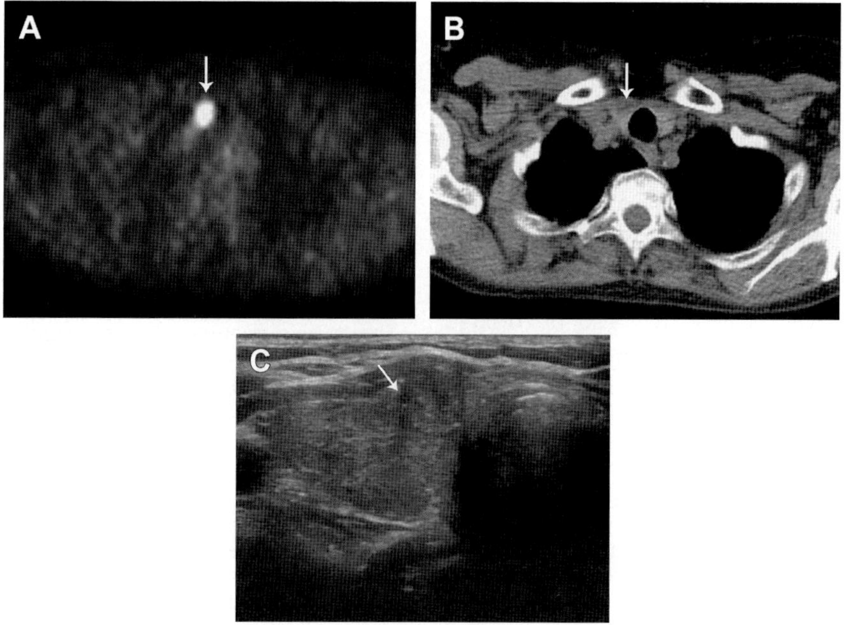

Fig. 1. A 63-year-old woman who had PET-CT for lymphoma surveillance and an incidental thyroid cancer detected on PET-CT. (*A*) PET image showing focal metabolic activity in the right lobe of thyroid (*arrow*). (*B*) Axial CT image at the same level shows a subtle thyroid nodule (*arrow*) measuring 1.3 cm in diameter. (*C*) Transverse ultrasonography image shows a solid hypoechoic nodule (*arrow*) measuring 1.5 cm with multiple hyperechoic foci representing microcalcifications. Fine-needle aspiration cytology revealed papillary thyroid cancer. She had a right partial thyroidectomy.

Recommendations

When interpreting the cervical spine CT in the 51-year-old woman, the radiologist can apply the 3-tiered system to the 1-cm ITN. If there are no other suspicious imaging features, the 1-cm nodule does not meet criteria for reporting the nodule in the impression section of the report and recommending subsequent evaluation with neck ultrasonography.

PROBLEM 2. GOITER FOR PREOPERATIVE PLANNING

A 64-year-old man has a goiter causing dysphagia. Thyroid function tests are within the normal range. On physical examination the inferior border of the thyroid could not be appreciated, suggesting a substernal component. He undergoes CT for surgical planning. What is the best approach to the CT scan interpretation?

Essential Facts and Updates

Goiter refers to abnormal growth and enlargement of the thyroid gland, which typically occurs over many years and is more common in women in their 50s and 60s.[25] Goiters can represent diffuse enlargement of the gland without nodules, or types with multinodular or uninodular patterns.

Approximately 20% to 25% of patients with goiters have evidence of either subclinical hyperthyroidism or overt hyperthyroidism.[26] Other symptoms relate to local mass effect on adjacent structures, particularly the trachea or esophagus. This condition is termed obstructive goiter and includes symptoms of discomfort or pressure, globus sensation, dyspnea, wheezing, cough, obstructive sleep apnea, dysphagia, and dysphonia (caused by pressure on the recurrent laryngeal nerve). Goiters can also be divided into those with or without substernal extension. There are also primary mediastinal goiters, which reside exclusively in the chest without any thyroid tissue in the neck.

Imaging Recommendations and Findings

Although sonography has the highest sensitivity for assessment of thyroid nodules within the goiter, CT plays a role in preoperative evaluation when there is clinical suspicion of substernal extension, if the goiter is massive with posterior and lateral extension, or if there is potential coexistence of cancer (**Fig. 2**). The approach to evaluation can follow 3 steps that cover the extent and effect of the goiter.

The first and most important feature to describe is the substernal extent because these goiters are most likely to cause respiratory symptoms and dysphagia. Substernal extent also affects surgical approach. Although most can still be resected from a cervical incision, a lower extent may require a partial or total sternotomy to facilitate complete resection. Sternotomy may also be required for excision of ectopic thyroid in the mediastinum. The radiologist should describe the lower extent of the goiter on each side and measure the distance from the sternal notch, which is best done on a sagittal reformatted image.

Next, evaluation should focus on the normal structures that are displaced and compressed by the goiter. These structures include central structures of the trachea, esophagus, larynx and pharynx, and recurrent laryngeal nerves. The radiologist should describe the direction and degree of displacement from the midline as well as effects of compression (see **Fig. 2**). The radiologist should evaluate for symmetry of the vocal cords and signs of vocal cord palsy. After evaluating central structures, attention should be directed to the upper extent of the goiter and structures immediately surrounding the thyroid gland, including the vascular structures, retropharyngeal space, and prevertebral space (see **Fig. 8**).

In the final step, the radiologist should question whether the imaging findings could represent malignancy or whether malignancy could coexist in the goiter. Clues of malignancy include invasion rather than compression of central and lateral structures and abnormal cervical lymph nodes.

Trap

The operative position is with arms down and neck extended. CT of the neck should not be performed with the arms up or the neck flexed. The thyroid assumes an apparently lower position in these positions, potentially misguiding the surgeon and resulting in unnecessary sternotomy rather than a simple low collar incision.[27]

Management Pearls

For many years the recommended surgical treatment of obstructive goiter was subtotal thyroidectomy to avoid postoperative hypothyroidism.[28] The main disadvantage of subtotal thyroidectomy is recurrence in up to 50% of patients.[29] In recent years, recommendations for symptomatic goiter have shifted toward total thyroidectomy. Lobectomy may be performed for unilocular goiter.

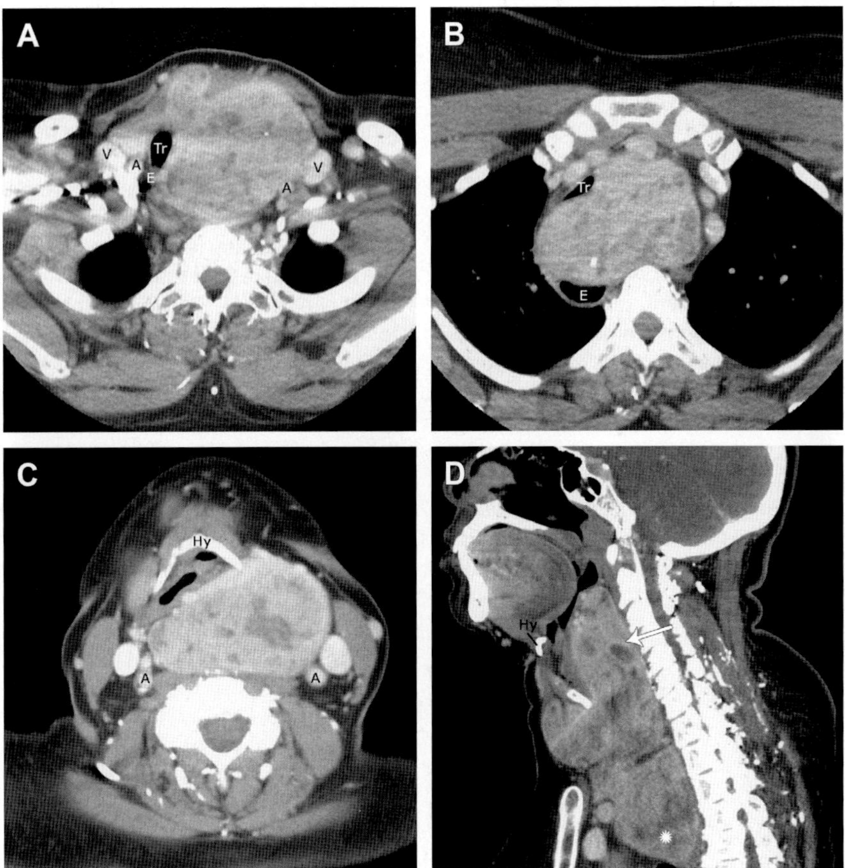

Fig. 2. A 57-year-old woman with 30-year history of large left-sided goiter and treatment with radioiodine presents with increased shortness of breath. (*A*) Axial enhanced CT image shows a goiter that compresses and displaces the trachea (Tr) and esophagus (E). The left common carotid artery (A) and internal jugular vein (V) are displaced laterally. (*B*) Axial enhanced CT image shows that the goiter extends into the mediastinum. The trachea (Tr) is displaced anteriorly and compressed. The esophagus is (E) is displaced to the right and posteriorly. (*C*) Axial enhanced CT image at the level of the hyoid bone (Hy) shows superior extension into the retropharyngeal space (between the internal carotid arteries [A]) where it has marked mass effect on the hypopharynx and supraglottic larynx. (*D*) Sagittal image shows the degree of substernal extension (*asterisk*) and the component extending superiorly in the retropharyngeal space (*arrow*). At total thyroidectomy was performed and a 555-g thyroid with marked nodular hyperplasia was removed.

Recommendations

This 64-year-old man has an obstructive goiter and concern for substernal extension. The approach to interpreting the CT should be a 3-step checklist evaluating mediastinal extent, assessing mass effect, and questioning if there is malignancy.

PROBLEM 3. HYPERTHYROIDISM

A 48-year-old woman presents with symptoms of hyperthyroidism and no palpable nodule. She has a suppressed thyroid-stimulating hormone (TSH) level and negative TSH-receptor antibodies. What is the next investigation and what are her treatment options?

Essential Facts and Updates

The most common cause of hyperthyroidism is Graves disease, followed by toxic multinodular goiter, toxic adenoma, and subacute thyroiditis.[30] Graves disease is an autoimmune thyroiditis that is characterized by autoantibodies to thyrotropin (TSH receptor). A toxic thyroid adenoma, or hot nodule, is an autonomously functioning nodule that accounts for 5% of patients with a solitary or dominant nodule.[20] Toxic multinodular goiter is an enlarged thyroid with multiple nodules in which 1 or more nodules are autonomously functioning; it is frequently seen in more mature patients.

Subacute thyroiditis is a transient inflammatory disorder of viral origin. It is also known as subacute granulomatous, nonsuppurative, and de Quervain thyroiditis. It presents with a characteristic history of painful thyroid mass and low-grade fever on a background of a preceding viral infection. Patients pass through a thyrotoxic phase, followed by a hypothyroid phase, and then resumption of normal thyroid function.

Rarer types of hyperthyroidism can be categorized as those caused by exogenous or ectopic thyroid hormone or TSH (factitious thyroid hormone ingestion, struma ovarii, choriocarcinoma), and diseases that produce inflammation in the thyroid gland (silent/painless thyroiditis, amiodarone-induced thyroiditis, and acute thyroiditis).

Approach to Imaging

The imaging investigation of choice for patients with hyperthyroidism is the radioactive iodine uptake (RAIU) scan.[20] The study comprises an uptake component that measures iodine uptake, and a scan component that produces a scintigraphic image of the thyroid.[30] The uptake component may use either iodine (I)-131 or I-123. I-123 has 2 main advantages: it has a shorter half-life, resulting in a lower radiation dose to the patient; and it has better resolution, which allows acquisition of the scan component with the uptake dose. When using I-131, a separate technetium-99m pertechnetate study is required for the scan component because a higher dose of I-131 would otherwise be required to obtain diagnostic scintigraphic images.[31]

Evaluating an RAIU scan involves 2 steps. The first step is to quantify uptake. Normal uptake is 10% to 30% at 24 hours. Uptake above and below this range is considered to be abnormal. The second step is to characterize the pattern of the scintigraphic image. A toxic adenoma has a high uptake, but it is localized to the hot nodule, and the remainder of the thyroid gland is suppressed

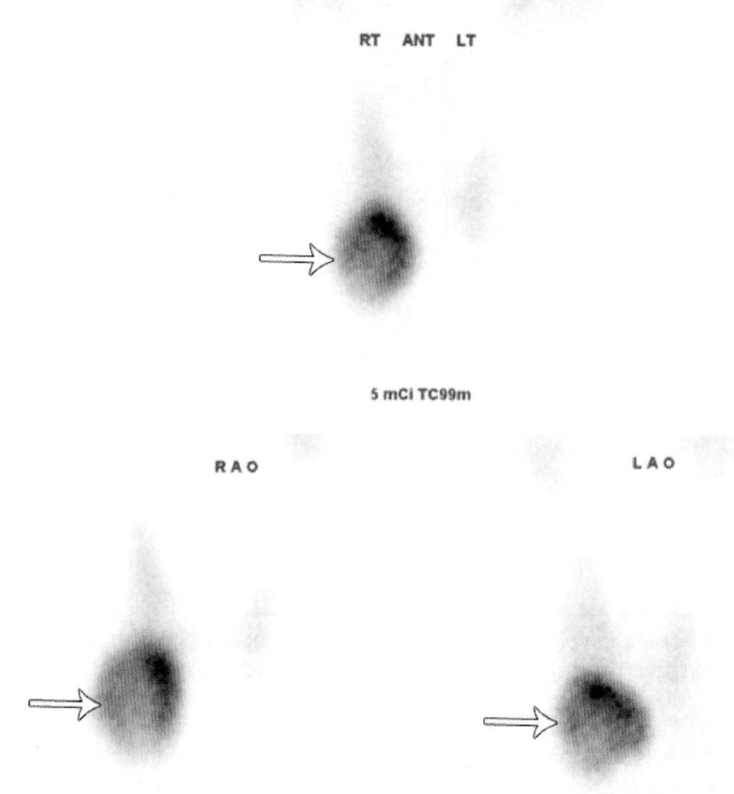

Fig. 3. A 72-year-old woman with a toxic adenoma. She had a low TSH level with thyroid hormones T3 and T4 at the upper normal range, but no symptoms aside from anxiety. A radioiodine uptake scan found increased uptake of 43%. The images show a pattern of a focal nodule in the right lobe (*arrows*) with suppression of the rest of the thyroid gland. The decision was made to treat because of concerns about the long-term detrimental effects of subclinical hyperthyroidism, and the patient was treated with 9.3 mCi of I-131. ANT, anterior; LAO, left anterior oblique; LT, left; RAO, right anterior oblique; RT, right.

(**Fig. 3**). Graves disease has high uptake, which is homogeneous in an enlarged gland (**Fig. 4**). Toxic multinodular goiter has high uptake, which is heterogeneous in an enlarged gland (**Fig. 5**). Subacute thyroiditis or exogenous thyroid hormone have low uptake of less than 10% (**Fig. 6**).

Tip

Proper preparation is essential for a useful RAIU scan. The Society of Nuclear Medicine and Molecular Imaging guidelines recommend avoidance of antithyroid drugs and various drugs and agents than can affect thyroid function and iodine metabolism.[31]

Tip

If the clinical presentation of hyperthyroidism is consistent with Graves disease and the patient has TSH-receptor antibodies, an RAIU scan is unnecessary.[30]

Management Pearls

Hyperthyroidism caused by Graves disease, toxic multinodular goiter, or toxic adenoma can be treated with medical therapy, surgery, or radioactive iodine (RAI) ablation. RAI ablation is most common in the United States.[32] Graves disease is treated a lower dose of RAI than toxic multinodular goiter and toxic adenoma.[30]

Surgery may be favored for the following indications: very large goiter, need for rapid correction, plans for pregnancy, concern for malignancy, severe Graves orbitopathy, or patient preference. Surgery has a lower rate of treatment failure of less than 1% compared with the RAI failure rate of 11% to 23%.[33,34] Patients having lobectomy for toxic adenoma are also less likely to have complications of hypothyroidism than patients receiving RAI, with rates of 2% and 60% at 20 years, respectively.[33,35]

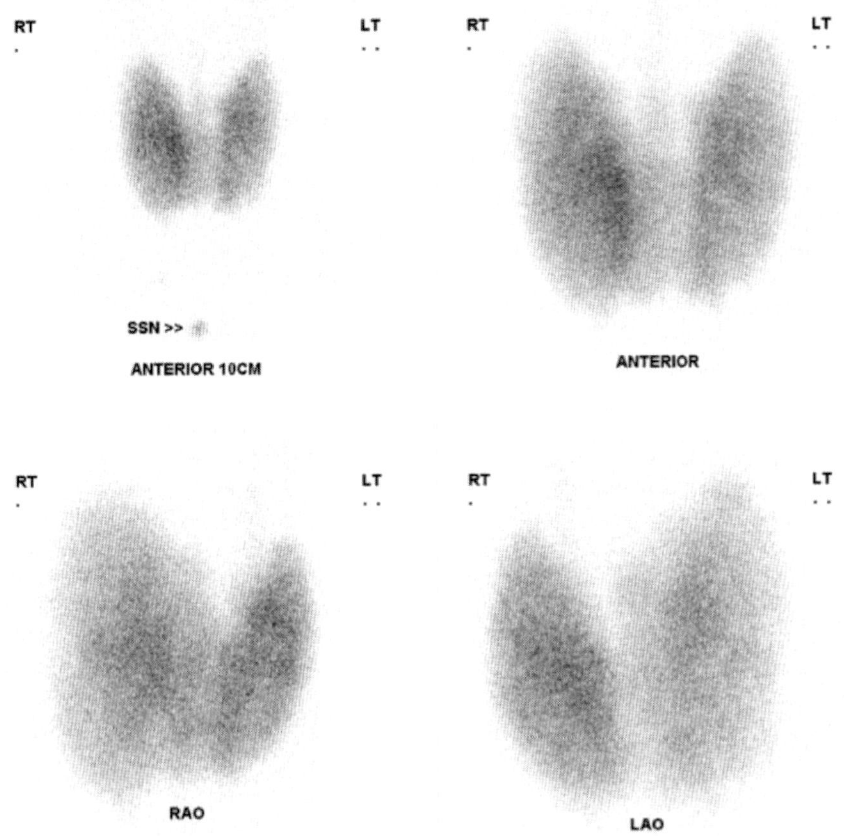

Fig. 4. A 21-year-old woman with Graves disease. She had symptoms of heat intolerance, jitteriness, and palpitations for several months. Thyroid function tests confirmed hyperthyroidism. RAIU scan found increased uptake of 90%. The scintigraphic images show a diffuse uptake pattern in keeping with Graves disease. The patient was treated with 8 mCi of I-131. SSN, suprasternal notch.

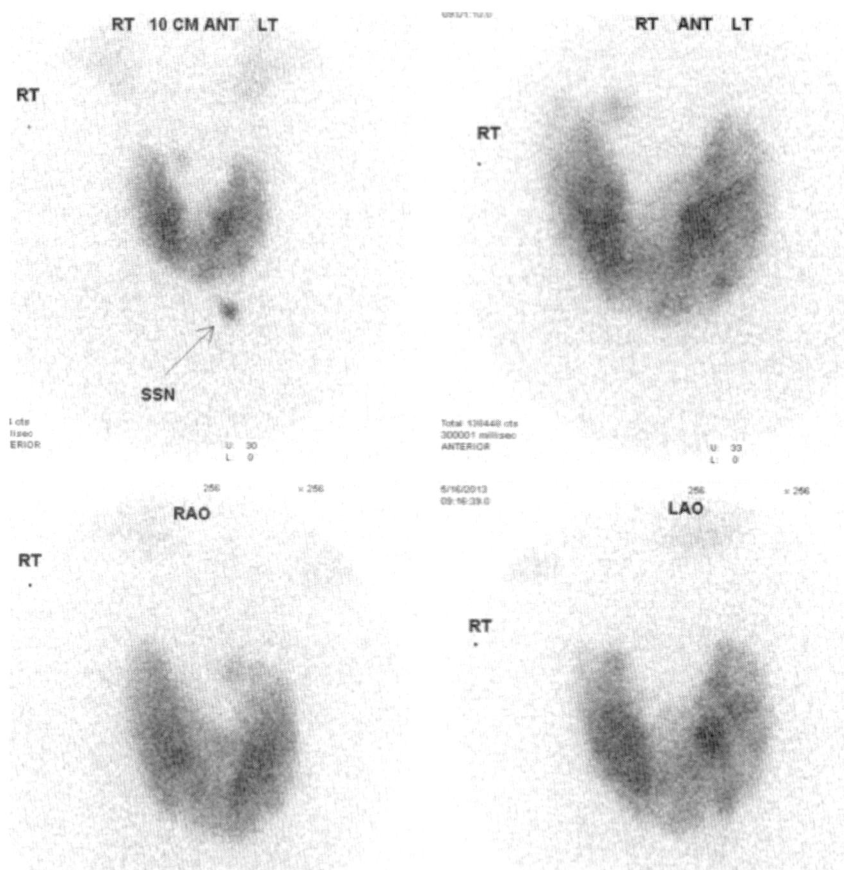

Fig. 5. A 20-year-old woman with toxic multinodular goiter. The patient had a history of central hypothyroidism following resection of a cerebellar pilocytic astrocytoma. She developed symptoms of hyperthyroidism and was found to have increased thyroid hormone levels. RAIU scan found mildly increased uptake of 35%. The scintigraphic images show a diffuse nodularity consistent with toxic multinodular goiter. Given the mild increase, the decision was made not to treat with radioiodine in this case.

Recommendations

The 48-year-old woman has symptoms of hyperthyroidism without TSH-receptor antibodies, which is not typical for Graves disease. The next investigation should be an RAIU scan. In her case, the uptake was increased and the scan showed a focal hyperintense abnormality consistent with a toxic adenoma. The treatment options are either RAI or thyroid lobectomy.

PROBLEM 4. PREOPERATIVE WORK-UP OF THYROID CANCER

A 75-year-old woman has a 4-cm mass in the left lobe of thyroid with tracheal deviation and fixation. The biopsy was positive for papillary thyroid cancer. Given the signs concerning for tracheal invasion, she requires CT for surgical planning. Should contrast be administered? What is the best approach to the CT scan interpretation?

Essential Facts and Updates

There are 4 main types of thyroid carcinomas. Papillary and follicular carcinomas (including the HÜrthle cell variant of follicular carcinoma) arise from the follicular epithelial cells and are known as differentiated thyroid carcinomas (DTC). They represent 88% and 8% of all thyroid malignancies, respectively.[10] DTC have an excellent prognosis, with a 10-year survival rate greater than 95% for papillary carcinoma and 85% for the follicular type.[36,37] Medullary thyroid carcinoma arises from neuroendocrine C cells and has a survival rate of 75% at 10 years.[36] Anaplastic carcinoma is an aggressive undifferentiated tumor typically occurring in the elderly with a median survival of 9 weeks and a 5-year survival of 7%.[38]

Risk factors for thyroid cancer depend on the histologic type and include childhood/adolescence head and neck irradiation, family history, and less commonly syndromes such as multiple

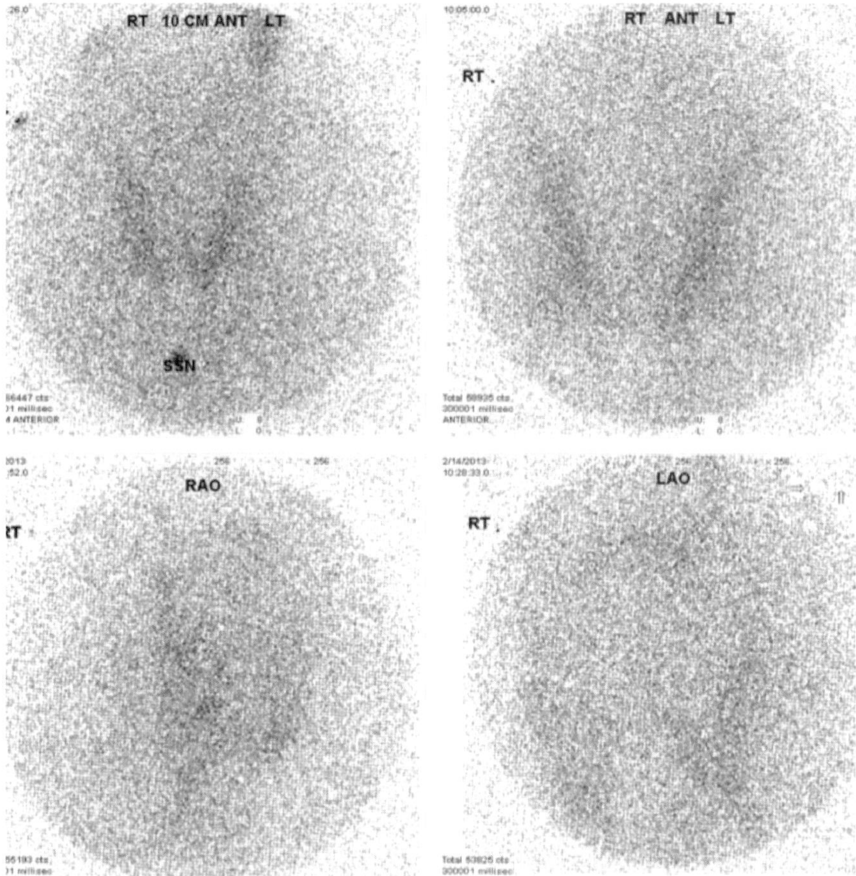

Fig. 6. A 64-year-old man with subacute thyroiditis. He presented with atrial flutter and was found to have a borderline low TSH level. RAIU scan found low uptake of 8% and images show no focal abnormality.

endocrine neoplasia 2 and familial medullary thyroid cancer. In most cases, thyroid cancer is sporadic, and there are no associated risk factors.

Imaging Recommendations and Findings

Role of ultrasonography

Sonography is the main imaging modality for thyroid lesion characterization and biopsy guidance. Once a diagnosis of malignancy is made on cytopathology, the American Thyroid Association (ATA) recommends preoperative neck ultrasonography for evaluation of extrathyroid extension, contralateral lobe disease, and cervical lymph nodes for all patients undergoing thyroidectomy.[20] Biopsy of sonographically suspicious lymph nodes should be performed under ultrasonography guidance if this would change the extent of neck dissection.[20]

Role of computed tomography and MR imaging, and approach to interpretation

Most patients do not have preoperative imaging with CT or MR imaging because ultrasonography adequately evaluates the primary tumor and nodal disease. The only reason to image with other cross-sectional modalities, such as CT and MR imaging, is concern for local invasion that may change the operative approach or preclude curative intent surgery. In these patients it is valuable for the radiologist to appreciate components of the American Joint Commission for Cancer (AJCC)/Union for International Cancer Control (UICC) tumor, node, metastasis (TNM) staging system (www.cancerstaging.org).[38]

The approach to evaluation can follow 3 steps that cover key sites for local invasion and metastatic disease. First, the radiologist should focus on central structures around which the thyroid normally drapes. These include the trachea, esophagus, larynx and pharynx, and recurrent laryngeal nerve. A thyroid mass that contacts the circumference of the airway or esophagus by 180° or more is suspicious for invasion, but other findings that are more specific are deformity of the lumen, focal mucosal irregularity, or mucosal thickening (**Figs. 7–9**).[39,40] Invasion of the

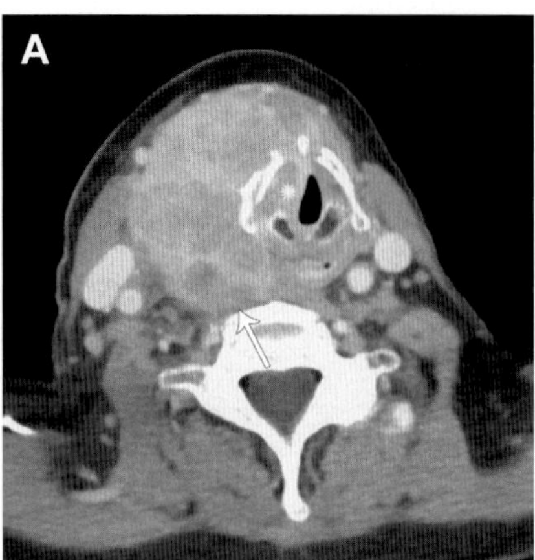

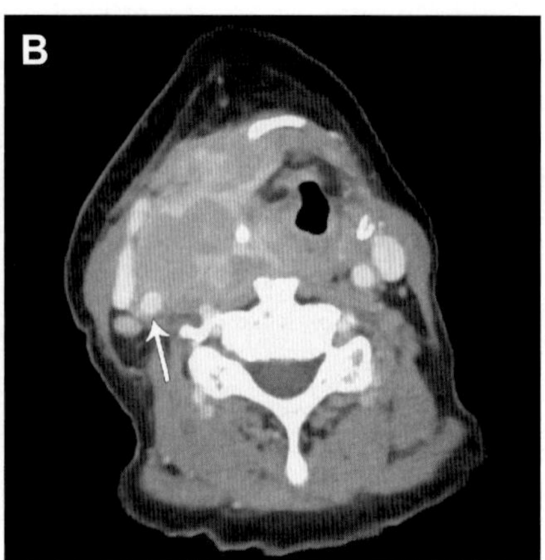

Fig. 7. A 78-year-old woman with locally invasive anaplastic thyroid carcinoma. (*A*) Axial enhanced CT shows a right thyroid mass invading through the larynx (*asterisk*) and contacting the hypopharynx with loss of fat plane. There is invasion through the strap muscles and tumor abutting the vertebra (*arrow*) compressing or invading the prevertebral muscles. (*B*) Axial enhanced CT at the level of the hyoid shows that the common carotid artery is encased by tumor (*arrow*) for almost 360°, which is concerning for carotid invasion. The patient was treated with chemotherapy and radiotherapy.

recurrent laryngeal nerve can be predicted by effaced fatty tissue in the tracheoesophageal groove for more than 3 axial images and signs of vocal cord dysfunction (see **Fig. 8**).[40,41] Invasion of the structures in step 1 constitutes T4a disease.

Step 2 turns to structures immediately surrounding the thyroid gland, which include the vascular structures, strap muscles, and prevertebral space. The internal jugular vein can be occluded or effaced by the tumor without invasion. Arteries are more resistant to compression so that deformity or narrowing of the artery is much more suspicious for invasion.[42] The other common, but less specific sign for invasion is tumor contacting the circumference of the artery by more than 180° (see **Fig. 7**).[40,42,43] Although the most common artery to be invaded is the carotid artery, mediastinal vessels should also be carefully assessed (**Fig. 10**). Arterial invasion meets criteria for T4b disease and may preclude curative surgery. The best sign of strap muscle invasion is asymmetry and tumor on the external surface of the muscle. Prevertebral musculature invasion is more difficult to evaluate because large tumors can compress the muscle and even result in signal changes on MR imaging without invasion.[44]

In addition, the 3-step approach requires assessment for metastatic disease. It is important to recognize the difference in the pattern of metastases for different tumor histologies. Papillary and medullary thyroid carcinomas commonly metastasize to regional lymph nodes (see **Figs. 8** and **10**). In contrast, the follicular subtype rarely involves lymph nodes, but more commonly metastasizes to lung and bone. Anaplastic carcinoma is locally aggressive, but can also metastasize to lymph nodes and the lung.

Thyroid nodal metastases commonly occur in the central compartment (level VI) followed by the lateral nodal groups (levels II–V) (see **Figs. 8** and **10**). Other nodal sites that should not be neglected are the lower paratracheal nodes in the superior mediastinum (level VII), and the retropharyngeal and retroesophageal groups.[45] The AJCC/UICC TNM staging system classifies nodal stage by site: N1a is level VI nodal disease (including pretracheal, paratracheal, and Delphian nodes), and N1b is involvement of unilateral or bilateral lateral cervical nodes, or superior mediastinal nodes.[38]

Tip

Morphologic findings of thyroid cancer nodal metastases include cystic components, calcification, intense enhancement, or proteinaceous or hemorrhagic content appearing as hyperdensity on CT and T1 hyperintensity on MR imaging.[45]

Tip

In the past there were concerns about iodinated contrast agents delaying subsequent whole-body scans or radioactive iodine, but these concerns have now been shown to be unfounded. Recent studies show that water-soluble iodinated contrast agents are generally cleared within 4 weeks in most patients, so postthyroidectomy patients requiring radioiodine therapy can be scanned with radioactive iodine within 1 month of the contrasted CT.[46,47]

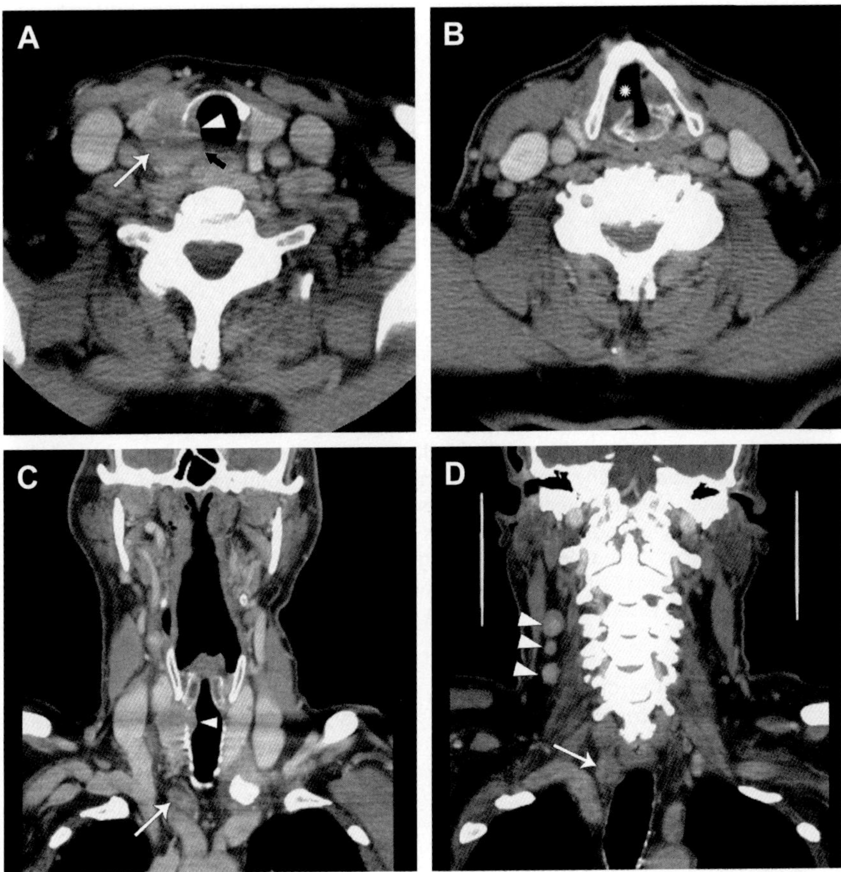

Fig. 8. A 72-year-old man with locally invasive papillary thyroid carcinoma and nodal metastases. The patient presented with hoarseness. (*A*) Axial enhanced CT image shows a right thyroid mass (*white arrow*) invading through the tracheal cartilage (*arrowhead*). The posteromedial border of the mass is separated from the esophagus by a thin fatty plane of cleavage (*black arrow*), but the tumor lies in the tracheoesophageal groove. (*B*) Axial enhanced CT image at the level of the vocal cords shows dilatation of the right laryngeal ventricle (*asterisk*), which is a sign of vocal cord palsy secondary to presumed local invasion of the right recurrent laryngeal nerve. (*C*) Coronal enhanced CT image shows the tumor invading through the upper tracheal rings (*arrowhead*). A level VI lymph node is enlarged (*arrow*). (*D*) Coronal enhanced CT shows abnormal central (level VI, *arrow*) and lateral cervical lymph nodes (*arrowheads*) in keeping with nodal metastases. The most superior lymph node has central calcifications. There were also left-sided abnormal lymph nodes (not shown). The patient underwent total thyroidectomy, bilateral lymph node dissection, and flap reconstruction of the tracheal defect, followed by ablative radioiodine therapy.

Management Pearls

Surgery remains the primary mode of treatment of DTC. Guidelines published by the ATA in 2009 recommend near-total or total thyroidectomy if the thyroid tumor is greater than 1 cm in diameter or if extrathyroidal extension or metastases are present.[20] The recommendation is for unilateral lobectomy and isthmusectomy when a unifocal tumor is less than 1 cm in diameter and confined to 1 lobe of the gland. Note that the ATA guidelines are in the process of undergoing revision and future recommendations may be less aggressive given recent epidemiologic studies of thyroid cancer incidence and survival.[10,11] Some centers are observing small papillary thyroid cancers without treatment.[9]

After surgery, RAI ablation is an option for remnant ablation and as an adjuvant therapy in patients with DTC. It is strongly recommended for patients who have known distant metastases, gross extrathyroidal disease extension, or primary tumor larger than 4 cm.[20]

Recommendations

The 75-year-old woman with a diagnosed 4-cm papillary thyroid cancer with tracheal deviation and fixation should undergo CT or MR imaging for surgical planning. Most practices and surgeons

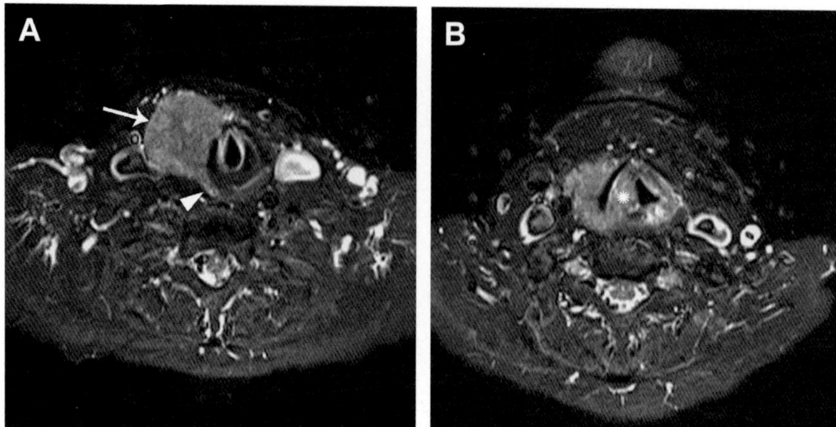

Fig. 9. An 81-year-old woman with locally invasive follicular thyroid carcinoma. She presented with palpable mass and hoarseness. Ultrasonography revealed a homogeneous, solid-appearing mass, and FNA showed irregular-appearing follicular cells. MR imaging was performed to evaluate for local invasion. (*A*) Axial short tau inversion recovery images show a right thyroid mass (*arrow*) that abuts the thyroid cartilage and the esophagus. The mass effaces the fat in the tracheoesophageal groove (*arrowhead*). (*B*) There is extension of the mass to the right true and false vocal cords (*asterisk*). The patient was not considered to be a good operative candidate and treatment proceeded with external beam radiation and radioiodine therapy.

prefer to perform CT. Iodinated contrast can be administered. The approach to interpreting the CT should encompass components on the 3-step checklist described earlier.

PROBLEM 5. SURVEILLANCE AND RECURRENT THYROID CANCER

A 65-year-old woman with T2N0M0 disease was treated 2 years ago for papillary thyroid cancer with total thyroidectomy followed by RAI remnant thyroid ablation. She returns for follow-up and is asymptomatic from the perspective of her thyroid cancer, but her serum thyroglobulin level is high and increasing. What is the significance of high thyroglobulin level in an asymptomatic patient? How should she be imaged?

Essential Facts and Updates

Rates of thyroid cancer recurrence range from 7% to 14%, usually with most occurring within the first decade.[48,49] The strongest predictor of tumor recurrence is large lymph node metastases

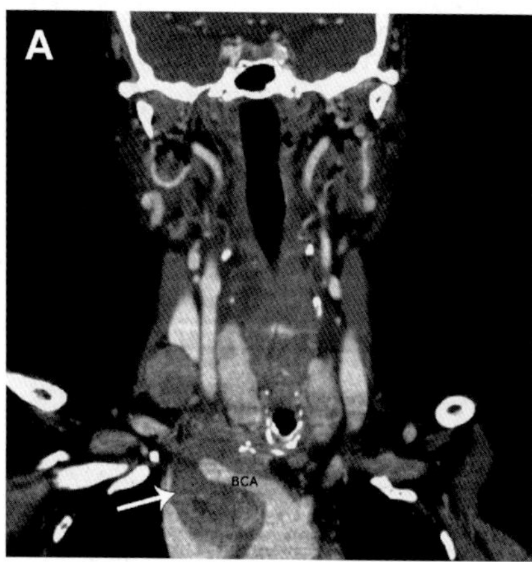

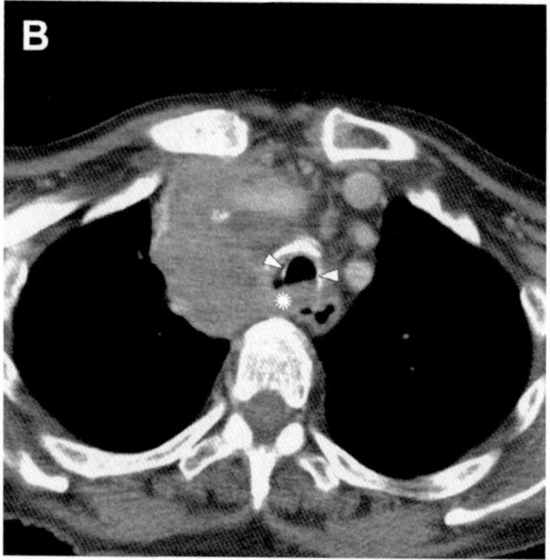

Fig. 10. A 68-year-old woman with micropapillary thyroid carcinoma and invasive metastatic nodal disease. (*A*) Coronal reformatted CT image shows the primary thyroid tumor is small and not appreciated as a dominant nodule. However, there is a large nodal metastasis (*arrow*) occupying right level VI and the mediastinum where there is encasement of the right brachiocephalic artery (BCA). (*B*) The nodal mass also invades the trachea (*asterisk*). Note that a tracheal stent (*arrowheads*) was placed 4 months earlier for treatment of hemoptysis. The tumor has invaded through the stent.

at initial diagnosis. In a study of recurrent papillary thyroid cancer, patients with lymph nodes greater than 3 cm at initial presentation were 6 times more likely to have nodal recurrence and more than 8 times more likely to have distant metastases.[48] Other predictors were older age, extrathyroidal extension, and primary tumor size greater than 2 cm.[48] The surveillance of all patients with thyroid cancer includes neck ultrasonography and serum measurements (thyroglobulin for DTC and calcitonin/carcinoembryonic antigen for medullary cancer). Increasing serum markers from baseline raise the question of persistent or recurrent disease.

Tumor recurrence with distant metastases reduces 10-year survival to 50%, but patients with locoregional recurrence may have no change in survival.[50] Some patients may have small nodal metastases that remain undetected on imaging and untreated for their lifetime.

Imaging Recommendation and Findings

Ultrasonography and radioiodine whole-body scintigraphy

Ultrasonography of the neck is the first imaging investigation for suspected tumor recurrence and includes evaluation of the thyroid bed and cervical nodes. If the ultrasonography is negative, radioiodine whole-body scintigraphy (WBS) is performed for DTC. WBS may also be performed as a first-line investigation in high-risk patients with DTC, such as those who initially had macroscopic invasion, gross residual disease, or distant metastases.

WBS can be performed with 2 isotopes of iodine. I-123 is a pure gamma emitter and has better imaging quality than I-131, but is more expensive. The study usually consists of whole-body images and pinhole images of the neck. Evaluation of a WBS requires knowledge of normal biodistribution of iodine and typical sites of metastases. There is normal activity in the salivary glands, stomach, and bladder (**Fig. 11**A). After surgery, uptake may initially be seen in the thyroid bed, but this should be absent after RAI ablation. Foci in lymph nodes, lungs, and bones are abnormal and are common sites for recurrence (**Fig. 11**B).

Tip

The preparation for WBS is coordinated by the endocrinologist. Imaging requires the patient to have a TSH level of 30 mIU/L or greater to have sufficient sensitivity. Patients are prepared either

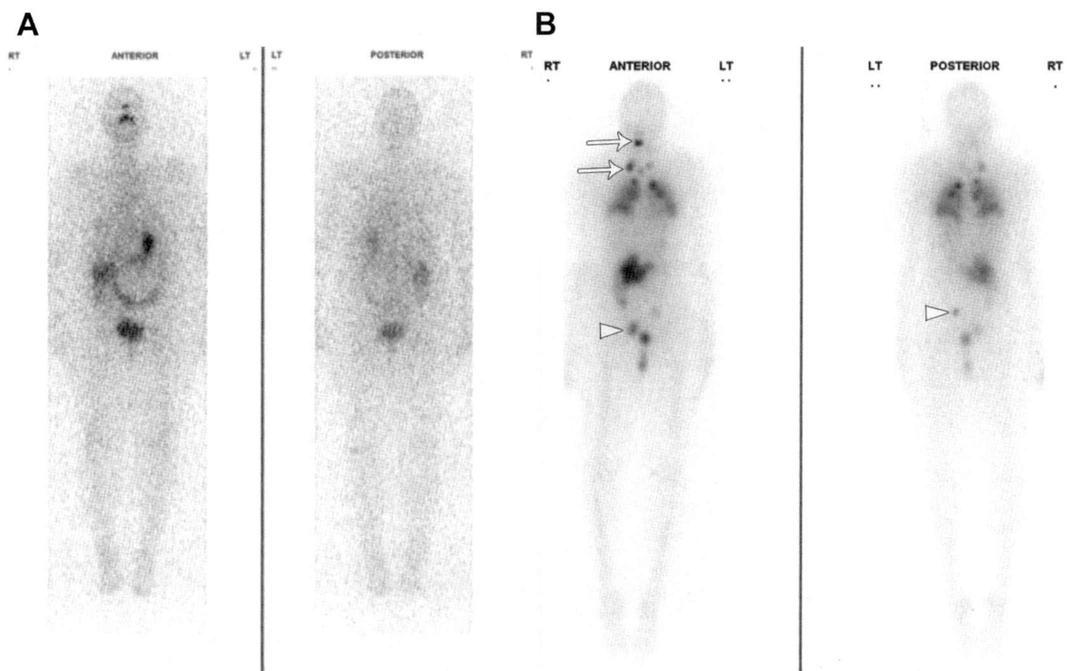

Fig. 11. (*A*) Normal postthyroidectomy and postablation radioactive iodine whole-body scan. Note the physiologic uptake in the nasal mucosa and salivary glands. Iodine is excreted from the stomach and kidneys so activity is also normally present in the stomach, bowel, and bladder. (*B*) A 23-year-old woman with metastatic papillary thyroid cancer to cervical nodes (*arrows*), lungs, and bones (*arrowheads*). Note the higher image quality compared with (*A*) because more iodine is retained in these areas.

by thyroid hormone withdrawal or by injection of the recombinant form of human TSH (Thyrogen).[31]

Fluorodeoxyglucose-PET

FDG-PET is performed if the ultrasonography and WBS are negative (**Fig. 12**). It is frequently positive when radioiodine uptake is negative, and vice versa, because radioiodine-negative tumor represents dedifferentiated disease. FDG-avid disease is typically not responsive to RAI and tends to have a worse prognosis.[51–53]

Trap

FDG-PET may be negative for medullary thyroid cancer. CT is most commonly performed for further imaging of recurrent disease after ultrasonography.

Management Pearls

Complete surgical resection of isolated symptomatic cervical metastases has been associated with improved survival, especially in patients less than 45 years of age.[20] Therefore, it is important for radiologists to correctly localize and estimate the burden of nodal disease. Smaller nodal metastases and distant metastases that are avid on WBS can be treated with RAI ablation. Typical doses may vary, but generally they are 100 to 150 mCi for nodal metastases and 100 to 200 mCi for distant metastases, compared with 30 to 100 mCi for thyroid bed remnants postoperatively.[20,54,55]

Recommendations

The 65-year-old woman has a high and increasing serum thyroglobulin level that is concerning for recurrent disease. Although she is not symptomatic, further imaging with ultrasonography must be performed. In her case, ultrasonography was negative and WBS was performed, which revealed metastatic disease throughout bones and lungs. The patient was treated with RAI with 200 mCi of I-131.

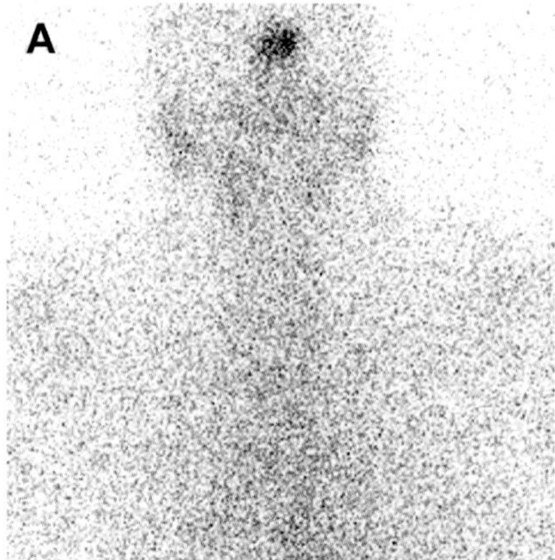

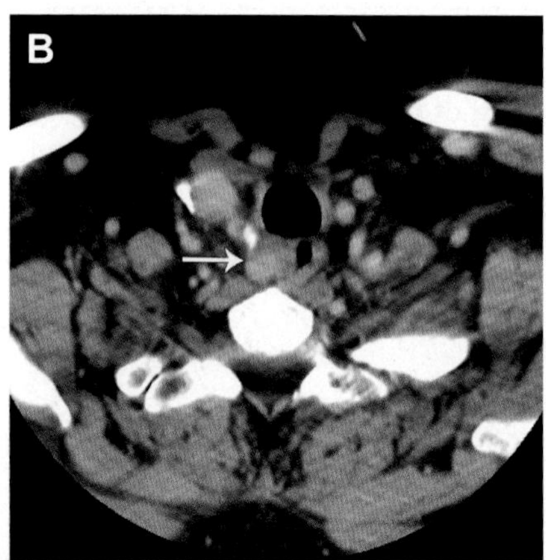

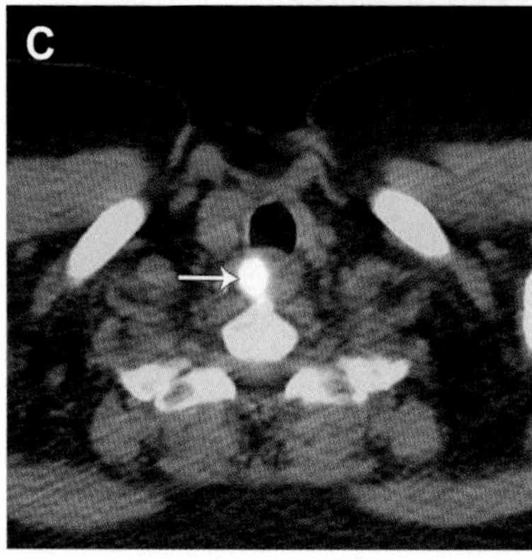

Fig. 12. A 66-year-old woman with history of T3N1M0 papillary thyroid cancer treated with total thyroidectomy, modified left neck dissection, and radioactive iodine ablation. Ten years later she was found to have an increased thyroglobulin level. (*A*) Magnified image from a radioactive iodine scan did not identify tumor in the neck. (*B*) Enhanced CT shows an enlarged lymph node in the paraesophageal location (*arrow*) that was FDG-avid (*C*) on the PET/CT scan (*arrow*). This mass and 2 other lymph nodes (not shown) were resected and confirmed to be nodal metastases.

SUMMARY

Diseases of the thyroid often require a multimodality, multidisciplinary, and collaborative approach across radiology, nuclear medicine, endocrinology, and endocrine surgery. Ultrasonography is ideal for characterizing thyroid nodules and guiding biopsy, but CT or MR imaging may be required preoperatively in cases of invasive thyroid cancer or substernal goiter. Imaging hyperthyroidism and recurrent thyroid cancer relies on nuclear medicine modalities. Excessive work-up of ITN and overdiagnosis of subclinical cancers is a costly health care problem.

REFERENCES

1. Nguyen XV, Choudhury KR, Eastwood JD, et al. Incidental thyroid nodules on CT: evaluation of 2 risk-categorization methods for work-up of nodules. AJNR Am J Neuroradiol 2013;34:1812–7.
2. Yoon DY, Chang SK, Choi CS, et al. The prevalence and significance of incidental thyroid nodules identified on computed tomography. J Comput Assist Tomogr 2008;32:810–5.
3. Yousem DM, Huang T, Loevner LA, et al. Clinical and economic impact of incidental thyroid lesions found with CT and MR. AJNR Am J Neuroradiol 1997;18:1423–8.
4. Harach HR, Franssila KO, Wasenius VM. Occult papillary carcinoma of the thyroid. A "normal" finding in Finland. A systematic autopsy study. Cancer 1985;56:531–8.
5. Hobbs HA, Bahl M, Nelson RC, et al. Journal club: incidental thyroid nodules detected at imaging: can diagnostic workup be reduced by use of the society of radiologists in ultrasound recommendations and the three-tiered system? AJR Am J Roentgenol 2014;202:18–24.
6. Bahl M, Sosa JA, Nelson RC, et al. Trends in incidentally identified thyroid cancers over a decade: a retrospective analysis of 2,090 surgical patients. World J Surg 2014;38(6):1312–7.
7. Bahl M, Sosa JA, Nelson RC, et al. Imaging-detected incidental thyroid nodules that undergo surgery: a single center's experience over one year. AJNR Am J Neuroradiol 2014. [Epub ahead of print].
8. Smith-Bindman R, Lebda P, Feldstein VA, et al. Risk of thyroid cancer based on thyroid ultrasound imaging characteristics: results of a population-based study. JAMA Intern Med 2013;173(19): 1788–96.
9. Ito Y, Miyauchi A, Inoue H, et al. An observational trial for papillary thyroid microcarcinoma in Japanese patients. World J Surg 2010;34: 28–35.
10. Hoang JK, Roy Choudhury K, Eastwood JD, et al. An exponential growth in incidence of thyroid cancer: trends and impact of CT imaging. AJNR Am J Neuroradiol 2014;35(4):778–83.
11. Davies L, Welch HG. Current thyroid cancer trends in the United States. JAMA Otolaryngol Head Neck Surg 2014;140(4):317–22.
12. Hoang JK, Lee WK, Lee M, et al. US Features of thyroid malignancy: pearls and pitfalls. Radiographics 2007;27:847–60.
13. Hoang JK, Riofrio A, Bashir MR, et al. High variability in radiologists' reporting practices for incidental thyroid nodules detected on CT and MRI. AJNR Am J Neuroradiol 2014;35(6):1190–4.
14. Hoang JK, Raduazo P, Yousem DM, et al. What to do with incidental thyroid nodules on imaging? An approach for the radiologist. Semin Ultrasound CT MR 2012;33:150–7.
15. Kang KW, Kim SK, Kang HS, et al. Prevalence and risk of cancer of focal thyroid incidentaloma identified by 18F-fluorodeoxyglucose positron emission tomography for metastasis evaluation and cancer screening in healthy subjects. J Clin Endocrinol Metab 2003;88:4100–4.
16. Cohen MS, Arslan N, Dehdashti F, et al. Risk of malignancy in thyroid incidentalomas identified by fluorodeoxyglucose-positron emission tomography. Surgery 2001;130:941–6.
17. Kim TY, Kim WB, Ryu JS, et al. 18F-fluorodeoxyglucose uptake in thyroid from positron emission tomogram (PET) for evaluation in cancer patients: high prevalence of malignancy in thyroid PET incidentaloma. Laryngoscope 2005; 115:1074–8.
18. Choi JY, Lee KS, Kim HJ, et al. Focal thyroid lesions incidentally identified by integrated 18F-FDG PET/CT: clinical significance and improved characterization. J Nucl Med 2006;47:609–15.
19. Shie P, Cardarelli R, Sprawls K, et al. Systematic review: prevalence of malignant incidental thyroid nodules identified on fluorine-18 fluorodeoxyglucose positron emission tomography. Nucl Med Commun 2009;30:742–8.
20. American Thyroid Association Guidelines Taskforce on Thyroid Nodules and Differentiated Thyroid Cancer, Cooper DS, Doherty GM, et al. Revised American Thyroid Association management guidelines for patients with thyroid nodules and differentiated thyroid cancer. Thyroid 2009; 19:1167–214.
21. Gharib H, Papini E, Paschke R, et al. American Association of Clinical Endocrinologists, Associazione Medici Endocrinologi, and European Thyroid Association medical guidelines for clinical practice for the diagnosis and management of thyroid nodules. Endocr Pract 2010;16(Suppl 1): 1–43.

22. NCC guidelines thyroid carcinoma - nodule evaluation version 2. 2013. 2013. Available at: http://www.nccn.org/professionals/physician_gls/f_guidelines.asp - thyroid.http://www.nccn.org/professionals/physician_gls/f_guidelines.asp#thyroid. Accessed May 7, 2013.
23. Frates MC, Benson CB, Charboneau JW, et al. Management of thyroid nodules detected at US: Society of Radiologists in Ultrasound consensus conference statement. Radiology 2005;237:794–800.
24. Bongiovanni M, Spitale A, Faquin WC, et al. The Bethesda system for reporting thyroid cytopathology: a meta-analysis. Acta Cytol 2012;56:333–9.
25. Katlic MR, Wang CA, Grillo HC. Substernal goiter. Ann Thorac Surg 1985;39:391–9.
26. Rieu M, Bekka S, Sambor B, et al. Prevalence of subclinical hyperthyroidism and relationship between thyroid hormonal status and thyroid ultrasonographic parameters in patients with non-toxic nodular goitre. Clin Endocrinol (Oxf) 1993;39:67–71.
27. Pollard DB, Weber CW, Hudgins PA. Preoperative imaging of thyroid goiter: how imaging technique can influence anatomic appearance and create a potential for inaccurate interpretation. AJNR Am J Neuroradiol 2005;26:1215–7.
28. Delbridge L. Total thyroidectomy: the evolution of surgical technique. ANZ J Surg 2003;73:761–8.
29. Rios A, Rodriguez JM, Galindo PJ, et al. Surgical treatment of multinodular goiter in young patients. Endocrine 2005;27:245–52.
30. Bahn Chair RS, Burch HB, Cooper DS, et al. Hyperthyroidism and other causes of thyrotoxicosis: management guidelines of the American Thyroid Association and American Association of Clinical Endocrinologists. Thyroid 2011;21:593–646.
31. American College of Radiology, Society of Nuclear Medicine, Society of Physics in Radiology. ACR–SNM–SPR practice guideline for the performance of thyroid scintigraphy and uptake measurements. 2009. Available at: http://snmmi.files.cms-plus.com/docs/Thyroid_Scintigraphy_1382732120053_10.pdf.http://snmmi.files.cms-plus.com/docs/Thyroid_Scintigraphy_1382732120053_10.pdf. Accessed March 19, 2014.
32. Burch HB, Burman KD, Cooper DS. A 2011 survey of clinical practice patterns in the management of Graves' disease. J Clin Endocrinol Metab 2012;97:4549–58.
33. Vidal-Trecan GM, Stahl JE, Eckman MH. Radioiodine or surgery for toxic thyroid adenoma: dissecting an important decision. A cost-effectiveness analysis. Thyroid 2004;14:933–45.
34. Nygaard B, Hegedus L, Nielsen KG, et al. Long-term effect of radioactive iodine on thyroid function and size in patients with solitary autonomously functioning toxic thyroid nodules. Clin Endocrinol (Oxf) 1999;50:197–202.
35. Ceccarelli C, Bencivelli W, Vitti P, et al. Outcome of radioiodine-131 therapy in hyperfunctioning thyroid nodules: a 20 years' retrospective study. Clin Endocrinol (Oxf) 2005;62:331–5.
36. Hundahl SA, Fleming ID, Fremgen AM, et al. A National Cancer Data Base report on 53,856 cases of thyroid carcinoma treated in the U.S., 1985–1995. Cancer 1998;83:2638–48.
37. Davies L, Welch HG. Increasing incidence of thyroid cancer in the United States, 1973–2002. JAMA 2006;295:2164–7.
38. Edge SB, American Joint Committee on Cancer. AJCC cancer staging manual. 7th edition. New York: Springer; 2010.
39. Wang JC, Takashima S, Takayama F, et al. Tracheal invasion by thyroid carcinoma: prediction using MR imaging. AJR Am J Roentgenol 2001;177:929–36.
40. Seo YL, Yoon DY, Lim KJ, et al. Locally advanced thyroid cancer: can CT help in prediction of extrathyroidal invasion to adjacent structures? AJR Am J Roentgenol 2010;195:W240–4.
41. Takashima S, Takayama F, Wang J, et al. Using MR imaging to predict invasion of the recurrent laryngeal nerve by thyroid carcinoma. AJR Am J Roentgenol 2003;180:837–42.
42. Yu Q, Wang P, Shi H, et al. Carotid artery and jugular vein invasion of oral-maxillofacial and neck malignant tumors: diagnostic value of computed tomography. Oral Surg Oral Med Oral Pathol Oral Radiol Endod 2003;96:368–72.
43. Yousem DM, Hatabu H, Hurst RW, et al. Carotid artery invasion by head and neck masses: prediction with MR imaging. Radiology 1995;195:715–20.
44. Loevner LA, Ott IL, Yousem DM, et al. Neoplastic fixation to the prevertebral compartment by squamous cell carcinoma of the head and neck. AJR Am J Roentgenol 1998;170:1389–94.
45. Hoang JK, Vanka J, Ludwig BJ, et al. Evaluation of cervical lymph nodes in head and neck cancer with CT and MRI: tips, traps, and a systematic approach. AJR Am J Roentgenol 2013;200:W17–25.
46. Sohn SY, Choi JH, Kim NK, et al. The impact of iodinated contrast agent administered during preoperative computed tomography scan on body iodine pool in patients with differentiated thyroid cancer preparing for radioactive iodine treatment. Thyroid 2014;24(5):872–7.
47. Padovani RP, Kasamatsu TS, Nakabashi CC, et al. One month is sufficient for urinary iodine to return to its baseline value after the use of water-soluble iodinated contrast agents in post-thyroidectomy patients requiring radioiodine therapy. Thyroid 2012;22:926–30.

48. Ito Y, Kudo T, Kobayashi K, et al. Prognostic factors for recurrence of papillary thyroid carcinoma in the lymph nodes, lung, and bone: analysis of 5,768 patients with average 10-year follow-up. World J Surg 2012;36:1274–8.
49. Hay ID, Thompson GB, Grant CS, et al. Papillary thyroid carcinoma managed at the Mayo Clinic during six decades (1940–1999): temporal trends in initial therapy and long-term outcome in 2444 consecutively treated patients. World J Surg 2002;26:879–85.
50. Ito Y, Higashiyama T, Takamura Y, et al. Clinical outcomes of patients with papillary thyroid carcinoma after the detection of distant recurrence. World J Surg 2010;34:2333–7.
51. Wang W, Larson SM, Tuttle RM, et al. Resistance of [18f]-fluorodeoxyglucose-avid metastatic thyroid cancer lesions to treatment with high-dose radioactive iodine. Thyroid 2001;11:1169–75.
52. Yoshio K, Sato S, Okumura Y, et al. The local efficacy of I-131 for F-18 FDG PET positive lesions in patients with recurrent or metastatic thyroid carcinomas. Clin Nucl Med 2011;36:113–7.
53. Schreinemakers JM, Vriens MR, Munoz-Perez N, et al. Fluorodeoxyglucose-positron emission tomography scan-positive recurrent papillary thyroid cancer and the prognosis and implications for surgical management. World J Surg Oncol 2012;10:192.
54. Silberstein EB, Alavi A, Balon HR, et al. The SNMMI practice guideline for therapy of thyroid disease with 131I 3.0. J Nucl Med 2012;53:1633–51.
55. Mallick U, Harmer C, Yap B, et al. Ablation with low-dose radioiodine and thyrotropin alfa in thyroid cancer. N Engl J Med 2012;366:1674–85.

Imaging of the Perivertebral Space

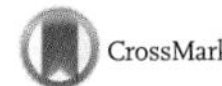

Megan K. Mills, MD*, Lubdha M. Shah, MD

KEYWORDS

- Perivertebral space • Prevertebral space • Paraspinal space • Deep cervical fascia
- Suprahyoid neck • Infrahyoid neck

KEY POINTS

- The perivertebral space is a complex compartment spanning the suprahyoid and infrahyoid neck and enveloped by the deep layer of the deep cervical fascia.
- By accurately localizing a disease process in this space and understanding the various tissue types contained within the prevertebral and paraspinal components, radiologists can provide meaningful differential diagnoses.
- Correct localization guides clinical decision making and treatment.

INTRODUCTION

The perivertebral space (PVS) lies deep within the neck surrounding the vertebral column, extending from the skull base to the mediastinum. The PVS is enveloped by the deep layer of the deep cervical fascia (DLDCF) and contains different tissue types, including muscles, bones, nerves, and vascular structures. Physical examination is of limited use in evaluating this space deeply located within the cervical soft tissues; therefore, imaging is important when interrogating for abnormalities.

This article defines the PVS anatomy, guides lesion localization, discusses different disease processes arising within this space, and reviews the best imaging approaches.

NORMAL ANATOMY

The PVS comprises the cervical soft tissues surrounding the vertebral column, traversing the suprahyoid and infrahyoid neck and extending from the skull base to the T4 level. The DLDCF encases the PVS and is interrupted only by traversing brachial plexus (BP) nerve roots.[1] The DLDCF divides the PVS into an anterior prevertebral space and posterior paraspinal space.[1] The anatomic landscape is formed by multiple other spaces in the suprahyoid and infrahyoid neck: the retropharyngeal space (RPS) anteriorly, carotid space laterally, and the posterior cervical space posterolaterally. Understanding the relationship of the PVS to adjacent spaces is key in disease localization.

FASCIAL LAYERS

The spaces of the suprahyoid and infrahyoid neck are defined by the layers of the deep cervical fascia (**Fig. 1**). The deep cervical fascia can be split into superficial, middle, and deep segments. Within the suprahyoid neck, the superficial layer of the deep cervical fascia (SLDCF) delineates the masticator space, parotid space, as well as a portion of the carotid sheath. Within the infrahyoid neck, the SLDCF encases the strap muscles, sternocleidomastoid muscles, and trapezius muscles.[2]

In the suprahyoid neck, the middle layer of the deep cervical fascia (MLDCF) defines the deep margin of the pharyngeal mucosa and gives contributions to the carotid sheath. The infrahyoid

Department of Radiology, University of Utah, 30 North 1900 East #1A071, Salt Lake City, UT 84132, USA
* Corresponding author.
E-mail address: megan.mills@hsc.utah.edu

Radiol Clin N Am 53 (2015) 163–180
http://dx.doi.org/10.1016/j.rcl.2014.09.008

radiologic.theclinics.com

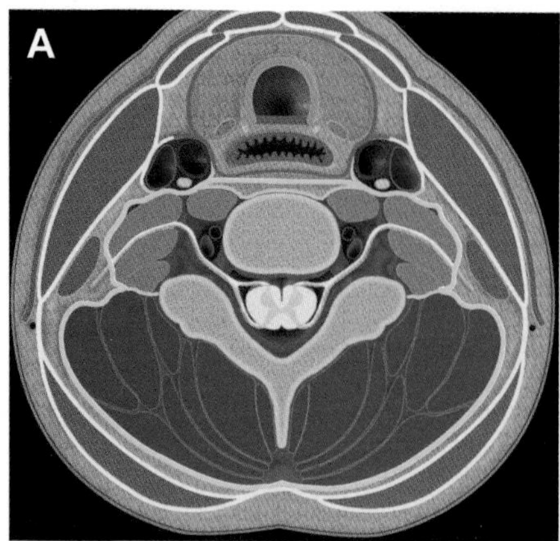

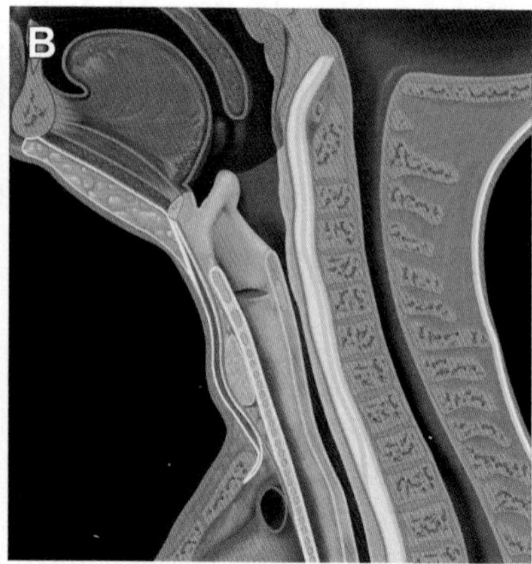

Fig. 1. (*A*) Axial graphic through the perivertebral space at the level of the infrahyoid neck. The perivertebral space is deep to the turquoise line representing the DLDCF. As the cervical fascia attaches to the transverse processes, it splits the perivertebral space into prevertebral and paraspinal components. The vertebral body, vertebral artery and vein, BP nerve roots, as well as multiple muscle of the neck are contained within this space. The relationship to the carotid space (anterior and lateral), the retropharyngeal space (anterior), as well as the posterior cervical space (superficial and posterior) are also defined. (*B*) Sagittal graphic through the midline of the cervical soft tissues delineates the craniocaudal extent of the perivertebral space. The attachment from the skull base to the posterior mediastinum is shown. The paraspinal space posteriorly is highlighted in purple and outlined by a turquoise line representing the DLDCF. The prevertebral space extends in a more transverse dimension, immediately abutting the anterior aspect of the cervical vertebral bodies. ([*B*] *Courtesy of* Amirsys, Salt Lake City, UT, USA, with permission.)

components of the MLDCF enclose the visceral space.[2]

The DLDCF surrounds the PVS and contributes to the carotid sheath in both the suprahyoid and infrahyoid neck. It has lateral openings for the BP nerve roots. The anterior portion of the DLDCF lies in front of the prevertebral muscles, extending to the transverse processes laterally. This anterior part serves as a barrier to infection, such as discitis-osteomyelitis, extending anteriorly from the spine into the retropharyngeal space. In contrast, it blocks pharyngeal lesions from penetrating posteriorly. The posterior part arches over the paraspinal muscles, attaching to the ligamentum nuchae.[2] In addition, there is inferior extension of the pharyngobasilar fascia from the superior pharyngeal constrictor muscle over the prevertebral space.[3]

A unique portion of the DLDCF is the alar fascia. This slip of fascia separates the danger space from the more anterior RPS, forms their lateral walls, and provides a portion of the carotid sheath. The RPS lies immediately anterior to the prevertebral space, extending variably from the clivus to the T1 to T6 levels. At its inferior extent, it fuses with the visceral space to obliterate the true RPS.[4] The danger space is posteriorly located and extends further inferiorly into the posterior mediastinum to the level of the diaphragm. The alar fascia is imperceptible on imaging; therefore, the danger space and the RPS cannot be distinguished in a healthy patient.[2,5]

PREVERTEBRAL SPACE

Muscles comprise most of the prevertebral space. Two major muscles of neck flexion are the longus capitis and longus colli (longus capitis/colli complex). The longus capitis defines the anterior prevertebral space, originating from the anterior tubercles of the C3 to C6 transverse processes and inserting on the basilar portion of the occipital bone (**Fig. 2**). The longer paired longus colli muscles originate on the anterior tubercle of the atlas and insert on the anterior tubercles of the upper cervical vertebral bodies to the T3 level (**Fig. 3**).[2] In addition, there are anterior and lateral rectus muscles that lie deep to the superior aspect of the longus capitis.

Along with the longus capitis/colli complex, the anterior, middle, and posterior scalene muscles also reside in the prevertebral space. The scalene muscles have an important role in inspiration, neck flexion, and laterally bending. The anterior scalene muscle lies deep to the sternocleidomastoid muscle, originating from the anterior tubercles of the C3 to C6 transverse processes and inserting on the scalene tubercle of the first rib.[6,7] Important anatomic features include its location between the subclavian vein and artery and anterior position relative to the BP nerve roots. The middle scalene muscle originates from the posterior tubercles of the C2 to C7 transverse processes and inserts on the upper surface of the first rib, posterior to the subclavian artery. The posterior

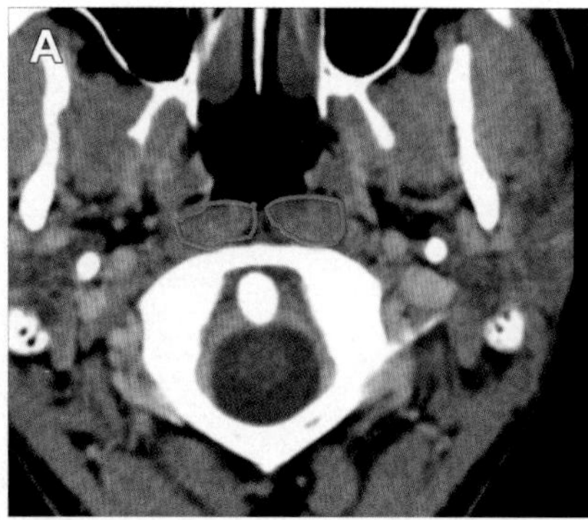

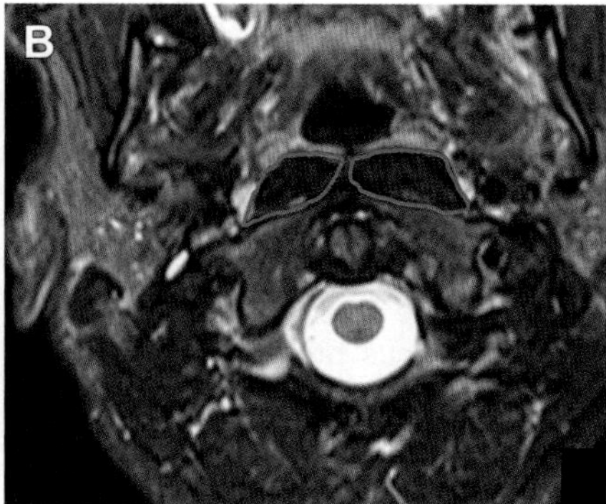

Fig. 2. Contrast-enhanced axial computed tomography (CT) (*A*) and axial T2-weighted (T2W) MR (*B*) images of the paired longus capitis muscles (outlined in *red*) at the level of C1. The longus capitis muscles originate from the anterior tubercles of the third to the sixth cervical vertebral bodies and insert on the basiocciput.

scalene muscle is the longest of the scalene muscles, originating from the posterior tubercles of the C5 to C7 transverse processes and inserting on the lateral surface of the second rib.[7]

Multiple nerve groups cross the prevertebral space en route to their respective end organs. The phrenic nerve is contained within the prevertebral space fascia from the C3 to the C5 level and crosses the anterior scalene muscle. The dorsal scapular nerve and the long thoracic nerve penetrate the belly of the middle scalene muscle. The BP nerve roots also traverse the prevertebral space and are a source of potential disorder. The BP is a somatic nerve plexus formed by intercommunications among the ventral rami of the C5 to T1 nerves, which form the roots of the BP. In addition to motor innervation to the muscles of the upper limb (except the trapezius and levator scapula), the BP supplies the cutaneous innervation to most of the upper limb (except the axilla and dorsal scapular area). The BP nerve roots lie deep to the posterior cervical space and posterior to the transverse processes. The roots further unite into trunks, which divide into divisions. The divisions unite into cords, which end in terminal branches, containing both sensory and motor axons.[8]

The vertebral body may be envisioned as the osseous scaffold on which the other contents of the PVS are supported. The vertebral arteries and veins are the major tributaries of the posterior circulation and travel in the transverse foramina of the vertebral bodies. The ventral rami of the C5 to T1 nerve roots of the BP are contained within the osseous spinal column. The muscles of neck flexion anchor their origins and insertions on the bony prominences of each vertebral body, as previously described. In addition, the discovertebral complex and supportive ligamentous structures, including the anterior and posterior longitudinal ligaments and the posterior ligamentous complex, provide biomechanical stability and functionality.

PARASPINAL SPACE

Similar to the prevertebral space, the bulk of the paraspinal space is composed of muscle tissue.

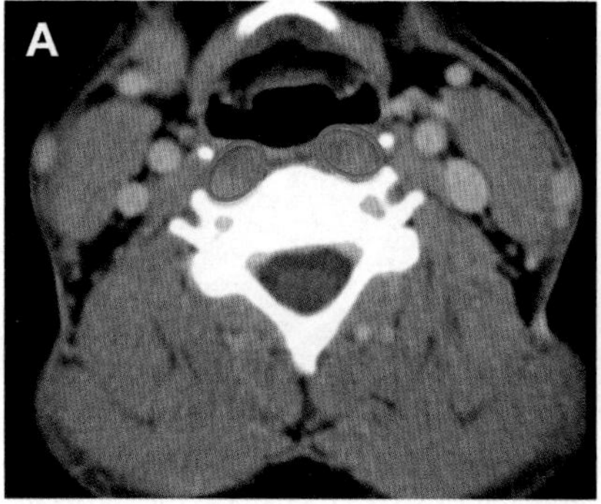

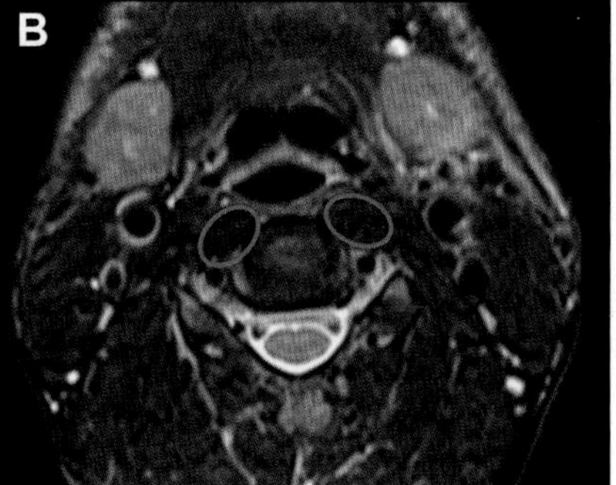

Fig. 3. Contrast-enhanced axial CT (*A*) and axial T2W MR (*B*) images of the paired longus colli muscles (outlined in *red*) at the level of the hyoid bone. The longus colli muscles extend cranially from the anterior tubercles of the atlas caudally to the T3 level and aid in neck flexion.

The paraspinal muscle groups are made up of multiple smaller individual muscles in an array of symmetric pairs separated by the spinous processes, interspinales muscles, and ligamentum nuchae (**Figs. 4** and **5**).

The major extensors of the head and neck are the splenius capitis, semispinalis capitis, and longissimus capitis. The large splenius capitis arises from the C3 to T3 spinous processes, and the splenius cervicis arises from the T3 to T6 spinous processes. They both course superiorly to insert on the superior nuchal line and the first 3 cervical transverse processes, respectively. The smaller semispinalis capitis and longissimus capitis lie immediately deep to the splenius capitis. More centrally located and smaller in size are the levator scapulae, multifidus, and interspinales muscles.[2,6] The SLDCF invests the trapezius muscles, which are part of the posterior cervical musculature and are separated from the paraspinal muscles by fat.

When reviewing cross-sectional imaging, the craniocaudal location may be helpful to identify which muscles are being evaluated. Images through the midcervical level show the longissimus capitis and cervicis and the more medial multifidi and semispinalis cervicis. In the lower cervical spine, the splenius capitis and the semispinalis capitis and cervicis are prominent, appearing as parallel muscle bundles deep to the trapezius muscles.[6] Also prominent in the lower cervical levels are the trapezius, levator scapulae, and sternocleidomastoid muscles.

The musculature may be the site of vascular malformations, inflammatory processes, or neoplastic processes. Soft tissue tumors with a predilection for the head and neck region include spindle cell lipoma, pleomorphic lipoma, and nuchal fibroma. In the setting of prior trauma, patients may develop a nonneoplastic, reactive fibrocartilaginous mass along the base of the neck, at the junction of the nuchal ligament and the deep cervical fascia. This nuchal fibrocartilaginous pseudotumor is considered analogous to fibrocartilage metaplasia seen in degenerated tendoligamentous structures.[9] The posterior elements of the vertebral body, including the lamina and spinous process, serve as the framework for the

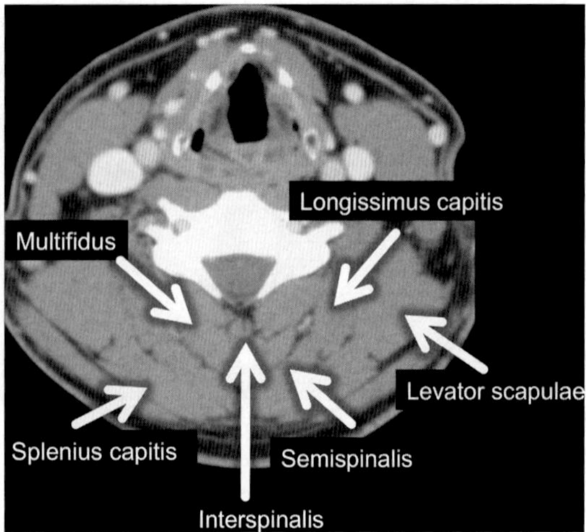

Fig. 5. Axial contrast-enhanced axial CT at the level of the infrahyoid neck shows the relationship of the deep paraspinal muscle groups. The paraspinal muscles primarily aid in neck extension and may be a potential source of disorder.

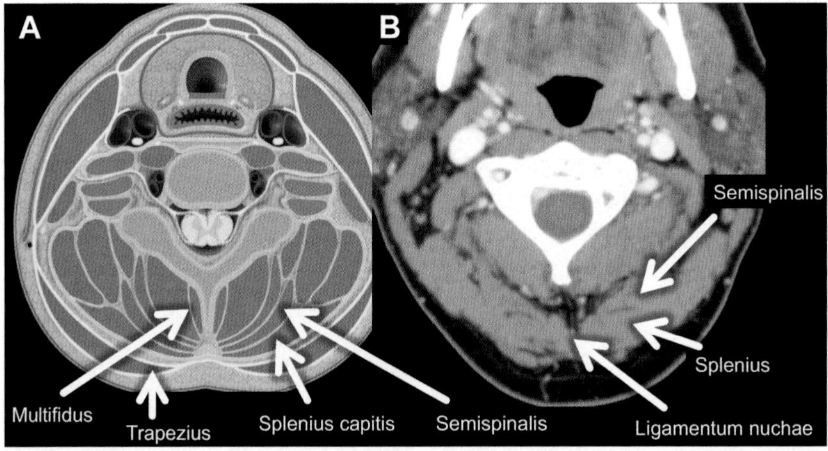

Fig. 4. Axial graphic (*A*) and contrast-enhanced axial CT (*B*) of the suprahyoid neck shows the relationship of the paraspinal muscle groups. Note the large paired splenius capitis muscles that make up the most superficial layer of the paraspinal space. These muscles abut the DLDCF and are separated from the posterior cervical space by the superficial layer of deep cervical fascia and fat. The delineation of the muscle groups depends on the level of the paraspinal space being evaluated.

muscles of neck extension. The osseous structures may also be the site of paraspinal disorders, such as fracture, interspinous degenerative change, and primary or secondary osseous neoplasm.

DISEASE LOCALIZATION

Because the PVS is surrounded by multiple other cervical spaces, understanding the anatomic landscape is key to lesion localization. For example, the position of the prevertebral muscles can be used to determine whether a lesion is in the prevertebral space or RPS. If the prevertebral muscles are lifted off the vertebral body, then the lesion is in the prevertebral space. In contrast, if the lesion pushes the prevertebral muscles posteriorly to the vertebral body, it is in the RPS (**Fig. 6**). Defining the origin of a pathologic process not only helps in narrowing the differential diagnosis but is also important in clinical management, especially when surgical intervention may be indicated.

The deep posterior cervical space is located posterolateral to the paraspinal space. The posterior cervical fat separates the two spaces and serves as an anatomic landmark to aid in disease localization. Lesions contained within the paraspinal space bow the cervical fat away from the spine and displace the posterior cervical space outward, whereas lesions in the posterior cervical space push the fat toward the central structures and cause mass effect on the paraspinal musculature (**Figs. 7** and **8**).[10]

IMAGING FINDINGS/PATHOLOGY

Infection and Inflammation

Infection is a common disease process involving the PVS and can arise hematogenously, iatrogenically, or through direct spread from adjacent spaces. Hematologic pathogens, such as *Staphylococcus aureus*, can seed the vertebral end plates and extend into the disc space, resulting in spondylodiscitis (**Table 1**). Atypical granulomatous osteomyelitis, such as tuberculosis, may have multilevel subligamentous spread. It is important to evaluate not only the prevertebral and paraspinal spaces but also the epidural space for abscess. Surgical intervention such as anterior cervical discectomy and fusion or percutaneous procedures such as selective nerve root injection are potential iatrogenic causes of infection. The aerodigestive tract is an uncommon source of infection spreading to the PVS given the distinctive protective fascial layers, described earlier.

Discitis/Osteomyelitis (Spondylodiscitis)

In adults, discitis/osteomyelitis describes infection of adjacent subchondral vertebral endplates extending into the intervertebral disc, usually from hematogenous seeding.[11] Although discitis/osteomyelitis commonly occurs in immunocompetent patients, chronic illness such as diabetes mellitus and risk factors such as intravenous drug use are predisposing conditions. It can be a challenging diagnosis because other disease processes, such as inflammatory discogenic endplate changes, can have similar imaging features.[11]

Computed tomography (CT) and MR imaging are complimentary modalities in evaluating suspected discitis/osteomyelitis. On CT, destructive endplates changes are a helpful clue. On MR imaging, hyperintensity on T2-weighted (T2W) and short tau inversion recovery (STIR) images, hypointensity on T1-weighted (T1W) images, and patchy enhancement in the vertebral endplates are characteristic findings (**Fig. 9**). The intervertebral disc may show T2W and STIR hyperintensity and typically shows rim enhancement rather than diffuse enhancement.[11] The DLDCF confines the PVS so that infection centered in the endplates and adjacent disc preferentially spreads centrally to the epidural space. Homogeneously enhancing

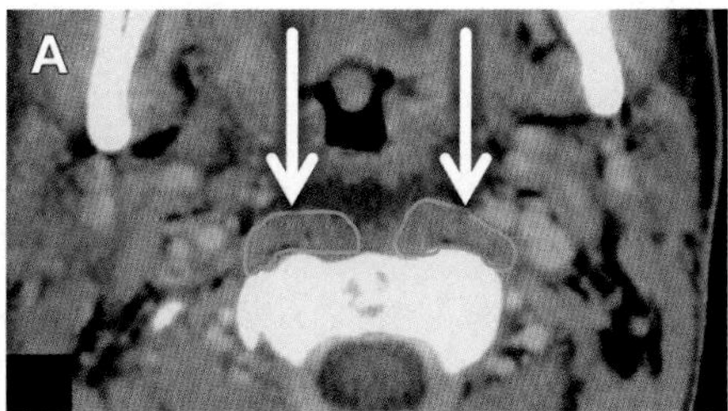

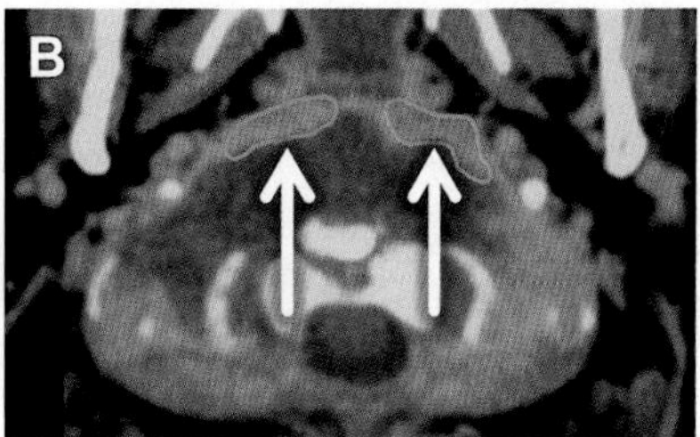

Fig. 6. (*A*) Contrast-enhanced axial CT shows fluid anterior to the prevertebral muscles with posterior displacement of the longus capitis muscles (*white arrows* and *orange outline*) confirming that hypodense fluid is within the retropharyngeal space. (*B*) Axial contrast-enhanced axial CT in a different patient shows elevation of the longus capitis muscles (*white arrows* and *orange outline*) away from the vertebral bodies caused by a hypodense fluid collection within the prevertebral space.

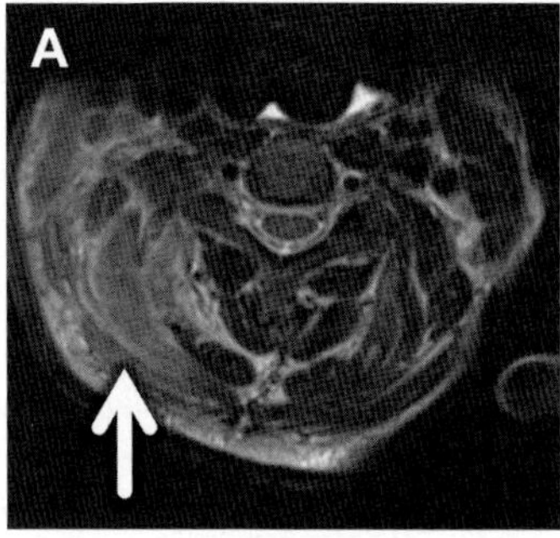

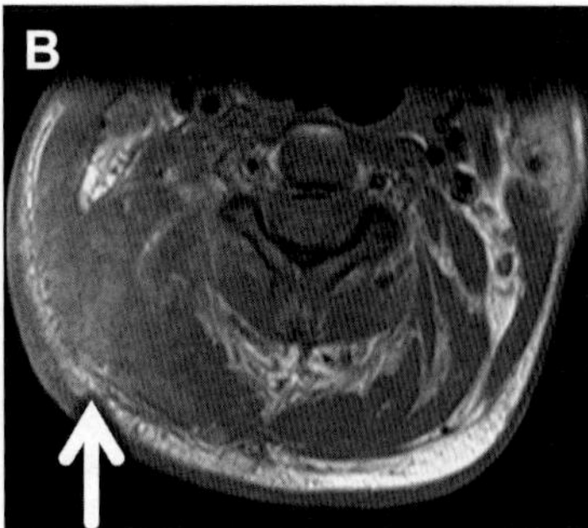

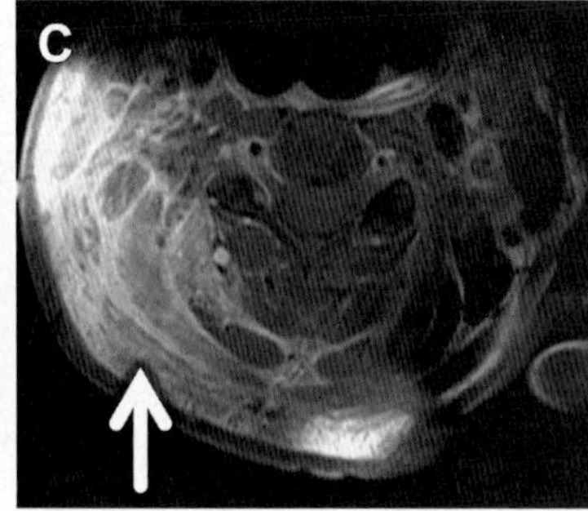

Fig. 7. (*A*) Axial T2W MR imaging shows hyperintensity in the right paraspinal muscles (*white arrow*) related to myofascitis in this patient with poorly controlled diabetes mellitus. (*B*) Axial T1-weighted (T1W) MR imaging reveals obscuration of the musculofascial planes in the right paraspinal space and infiltration of the phlegmon into the posterior cervical fat (*white arrow*). (*C*) Axial T1W + contrast MR imaging shows mild enlargement and enhancement of the right paraspinal muscles (*white arrow*). No focal fluid collection to suggest abscess is identified.

epidural phlegmon may extend several cervical levels and can encroach on the spinal cord and nerve roots leading to acute myelopathy or radiculopathy.[12,13] A central T1 hypointense fluid collection with rim enhancement is compatible with abscess formation. There may be perivertebral extension into the longus colli-capitis complex and paraspinal muscles (**Fig. 10**). The involved musculature becomes edematous with T2 hyperintensity, enlarges, and shows abnormal enhancement. Focal abscesses may form in the paraspinal muscles, showing central T1 hypointensity, T2 hyperintensity, and peripheral enhancement.[14]

Initial treatment of discitis/osteomyelitis is conservative management with an extended course antimicrobial therapy and nonpharmacologic treatments such as physiotherapy and immobilization. Immobilization is advocated when pain is significant or when there is a risk of spinal instability.[15] The formation of perivertebral abscess may require surgical intervention, particularly if there are neurologic deficits. Surgical intervention is indicated if there is compression of neural elements, spinal instability caused by extensive bony destruction, severe kyphosis, or failure of conservative management (**Table 2**).[15]

Fig. 8. Contrast-enhanced axial CT of the neck reveals a multiloculated venolymphatic malformation centered in the posterior cervical space (*white arrows*). It effaces the adjacent fat.

Lemierre Syndrome

Acute oropharyngeal infection can rarely result in secondary septic thrombophlebitis of the internal jugular vein and possible septic metastasis. This soft tissue infection, known as Lemierre

Table 1
Diseases of the perivertebral space

Common Diseases	Uncommon Diseases
Infection/Inflammation	
Discitis/osteomyelitis (spondylodiscitis)	Lemierre syndrome
	Longus colli tendinitis
Postoperative infection	
Tumor	
Metastatic disease	Chordoma
Multiple myeloma	Chondrosarcoma
	Aneurysmal bone cyst
	Giant cell tumor
	Schwannoma
	Neurofibroma
	Malignant nerve sheath tumor
Vascular	
Atherosclerotic disease	Vascular malformation
Dissection	Hemangioma
Hematoma	Venolymphatic malformation

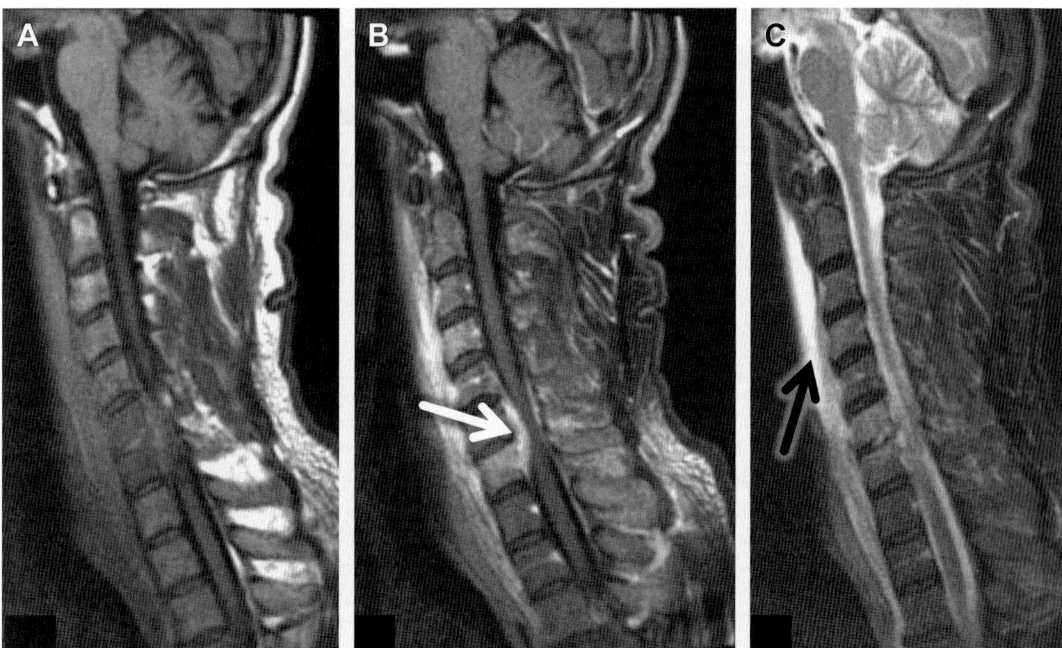

Fig. 9. Sagittal T1W (*A*), T1W +C with fat saturation (*B*), and STIR (*C*) MR images of the cervical spine show confluent low T1 signal, high STIR signal, and abnormal diffuse enhancement in the C6 and C7 vertebral bodies. There is corresponding high STIR signal in the C6 to C7 disc space as well as throughout the prevertebral soft tissues. Fluid is also noted in the retropharyngeal space (*black arrow*). A lentiform enhancing collection (*white arrow*) posterior to the vertebral bodies creates mass effect on the spinal cord and is consistent with epidural phlegmon.

syndrome, is almost always caused by *Fusobacterium necrophorum*. Infection spreads by local invasion into the lateral pharyngeal space with seeding of the internal jugular vein. The venous system serves as the route of spread to the rest of the body. Neck swelling and tenderness may be the earliest signs that uncomplicated pharyngitis has extended beyond the oropharynx. The typical clinical triad includes pharyngitis, a tender/swollen neck, and noncavitating pulmonary infiltrates. Contrast-enhanced CT shows tonsillar and peritonsillar edema, phlegmon, and abscess associated with the primary site of infection and reveals the internal jugular vein thrombosis and perivascular edema (thrombophlebitis). The soft tissue infection can spread into the RPS and PVS (**Fig. 11**). Several series have described Lemierre syndrome to primarily affect previously healthy children, adolescents, and young adults, with an equal to slightly increased male-to-female predominance.[16,17] Patients with recurrent pharyngitis may be at an increased risk. Antibiotics markedly decrease the rate of metastatic complications but, if left untreated, septic metastases may progress to cavitating pneumonia and septic arthritis.[18]

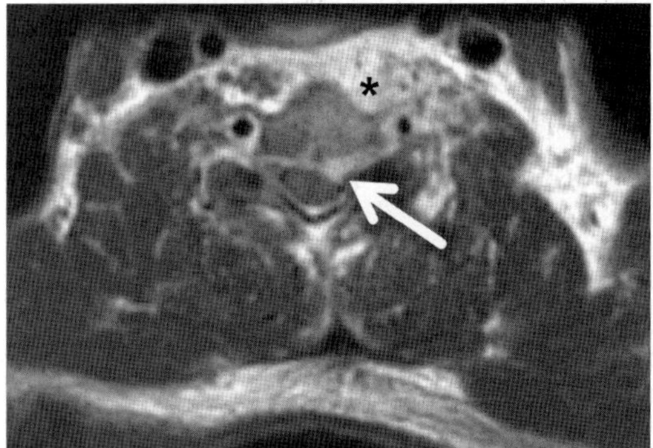

Fig. 10. The epidural extent of disease and mass effect on the spinal cord is better seen on the enhanced axial T1W MR image (*white arrow*). Abnormal enhancement of the endplates as well as of the prevertebral soft tissues is seen. Note that the longus colli muscles are enlarged and show diffuse enhancement, greater on the left (*black asterisk*). They are slightly lifted off the anterior aspect of the vertebral body because of prevertebral edema.

Longus Colli Tendinitis

Inflammatory processes, such as longus colli tendinitis (LCT), can cause acute pain, clinically mimicking more serious diseases (**Table 3**). In

Table 2
Imaging features of discitis/osteomyelitis and abscess

		MR Imaging Findings		
	CT Findings	T1	T2/STIR	T1 +C
Discitis/ Osteomyelitis	Endplate erosions	Hypointensity	Hyperintensity	Diffuse endplate and rim enhancement of the disc
Abscess	Hypodense fluid collection with hyperdense, enhancing rim	Intermediate	Hyperintense fluid with hypointense rim	Rim enhancement

LCT, or acute calcific prevertebral tendinitis, rupture of calcium hydroxyapatite deposits within the longus colli tendon provokes an inflammatory response and results in acute neck pain and RPS edema.[5] Similar to discitis/osteomyelitis and retropharyngeal abscess, patients with LCT may present with neck pain, fever, odynophagia, and dysphagia.

On imaging, there is calcification in the longus capitis-colli tendinous insertions, usually at the C1/C2 level. Edema in the adjacent RPS is typically present. The tendinous calcifications can be detected on radiographs but are best seen on CT (**Figs. 12**). These calcifications are hypointense on all MR imaging sequences and usually do not enhance.[19,20] Helpful imaging clues to suggest an inflammatory process rather than a potential infectious process include the absence of lymphadenopathy and the preservation of the osseous structures. Enlargement and inflammation of the longus capitis-colli muscle bellies may be seen in LCT and may mimic the imaging appearance of a neoplasm. The presence of normal muscle striations in this inflammatory condition is a helpful imaging feature to differentiate it from a neoplastic process.

Treatment of this self-limited inflammatory process is supportive. Imaging can be key in distinguishing inflammatory tendinitis from infectious retropharyngeal abscess because both conditions

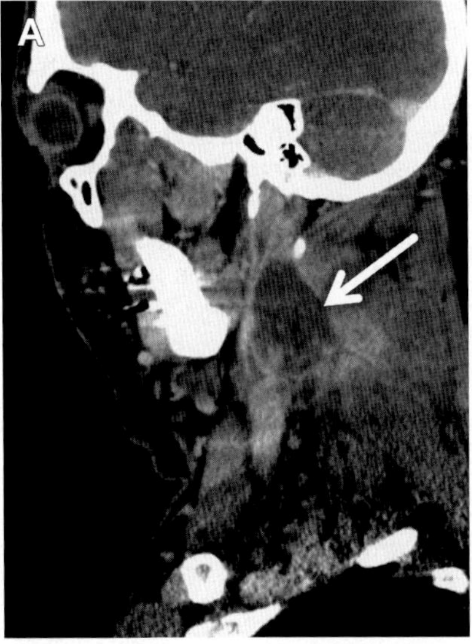

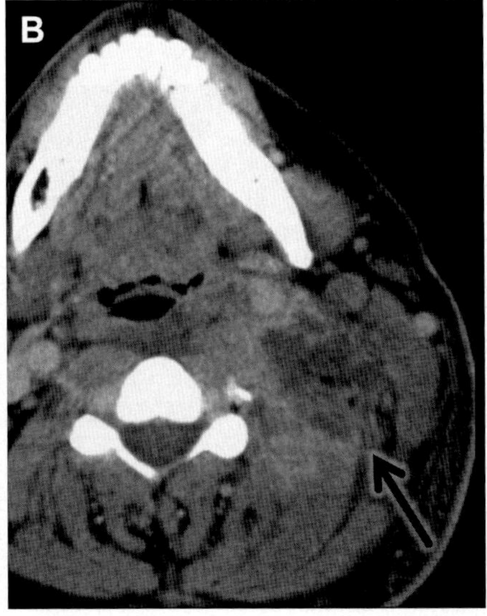

Fig. 11. Sagittal (*A*) and axial (*B*) contrast-enhanced CT images of the neck soft tissues show a trans-spatial infectious process originating from a pharyngeal infection. There is a large, ill-defined, hypoattenuating collection with internal foci of gas and patchy peripheral enhancement involving the left carotid space (*white arrow*) with thrombophlebitis of the internal jugular vein. The inflammatory process infiltrates into the perivertebral space and posterior cervical fat (*black arrow*).

Table 3
Features of inflammatory/infectious diseases of the perivertebral space

LCT	Discitis/Osteomyelitis	Retropharyngeal Abscess
Calcification of the tendons at C1/C2	Osseous destruction	—
Preservation of muscle striations	Abscess in perivertebral soft tissues or epidural space	Peripheral enhancement
No lymphadenopathy	Lymphadenopathy	Suppurative retropharyngeal lymph nodes
Possible bone marrow edema	Bone marrow edema	—
Perivertebral muscle edema, enlargement	Perivertebral muscle edema, enlargement	—
Fluid in retropharyngeal space without rim enhancement	—	Fluid in retropharyngeal space

can show abnormal laboratory studies, such as increase in erythrocyte sedimentation rate and leukocytosis.[21]

TUMORS OF OSSEOUS ORIGIN

When multiple destructive osseous lesions are present, metastases and multiple myeloma should be leading differential considerations. When a single destructive lesion is present in a vertebral body, the differential diagnosis includes infection and primary bone neoplasms.[22] Because of the various tissue types contained within the PVS, a variety of primary neoplasms can be seen in this location. Most are rare, but understanding the anatomy and imaging features is important when these uncommon lesions arise.

Metastatic Disease

The most common disease of the PVS is metastatic disease. Any neoplasm that has a propensity for osseous metastasis can involve the vertebrae of the PVS. Sclerotic osseous lesions are commonly seen in metastatic prostate, bladder, and carcinoid tumors, whereas lytic metastases

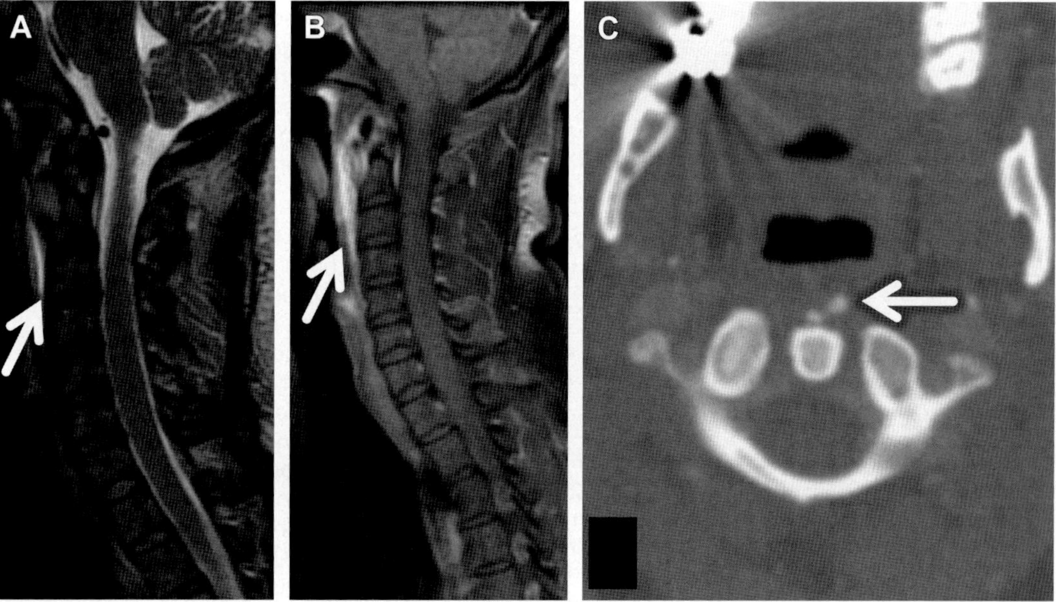

Fig. 12. (*A*) Sagittal STIR MR image shows fluid in the retropharyngeal space (*white arrow*). (*B*) Sagittal T1W +C MR image with fat saturation shows homogeneous enhancement (*white arrow*) of this retropharyngeal fluid. (*C*) Axial CT image in bone algorithm reveals calcification of the tendons of the longus colli/capitis complex (*white arrow*). (*Courtesy of* Chris Harker, MD, Medical Imaging Associates, Idaho Falls, ID.)

are observed with renal and thyroid carcinoma **Fig. 13**. Primary carcinomas of lung and breast origin can present with sclerotic, lytic, or mixed osseous metastases.

One imaging features that may aid in distinguishing a metastasis from other disease processes is vertebral body destruction with sparing of the disc space. Unlike discitis/osteomyelitis, in which infection is centered in the end plates and adjacent disc spaces, metastases are centered in the vertebral body or posterior elements and typically spare the disc spaces.

Chordoma

Chordoma should be considered when a midline destructive osseous lesion is present in the spine. Although the sacrococcygeal and sphenooccipital locations are more common, vertebral body chordomas do occur, and, when present, they have a predilection for the C2 vertebral body.[23] These lesions arise from notochordal remnants and spread via local invasion with destruction of adjacent osseous structures. The typical imaging appearance is a solid destructive mass centered within the vertebral body. Extension may continue into the disc, epidural space, adjacent vertebral bodies, and/or along nerve roots. Chordomas characteristically show T2/STIR hyperintensity relative to the adjacent disc and similar to cerebrospinal fluid. There may be internal septae, and the enhancement may vary from patchy to intense, solid enhancement (**Fig. 14**).[24,25]

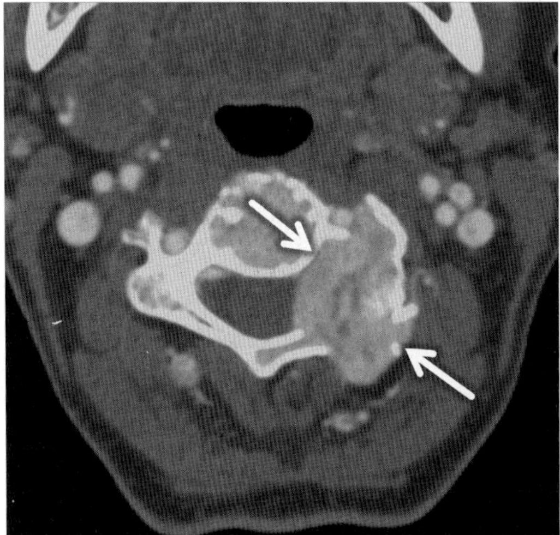

Fig. 13. Axial contrast-enhanced CT shows a hypervascular metastasis (*white arrows*) from thyroid carcinoma. Metastases usually show aggressive features with cortical breakthrough and extension into the adjacent soft tissues. Although metastases may vary in their imaging appearance depending on the primary carcinoma, metastases almost always have an aggressive imaging appearance with osteolysis and narrow zone of transition.

Osteochondroma/Chondrosarcoma

Sessile or pedunculated osteochondromas arising from the vertebral column can involve the PVS. Vertebral column involvement is uncommon, comprising less than 5% of cases.[26] On CT and MR imaging, osteochondromas have a cauliflower appearance and are contiguous with the medullary cavity of the parent vertebral body. A benign osteochondroma is T1 and T2 isointense/hyperintense (similar to bone marrow) and is surrounded by hypointense cortex. The lesions have a T1 hypointense/isointense and T2 hyperintense cartilaginous cap, which is the site of growth during skeletal development. After skeletal maturity, a cartilaginous cap measuring greater than 1.5 cm and/or showing rapid growth may indicate potential malignant degeneration into chondrosarcoma (**Fig. 15**).[26]

A destructive lytic osseous lesion with internal chondroid matrix in the PVS raises the possibility of a chondrosarcoma. These tumors of connective tissue may arise in the posterior elements (40%), the vertebral body (15%), or both (45%).[27] Chondrosarcomas may be primary lesions and can arise as a sequela of radiation therapy. Secondary lesions can arise from malignant degeneration of an osteochondroma or enchondroma. Malignant degeneration occurs in less than 1% of osteochondromas and in up to 3% to 5% in patients with multiple hereditary enchondroma syndrome.[26,27] CT is helpful to evaluate for chondroid matrix, cortical destruction, intraosseous extension, and extraosseous extension. MR imaging is better for delineating the extent of tumor within bone and into the adjacent soft tissues.[28]

Aneurysmal Bone Cyst

An aneurysmal bone cyst (ABC) is a benign, expansile, multiloculated cystic lesion with a predilection for the spinal posterior elements and thus can be found in the PVS. Between 10% and 30% of ABCs arise from the spine and sacrum.[29] These lesions commonly extend into the vertebral body (75%–90%) and may extend beyond the osseous structures to involve the PVS and epidural space. ABCs cause balloonlike, expansile remodeling of bone with thinning of the cortex and internal cysts with fluid-fluid levels. Multiple cystic locules with fluid-fluid levels caused by hemorrhage and sedimentation of blood products are better delineated on MR imaging than on CT (**Fig. 16**). On CT, ABCs may reveal some seemingly aggressive features, such as cortical

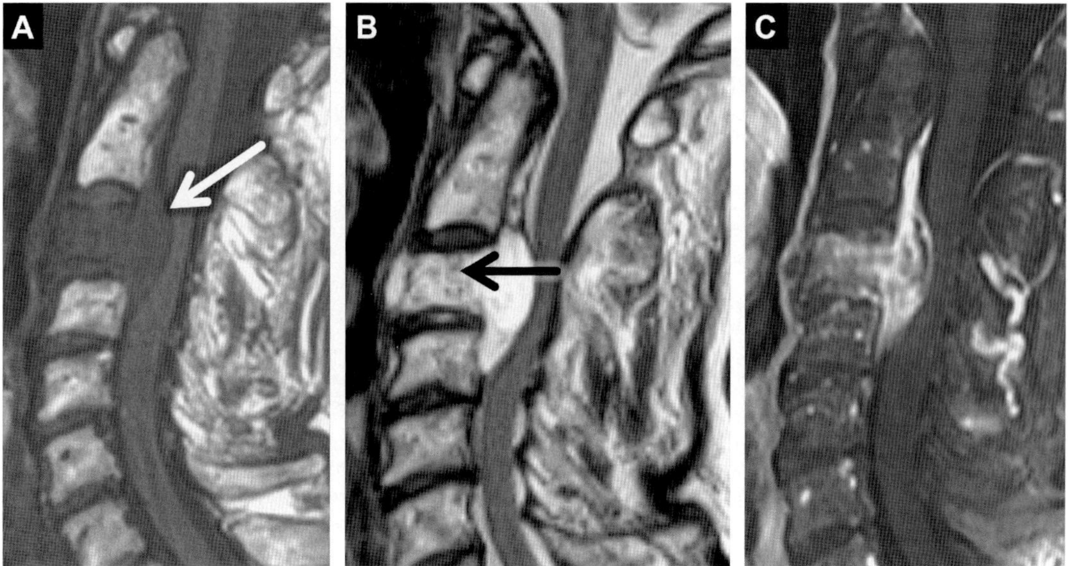

Fig. 14. (*A*) Midline sagittal T1W MR image through the cervical spine shows a hypointense lesion completely replacing the C3 vertebral body. The lesion has broken through the anterior cortex into the prevertebral space and through the posterior cortex to extend into the ventral epidural space (*white arrow*). (*B*) On the T2W MR image, the lesion is hyperintense with subtle internal hypointense septae (*black arrow*). (*C*) On the T1W +C MR image, the lesion shows heterogeneous enhancement with craniocaudal epidural extension from C2 to C4. This lesion is a pathologically proven chordoma.

breakthrough into the surrounding soft tissues and indistinct margins. When faced with an expansile osseous lesion with fluid-fluid levels, ABC is a leading consideration. A preexisting lesion can be identified in 29% to 35% of cases; the most common of these is giant cell tumor, accounting for 19% to 39% of cases in which a preexisting lesion is found. Other common precursor lesions

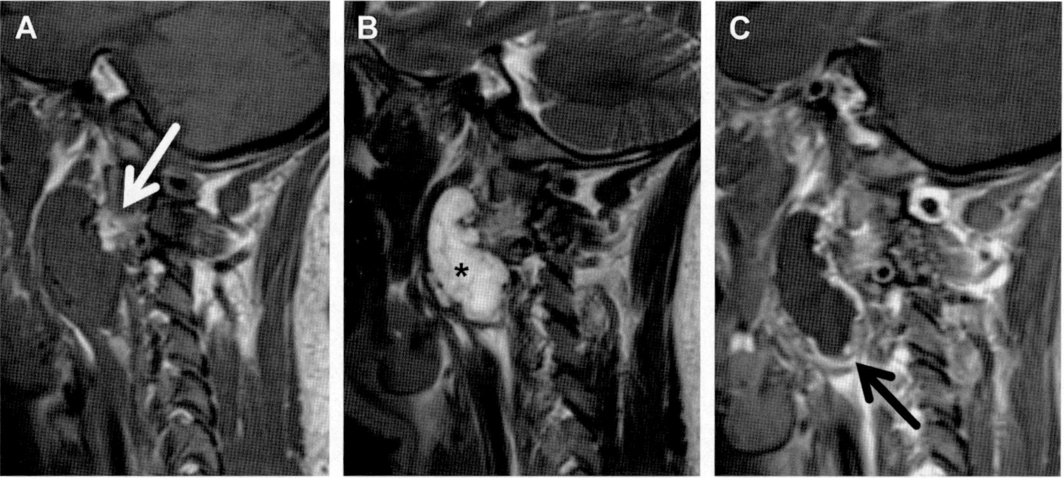

Fig. 15. Sagittal T1W (*A*) MR image show an exophytic lesion arising from the C2 vertebral body in this patient, who presented with a neck mass. A T1 isointense to marrow lesion is exophytic from the C2 vertebral body and shows the characteristic medullary continuity (*white arrow*) seen with osteochondromas. Sagittal T2W (*B*) MR image shows the large, pedunculated, T2 hyperintense component extending into the prevertebral space (*black asterisk*). Sagittal T1W +C (*C*) MR image shows peripheral enhancement of the cartilaginous cap (*black arrow*). Although the medullary continuity can be seen in the setting of benign osteochondroma, a cartilaginous cap greater than 1.5 cm suggests sarcomatous transformation, as is present in this case of pathologically proven chondrosarcoma.

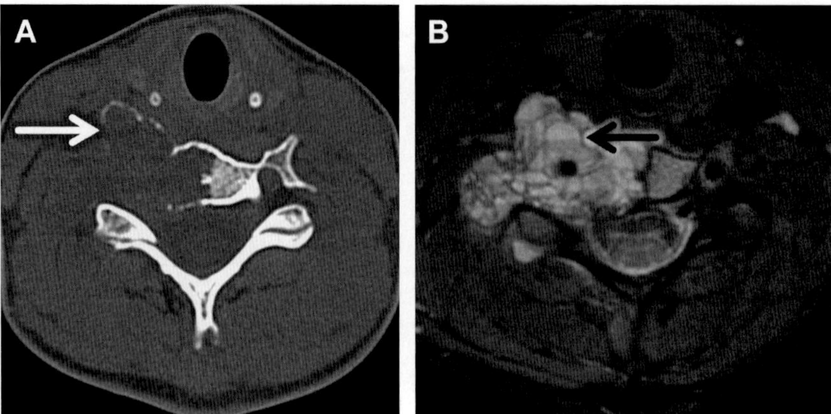

Fig. 16. Axial CT (*A*) and T2W MR with fat saturation (*B*) images through the cervical spine show the characteristic features of an ABC. The expansile nature of the ABC and thinned cortex (*white arrow*) is easily appreciated on the CT examination, whereas the characteristic fluid-fluid levels (*black arrow*) are readily apparent on MR imaging. Although ABCs typically arise in the posterior elements, extension into the vertebral body is common.

include osteoblastoma, angioma, and chondroblastoma.[30,31] A potential mimicker of an ABC is an aggressive, telangiectatic osteogenic osteosarcoma. The two lesions must be distinguished because of the discordance in aggressiveness and differences in management. Although these lesions can appear similar on MR imaging, osteogenic sarcomas show more aggressive features, including a wider zone of transition, bone destruction, and soft tissue infiltration.

Giant Cell Tumor

An additional, lytic expansile bone lesion that may be identified in the PVS in skeletally mature patients is a giant cell tumor (GCT). In contradistinction to the ABC, a GCT is usually centered in the vertebral body, although there is frequent involvement of the posterior arch. In 79% of cases, there is extraosseous extension into the soft tissues.[32] These lesions have benign radiographic features with a narrow zone of transition and well-defined, nonsclerotic margins (**Fig. 17**). Although residual bone fragments can be present in a GCT, there is no true matrix formation. Approximately 10% to 15% of GCTs have an ABC component.[31] Because the lesions contain collagen, hemosiderin, and necrosis, they show variable signal intensities on MR imaging. GCTs typically show low to intermediate T1 signal intensity and intermediate to high T2 signal intensity, the latter caused by collagen-containing components. Despite their nonaggressive appearance, GCTs can invade local structures, and recurrence after surgical

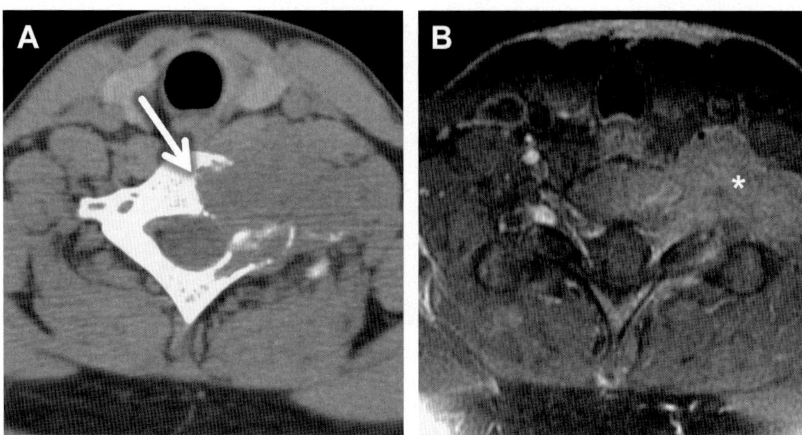

Fig. 17. (*A*) Axial CT shows that an expansile mass is centered within the subaxial cervical vertebral body. There is osseous destruction with a sharp zone of transition and without matrix formation (*white arrow*). (*B*) Axial T1W +C MR image with fat saturation better delineates this mildly enhancing lesion, particularly the extraosseous extension (*white asterisk*).

excision is seen in 12% to 50% of cases.[33] Although GCTs are benign lesions, there is a 10% risk of sarcomatous transformation, either spontaneously or in response to radiation therapy.[33] Primary malignant GCTs are rare and may metastasize to lung, liver, and bone.[34]

TUMORS OF NERVOUS TISSUE ORIGIN

Schwannoma

Together with neurofibromas, schwannomas make up most intradural extramedullary tumors that may be detected when evaluating the PVS. Schwannomas arise from Schwann cells, and loss of heterozygosity on chromosome 22 is a frequent event in the tumorigenesis of sporadic schwannoma.[35] Although most (~70%) schwannomas are intradural, a small percentage (15%) is entirely extradural or can be both intradural and extradural (15%), giving rise to the classic dumbbell shape.[36] These well-circumscribed lesions can vary in size from small intradural lesions to large intraspinal and paraspinal giant schwannomas, which may span multiple vertebral levels. On CT, schwannomas are isodense to the spinal cord and may show internal cystic change and, rarely, calcification. These slow-growing lesions may show adjacent bone remodeling and neural foraminal enlargement. On MR imaging, most schwannomas are T1 isointense/hypointense and T2 hyperintense to the spinal cord (**Fig. 18**). They may reveal cystic or fatty degeneration and even hemorrhage in some cases. The enhancement pattern is variable from uniform to heterogeneous to peripheral.[37] Schwannomas may show central T2 hypointensity with peripheral T2 hyperintensity, the so-called target sign, but less commonly than neurofibromas.[38] Schwannomas most often occur sporadically but can also be seen in genetic conditions, such as neurofibromatosis type 2, schwannomatosis, and the Carney complex. It can be difficult to distinguish a solitary, well-circumscribed peripheral nerve lesion in the PVS as a schwannoma or neurofibroma because of the overlapping imaging features. Clinical history of a genetic predisposition, such as neurofibromatosis type 2, may help guide the diagnosis to schwannoma.[39]

Neurofibroma

A circumscribed lesion arising from the cervical nerve roots may be a neurofibroma. Neurofibromas are spontaneous in 30% to 50% of cases, likely because of alteration of the neurofibromin gene on chromosome 17.[40] Although often spontaneous, neurofibromas, particularly plexiform neurofibromas, can be associated with neurofibromatosis type 1 (NF-1).[41] These nonencapsulated lesions of peripheral nerves contain elements of the parent peripheral nerve with proliferation of Schwann cells, fibroblasts, myxoid material, and nerve fascicles.[42] Neurofibromas are typically intradural extramedullary lesions but can be extradural in location. They can range in size from small, well-circumscribed lesions to large, lobulated, plexiform masses or diffuse infiltrative tumors. On CT, neurofibromas may be isodense or hypodense to the spinal cord, with variable enhancement. Because they are benign, slow-growing masses, they may cause adjacent bone remodeling.[43] On MR imaging, neurofibromas are T1 isointense and T2 isointense/hyperintense to the spinal cord and show variable enhancement (**Fig. 19**). The target sign of central T2 hypointensity with a rim of hyperintensity suggests, but is not pathognomonic for, a neurofibroma.[44] The

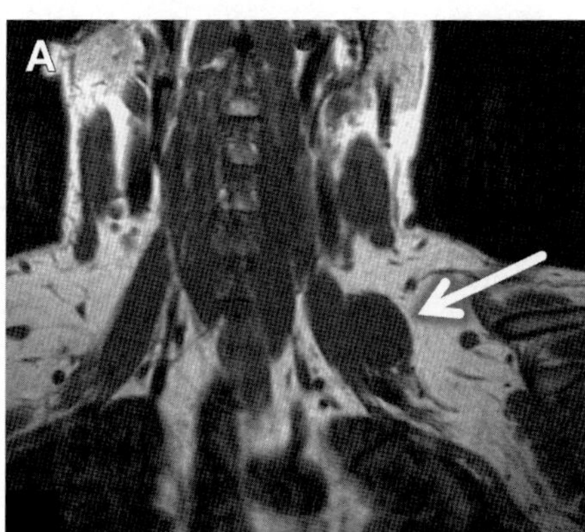

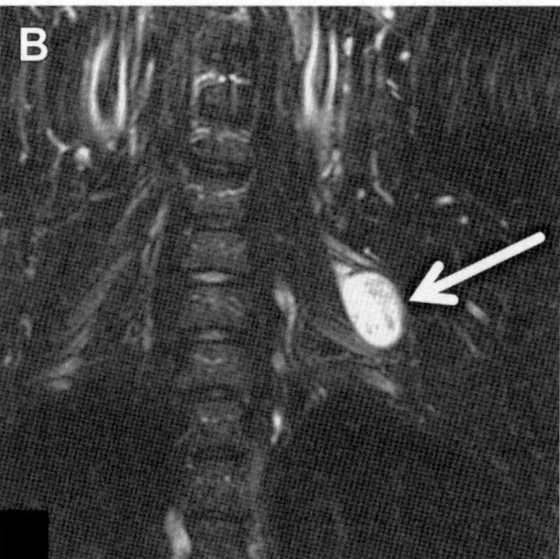

Fig. 18. Coronal T1W (*A*) and coronal STIR (*B*) MR images reveal a T1 isointense and STIR hyperintense ovoid lesion (*white arrows*) arising from the left BP nerve roots, traversing the perivertebral space. This well-delineated lesion represents a benign schwannoma and can be difficult to distinguish from other nerve sheath tumors, such as neurofibromas.

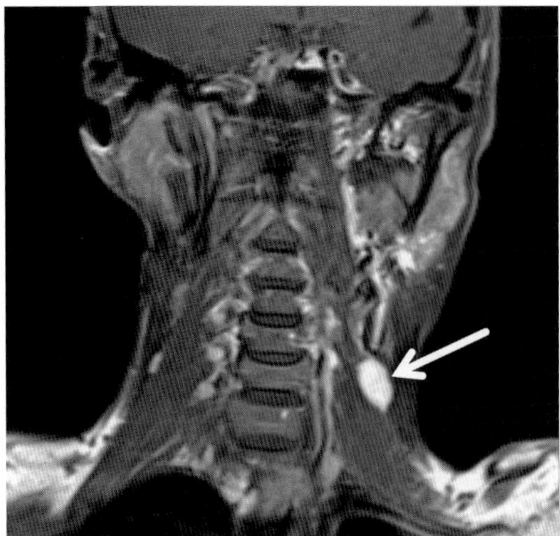

Fig. 19. Coronal T1W +C MR image with fat saturation shows a well-circumscribed neurofibroma (*white arrow*) that shows fusiform focal enlargement of a BP nerve. It enhances avidly without infiltration into the surrounding paraspinal muscles.

more complex plexiform neurofibromas can show a bag-of-worms appearance, with multinodular nerve enlargement interdigitating within the surrounding soft tissues (Fig. 20).

Malignant Peripheral Nerve Sheath Tumor

Malignant peripheral nerve sheath tumors (MPNSTs) are soft tissue sarcomas arising spontaneously from cells differentiating toward Schwann cells, perineural cells, or fibrocytes.[45] MPNSTs may alternatively result from the malignant degeneration of a preexisting neurofibroma, particularly in patients with NF-1 with plexiform neurofibromas. Approximately 50% to 60% of MPNSTs are associated with NF-1.[43] On both CT and MR imaging, MPNSTs show marked heterogeneity secondary to hemorrhage, calcification, cystic degeneration, and necrosis. The adjacent osseous structures may show foraminal enlargement and vertebral scalloping as well as bone destruction. These hypervascular masses are T1 isointense to muscle and heterogeneously T2 hyperintense. Avid to heterogeneous enhancement may be seen depending on the degree of internal hemorrhage, necrosis, and cystic degeneration (Fig. 21). Invasion into the surrounding soft tissues and parenchymal heterogeneity are helpful clues to diagnosing a MPNST in a patient with an enlarging, painful peripheral mass. In questionable cases of MPNST,[18] [F] 2-fluoro-2-deoxy-D-glucose (FDG) PET imaging may aid in differentiation because metabolically active MPNST shows increased FDG uptake (Fig. 22).[46]

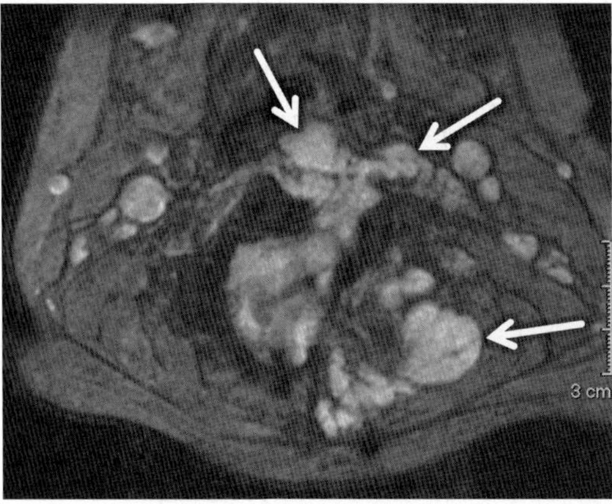

Fig. 20. Axial T2W MR image with fat saturation of a plexiform neurofibroma shows the bag-of-worms appearance with tendrils of the mass insinuating through the prevertebral and paraspinal spaces (*white arrows*).

VASCULAR LESIONS

Vascular lesions comprise the last major category of PVS lesions, with injury being the most common disorder. The vertebral arteries (VAs) are

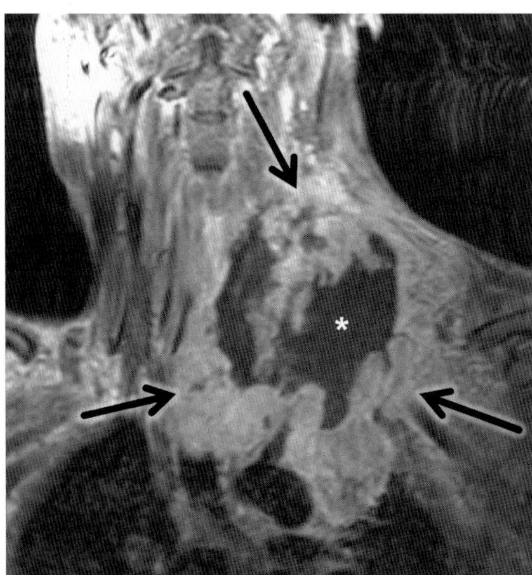

Fig. 21. Coronal T1W +C MR image with fat saturation shows the aggressive imaging appearance of a MPNST, which infiltrates into the surrounding structures with obscuration of musculofascial planes. It shows intense, heterogeneous enhancement along its irregular margins (*black arrows*) surrounding a necrotic core (*white asterisk*). Although it is not difficult to distinguishing this lesion from a benign neurofibroma, other cases of malignant degeneration can be difficult on imaging.

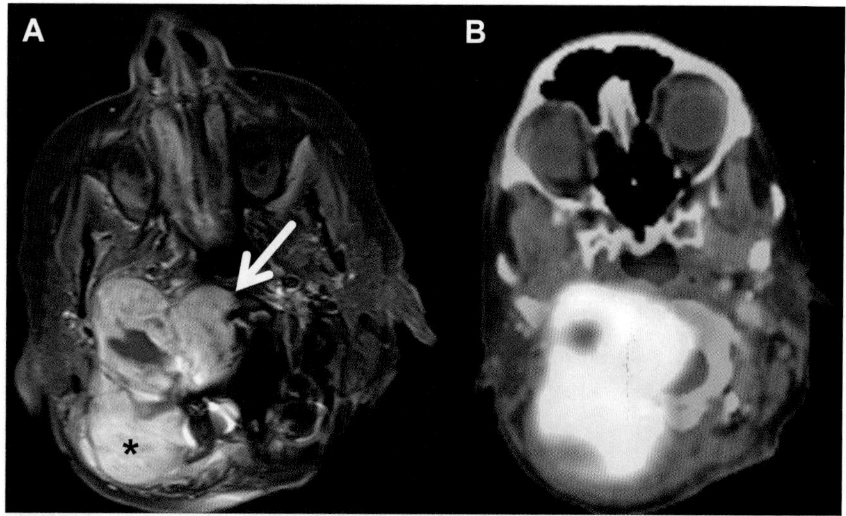

Fig. 22. This 33 year-old woman with NF-1 and history of a right cervical plexiform neurofibroma complains of increasing right neck and shoulder pain. (*A*) Axial T1W +C MR image with fat saturation shows a heterogeneously enhancing malignant nerve sheath tumor in the superior cervical perivertebral space. The lesion infiltrates into the prevertebral space (*white arrow*) as well as the paraspinal muscles (*black asterisk*). (*B*) Axial FDG-PET image shows intense uptake in this heterogeneous mass, which is consistent with malignant transformation of the plexiform neurofibroma into a MPNST. (*Courtesy of* Justin B. Sims, MD, Indiana University Health.)

the major vascular conduit in this space and have the highest injury rate between the mobile and immobile segments.[47] Blunt trauma can result in a spectrum of vascular injuries, including dissection, aneurysm, pseudoaneurysm, occlusion, and arteriovenous fistula formation. In high-energy mechanisms, multivessel injury is common, occurring in 18% to 38% of patients.[47] Blunt injury to the VAs carries a high rate of morbidity and mortality, and early injury detection is critical in preventing severe complications, such as stroke. Although digital subtraction angiography (DSA) remains the gold standard in detecting vascular injury, MR angiography (MRA) and CT angiography (CTA) both have high sensitivity and specificity for detecting vascular injury.[48] CTA has been shown to be concordant with DSA.[49] MR flow-sensitive sequences show the patency of cervical vessels, and the superb soft tissue resolution of MR imaging may also reveal a dissection flap with mural thrombus.

Dissection

A common vascular injury in the setting of blunt cervical trauma is VA dissection. Most of the traumatic dissections involve the V3 segment of the artery, which is anchored between the C2 foramen transversarium and the dura.[50] Although trauma is the usual antecedent event for vascular injury, dissection can arise spontaneously, particularly if the patient has a predisposition such as fibromuscular dysplasia or in the setting of hypertension.

A tear of the vessel intima can lead to intramural hematoma with partial or complete luminal occlusion. On MR imaging, the intraluminal hematoma of a VA dissection shows crescentic T1 and T2 hyperintense mural hematoma and a narrowed flow-void of the parent vessel. Fat-saturated, proton density, and magnetization-prepared 180° radiofrequency pulses and rapid gradient-echo sequences can increase the conspicuity of mural hematoma. However, CTA has the advantage of higher spatial resolution than MR imaging/MRA and is not affected by flow-related artifacts. CTA can show subtle vessel irregularity and areas of tapering (**Fig. 23**). Focal dilatation and focal narrowing may produce a pearl-and-string appearance. Increased external diameter and crescent-shaped mural thickening have been shown to be the most suggestive CTA findings.[51] DSA remains the gold standard because of its ability to detect a miniscule residual lumen that may not be apparent on CTA; however, CTA and MR imaging/MRA have replaced DSA as an initial screening tool. Although large-vessel dissections may show the typical intimal flap on DSA, small-caliber VA dissections rarely present with a visible flap.[52] DSA may reveal stenotic, occlusive, and aneurysmal types of VA dissections. DSA is usually reserved for vascular lesions that may potentially undergo intervention.[53]

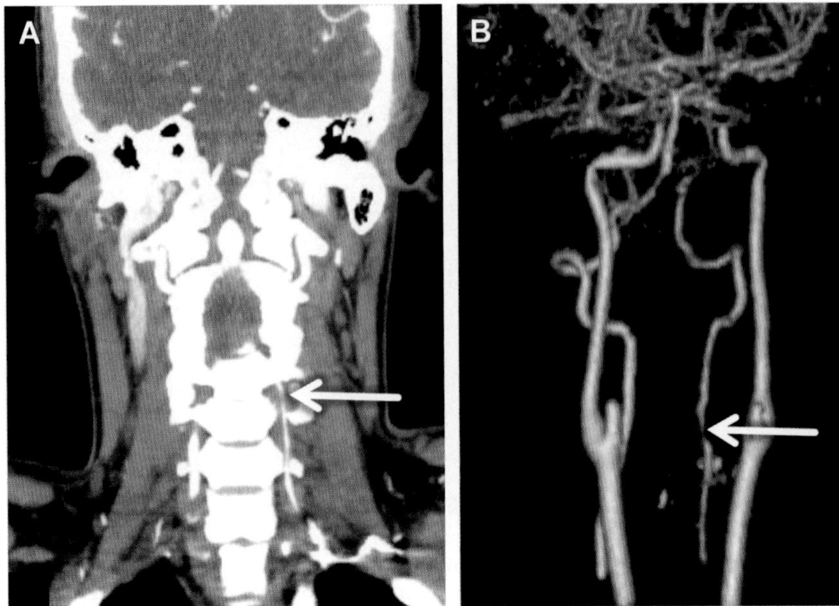

Fig. 23. Coronal CTA reconstruction (*A*) and three-dimensional surface-rendered reformation (*B*) show an acute left vertebral artery dissection (*white arrows*). Note the irregularity of the vessel lumen as well as the abrupt caliber change. An intimal flap may be difficult to identify in the setting of acute dissection secondary to the small caliber of the vertebral artery.

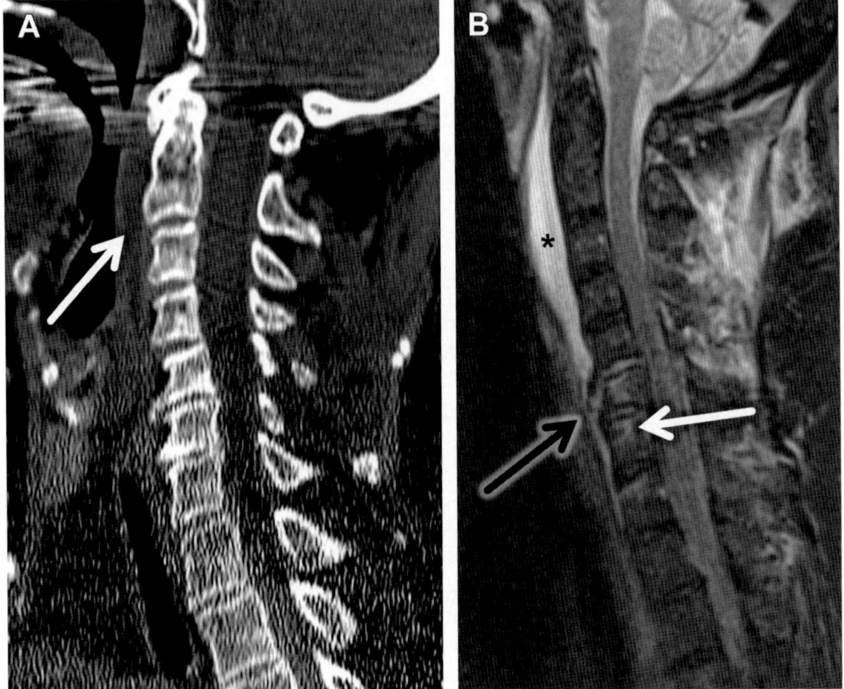

Fig. 24. (*A*) Sagittal CT reconstruction of the cervical spine in a patient with trauma shows a small prevertebral hematoma extending from C1 to C5 (*white arrow*). The presence of a hematoma in this region should raise the concern for a coexisting soft tissue or osseous injury. (*B*) Sagittal STIR MR image confirms not only the presence of the hyperintense prevertebral hematoma (*black asterisk*) but also reveals focal disruption of the anterior longitudinal ligament (*black arrow*) and marrow edema in the C6, C7 (*white arrow*), and T1 vertebral bodies.

Hematoma

Blunt trauma often results in multiple injuries not only involving the arteries but also the veins, osseous, and soft tissue structures. Traumatic retropharyngeal and prevertebral hematomas occasionally occur in isolation.[54] The hematoma itself may have little clinical significance, but its presence may herald a more severe osseous or soft tissue injury (ligamentous/spinal cord). Therefore, clinicians should scrutinize not only the cervical arterial structures but also the osseous and venous structures for potential disorders. A prevertebral hematoma is likely caused by disruption of the vessels overlying the anterior vertebral column and is associated with fracture and injury to the anterior longitudinal ligament and prevertebral fascia (**Fig. 24**).[55] Although a small hematoma can be associated with fractures of the odontoid process and compression fractures of the subaxial vertebral bodies, large prevertebral hematomas are more commonly seen with high-energy hyperextension mechanisms and injury to the anterior soft tissues. Most prevertebral hematomas resolve within 2 weeks of injury.[55]

SUMMARY

The PVS is complex compartment spanning the suprahyoid and infrahyoid neck and enveloped by the DLDCF. By accurately localizing a disease process in this space and understanding the various tissue types contained within the prevertebral and paraspinal components, radiologists can provide a meaningful differential diagnosis. Furthermore, correct localization guides clinical decision making and treatment.

REFERENCES

1. Harnsberger H. Perivertebral space anatomy - Imaging Issues. Diagnostic imaging. III-10-2-3. Diagnostic Imaging Head and Neck. Manitoba (Canada): Amirsys Publishing; 2004.
2. Hutchins T. Perivertebral space overview. 2nd edition. Manitoba (Canada): Amirsys Publishing; 2012.
3. Bohman L, Mancuso A, Thompson J, et al. CT approach to benign nasopharyngeal masses. AJNR Am J Neuroradiol 1980;1:513–20.
4. Davis WL, Harnsberger HR, Smoker WR, et al. Retropharyngeal space: evaluation of normal anatomy and diseases with CT and MR imaging. Radiology 1990;174(1):59–64.
5. Hoang JK, Branstetter BF 4th, Eastwood JD, et al. Multiplanar CT and MRI of collections in the retropharyngeal space: is it an abscess? AJR Am J Roentgenol 2011;196(4):W426–32.
6. Osborn AG, Koehler PR. Computed tomography of the paraspinal musculature: normal and pathologic anatomy. AJR Am J Roentgenol 1982;138(1):93–8.
7. Albertine KH, Morton DA, Foreman KB. Chapter 25: overview of the neck, muscles of the neck. New York: McGraw-Hill; 2011.
8. Mukherji SK, Castillo M, Wagle AG. The brachial plexus. Semin Ultrasound CT MR 1996;17(6): 519–38.
9. O'Connell JX, Janzen DL, Hughes TR. Nuchal fibrocartilaginous pseudotumor: a distinctive soft-tissue lesion associated with prior neck injury. Am J Surg Pathol 1997;21(7):836–40.
10. Davis WL, Harnsberger HR. CT and MRI of the normal and diseased perivertebral space. Neuroradiology 1995;37(5):388–94.
11. Ledermann HP, Schweitzer ME, Morrison WB, et al. MR imaging findings in spinal infections: rules or myths? Radiology 2003;228(2):506–14.
12. Ross JS. Pathways of spread. 2nd edition. Manitoba (Canada): Amirsys Publishing; 2010.
13. Shah LM. Epidural abscess. 2nd edition. Manitoba (Canada): Amirsys Publishing; 2010.
14. Shah LM. Paraspinal abscess. 2nd edition. Manitoba (Canada): Amirsys Publishing; 2010.
15. Quinones-Hinojosa A, Jun P, Jacobs R, et al. General principles in the medical and surgical management of spinal infections: a multidisciplinary approach. Neurosurg Focus 2004;17(6):E1.
16. Wright WF, Shiner CN, Ribes JA. Lemierre syndrome. South Med J 2012;105(5):283–8.
17. Karkos PD, Asrani S, Karkos CD, et al. Lemierre's syndrome: a systematic review. Laryngoscope 2009;119(8):1552–9.
18. Chirinos JA, Lichtstein DM, Garcia J, et al. The evolution of Lemierre syndrome: report of 2 cases and review of the literature. Medicine 2002;81(6):458–65.
19. Eastwood JD, Hudgins PA, Malone D. Retropharyngeal effusion in acute calcific prevertebral tendinitis: diagnosis with CT and MR imaging. AJNR Am J Neuroradiol 1998;19(9):1789–92.
20. Phillips CD. Acute calcific longus colli tendonitis. 2nd edition. Manitoba (Canada): Amirsys Publishing; 2012.
21. Ring D, Vaccaro AR, Scuderi G, et al. Acute calcific retropharyngeal tendinitis. Clinical presentation and pathological characterization. J Bone Joint Surg Am 1994;76(11):1636–42.
22. Phillips CD. Vertebral body metastasis in perivertebral space. 2nd edition. Manitoba (Canada): Amirsys Publishing; 2012.
23. Sciubba DM, Chi JH, Rhines LD, et al. Chordoma of the spinal column. Neurosurg Clin N Am 2008; 19(1):5–15.
24. Wippold FJ 2nd, Koeller KK, Smirniotopoulos JG. Clinical and imaging features of cervical chordoma. AJR Am J Roentgenol 1999;172(5):1423–6.

25. Phillips CD. Chordoma in perivertebral space. 2nd edition. Manitoba (Canada): Amirsys Publishing; 2012.
26. Murphey MD, Choi JJ, Kransdorf MJ, et al. Imaging of osteochondroma: variants and complications with radiologic-pathologic correlation. Radiographics 2000;20(5):1407–34.
27. McLoughlin GS, Sciubba DM, Wolinsky JP. Chondroma/chondrosarcoma of the spine. Neurosurg Clin N Am 2008;19(1):57–63.
28. Murphey MD, Walker EA, Wilson AJ, et al. From the archives of the AFIP: imaging of primary chondrosarcoma: radiologic-pathologic correlation. Radiographics 2003;23(5):1245–78.
29. Murphey MD, Andrews CL, Flemming DJ, et al. From the archives of the AFIP. Primary tumors of the spine: radiologic pathologic correlation. Radiographics 1996;16(5):1131–58.
30. Kransdorf MJ, Sweet DE. Aneurysmal bone cyst: concept, controversy, clinical presentation, and imaging. AJR Am J Roentgenol 1995;164(3):573–80.
31. Rodallec MH, Feydy A, Larousserie F, et al. Diagnostic imaging of solitary tumors of the spine: what to do and say. Radiographics 2008;28(4):1019–41.
32. Hart RA, Boriani S, Biagini R, et al. A system for surgical staging and management of spine tumors. A clinical outcome study of giant cell tumors of the spine. Spine (Phila Pa 1976) 1997;22(15):1773–82 [discussion: 1783].
33. Crim J. Giant cell tumor. 2nd edition. Manitoba (Canada): Amirsys Publishing; 2010.
34. Meis JM, Dorfman HD, Nathanson SD, et al. Primary malignant giant cell tumor of bone: "dedifferentiated" giant cell tumor. Mod Pathol 1989;2(5):541–6.
35. Bian LG, Sun QF, Tirakotai W, et al. Loss of heterozygosity on chromosome 22 in sporadic schwannoma and its relation to the proliferation of tumor cells. Chin Med J 2005;118(18):1517–24.
36. Borg B. Schwannoma. 2nd edition. Manitoba (Canada): Amirsys Publishing; 2010.
37. Parmar HA, Ibrahim M, Castillo M, et al. Pictorial essay: diverse imaging features of spinal schwannomas. J Comput Assist Tomogr 2007;31(3):329–34.
38. Jee WH, Oh SN, McCauley T, et al. Extraaxial neurofibromas versus neurilemmomas: discrimination with MRI. AJR Am J Roentgenol 2004;183(3):629–33.
39. Phillips CD. Brachial plexus schwannoma in perivertebral space. 2nd edition. Manitoba (Canada): Amirsys Publishing; 2012.
40. Viskochil D. Genetics of neurofibromatosis 1 and the NF1 gene. J Child Neurol 2002;17(8):562–70 [discussion: 571–2, 646–51].
41. Woertler K. Tumors and tumor-like lesions of peripheral nerves. Semin Musculoskelet Radiol 2010;14(5):547–58.
42. Levy AD, Patel N, Dow N, et al. From the archives of the AFIP: abdominal neoplasms in patients with neurofibromatosis type 1: radiologic-pathologic correlation. Radiographics 2005;25(2):455–80.
43. Borg B. Neurofibroma. 2nd edition. Manitoba (Canada): Amirsys Publishing; 2010.
44. Varma DG, Moulopoulos A, Sara AS, et al. MR imaging of extracranial nerve sheath tumors. J Comput Assist Tomogr 1992;16(3):448–53.
45. Gupta G, Mammis A, Maniker A. Malignant peripheral nerve sheath tumors. Neurosurg Clin N Am 2008;19(4):533–43, v.
46. Ferner RE, Golding JF, Smith M, et al. [18F]2-fluoro-2-deoxy-D-glucose positron emission tomography (FDG PET) as a diagnostic tool for neurofibromatosis 1 (NF1) associated malignant peripheral nerve sheath tumours (MPNSTs): a long-term clinical study. Ann Oncol 2008;19(2):390–4.
47. Sliker CW, Mirvis SE. Imaging of blunt cerebrovascular injuries. Eur J Radiol 2007;64(1):3–14.
48. Provenzale JM, Sarikaya B. Comparison of test performance characteristics of MRI, MR angiography, and CT angiography in the diagnosis of carotid and vertebral artery dissection: a review of the medical literature. AJR Am J Roentgenol 2009;193(4):1167–74.
49. Eastman AL, Chason DP, Perez CL, et al. Computed tomographic angiography for the diagnosis of blunt cervical vascular injury: is it ready for primetime? J Trauma 2006;60(5):925–9 [discussion: 929].
50. Bruneau M, Cornelius JF, George B. Anterolateral approach to the V1 segment of the vertebral artery. Neurosurgery 2006;58(4 Suppl 2):ONS-215–9 [discussion: ONS-219].
51. Chen CJ, Tseng YC, Lee TH, et al. Multisection CT angiography compared with catheter angiography in diagnosing vertebral artery dissection. AJNR Am J Neuroradiol 2004;25(5):769–74.
52. Provenzale JM. Dissection of the internal carotid and vertebral arteries: imaging features. AJR Am J Roentgenol 1995;165(5):1099–104.
53. Phillips CD. Vertebral artery dissection in neck. 2nd edition. Manitoba (Canada): Amirsys Publishing; 2012.
54. Anagnostara A, Athanassopoulou A, Kailidou E, et al. Traumatic retropharyngeal hematoma and prevertebral edema induced by whiplash injury. Emerg Radiol 2005;11(3):145–9.
55. Penning L. Prevertebral hematoma in cervical spine injury: incidence and etiologic significance. AJR Am J Roentgenol 1981;136(3):553–61.

Common Pediatric Head and Neck Congenital/ Developmental Anomalies

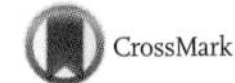

Justin K. LaPlante, MD, MS[a,*], Nicholas S. Pierson, MD[a], Gary L. Hedlund, DO[b]

KEYWORDS

• Congenital • Developmental • Neuroradiology • Pediatric • Genetic • Head & neck

KEY POINTS

- Identifying the location of pathologic entities relative to normal anatomic structures helps hone differential diagnosis and guides surgical approach.
- Clinical history, patient age, entity location, and the presence of associated anomalies all play important roles in refining a differential diagnosis.
- Many congenital pediatric head and neck disorders have pathognomonic imaging features which allow an interpreter to virtually make a diagnosis prior to biopsy.
- Although some lesions may seem aggressive, such as fibromatosis colli, they are considered to be do-not-touch lesions.
- A thorough understanding of pathologic entities is necessary to know when additional imaging studies are prudent.

INTRODUCTION

The complex nature of head and neck anatomy, in conjunction with the myriad of neonatal and early childhood head and neck disorders, often creates a diagnostic dilemma for primary pediatric care providers. Although adult head and neck disorders are primarily neoplasms such as squamous cell carcinoma, lymphoma, or melanoma, pediatric disorders are more often congenital/developmental anomalies such as infantile hemangioma, fibromatosis colli, thyroglossal duct cysts, or branchial apparatus anomalies. Clinicians are often able to determine with a high degree of certainty what a lesion may represent based on presentation and location. For instance, a warm, red or strawberrylike cutaneous discoloration most likely represents a benign infantile hemangioma, in which case watchful waiting or a simple ultrasonography (US) is all that may be needed. However, if a child presents with asymmetric cervical soft tissues, enlarging neck mass, or changes in feeding, a more rigorous diagnostic imaging work-up may be warranted.

When possible, most head and neck diagnostic evaluations in neonates, infants, and young children begin with US. This modality provides real-time information about blood flow direction and velocity, in addition to characteristic of the disorder and its relationship to adjacent structures. In addition, US is a cost-effective, readily available, and quick diagnostic imaging modality. In cases in which US does not completely characterize a lesion, or if the suspected entity is thought to

Disclosure: The authors have nothing to disclose.

[a] Department of Neuroradiology, University of Utah, 30 North 1900 East, #1A071, Salt Lake City, UT 84132, USA; [b] Department of Pediatric Medical Imaging, Primary Children's Hospital, Intermountain Healthcare, 100 No. Mario Capecchi Drive, Salt Lake City, UT 84113, USA
* Corresponding author.
E-mail address: justinklaplante@gmail.com

Radiol Clin N Am 53 (2015) 181–196
http://dx.doi.org/10.1016/j.rcl.2014.09.006

originate within the deep cervical soft tissues, a computed tomography (CT) scan or MR imaging scan may be needed.

Although CT exposes patients to ionizing radiation, it is a more cost-effective and a faster imaging technique than MR imaging. In addition, it provides exquisite detail of involved osseous structures. MR imaging provides greater soft tissue evaluation and allows the determination of subtle soft tissue findings such as perineural tumor spread. However, patients may be subjected to conscious or full sedation, which have inherent risks. Radiologists and clinicians should work together to determine the most efficacious diagnostic work-up. This article reviews some of the commonly encountered pediatric head and neck anomalies, how to use a prudent diagnostic work-up, relevant anatomy, treatment options, and pearls that referring physicians should consider.

PATHOLOGY

Thyroglossal Duct Cyst

Thyroglossal duct cyst (TGDC) is a benign cystic mass occurring in the midline between the foramen cecum at the base of the tongue and the thyroid bed in the infrahyoid neck. It is the most common congenital neck malformation and is found in 5% to 10% of the population at autopsy. Presence represents failure of involution of the thyroglossal duct with persistent secretion via the epithelial lining. Most cases are spontaneous without a significant gender predilection. However, a rare autosomal dominant form, occurring most commonly in women, has a strong association with developmental thyroid anomalies.[1–3]

TGDC usually presents before 10 years of age as recurrent, intermittent swelling following recent respiratory infection. In rare cases, a lingual TGDC may lead to airway obstruction in the neonate. Differential considerations are broad and include additional cystic neck masses such as abscess, venolymphatic malformation, dermoid/epidermoid, or laryngocele.[4,5]

Physical examination shows a midline or paramedian palpable and compressible mass along the ventral neck. Approximately 25% occur in the suprahyoid neck, 25% in the infrahyoid neck, and nearly 50% at the hyoid bone. Treatment is via complete surgical resection. Location relative to the hyoid bone guides surgical approach. In most cases, a small section of the midline hyoid bone is resected to minimize recurrence.[6,7]

US is the imaging modality of choice for initial evaluation (see **Box 5**). A typical TGDC is midline along the ventral neck, well circumscribed, has anechoic internal echoes representing simple fluid, and thin walls. Its relationship to the hyoid bone should be noted (**Fig. 1**). If atypical features such as calcification, thick wall, isoechoic/hyperechoic internal echoes, or prominent adjacent vascularity are present, additional imaging with CT or MR should be pursued. Given the rare occurrence of associated thyroid anomalies, localization of normal thyroid tissue should be performed at the time of initial examination. If a normal thyroid gland is absent, nuclear scintigraphy aids in further evaluation. Please refer to **Table 1** and **Boxes 1** and **2** for additional diagnostic imaging findings.[2,3,5]

Branchial Apparatus Anomalies

Although the detailed embryology of the formation and development of the branchial (pharyngeal) apparatus is beyond the scope of this article, a basic understanding of the organization of the branchial arches, pouches, and clefts and their derivatives is helpful in understanding the pathogenesis of some important congenital head and neck masses.[8] Knowing the relationship of branchial remnants to normal anatomic structures is important in defining the anomaly and its point of origin,[9,10] which becomes clinically relevant in avoiding operative complications related to damaging adjacent structures during complete resection of these anomalies, which is the treatment of choice. The branchial anomaly and its associated tract typically are present inferior to the derivatives of its own arch and superior to the derivatives of the adjacent arch.[11,12] A simplified summary of branchial arch, pouch, and cleft derivatives are contained in **Table 2** and imaging recommendations of suspected lesions are shown in **Box 3**.

The most common branchial apparatus anomalies involve the first and second branchial clefts, whereas anomalies of the third and fourth apparatuses are rare. Approximately 95% of branchial cleft anomalies are related to the second branchial cleft, which also represents the second most commonly encountered congenital neck mass behind the thyroglossal duct cyst.[13] Between 1% and 4% of branchial anomalies can be attributed to the first branchial cleft. The first and second branchial cleft cysts are discussed here. Cervical thymic remnants, which are anomalies of derivatives of the third branchial apparatus, are discussed separately.

First branchial cleft cysts can present as masses within the region extending from the external auditory canal to the angle of the jaw, including the parotid gland.[2] Lesions associated with the external auditory canal may present auricular swellings, fistulas, or otorrhea, and may be

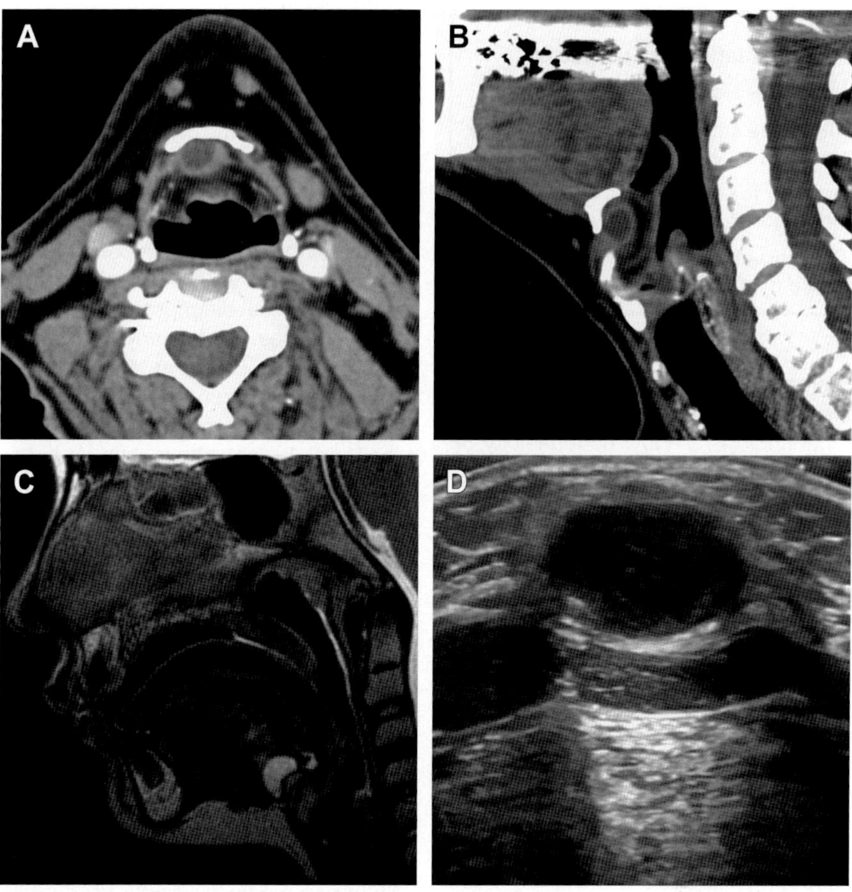

Fig. 1. Thyroglossal duct cyst. (*A*) Axial contrast-enhanced CT (CECT) shows a fluid-attenuating central neck mass closely associated with the hyoid bone. (*B*) The same lesion in the sagittal plane. (*C*) Fluid-weighted MR imaging shows the cystic nature of the mass. (*D*) Axial US shows a low-echogenicity lesion with increased through-transmission at the level of the hyoid. No internal flow was seen on Doppler interrogation (not shown).

confused clinically for preauricular pits or sinuses. When involving the parotid gland, the presenting symptom may be superinfection with abscess or parotitis. The differential diagnosis of a pediatric cystic mass of the parotid including neoplasm, lymphoepithelial cysts, and sialoceles makes correct identification of the anomaly difficult by imaging alone.[14] On any imaging modality the lesions

Table 1
Imaging characteristics of thyroglossal duct cysts

Imaging Technique	Imaging Findings
US	Circumscribed, anechoic, or hypoechoic midline ventral neck mass without significant adjacent vascularity. Internal echoes may represent hemorrhage or infectious material
CT	Hypoattenuating midline ventral neck mass with a thin peripheral rim of enhancement. Thick wall with central more isoattenuating/hyperattenuating material may represent hemorrhage or superimposed infection
MR imaging	T1: hypointense (simple fluid); hyperintense (proteinaceous/hemorrhagic fluid) T2: homogeneously hyperintense T1 with contrast: cystic component should not enhance. Peripheral/rim enhancement when infected
Nuclear scintigraphy	Only used if ectopic thyroid is suspected

Box 1
Imaging recommendations for suspected thyroglossal duct cysts

- US for initial assessment and to evaluate for normal thyroid tissue
- CT/MR reserved for suspected infection, or if US is nondiagnostic
- Nuclear scintigraphy to evaluate for ectopic thyroid tissue (if suspected)

show the characteristics of a simple or complicated cyst depending on the contents of the fluid (**Fig. 2**). Typical findings are low echogenicity on US, low attenuation on CT, and variable signal on MR imaging. Thickened enhancing walls on cross-sectional imaging are typically only seen if infection is present (**Table 3**). The relationship of the lesion to the facial nerve on imaging and at surgery is important.

Second branchial cleft cysts typically present as painless, fluctuant, lateral neck masses unless infected. A history of repeated soft tissue infections of the lateral neck suggests the diagnosis.[14] Location is key in identification, with the most common being dorsal to the submandibular gland, lateral to the carotid space, and anteromedial to the sternocleidomastoid (SCM) muscle. These masses can be classified into 4 types and are found anywhere from the parapharyngeal space to superficial to the SCM deep to the platysma. Although the imaging characteristics are similar to those of the first branchial cleft cyst as previously described, location is the discriminating feature (**Fig. 3**). Differential considerations of cystic masses within the region in which second branchial cleft cysts are found may include lymphatic malformation, thymic cyst, or suppurative nontuberculous mycobacterial adenitis. Beware of new diagnoses of cystic neck mass in adult patients because this may represent the initially presentation of squamous cell carcinoma (**Box 4**).

Box 2
Thyroglossal duct cyst: pearls for the referring physician

- Commonly presents as a midline ventral neck mass/swelling following minor respiratory infection.
- If nodularity or calcification is present, further evaluation for associated thyroid carcinoma should be undertaken.
- Perform thyroid imaging (US or scintigraphy) to ensure that normal thyroid tissue is present.

Cervical Thymic Remnants

The thymus plays an important role as a lymphoid organ in infants and young children and is integral in cell-mediated immunity. Cervical thymic remnants, although rare, represent a category of neck masses that radiologists should consider in their differential diagnoses of both cystic and solid neck masses, particularly in newborns, infants, and young children (**Fig. 4**).

The embryologic origin of the thymus is predominantly from the third and, to a lesser extent, the fourth branchial pouches. At birth, the thymus normally resides within the superior mediastinum (prevascular space). The embryonic pathway of migration of the thymus is in the neck along the guide paths of the thymopharyngeal ducts, ventral to the carotid spaces. Arrest in normal thymic migration (descent) around the ninth week of gestation leads to ectopic cervical thymic remnants. The degeneration of Hassall corpuscles within the ectopic thymic tissue is a proposed mechanism of cystic change. The cervical thymic remnant could occur anywhere from the angle of the mandible to the cervicomediastinal junction. The cervical remnants are more common within the left neck (60%–70%) and cystic. Solid and cystic remnants have, rarely, been detected in unusual unpredictable locations such as the retropharynx. The diagnosis of cervical thymic remnants is rarely made preoperatively (~15%).[15,16]

For the parents of a child with a newly discovered neck mass, the concern over neoplasia looms large in the background. The clinical presentation of a cervical thymic remnant varies with patient age, size of the lesion, and whether the lesion is cystic (most common) or solid (less common). US may be the best initial modality to make this distinction (**Box 5**). Most often, the patient is asymptomatic and the mass is incidentally discovered. Stridor, dyspnea, and dysphagia caused by mechanical compression are uncommon. The cystic thymic remnant may become complicated by infection or hemorrhage and thus present more acutely. In a study by Statham and colleagues[17] of 20 pediatric patients with resected cervical thymic remnants, 14 were cystic and 6 solid, and the cystic lesions were most commonly located within the lower neck or cervicomediastinal region.

In newborns, infants, or young children, the cervical cystic thymic remnant is often fusiform or cigar shaped, with the rostral portion extending

Table 2
Derivatives of the branchial apparatus

Level	Cleft	Arch	Pouch
1	External auditory canal	Malleus, incus, auricle, mandible, V3 segment of the trigeminal nerve (cranial nerve V), muscle of mastication	Mastoid air cells, tympanic cavity, eustachian tube
2	Obliterated cervical sinus	Lesser horn and upper body of hyoid, CN VII, facial musculature	Palatine tonsils
3	Obliterated cervical sinus	Greater horn and inferior body of hyoid, CN IX, pharyngeal constrictors, internal carotid arteries	Inferior parathyroid glands, thymus, pyriform sinus
4	Obliterated cervical sinus	Thyroid cartilage, CN X, Laryngeal muscles, aortic arch, and right subclavian	Superior parathyroid glands, pyriform sinus
5 + 6	—	Arytenoid and cricoid cartilage, recurrent laryngeal nerves, intrinsic laryngeal musculature	Parafollicular cells of the thyroid gland

Abbreviation: CN, cranial nerve.

toward the angle of the mandible or skull base and the caudal aspect of the mass often extending with a tail toward the superior mediastinum. The less common solid cervical thymic remnant is typically homogeneous and shows sonographic (US), attenuation (CT), and signal features (MR imaging) identical to mediastinal thymic tissue.[17]

The more common cystic thymic remnant is fusiform, found ventral and closely approximated to the carotid space, and often extends caudally into the cervicomediastinal region. US of the cystic remnant shows an anechoic or hypoechoic (if internal debris is present) mass that may be unilocular or contain internal septations. Contrast-enhanced CT (CECT) may show subtle marginal rim enhancement. MR imaging shows a cystic mass with internal fluid signal often slightly greater in signal than cerebrospinal fluid (CSF) on T1-weighted imaging and hyperintense on T2-weighted imaging (**Table 4**). The lesions lack diffusion restriction and show thin marginal wall enhancement following intravenous contrast.[2,17]

Box 3
Imaging recommendations for suspected branchial apparatus anomalies

- US for initial assessment.
- Contrast-enhanced CT (CECT) reserved for suspected superimposed infection or acute change in size. Often satisfactory for characterization and surgical planning.
- MR imaging plus intravenous (IV) contrast for definitive characterization and surgical planning.

The solid thymic remnants show sonographic, CT, and MR imaging features that are identical to orthotopic thymic tissue within the mediastinum (see **Table 4**). The investigation of all solid cervical masses in a child warrant intravenous contrast. Therefore, it is helpful when evaluating a solid cervical neck mass in a child to judge the imaging characteristics to the internal standard of the orthotopic mediastinal thymus (**Box 6**).[2]

Fibromatosis Colli (Sternocleidomastoid Pseudotumor, Congenital Muscular Torticollis)

Fibromatosis colli is a benign solid mass lesion (pseudotumor) of the neck that may be noted at birth or within the first few weeks of life and is intrinsic to the SCM muscle; often associated with torticollis. This neck mass may result from birth trauma, fetal intrauterine malposition (packing), or ischemia from fetal vascular compromise. The affected SCM contains localized fibrous tissue; some investigators consider fibromatosis colli to be a form of benign infantile fibrosis. Hemorrhagic elements intermixed with the fibrosis have also been reported.[18,19]

Most often, a parent or caretaker has become alarmed after palpating a hard neck mass in the young infant (typically around 4–6 weeks of age). This benign condition occurs with equal frequency on the right and left sides. Torticollis is often part of the clinical picture with the head tilted toward the involved side, and the chin rotated away from the lesion. Based on health history and detailed physical examination, the clinician often has a strong suspicion of the diagnosis of fibromatosis colli. An imaging request, if forthcoming, serves not only to improve the

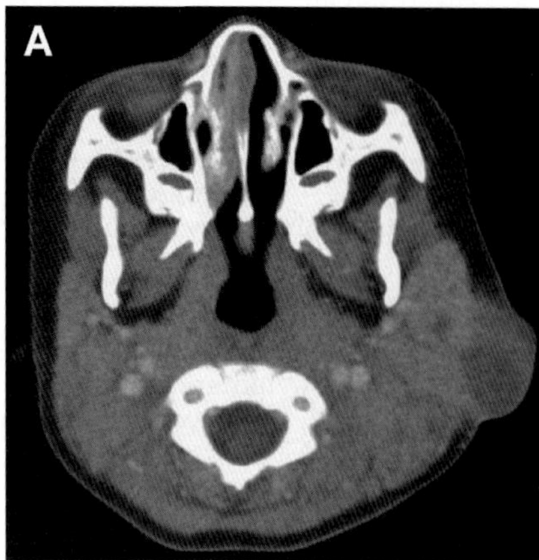
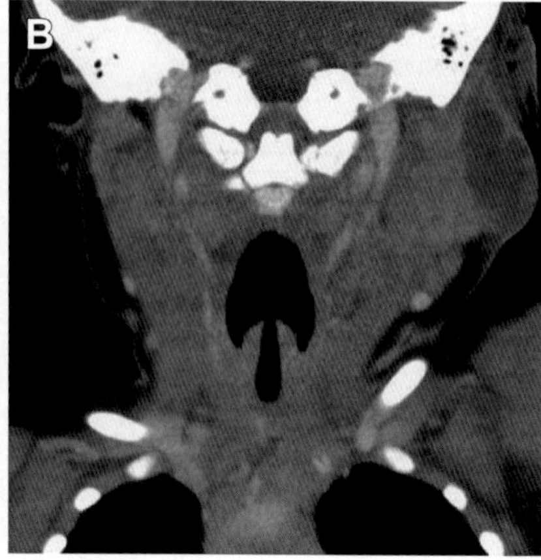

Fig. 2. First branchial cleft anomaly. (*A*) Axial CECT through the parotid. (*B*) The same lesion in the sagittal plane.

specificity of the clinician's differential diagnosis but more importantly may bring relief to the worried family. This benign condition is self-limited, usually resolving within 6 to 8 months. Therapy is conservative with active and passive exercises often performed under the direction of a physiotherapist in order to prevent a permanent muscle contracture and associated plagiocephaly. Important associations that have been described with fibromatosis colli include clubfoot, Erb palsy, and hip dysplasia. With regard to the association with hip dysplasia, many pediatric centers on confirming the characteristic US findings of fibromatosis colli move on to scan the hips to pick up occult dysplasia.[18]

The key to accurately imaging fibromatosis is to focus on high-resolution neck sonography and to avoid the modalities of CECT and MR imaging, which may only serve to confound the diagnosis (**Box 7**). Thus, when imaging is requested in the context of suspected fibromatosis colli, US is the imaging test of choice. The most important responsibility of the sonographer and radiologist is to confidently decide whether the mass is intrinsic to the SCM or not (**Fig. 5**). The US features of fibromatosis colli are those of focal or fusiform enlargement of the SCM, and variable intrinsic echotexture (hyperechoic, mixed, or hypoechoic). With sonography, the cranial aspect of the SCM can be traced to the muscle's origin at the skull base and the caudal sternal and clavicular heads can be identified. The adjacent paramuscular soft tissues are typically normal. If sonography shows the mass to be solid and extrinsic to the SCM, then further cross-sectional MR imaging is warranted. If CECT and or MR imaging are performed as the initial imaging studies in the clinical context of fibromatosis colli, they may suggest that the SCM mass is indeterminate or, worse, suggest the possibility of soft tissue sarcoma (rhabdomyosarcoma) (**Table 5**). Such an interpretation can lead to unnecessary biopsy and/or surgery. Unnecessary surgery should be avoided at all costs (**Box 8**).[19–21]

Table 3
Imaging characteristics of branchial apparatus anomalies

Imaging Technique	Imaging Findings
US	Anechoic, hypoechoic with internal debris, or heterogeneous, depending on content and whether infected
CECT	Typically presents as a thin-walled cyst with similar density to water. Can have thickened enhancing walls and increased density when complicated by infection and or hemorrhage
MR imaging	Typically presents as a thin-walled cyst with characteristic fluid signal on T2-weighted and T1-weighted sequences. Thickened enhancing walls and altered internal T1/T2 characteristics are seen in the setting of infection or hemorrhage

Abbreviation: CECT, contrast-enhanced CT.

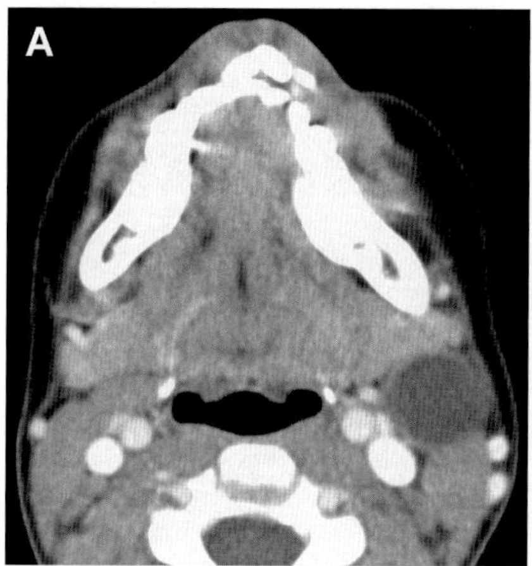

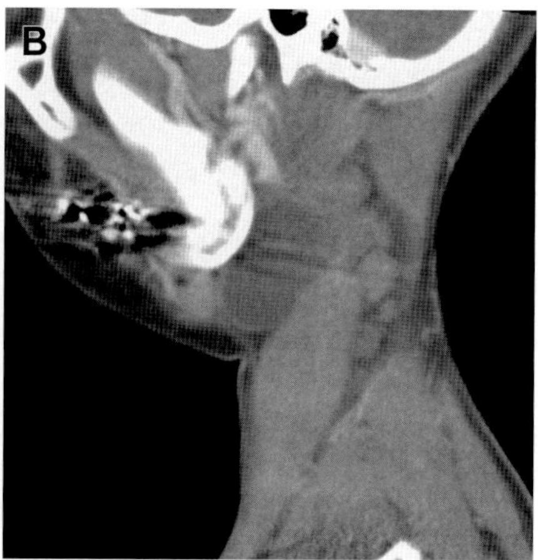

Fig. 3. Second branchial cleft anomaly. (*A*) Axial CECT shows a cystic left neck mass anterior to the SCM muscle and lateral to the carotid space. Wall thickening and enhancement is present, suggesting superinfection. (*B*) The same lesion in the sagittal plane, seen at the angle of the jaw, displacing the submandibular gland.

Infantile Hemangioma (Proliferative Hemangioma)

Infantile or proliferative hemangioma is a vascular anomaly and more specifically a vascular tumor. It is characterized by high endothelial cell turnover and glucose transporter 1 (GLUT1) positivity. Other less common pediatric vascular tumors include hemangioendothelioma and angiosarcoma. The other main subdivisions of vascular anomalies are the vascular malformations, which include slow-flow (capillary, venous, and lymphatic), fast-flow (arterial), and combined lesions. These vascular malformations are GLUT1 negative.[22]

Infantile or proliferative hemangioma is a common tumor of infancy and early childhood. It is particularly common among preterm newborns weighing less than 1000 g, and the incidence is approximately 23%. Multiple hemangiomas are found 20% of the time. The head and neck regions are most commonly involved, followed by the trunk and extremities. These lesions are not usually detected at birth (roughly one-third present at birth with a reddish macule or telangiectasia). The hemangioma proliferates rapidly (for 8–12 months), followed by a prolonged phase of involution (1–12 years), and finally the hemangioma shows a fibrofatty residuum as an end stage. Common head and neck locations include the parotid gland, orbit, frontonasal region, and scalp. The decision to treat these tumors is based on local mass effect (eg, visual impairment, airway compression), ulceration and bleeding, congestive heart failure, and platelet consumption. Medical arms of therapy include corticosteroids, propranolol, interferon, and vincristine. Surgical and laser excision options are also considerations.[22–24]

Most patients with infantile hemangioma are nonsyndromic; however, some hemangiomas (periorbital lesions larger than 5 cm, and hemangiomas in a bearded or dermatomal distribution) may be associated with the neurocutaneous syndrome PHACES (posterior fossa brain anomalies [eg, Dandy Walker malformation], large facial/orbital hemangiomas, arterial anomalies [aneurysms, absent vessels], aortic and cardiac abnormalities, eye anomalies, and sternal defects).[25]

Infantile or proliferative hemangioma has characteristic imaging features (**Box 9**, **Table 6**). US with color flow and pulsed Doppler shows a solid vascular lesion with high diastolic flow. Pediatric soft tissue sarcomas such as rhabdomyosarcoma typically show low diastolic flow. CECT shows a

> **Box 4**
> **Branchial anomalies: pearls for the referring physician**
>
> - Understanding of embryology of the head and neck region is key in understanding pathogenesis and in correctly identifying a branchial apparatus anomaly.
> - Although having similar imaging appearance, the discriminating feature between first and second branchial cleft cysts is location.
> - Always include an age-appropriate differential diagnosis of a cystic neck mass. Beware of a new diagnosis of a branchial cleft cyst in an adult because this may represent the initial presentation of squamous cell carcinoma.

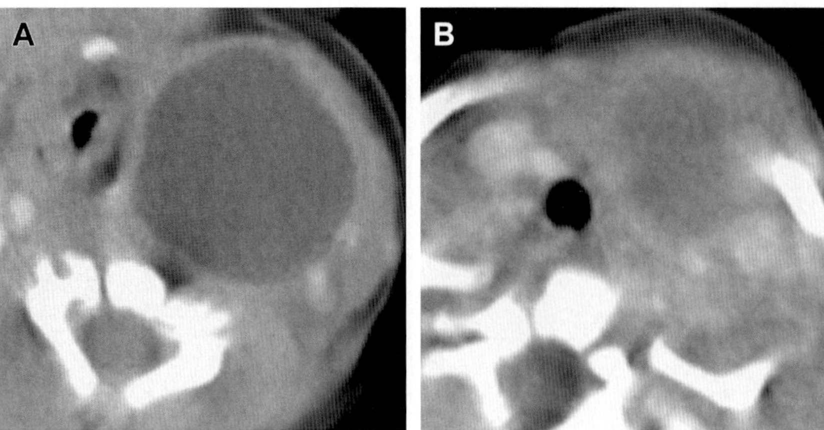

Fig. 4. Cervical thymic remnant. (*A*) Axial CECT shows a large fluid-attenuating left neck mass ventral and medial to the carotid space. (*B*) Caudal CECT at the cervicomediastinal inlet shows the mass extending into the superior mediastinum.

Box 5
Imaging recommendations for suspected thymic remnants

- US for initial assessment. If solid, compare with mediastinal thymus.
- CECT reserved for suspected infection/hemorrhage, or if US is nondiagnostic.
- MR imaging plus IV contrast for comprehensive characterization and surgical planning.

well-demarcated lobulated mass similar to regional musculature in attenuation before intravenous (IV) contrast and robust enhancement following IV contrast. Detecting internal vessels is common. MR is the preferred imaging test for comprehensive characterization of the mass, definition of the tumor extent, and the identification of other lesions that might exist in the setting of PHACES syndrome (**Fig. 6**). On T1-weighted MR imaging, the lesion is well defined, often lobular, and typically contains subtle internal regions of

Table 4
Imaging characteristics of thymic remnants

Imaging Technique	Imaging Findings
Conventional radiography	Nonspecific mass effect on the trachea either confined to the neck or neck and upper chest
US	Cystic remnant: hypoechoic to anechoic. Unilocular or septated, fusiform, and typically arises somewhere between the pyriform recesses and the thoracic inlet. The mass resides ventral to the carotid space Solid remnant: is noncalcified, homogeneous, and mirrors the US features of the orthotopic thymic tissue
CECT	Cystic remnant: hypoattenuating centrally. Rarely exhibits a fluid debris level (only if infected or has hemorrhaged) with or without a thin marginal rim of enhancement Solid remnant: homogeneous, noncalcified mass with imaging characteristics identical to thymus tissue. Enhances like thymic tissue
MR imaging	Cystic remnant: unilocular or septated cystic mass. Predilection for the lower neck and cervicomediastinal junction. Fluid may mirror CSF signal or show slight increase in T1 signal because of protein content within the fluid. Thin marginal enhancement may be seen following IV contrast Solid remnant: homogeneous and mirrors orthotopic thymus on all pulse sequences

Abbreviation: IV, intravenous.

Box 6
Thymic remnants: pearls for the referring physician

- Consider cystic thymic remnant for all cystic pediatric neck masses, particularly those that reside anterior to the carotid space and are fusiform in shape.
- When a solid cervical neck mass is detected in a child, always assess the characteristics of the tumor against the orthotopic thymic tissue in the mediastinum.
- The presence of Ca^{++} within the mass mitigates against the diagnosis of cervical thymic remnant.

Box 7
Imaging recommendations for suspected fibromatosis colli

- US. If findings are consistent with fibromatosis colli, stop. Only proceed to MR imaging or CECT if the mass is extrinsic to the SCM.
- CECT. Avoid because results are inconclusive and may lead to unnecessary biopsy or surgery.
- MR imaging. Avoid because results are inconclusive and may lead to unnecessary biopsy or surgery.

T1 shortening (hyperintensity) as a result of flow-related enhancement or fatty striations. The lesion overall is similar to the T1 signal intensity of regional facial musculature. T2-weighted images show the mass to be hyperintense with tubular internal vascular hypointensities (flow signal loss). Vibrant enhancement is shown following IV contrast and vascular imaging sequences following IV contrast depict internal vessels. These US, CECT, and MR imaging characteristics support the hypervascular nature of this proliferative tumor (**Box 10**).[22,25]

Neurofibromatosis Type 1

Neurofibromatosis can be separated into 2 distinct forms, type I and type II, depending on the tumor suppressor gene that is affected. Given the predilection of neurofibromatosis type II manifestations to occur intradurally, only neurofibromatosis type I (NFI) is discussed here.

NFI, formerly known as von Recklinghausen disease, is an autosomal dominant neurocutaneous phakomatosis. NFI is one of the most common autosomal dominant inherited disorders, occurring in approximately 1 in 2500 to 1 in 3000 births. It is typically caused by a mutation in the NFI gene locus on chromosome 17. This locus encodes a tumor suppressor gene called neurofibromin, which participates in cell signaling and cell growth regulation.[26,27] Once altered, a myriad of manifestations affecting everything from the skin to nerves to the skeleton may present. At least 2 of 7 criteria, as detailed by the National Institutes of Health, must be met in order to receive a diagnosis of NFI (**Box 11**).

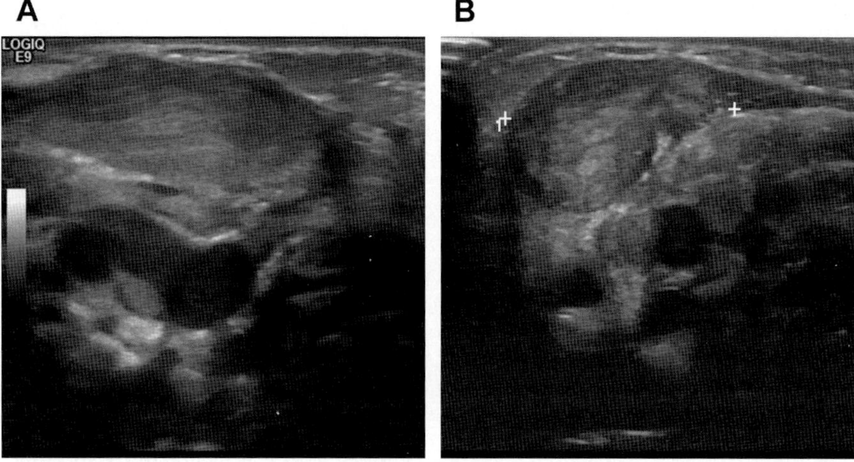

Fig. 5. Fibromatosis colli. (*A*) Longitudinal sonographic image of the right neck in a 6-week-old boy with a firm palpable neck mass shows the characteristic fusiform enlargement of the SCM consistent with the diagnosis of fibromatosis colli. Heterogeneous internal echoes are common in fibromatosis colli. (*B*) Transverse US image of the lower neck confirms the intramuscular location of the mass. Caudal imaging of the neck shows the divisions of the muscle into the clavicular and sternal heads and their insertions.

Table 5
Imaging characteristics of fibromatosis colli

Imaging Technique	Imaging Findings
US	Focal or fusiform mass of the SCM. The echotexture of the fibromatosis colli lesion can vary considerably ranging from hyperechoic to mixed to hypoechoic. The resistive index of the mass on Doppler may be increased. The adjacent tissues are typically normal. The goal with US in this clinical setting is to decide whether the lesion is within or external to the SCM
CECT	Avoid performing CECT in the clinical setting of suspected fibromatosis colli. The imaging findings are indeterminate, showing SCM enlargement and varied internal attenuation based on the constituents of edema, fibrosis, and hemorrhage
MR imaging	Avoid performing MR imaging in the clinical setting of suspected fibromatosis colli. The imaging findings are indeterminate, showing SCM enlargement and varied internal muscle signal intensity based on constituents of edema, fibrosis, and hemorrhage
***CECT and MR imaging	Should be reserved for masses extrinsic to the SCM

Although NFI may present at any age, it is most common in late childhood or early adulthood. Physical examination findings are highly variable and depend on the phenotypic expression of the disease. Given the diverse collection of manifestation, individuals within the same family may have variable expressivity. This variation makes determining prognosis difficult and patient specific. Although one patient may have cutaneous lesions and a few nonburdensome neurofibromas, another may have profound cognitive and learning deficits.

At present, there is no consensus guideline regarding screening imaging studies once a diagnosis of NFI has been made (**Box 12**). In the past, clinicians routinely ordered CT and/or MR imaging for patients with a new diagnosis of NFI. However, given the effects of radiation and concerns of health care costs, this has fallen out of favor. Although some clinicians still order

Box 8
Fibromatosis colli: pearls for the referring physician

- Consider the diagnosis of fibromatosis colli in infants 4 to 6 weeks old with a hard neck mass that seems clinically to be confined to the SCM.
- US is the modality of choice for determining the diagnosis of fibromatosis colli. Diagnostic US is a reasonable way to begin the imaging evaluation of any neck mass in a neonate or infant. No other imaging is necessary.
- The echotexture features of fibromatosis colli are variable so focus on whether the mass is intrinsic to the SCM or not. That is the key observation in making the diagnosis of this benign condition.
- Avoid CECT and MR imaging in this setting because they may confuse the diagnosis. Reserve them for masses that reside outside the SCM.

Box 9
Imaging recommendations for suspected infantile hemangioma

- MR imaging. The preferred modality, and the best assessment of mass extent and PHACES association. For the evaluation of suspected PHACES syndrome, include comprehensive brain imaging with IV contrast and aortic arch through circle of Willis MR angiography (MRA) for the detection of vascular anomalies. Disadvantage: requires sedation or general anesthesia, and is a lengthy examination.
- CECT. Fast, may require no sedation, shows location and extent of the tumor and adjacent structures. Shows strong enhancement. Disadvantage: ionizing radiation.
- US. Useful to characterize internal flow features (Doppler). US with Doppler and color flow represent a useful adjunct to cross-sectional imaging in the evaluation of vascular anomalies.

Table 6
Imaging characteristics of infantile hemangioma

Imaging Technique	Imaging Findings
US	Doppler shows a hypervascular mass with high diastolic flow
CECT	Lobulated, noncalcified, strongly enhancing mass
MR imaging	Isointense to hypointense lobulated mass compared with regional musculature, hyperintense on T2-weighted imaging, flow voids within the mass detected on T1 and T2 sequences before IV contrast. Vibrant enhancement following IV contrast. Include pre-IV and post-IV enhanced imaging of the whole brain when PHACES is suspected
MRA	When PHACES syndrome is a consideration include arterial imaging from aortic arch through circle of Willis to assess for vessel anomalies to include aneurysms

Abbreviation: MRA, MR angiography.

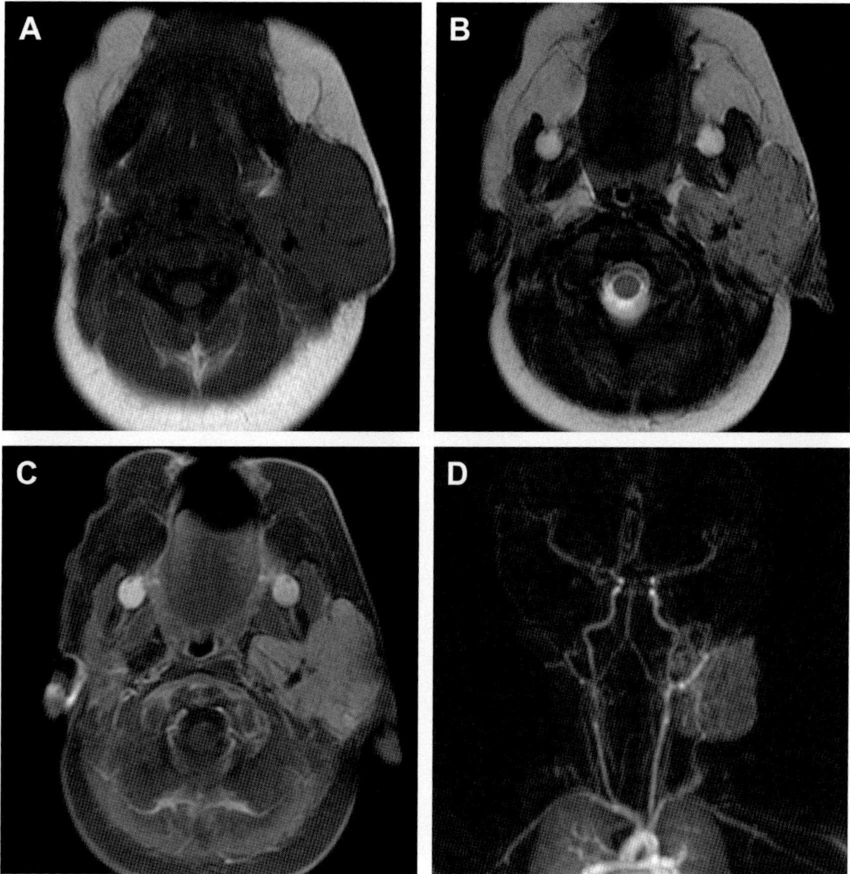

Fig. 6. Infantile hemangioma. (*A*) Axial T1-weighted image through the face shows a large well-demarcated left parotid space mass occupying deep and superficial parotid lobes, showing internal flow voids. (*B*) Axial T2-weighted MR image through the face shows hyperintensity of the left parotid space mass with numerous tubular hypointense internal flow voids. (*C*) Axial T1 MR image following IV contrast shows strong tumor enhancement. (*D*) Coronal projection from IV contrast-enhanced magnetic resonance angiography (MRA) shows the hypervascular left parotid space mass, internal vessels, and enlargement of the left external carotid artery.

Box 10
Infantile hemangioma: pearls for the referring physician

- Infantile hemangioma is a common head and neck tumor of infancy and childhood
- High diastolic flow is a typical Doppler US finding
- MR imaging including IV contrast is the preferred imaging tool, usually requiring sedation
- Large tumors and those in dermatomal distribution may be associated with PHACES
- When PHACES is considered, MR imaging should include whole-brain MR imaging with IV contrast and aortic arch to circle of Willis MRA imaging

Box 12
Imaging recommendations for NFI

- US has minimal role in neurofibromatosis diagnosis or mass evaluation.
- CT/MR reserved for new or changing symptoms. If there is concern for orbital or intracranial involvement this may be used, although the previous model of imaging all new NFI diagnoses is no longer supported.
- Little role for nuclear scintigraphy.

baseline brain MR imaging or CT of the head and neck, these studies are usually reserved for patients with new or changing symptoms. By far the most common 2 imaging diagnoses that neuroradiologists encounter are neurofibromas (including plexiform neurofibroma) and optic pathway gliomas.[27,28]

Neurofibromas present as circumscribed, dumbbell-shaped, or spindle-shaped masses centered within the neuroforamen or along peripheral nerves (**Table 7**). If present within a neuroforamen, there may be associated expansion of the foramen. CT shows a central region of hypoattenuation (5–30 HU) that enhances relative to the periphery, referred to as the target sign. MR shows a peripherally T2 hyperintense mass with central T2 hypointensity. Avid, homogeneous enhancement is present on postgadolinium images unless large, when it may be heterogeneous. Plexiform neurofibromas are an aggressive form of neurofibroma that are usually multilevel in origin, tortuous, and have ropelike extensions along the course of the nerve. When neurofibromas degrade to malignant forms, they are often large (>5 cm), heterogeneously enhancing with central regions of necrosis, and may appear infiltrative or rapidly enlarging (**Fig. 7**).[28,29]

Neurofibroma differential considerations are broad and depend on location. Within the neuroforamen, neurofibroma, schwannoma, or potentially meningioma should be considered. However, in the carotid space, paraganglioma, schwannoma, pseudoaneurysm, or branchial cleft

Box 11
Diagnostic NFI criteria (2 or more must be present)

- More than 6 cafe-au-lait spots greater than 5 mm if prepubertal or greater than 15 mm if postpubertal
- One plexiform neurofibroma or 2 or more neurofibromas
- Axillary or inguinal freckling
- Optic pathway glioma
- Two or more retinal hamartomas
- Osseous lesions such as kyphoscoliosis, sphenoid wing dysplasia, thinning of long bone cortex with or without pseudoarthrosis
- First-degree relative with NFI based on these criteria

Table 7
Imaging characteristics of NFI

Imaging Technique	Imaging Findings
CECT	Circumscribed, hypoattenuating lesion that may mimic a lymphatic malformation. Paraspinal lesions often show a dumbbell shape
MR imaging	Hyperintense T2 signal with a target sign represented by central hypointensity and peripheral hyperintensity. Heterogeneous/ homogeneous enhancement depending on lesion size

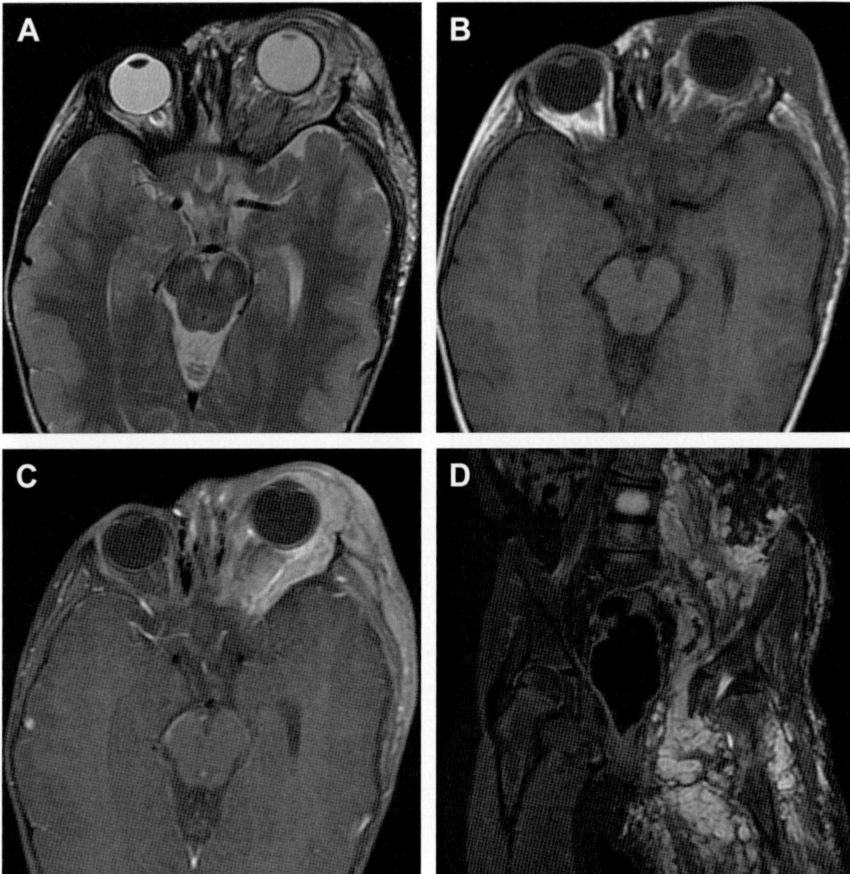

Fig. 7. Neurofibromatosis type 1. (*A*) Infiltrative T2 hyperintense plexiform neurofibroma that extends into the orbit, overlying periorbital soft tissues and suprazygomatic masticator space. (*B*) The same neurofibroma shows T1 hypointensity. (*C*) Avid homogeneous postcontrast enhancement is seen on enhanced images. (*D*) Although some plexiform neurofibromas involve the head and neck, others may be more trans-spatial, extending from the retroperitoneum into the lower extremity, as shown in images with hyperintense T2 signal.

cyst are considerations depending on imaging characteristics.

NFI: pearls for the referring clinician

- Combination of physical examination and diagnostic imaging findings may be necessary to make the diagnosis of NFI
- Cognitive and learning disabilities may be the first manifestations of the disease and have a significant impact on development
- Prognosis is difficult to predict and is based on physical and psychological manifestations of the disease

Retinoblastoma

Retinoblastoma (RB) is a malignant neoplasm arising from neuroectodermal cells in the globes of neonates. It is considered the most common malignant intraocular neoplasm of childhood. Approximately 60% are considered sporadic nonfamilial forms requiring 2 spontaneous mutations in the RB1 gene locus on chromosome 13. The remaining 40% are hereditary (autosomal dominant), requiring only a single spontaneous mutation in addition to the inherited germline defect. Nonfamilial and familial forms usually occur unilaterally and bilaterally respectively. RB1 encodes a tumor suppressor gene responsible for regulating cell growth, apoptosis, and division.[30]

In patients with a known family history, detection occurs earlier given rigorous screening. Average age of diagnosis is 13 months with greater than 95% detection by 5 years of age. Common presenting symptoms include leukocoria (white pupil reflex), strabismus, changes in vision, or inflammatory eye disease. RB accounts for 5% of childhood blindness and occurs in approximately 1 in 18,000 to 1 in 30,000 births. Treatments include a

Table 8
Therapeutic options in retinoblastoma treatment

Therapy	Indication
Chemotherapy	Low-grade tumors, in conjunction with EBRT
EBRT	Large, aggressive tumors with seeding
Enucleation	Indicated when there is no chance of preserving vision
Cryotherapy	Limited use as primary local therapy in small anterior tumors
Photocoagulation	Limited use as primary local therapy in small posterior tumors

Abbreviation: EBRT, external beam radiation therapy.

Box 13
Imaging recommendations for retinoblastoma

US may serve as the initial tool for evaluation of intraocular mass in conjunction with ophthalmologic examination.

CT helps delineate the calcified components of the masses.

MR is the imaging modality of choice to determine growth pattern and relation of mass to optic disc, anterior chamber, intracranial disease, and extraocular extent of disease.

combination of chemotherapy, external beam radiation, enucleation, cryotherapy, or photocoagulation (**Table 8**).[30–32]

Retinoblastomas present as mixed calcified and noncalcified intraocular soft tissue masses (**Table 9**). They may show an endophytic, exophytic, or diffuse growth pattern. Exophytic refers to an outward growth between the pigmented retinal epithelium and sensory retina leading to a detached retina. With associated retinal detachment, this may clinically resemble Coats disease, which involves retinal telangiectasias and exudative retinopathy. Endophytic growth extends inward toward the vitreous cavity and is readily apparent on ophthalmologic examination. This form may seed the vitreous cavity or anterior chamber, thus mimicking an endophthalmitis toxocariasis infection. Diffuse growth extends along the entire retina without focal discrete mass formation.[30] Diffuse growth is a rare form that clinically mimics endophthalmitis.

CT imaging shows variable enhancement and mildly hyperdense vitreous. MR imaging shows a mildly hyperintense T1 mass relative to the vitreous with corresponding T2 hypointensity (**Box 13**, see **Table 9**). Moderate to avid enhancement is noted on postgadolinium imaging (**Fig. 8**). Local extent of disease in relation to the optic nerve and sclera, laterality within the globe, and associated retinal detachment should be discussed. All initial diagnostic work-ups should include whole-brain T2, T1 precontrast sequences, and T1 postcontrast sequences to evaluate for CSF seeding, pineal involvement, or suprasellar involvement because this guides treatment objectives (see **Table 8**).[33–35]

Differential considerations include Coats disease, ocular toxocariasis, astrocytic hamartoma, medulloepithelioma, or choroidal hemangioma.

Table 9
Imaging characteristics of retinoblastoma

Imaging Technique	Imaging Findings
US	Amplitude modulation scan is used to detect flaws in a material in 1 dimension, such as highly reflective spikes from calcifications Brightness scan is a two-dimensional evaluation that can show an echogenic, irregular mass Limited utility in determining extraocular extent
CECT	90%–95% show a calcified intraocular mass. Variable enhancement of noncalcified portion
MR imaging	Variable T1 signal with hypointense T2 signal relative to vitreous. Moderate to marked heterogeneous enhancement. Evaluate for trans-scleral extension, relationship to optic nerve, anterior chamber, and extraocular involvement

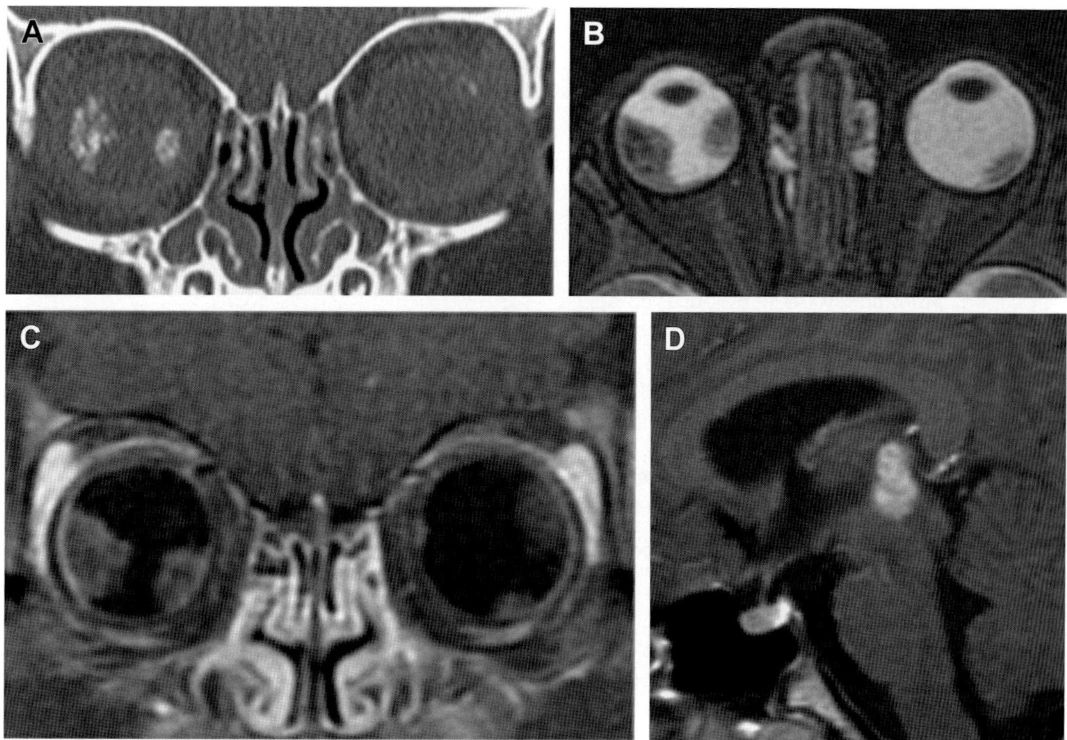

Fig. 8. Retinoblastoma. (*A*) Note the bilateral intraocular calcifications, which are highly suggestive of retinoblastoma. (*B*) The masses show T2 hypointense signal relative to the vitreous. (*C*) Moderate postgadolinium enhancement is shown. (*D*) It is always critical to evaluate for intracranial metastatic disease, as shown in this case by an enhancing pineal mass that turned out to be trilateral retinoblastoma. Quadrilateral disease also involves the suprasellar region (not shown here).

Coats usually presents with retinal detachment and subretinal exudate. If retinal astrocytic hamartoma is of consideration, sequelae of tuberous sclerosis are usually present. Medulloepithelioma arises from the ciliary neuroepithelium and usually presents with cystic component without internal calcifications. Choroidal hemangiomas have the characteristic T1/T2 hyperintense signal and avid postcontrast enhancement (**Box 14**).[33–35]

Box 14
Retinoblastoma: pearls for the referring physician

- Consider the diagnosis of retinoblastoma in any neonate or child less than 5 years old presenting with vision changes or leukocoria
- Close follow-up until the age of 7 years is recommend to exclude metachronous tumors
- Diagnosis should be made with imaging to avoid unnecessary biopsy to reduce the risk of seeding
- If present, evaluate contralateral globe, pineal region, and suprasellar region for additional sites of disease

SUMMARY

Most pediatric head and neck anomalies can be delineated with a high degree of certainty through the combination of clinical examination and prudent diagnostic imaging. Evaluation and clinical management depend on the specific cause, its location, and the involvement of adjacent structures. Although some lesions or pseudolesions resolve or involute over time, others necessitate surgical management. Understanding each clinical entity and its association with other malformations determines whether further diagnostic imaging is warranted. Radiologists serve an important role not only in diagnosis but also in recommending appropriate referral and participating in treatment.

REFERENCES

1. Gaddikeri S. Congenital cystic neck masses: embryology and imaging appearances, with clinicopathological correlation. Curr Probl Diagn Radiol 2014; 43(2):55–67.
2. Koch BL. Cystic malformations of the neck in children. Pediatr Radiol 2005;35(5):463–77.
3. Ibrahim M. Congenital cystic lesions of the head and neck. Neuroimaging Clin N Am 2011;21(3):621–39.
4. Diaz MC. A thyroglossal duct cyst causing apnea and cyanosis in a neonate. Pediatr Emerg Care 2005;21(1):35–7.
5. Lin ST. Thyroglossal duct cyst: a comparison between children and adults. Am J Otolaryngol 2008; 29(2):83–7.
6. Marianowski R. Risk factors for thyroglossal duct remnants after Sistrunk procedure in a pediatric population. Int J Pediatr Otorhinolaryngol 2003; 67(1):19–23.
7. Dedivitis RA. Thyroglossal duct: a review of 55 cases. J Am Coll Surg 2002;194(3):274–7.
8. Sadler TW. Langman's medical embryology with CD. Philadelphia: Wolters Kluwer Lippincott Williams & Wilkins; 2010.
9. Waldhausen JH. Branchial cleft and arch anomalies in children. Semin Pediatr Surg 2006;15(2):64–9.
10. Acierno SP, Waldhausen JH. Congenital cervical cysts, sinuses and fistulae. Otolaryngol Clin North Am 2006;40(1):161–76.
11. Bajaj Y, Ifeacho S, Tweedie D. Branchial anomalies in children. Int J Pediatr Otorhinolaryngol 2011; 75(8):1020–3.
12. Schroeder JW Jr, Mohyuddin N, Maddalozzo J. Branchial anomalies in the pediatric population. Otolaryngol Head Neck Surg 2007;137(2):289–95.
13. LaRiviere CA, Waldhausen JH. Congenital cervical cysts, sinuses, and fistulae in pediatric surgery. Surg Clin North Am 2012;92(3):583–97.
14. Lev S, Lev MH. Imaging of cystic lesions. Radiol Clin North Am 2000;38(5):1013–27.
15. Tovi F. The aberrant cervical thymus. Embryology, pathology, and clinical implications. Am J Surg 1978;136(5):631–7.
16. Tunkel DE. Ectopic cervical thymic tissue. Arch Pathol Lab Med 2001;125:278–81.
17. Statham MM. Cervical thymic remnants in children. Int J Pediatr Otorhinolaryngol 2008;72(12):1807–13.
18. Walsh S. Torticollis in infancy. J Pediatr Health Care 1997;11(3):138, 151–2.
19. Steven M. Sonographic diagnosis of fibromatosis colli. J Diagn Med Sonogr 2006;22(6):339–402.
20. Crawford S. Fibromatosis colli of infancy: CT and sonographic findings. AJR Am J Roentgenol 1988; 151(6):1183–4.
21. Ablin DS. Ultrasound and MR imaging of fibromatosis colli (sternomastoid tumor of infancy). Pediatr Radiol 1998;28(4):230–3.
22. Eivazi B. Update on hemangiomas and vascular malformations of the head and neck. Eur Arch Otorhinolaryngol 2009;266(2):187–97.
23. Finn MC. Congenital vascular lesions: clinical application of a new classification. J Pediatr Surg 1983; 18(6):894–900.
24. Margileth AM. Cutaneous hemangiomas in children. Diagnosis and conservative management. JAMA 1965;194(5):523–6.
25. Metry DW. The many faces of PHACE syndrome. J Pediatr 2001;139(1):117–23.
26. Ferner RE. Guidelines for the diagnosis and management of individuals with neurofibromatosis 1 (NF1). J Med Genet 2007;44(2):81–8.
27. Williams VC. Neurofibromatosis type 1 revisited. Pediatrics 2009;123(1):124–33.
28. Mautner VF. MRI growth patterns of plexiform neurofibromas in patients with neurofibromatosis type 1. Neuroradiology 2006;48(3):160–5.
29. Fortman BJ. Neurofibromatosis type 1: a diagnostic mimicker at CT. Radiographics 2001;21(3):601–12.
30. Villegas VM. Retinoblastoma. Curr Opin Ophthalmol 2013;24(6):581–8.
31. de Potter P. Current treatment of retinoblastoma. Curr Opin Ophthalmol 2002;13(5):331–6.
32. Mallipatna AC. Management and outcome of unilateral retinoblastoma. J AAPOS 2009;13(6):546–50.
33. de Graaf P. Eye size in retinoblastoma: MR imaging measurements in normal and affected eyes. Radiology 2007;244(1):273–80.
34. de Graaf P. Retinoblastoma: MR imaging parameters in detection of tumor extent. Radiology 2005;235(1):197–207.
35. de Jong MC. Diagnostic performance of magnetic resonance imaging and computed tomography for advanced retinoblastoma: a systematic review and meta-analysis. Ophthalmology 2014;121(5):1109–18. S0161-6420(13)01087-7.

Imaging of Vascular Lesions of the Head and Neck

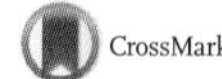

Julius Griauzde, MD, Ashok Srinivasan, MBBS, MD*

KEYWORDS

• Vascular malformation • Head and neck • Hemangioma • Carotid body tumor • Glomus jugulare • Juvenile nasopharyngeal angiofibroma

KEY POINTS

- Vascular lesions of the head and neck are classified based on their endothelial cell turnover as either malformations or tumors.
- Further subclassification based on flow characteristics helps to direct diagnosis and treatment.
- Imaging plays a key role in the diagnosis of most vascular lesions of the head and neck.
- Ultrasonography is an appropriate screening tool, with MRI providing more details about lesion characteristics and extent.
- Many vascular lesions are treated with sclerosants or embolization as either primary or adjunct therapies.

INTRODUCTION

Vascular lesions of the head and neck represent a challenging pathologic subset for the clinician and the radiologist. The classification system described by Mulliken and Glowacki[1] separates the lesions into 2 groups: Those that are vascular malformations, with normal endothelial cell turnover, and those that are vascular tumors, with high endothelial cell turnover (**Box 1**). Further stratification of these lesions is achieved by evaluating the imaging characteristics and clinical presentation; this allows for an accurate diagnosis and choosing appropriate therapeutic management (**Box 2**). Important imaging features that help to narrow the differential diagnosis include lesion flow characteristics, internal tissue characteristics, anatomic location, and extent. Because the literature has been abundant with confusing terms (such as cavernous hemangioma (HM), which truly are venous vascular malformations), it is important to understand which terms are interchangeable, and to move toward more consistent terminology (**Box 3**).

Vascular malformations of the head and neck include capillary malformations (CM), venous malformations (VM), lymphatic malformations (LM), arteriovenous malformations (AVM), and mixed-type lesions. Because vascular malformations are nonneoplastic, their growth is proportional to body size.[1] Vascular tumors, on the other hand, are neoplastic, so their growth is independent of body size. Although the list of vascular tumors of the head and neck can be quite long, we discuss some of the common lesions in this article, including HM, carotid body tumors (CBTs), glomus jugulare tumors (GJTs), and juvenile nasopharyngeal angiofibromas (JNA). In this review, we address clinical presentation, differential diagnosis, differentiating features, characteristic imaging findings, as well as a brief discussion of treatment options of these lesions.

Department of Radiology, University of Michigan Health System, 1500 E Medical Center Drive, Ann Arbor, MI 48109, USA
* Corresponding author.
E-mail address: ashoks@med.umich.edu

Radiol Clin N Am 53 (2015) 197–213
http://dx.doi.org/10.1016/j.rcl.2014.09.001
0033-8389/15/$ – see front matter

Box 1
Lesion classification

Vascular Malformations	Vascular Tumors
Capillary malformation	Hemangioma
Venous malformation	Carotid body tumor
Lymphatic malformation	Glomus jugulare tumor
Arteriovenous Malformation	Juvenile nasopharyngeal angiofibroma
Mixed type lesion	

IMAGING TECHNIQUES

Several imaging modalities play an integral role in the diagnosis and treatment planning of vascular lesions of the head and neck. These include ultrasonography (US), computed tomography (CT), MRI, as well as cross-sectional angiography and catheter-guided angiography (magnetic resonance angiography, CT angiography, digital subtraction angiography). In some instances, plain radiography can also contribute to the diagnosis. Because these lesions occur most commonly in pediatric and adolescent patients, judicious use of radiation is paramount.

US is an appropriate initial screening modality, particularly in superficial lesions.[2] US can help to identify rudimentary characteristics of the lesion, delineate lesion depth, characterize cystic/solid spaces, and identify the lesion's flow characteristics.[3] MRI is often used for further characterization because it is the best modality for delineating lesion extent and determining the involvement of soft tissue structures.[2,4] When available, dynamic magnetic resonance angiography (such as 4D-TRAK) can noninvasively determine the flow pattern within a lesion and thereby help in the diagnosis.[5] CT can also provide a wealth of diagnostic information and is particularly valuable in determining bony involvement, vascularity, and in evaluating for the presence of phleboliths (also identified on plain radiography).[2] However, CT use should follow the "as low as reasonably achievable" principles to minimize radiation exposure, especially in pediatric patients. Catheter angiography plays a limited role and is mainly employed when embolization therapy is a consideration. In many cases, characterization of the intralesional components and anatomic location allows for a definitive diagnosis.

Box 2
Flow characteristics

High Flow	Low Flow
Arteriovenous malformation	Capillary malformation
Hemangioma (proliferative phase)	Venous malformation
Carotid body tumor	Lymphatic malformation
Juvenile nasopharyngeal angiofibroma	

Box 3
Terminology: new and old

New	Old
Hemangioma	Capillary hemangioma
Capillary malformation	Port wine stain
Venous malformation	Cavernous hemangioma
Lymphatic malformation	Lymphangioma; cystic hygroma

IMAGING FINDINGS/PATHOLOGY

Vascular Malformations

Capillary malformations

CM in the head and neck present as a "port wine stain" cutaneous lesion. These lesions follow a dermatomal pattern of the trigeminal nerve in 23% to 43% of patients, but can be much more extensive in other cases.[6,7] Sturge–Webber syndrome, a congenital cutaneous and neurologic disorder, affects 3% of patients presenting with a port wine stain.[6] Imaging plays a limited role in evaluation of CM because diagnosis can often be made based on clinical characteristics. However, it can provide value in patients with Sturge–Webber syndrome or in those where the clinical presentation is equivocal. Key differential considerations of CM include superficial HM, VM, and AVM.

On US, CMs are usually located in the dermis and appear isoechoic.[8] Even though they are generally considered low flow, Doppler signal can be identified in up to 29%.[8] When Sturge–Webber syndrome is suspected, MRI or CT can be used to evaluate for disease sequelae, including ipsilateral leptomeningeal vascular anomalies.[7] These modalities also aid in the differentiation of CM from other vascular lesions, which commonly extend deeper into the tissues, involve bony structures, and have more robust internal flow.

CMs are generally benign lesions. They can become darker and more obvious with time, however, which makes them cosmetically bothersome to many patients. In these cases, the treatment of choice is laser therapy.[9] In recurrent, extensive, or hypertrophic and nodular lesions, wide surgical excision and reconstruction is an additional consideration.[10]

Venous malformations

VM are the most common low-flow vascular malformations.[8] They often occur in the head and neck, presenting with facial deformity and pain secondary to local inflammatory changes or compressive effects.[11–14] Up to 50% of head and neck VM are noted at birth.[11] Upon inspection, VM are soft bluish masses that undergo expansion with compression of the ipsilateral jugular vein, with Valsalva maneuvers, and with dependent positioning.[15] Their growth is proportional to body size and they are responsive to hormonal changes. Differential considerations of VM include HM, AVM, mixed vascular malformations, and dermoids.

The key imaging feature of VM is the presence of phleboliths, which can be seen in up to 48% of cases.[11,16] On US, these lesions commonly have a hypoechoic, heterogeneous appearance with phleboliths appearing hyperechoic and demonstrating acoustic shadowing.[8,17] Doppler flow is identified in up to 37%.[8] On CT, VM have soft tissue attenuation, show variable contrast enhancement (**Fig. 1**) and phleboliths are again identified.[16] Bony involvement also occurs and is best characterized by CT.[4] Bone changes can include osteolysis, demineralization, hypoplasia, and cortical thickening.[18,19]

MRI is the most important modality for evaluating VM because it clearly delineates the spatial extent of the lesion. These lesions are generally isointense on T1 weighted imaging (T1WI), hyperintense on T2 weighted imaging (T2WI), and show a heterogeneous enhancement pattern after contrast administration (**Fig. 2**).[4,15,16,20,21] Discrete areas of high T2 signal can be seen, which correspond with venous lakes.[4] Phleboliths are identified as signal voids on both T1WI and T2WI (**Fig. 3**).[4] On catheter angiography, these lesions have slow flow and arterial supply is often not definitely identified. With direct percutaneous injection, contrast can be seen pooling in dilated venous channels (**Fig. 4**).

Decision to treat VM depends on the size of the lesion and the functional impact on the patient. Conservative management is preferred, if possible. It should be noted that diffuse lesions are more likely to progress and therefore may be more likely to need treatment.[12] Treatment generally includes percutaneous sclerotherapy with ethanol or sodium tetradecyl sulfate (Sotradecol) with 76% to 93% of patients being cured or having significant improvement.[11,14] If the lesion is large and difficult to delineate, sclerotherapy is used in combination with reconstructive surgery.[11,13] However, recurrence has been noted to occur in up to 35% of patients and is possibly owing to incomplete initial therapy or hormonal influences.[11]

Lymphatic malformations

The typical presentation of a LM is a soft, colorless mass, most commonly occurring in the head and neck.[22] Up to 90% of these lesions are diagnosed by age 5.[23] There are 2 types of LM, macrocystic and microcystic. Macrocystic lesions more commonly originate below the mylohyoid in the anterior or posterior triangles of the neck

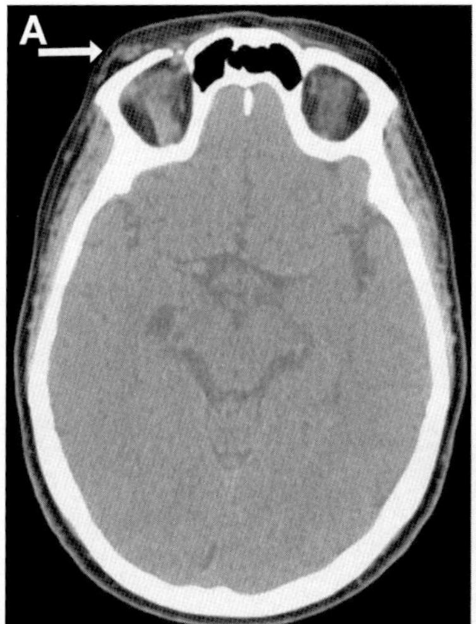

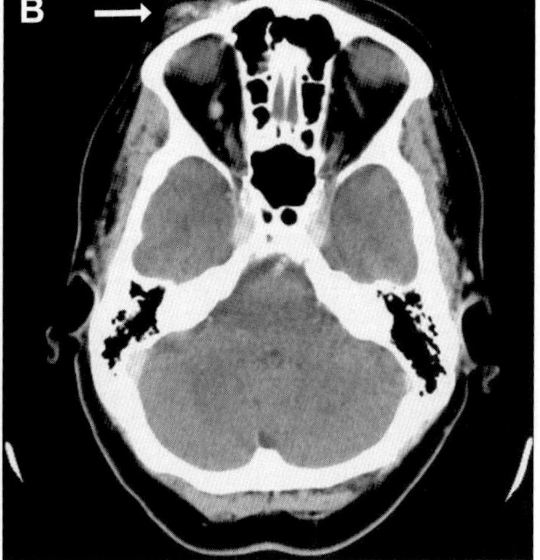

Fig. 1. (*A*) Noncontrast axial computed tomography (CT) of the head demonstrates a soft tissue attenuation lesion in the subcutaneous tissue of the right face (*arrow*). (*B*) Contrast-enhanced axial CT shows the lesion (*arrow*) demonstrating heterogeneous marked contrast enhancement.

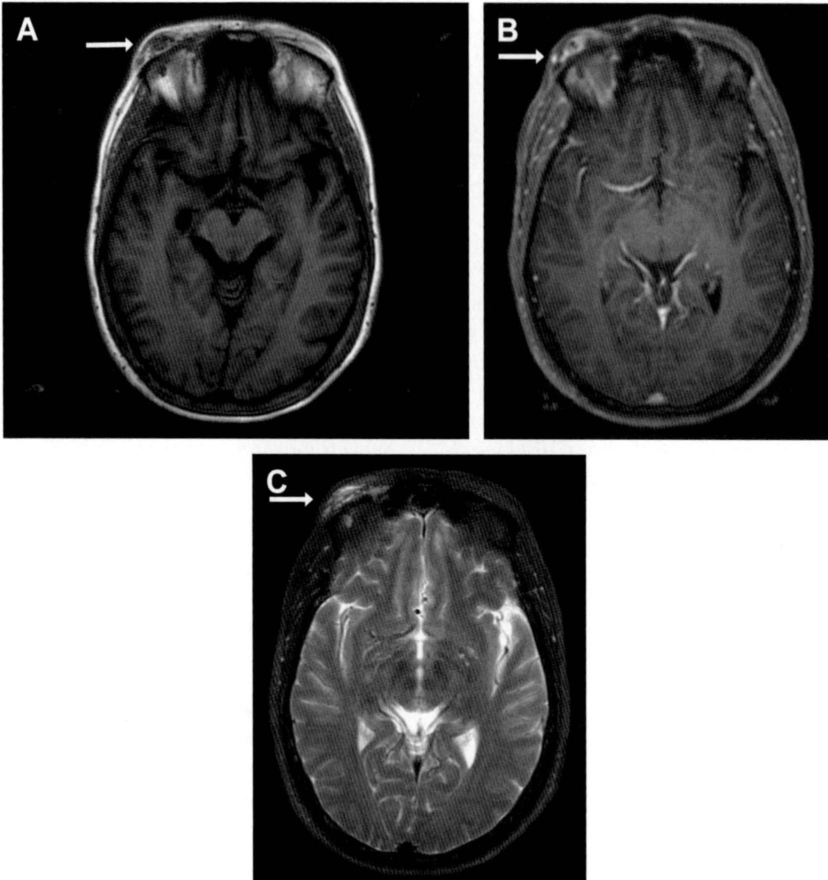

Fig. 2. (*A*) Axial T1 weighted image (WI) without contrast shows an isointense venous malformation (VM; *arrow*). (*B*) With contrast administration, the VM demonstrates significant contrast enhancement (*arrow*). (*C*) Axial T2WI demonstrates a hyperintense VM (*arrow*).

(historically termed cystic hygromas). Microcystic lesions commonly occur above the mylohyoid involving oral/perioral structures as well as the parotid gland (historically termed lymphangiomas). Differential diagnoses of LM include venous malformations, mixed malformations, branchial cleft cysts, and thyroglossal duct cysts.

On US, LMs are usually hypoechoic and Doppler flow is uncommon.[8] On CT, these lesions are seen as an unilocculated or multiloculated cystic mass with low density and may be poorly circumscribed. Fluid–fluid levels can be identified, particularly in cases of prior internal hemorrhage or debris from infection.[4,20] Absence of contrast enhancement

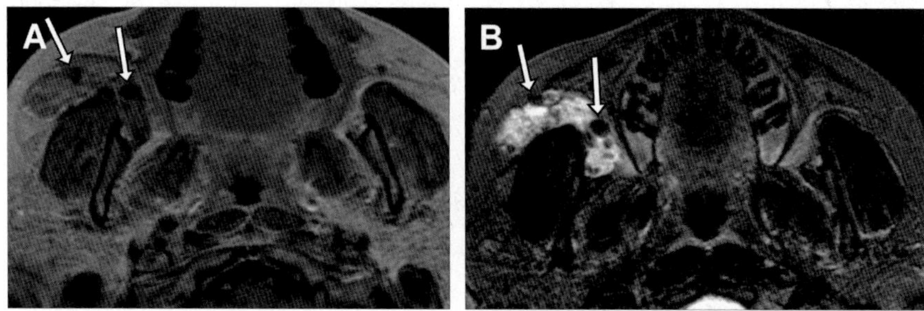

Fig. 3. (*A*) Axial T1 weighted image (WI) demonstrates an isointense venous malformation (VM) in the right buccal space, which displays punctate foci of signal void consistent with phleboliths (*arrows*). (*B*) Axial T2WI demonstrates a hyperintense VM with foci of signal drop out consistent with phleboliths (*arrows*).

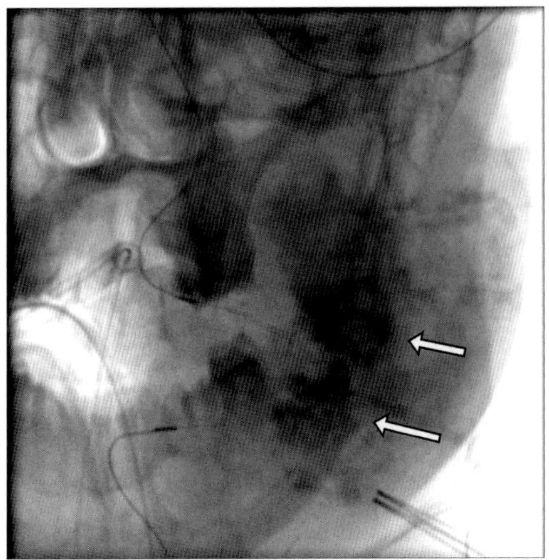

Fig. 4. Direct percutaneous injection under fluoroscopy shows contrast pooling within dilated venous channels (*arrows*) of a venous malformation.

is considered an important feature of a simple LM (**Fig. 5**).[16] On MRI, LMs are hypointense on T1WI, hyperintense on T2WI, and show no contrast enhancement (**Fig. 6**).[15,16,20,24] MRI is integral in preoperative planning and determining lesion extent because LMs can be locally aggressive, engulfing and encasing adjacent structures.[24] In mixed venolymphatic malformations, the venous portions are commonly seen admixed with the lymphatic components and these typically show enhancement (**Fig. 7**).

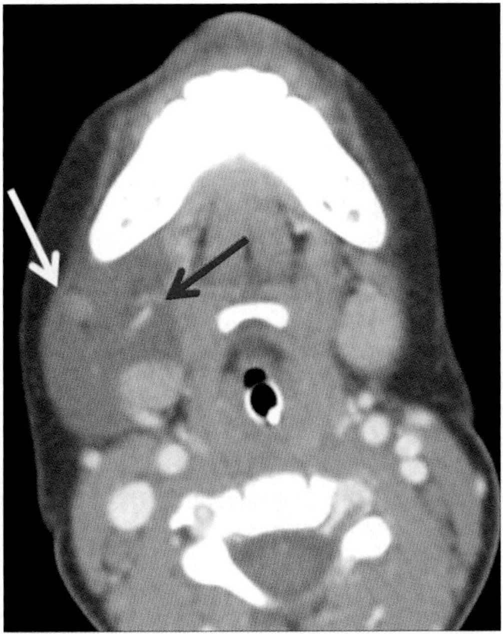

Fig. 5. Enhanced computed tomography demonstrating a nonenhancing cystic lymphatic malformation in the right neck extending into the lateral tongue (*arrows*).

The treatment of choice for LM is surgical excision.[22] In extensive or complex lesions, however, sclerotherapy alone or in combination with surgical excision can be employed (**Fig. 8**). Although successful sclerosant materials include alcohol, doxycycline, picibanil, or bleomycin, sclerotherapy has limited efficacy in microcystic lesions.[22,23,25–27] Regardless of therapy, recurrence rates can be high (particularly in microcystic lesions) and more than 1 procedure is often necessary for successful therapy.[22,25–27]

Arteriovenous malformations

AVM of the head and neck commonly manifest later in childhood or in adolescence.[28] These lesions often present with cosmetic deformity, skin discoloration, and/or an underlying pulsatile bruit.[29] Additional presenting characteristics include pain, bleeding, or ulceration.[28,29] Key differential considerations include HM and VMs.

Color Doppler US aids in basic characterization of these lesions as high flow and in characterizing microscopic or macroscopic intralesional arteriovenous fistulas (**Box 4**).[30] CT is often employed to determine skeletal involvement, which is not uncommon (**Fig. 9**).[28] An additional CT finding is large, dilated, serpiginous enhancing structures, often indistinguishable as arterial or venous in origin (**Fig. 10**). MRI is integral to determining lesion extent and soft tissue involvement and distortion.[28,31] MRI shows enlarged serpiginous flow voids on both T1WI and T2WI with a soft tissue infiltrating component.[15,31,32] Angiographically, these lesions demonstrate rapid flow with enlarged, tortuous arteries, and dilated draining veins (**Fig. 11**). Angiography helps in characterizing extent of the lesion as well as in directing therapeutic embolization.[30]

AVM of the head and neck can be difficult to treat. Treatment varies and includes complete surgical resection, embolization, or combined therapy.[28,31] In cases undergoing embolization, selective embolization using embolic materials or coils can be used (**Fig. 12**) with subsequent surgical resection performed within 24 to 48 hours.[30]

VASCULAR TUMORS

Hemangioma

HM are benign vascular neoplasms that occur most commonly in the head and neck.[33] HMs represent one of the most common tumors of infancy with up to 70% present at birth and 87%

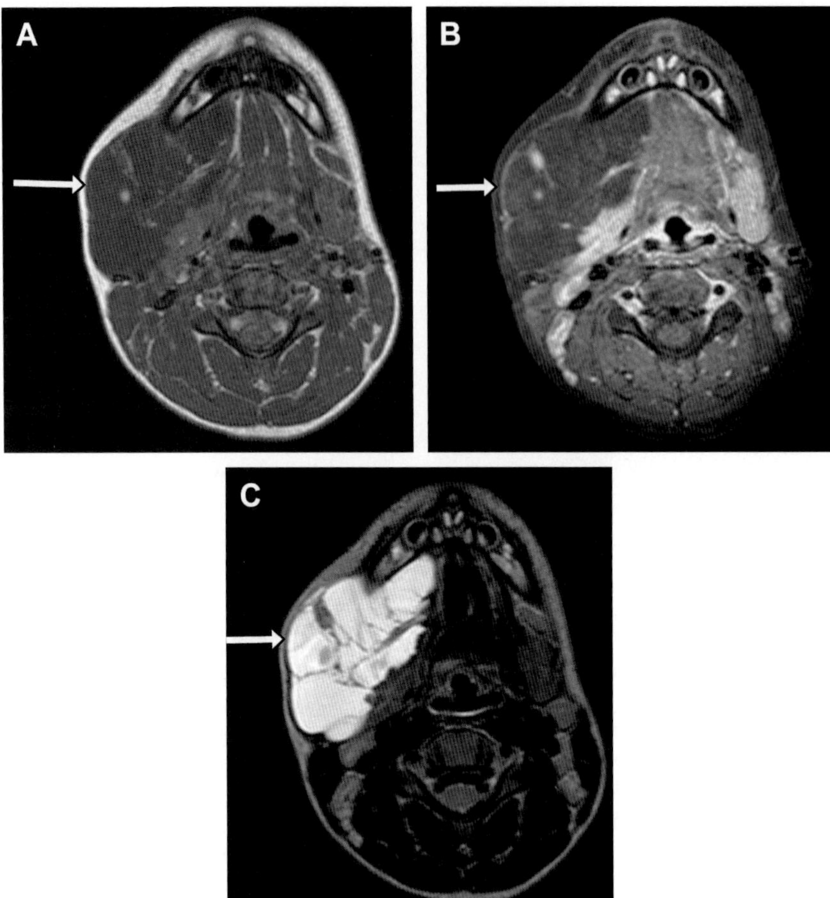

Fig. 6. (*A*) Axial TI weighted image (WI) demonstrates a hypointense venous malformation (VM) in the right neck (*arrow*). (*B*) After contrast administration, there is no enhancement (*arrow*). (*C*) T2WI demonstrates multiple locules and fluid intensity in the lymphatic malformation (*arrow*).

diagnosed by 1 month of age.[33] They often present as a red, superficial skin lesion that undergoes rapid enlargement during the proliferative phase. Deeper lesions without a cutaneous component are rarer and present as a painless, enlarging mass in adult patients.[34] When clinical examination is equivocal, imaging can be used for confirmation of the diagnosis of HM. Key differential considerations include VM, AVM, mixed malformation, and malignant lesions, like rhabdomyosarcomas.

Imaging plays a key role in the evaluation of HM (**Box 5**). It aids with anatomic localization and in delineating lesion extent.[35] On US, HMs seem to be heterogeneous, although the grayscale appearance is nonspecific.[36] They display high vascular flow, particularly in the proliferative phase.[36] On CT, HMs are isoattenuating to muscle on noncontrast scans, which makes them difficult to delineate. They do, however, avidly enhance with contrast, which aids in differentiation from surrounding structures (particularly in the proliferative phase; **Fig. 13**).[16] On MRI, HMs are isointense to slightly hyperintense on T1WI, hyperintense on T2WI, and demonstrate avid contrast enhancement (**Fig. 14**).[4,15,20,32,34] On catheter angiography, these lesions show high flow, an arterial blush, and persistent tissue staining (**Fig. 15**).[16]

Because HM are often small and self-involuting, the first step in therapy is expectant management.[35] Lesions that require intervention are generally either cosmetically bothersome or they compromise function of important anatomic structures.[37] The first line of therapy in these cases is systemic propranolol, which leads to improvement in 97% of cases with about one half showing an excellent response.[37] Significant improvement generally occurs during the first week of therapy.[38] In persistent lesions, additional treatment modalities include surgery, laser therapy, intralesional steroids, or chemotherapeutic agents.[33,35,37]

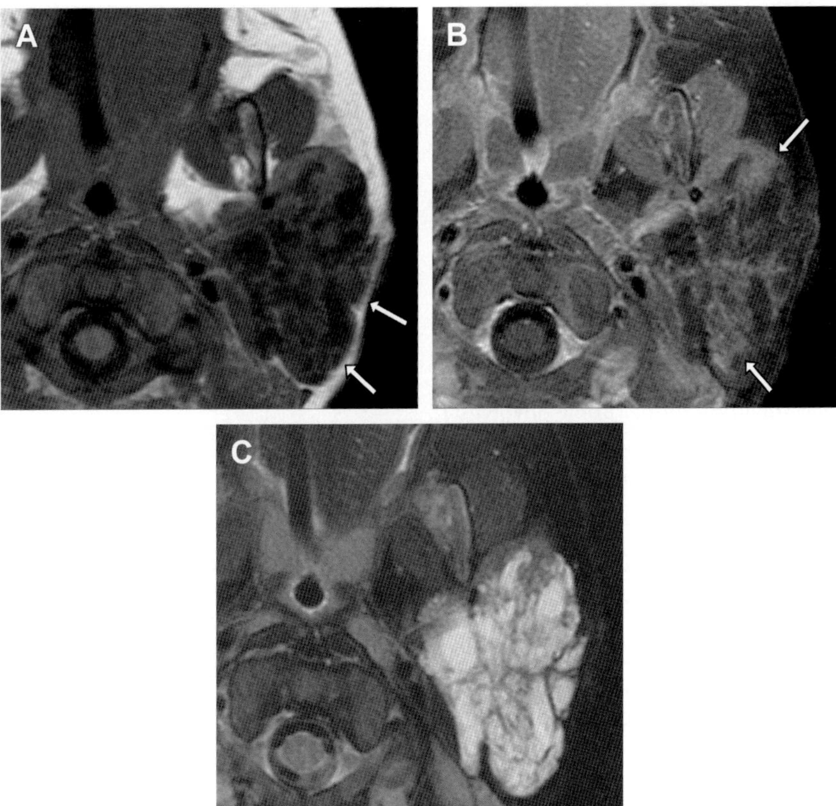

Fig. 7. (*A*) Axial TI weighted image (WI) demonstrates a heterogenous venolymphatic malformation in the left parotid region (*arrows*). (*B*) After contrast administration, there are scattered areas of enhancement representing the venous components (*arrows*). (*C*) T2WI demonstrates multiple locules and fluid intensity in this mixed malformation.

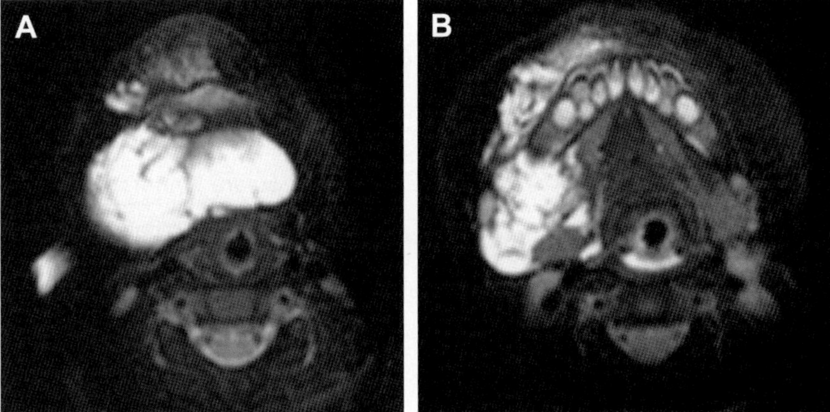

Fig. 8. (*A*) Presclerotherapy axial T2 weighted image (WI) demonstrates a multispatial lymphatic malformation. (*B*) Postsclerotherapy axial T2WI shows significant reduction in lesion size, which improves surgical results.

Box 4
Imaging pearls: vascular malformations

Capillary malformations: Imaging used to exclude more extensive differentials and in the workup of Sturge-Webber syndrome.

Venous malformation: Phleboliths are a differentiating feature and can be seen on ultrasonography, computed tomography (CT), MRI, and radiography.

High T2 areas represent venous lakes

Lymphatic malformation: No contrast enhancement. Fluid–fluid levels.

Arteriovenous malformation: Bony involvement evaluated with CT.

MRI shows flow voids on T1 and T2 and delineates lesion extent.

Mixed lesion: Areas of fluid signal and heterogenous contrast enhancement on MRI and CT.

Carotid Body Tumors

CBT are the most common paragangliomas of the head and neck.[39,40] They characteristically present as a painless, enlarging neck mass.[41–43] CBTs are generally benign, but can have malignant features.[43] Key differential considerations include schwannoma, neurofibroma, carotid artery aneurysm, or other glomus tumors. Imaging and anatomic location play a key role in differentiation.

On US, these lesions seem to be hypoechoic and solid.[42] They are hypervascular and splay the internal and external carotid arteries.[42] On CT, they have a heterogeneous and lobular appearance and show hyperenhancement (**Fig. 16**).[42] On MRI, CBTs display a characteristic heterogeneous "salt-and-pepper" appearance on T1WI.[44] The "salt" represents areas of subacute hemorrhage or slow flowing blood, whereas the "pepper" represents hypointense areas of serpiginous flow voids (**Fig. 17**A).[44] These lesions display intense enhancement with administration of gadolinium. On T2WI, CBTs are mildly hyperintense (see **Fig. 17**B). Angiographic imaging (digital subtraction angiography and reformatted CT angiography/magnetic resonance angiography) shows the classic "lyre sign" of a hypervascular mass splaying the internal and external carotids (**Fig. 18**A).[42] Additionally, a prolonged tumor blush is seen on catheter angiography (see **Fig. 18**B).

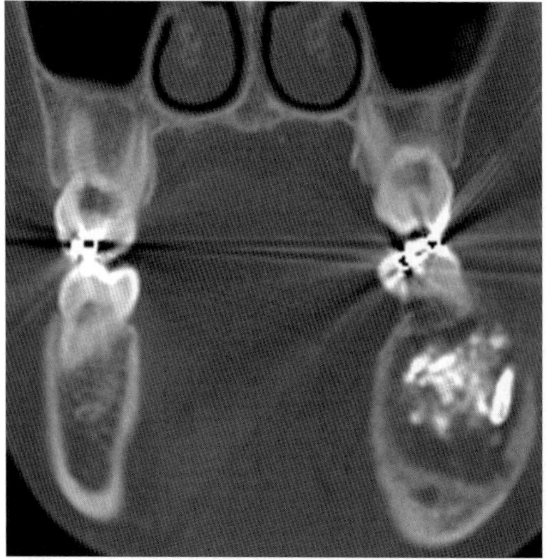

Fig. 9. Coronal contrast-enhanced computed tomography demonstrates contrast pooling within a left mandibular arteriovenous malformation.

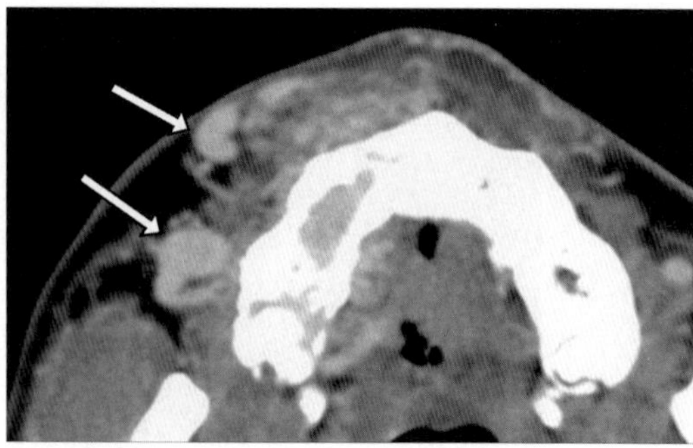

Fig. 10. Axial contrast-enhanced computed tomography demonstrates an abnormal nidus of vessels along the right face with dilated vascular channels, likely draining veins (*arrows*).

CBTs are generally treated because of their potential to be locally aggressive, malignant, or cause functional impairment.[41] Surgical resection is considered the treatment of choice.[45] Preoperative embolization is beneficial because it decreases operative blood loss.[46] Embolization can be achieved transarterially, percutaneously (with direct CBT puncture), or with a combined approach and is generally performed 24 to 48 hours before operative resection (**Fig. 19**).[47,48]

Glomus Jugulare Tumors

GJT are vascular paragangliomas that represent the most common tumor arising in the jugular foramen.[49] They are generally benign; however, they can be locally aggressive or invasive and can metastasize. The most common presenting symptoms of GJT include pulsatile tinnitus, with possible conductive hearing loss, as well as cranial nerve IX and X palsies.[43,50] Key differential considerations for these lesions include jugular

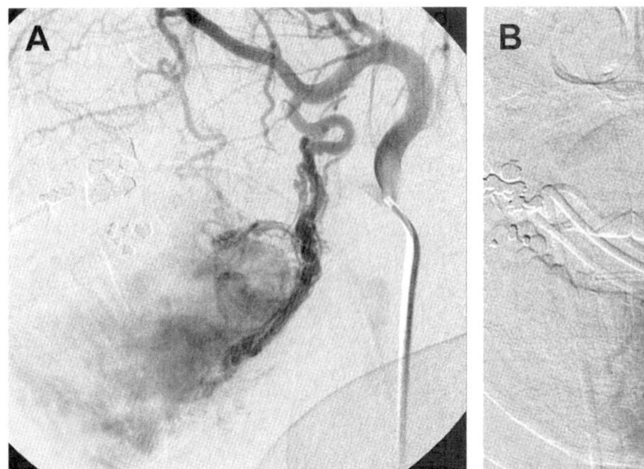

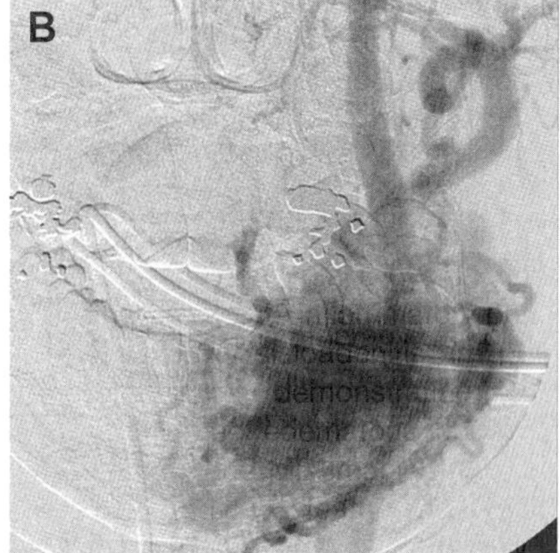

Fig. 11. (*A*) Angiographic image shows enlarged, tortuous arteries and dilated veins. (*B*) Delayed angiographic image demonstrates an intense vascular blush.

schwannomas and meningiomas with imaging and anatomic location again paramount to achieving the correct diagnosis.[51,52]

Noncontrast CT shows a poorly defined soft tissue mass with permeative and destructive bony changes along the jugular foramen.[50–54] These lesions show diffuse contrast enhancement (**Fig. 20**).[50–54] MRI is highly beneficial in delineating the lesion and evaluating intracranial extent.[54] On T1WI, these lesions have a "salt-and-pepper" appearance (with dark vascular flow voids) and show intense contrast enhancement (**Fig. 21**A, B).[49,51–54] On T2WI, GJT are heterogeneous with dark flow voids (see **Fig. 21**C).[51,53,54] Angiographic imaging shows a hypervascular mass with primary blood supply from the ascending pharyngeal artery (often hypertrophied) or other external carotid artery branches.[49,51] Catheter-based angiography (often employed in operative planning and embolization) additionally shows a rapid arterial brush and in some cases, invasion of the internal carotid artery.[49,52] Venographic imaging, shows enlarged veins as well as possible compression or invasion of the jugular vein.[51] Extension into the middle ear is important to identify, because it alters surgical management. If a lesion is seen in the middle ear without extension beyond, a glomus tympanicum tumor becomes a primary consideration.

In small GJT, the treatment of choice is surgical removal.[49,53] Patients with larger lesions usually undergo preoperative embolization because of their high vascularity.[53] In patients with extensive, malignant, or subtotally resected GJT (as well as in poor surgical candidates), radiotherapy is a primary consideration in tumor control and symptomatic treatment.[55,56]

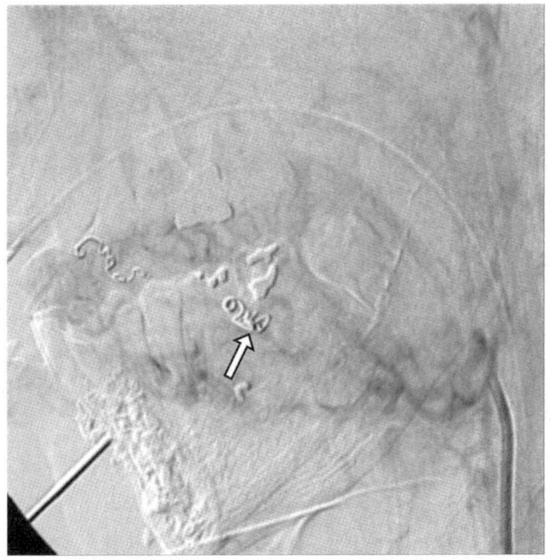

Fig. 12. Endovascular coil embolization of inferior alveolar artery with successful total occlusion of mandibular arteriovenous malformation. Coil is identified by an *arrow*.

Box 5
Imaging pearls vascular tumors

Hemangioma: High flow and contrast enhancing in proliferative phase.

Carotid body tumor: Splay internal and external carotids.

Glomus jugulare tumors: Destructive and permeative lesion in the jugular foramen. Middle ear extension alters therapy.

Juvenile nasopharyngeal angiofibroma: Heterogenous vascular soft tissue mass of the nose/nasopharynx in an adolescent male presenting with epistaxis.

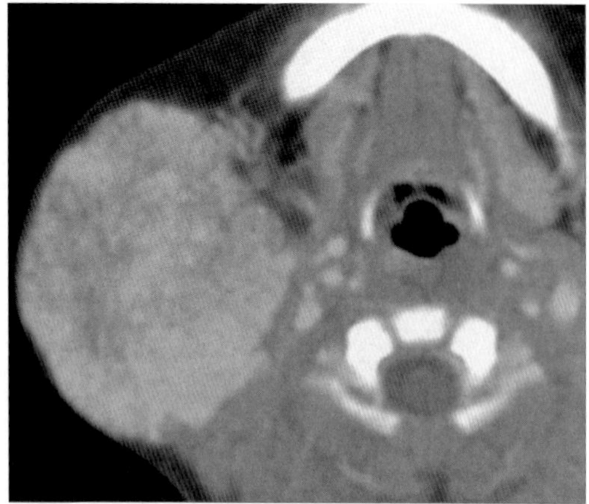

Fig. 13. Contrast-enhanced computed tomography shows an enhancing right neck mass that was progressively getting larger since birth.

Juvenile Nasopharyngeal Angiofibroma

JNA is a rare vascular neoplasm with a predilection for adolescent males.[57] The most common presenting symptoms are nasal obstruction and epistaxis.[57] Biopsy is generally avoided secondary to high tumor vascularity; therefore, clinical presentation and imaging play a key role in diagnosis. Key differential considerations include squamous cell carcinoma, rhabdomyosarcoma, and HM.

On plain radiography, JNA is seen as a soft tissue mass in the nose or nasopharynx that bows the posterior wall of the maxillary sinus.[58] If US is employed, high vascularity is a characteristic finding.[59] Unenhanced CT shows a heterogeneous soft tissue attenuation mass in the nose, nasopharynx, or pterygopalatine fossa.[60] With contrast

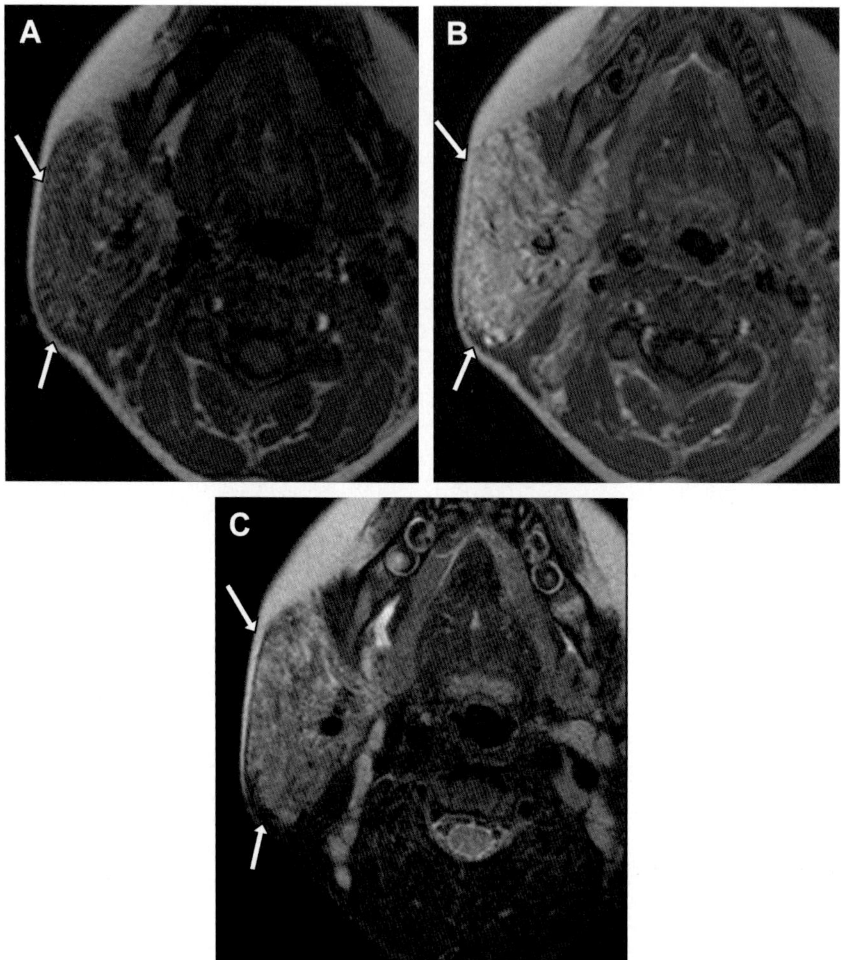

Fig. 14. (*A*) Axial T1 weighted image (WI) demonstrates a heterogeneous isointense to slightly hyperintense hemangioma (HM) in the right neck (*arrows*). (*B*) There is significant contrast enhancement (*arrows*) of the HM. (*C*) Axial T2W1 demonstrates heterogeneous high T2 signal (*arrows*) in the HM.

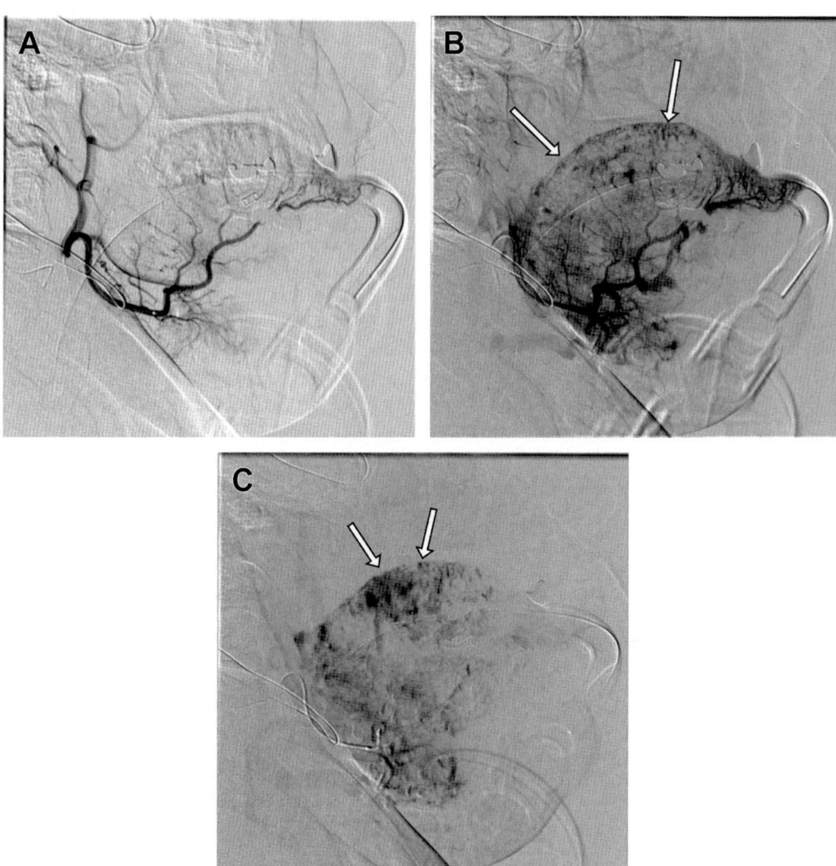

Fig. 15. (*A*) Early arterial phase angiography shows a high flow hemangioma (HM). (*B*) Later arterial phase angiographic image shows lobular intense enhancement of the HM (*arrows*). (*C*) Delayed angiographic image shows persistent tissue staining of the HM (*arrows*).

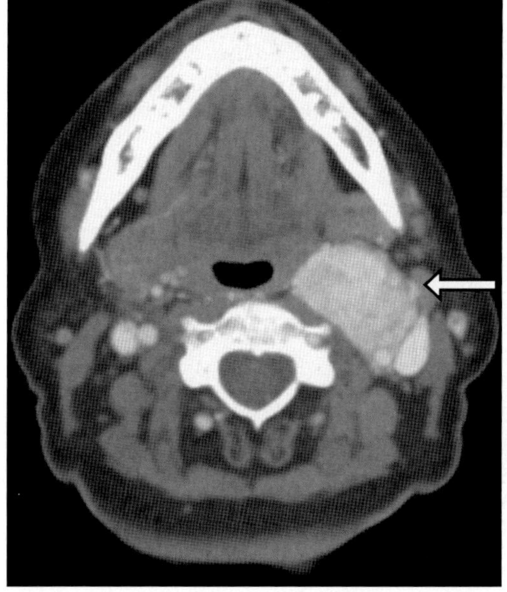

Fig. 16. Axial contrast-enhanced computed tomography demonstrates a lobular avidly enhancing mass in the left carotid space (*arrow*).

administration, intense enhancement is seen.[60,61] Erosion and expansion of the surrounding bony structures of the skull base is common.[60–63] The mass is heterogeneous and isointense to hyperintense on T1WI and T2WI with intense contrast enhancement (**Fig. 22**).[60,64] On angiography, these tumors show an intense capillary blush with the internal maxillary artery identified as a common feeding artery (**Fig. 23**).[58,63]

The treatment of choice for JNA is surgical resection.[57,65,66] Endoscopic surgery may decrease blood loss and have better cosmetic outcomes.[57,65] Similarly, preoperative embolization can decrease operative blood loss and operative transfusion requirements and is generally performed 24 to 48 hours before resection.[57,65–67] Embolization is performed transarterially or via direct puncture with liquid embolic agents (**Fig. 24**).[68] In extensive or unresectable lesions, radiation therapy can be used alone or

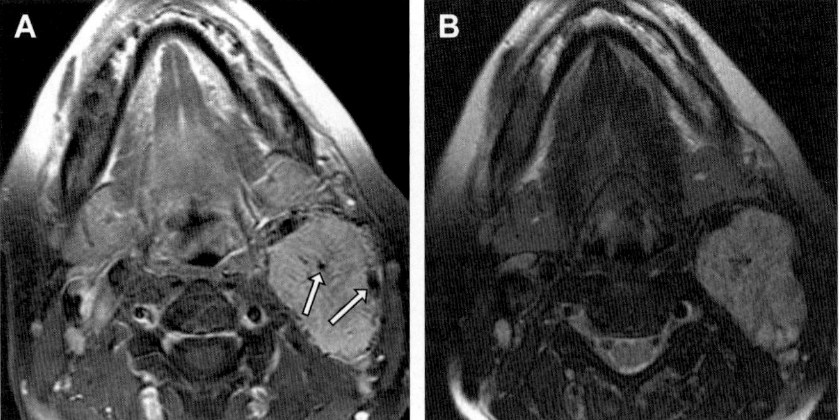

Fig. 17. (*A*) Axial T1 weighted image (WI) demonstrates a heterogenous carotid body tumor (CBT) in the left carotid space. Dark areas represent flow voids (*arrows*). (*B*) Axial T2WI demonstrates a mildly hyperintense left carotid space CBT.

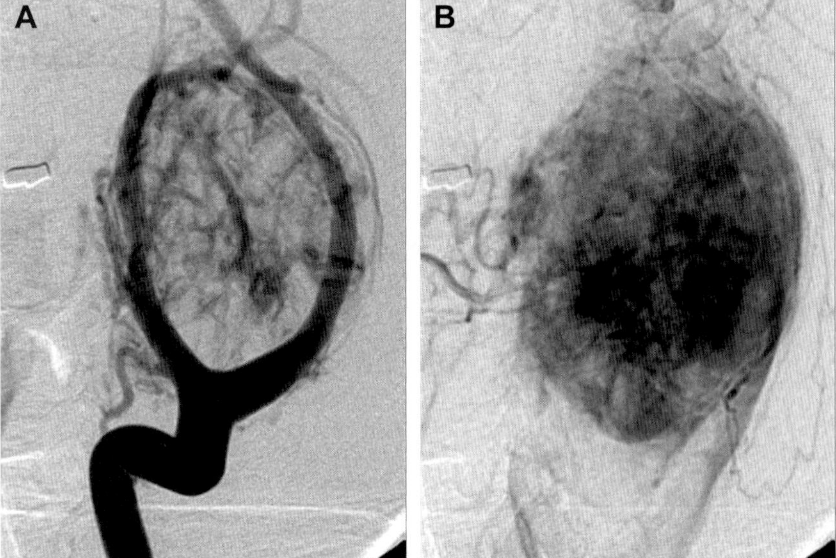

Fig. 18. (*A*) Angiographic images demonstrating a hypervascular mass splaying the internal and external carotids. (*B*) Delayed angiographic image shows a carotid body tumor with intense, prolonged tumor blush.

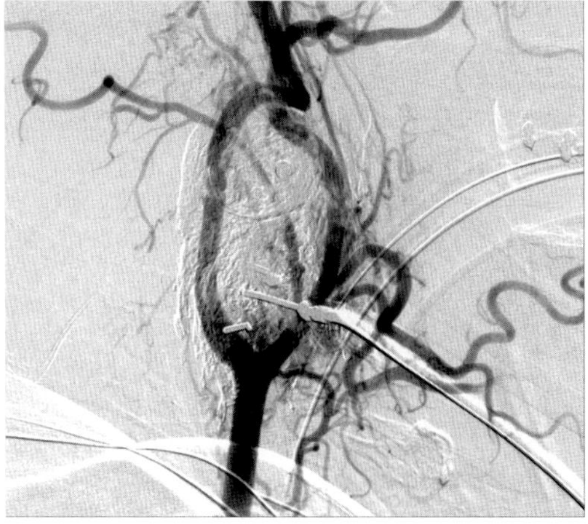

Fig. 19. Angiographic image after percutaneous liquid embolization shows complete devascularization of the carotid body tumor.

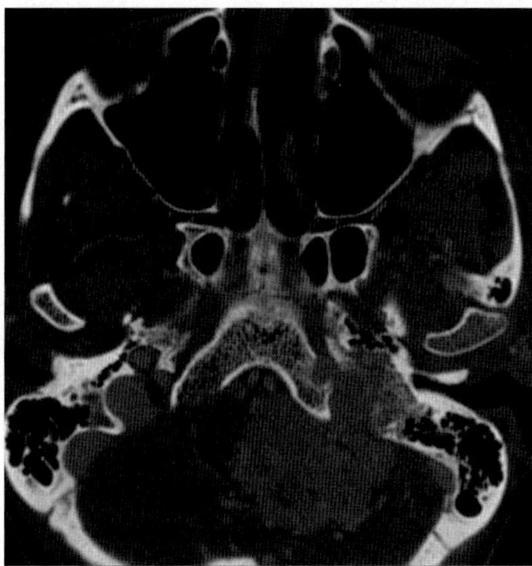

Fig. 20. Axial contrast-enhanced computed tomography demonstrates a glomus jugulare tumor displaying diffuse enhancement and bony erosion.

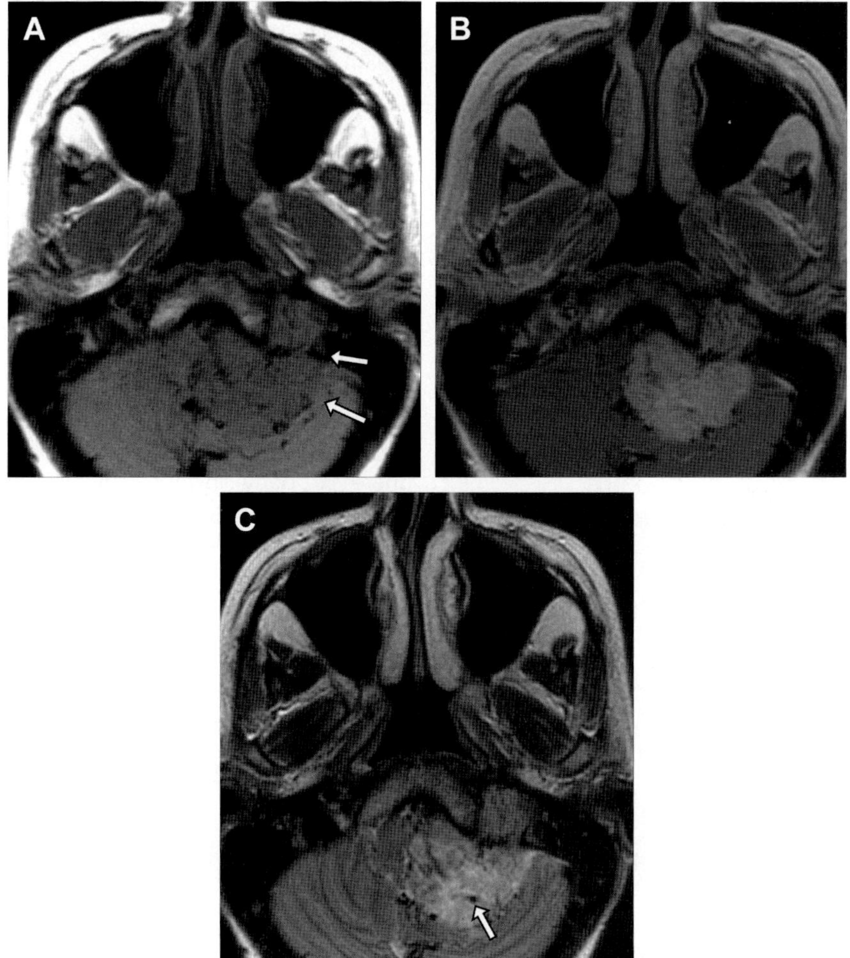

Fig. 21. (*A*) Axial T1 weighted image (WI) demonstrates an isointense glomus jugulare tumor (GJT) extending posteriorly from the region of the left jugular foramen (*arrows*). (*B*) The GJT demonstrates intense contrast enhancement on post T1WI. (*C*) On axial T2W1 the GJT is heterogeneous and mildly hyperintense with a dark internal flow void (*arrow*).

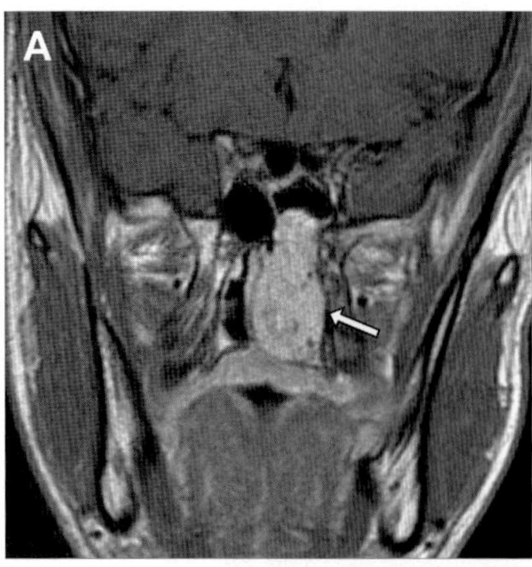

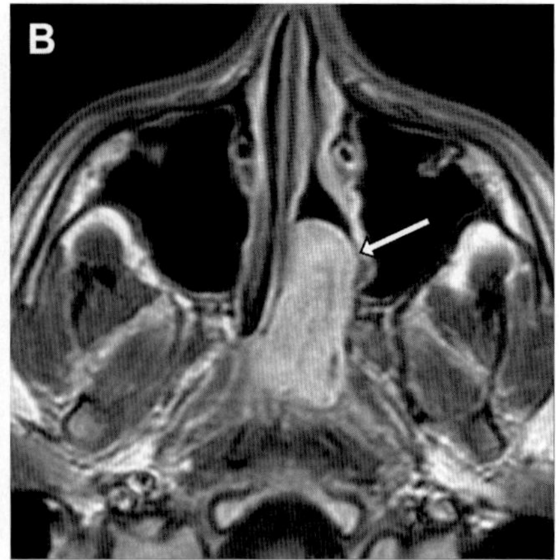

Fig. 22. (*A*) Coronal T1 weighted image (WI) demonstrates a mildly hyperintense juvenile nasopharyngeal angiofibroma (JNA) in the left nasal cavity (*arrow*). (*B*) On axial post contrast T1WI the JNA demonstrates enhancement (*arrow*).

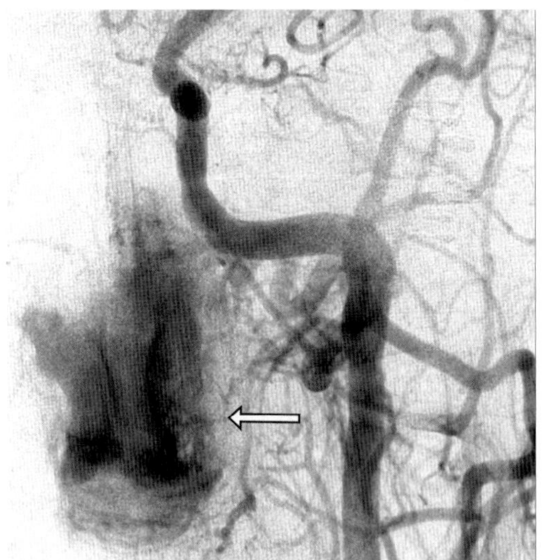

Fig. 23. Angiographic image shows a juvenile nasopharyngeal angiofibroma with intense tumor blush secondary to vascularity (*arrow*).

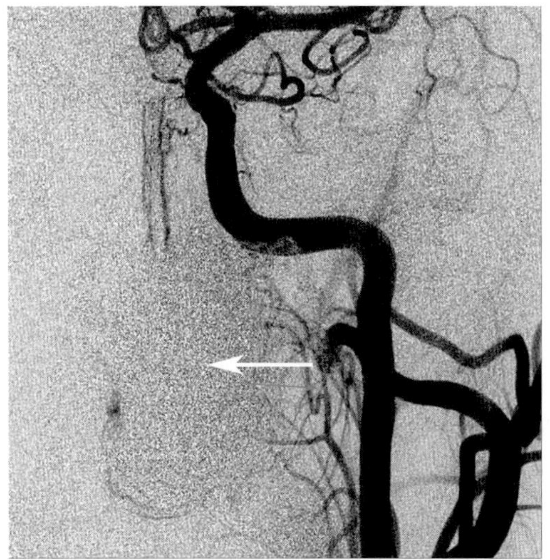

Fig. 24. Angiographic image after liquid embolization shows no residual tumor blush (*arrow*).

in combination with surgery.[69] Recurrence has been noted to occur in 20% to 50% and postoperative radiation therapy can be effective in delaying or preventing recurrence.[65,67,70,71] Risk factors for recurrence include younger age at diagnosis, larger tumor size, and higher stage lesion.[71]

SUMMARY

The diagnosis of vascular lesions of the head and neck should be directed by classifying the lesions as tumors or malformations and by determining their flow characteristics (**Box 6**). Location of the lesion is key when differentiating between vascular neoplasms. US is an appropriate screening tool; MRI is often used to confirm the diagnosis. CT can be used for further characterization of the lesion, particularly when there is bony involvement. In many cases, vascular lesions grow to be extensive. In these cases, percutaneous sclerotherapy or embolization therapy can be employed to aid in surgical resection.

Box 6
What the referring physician needs to note

Ultrasonography is a high-value screening method for evaluating superficial vascular lesions.

MRI is the most important modality for determining lesion extent and its involvement with soft tissues.

Computed tomography should be used judiciously, but is integral in evaluating bony involvement.

REFERENCES

1. Mulliken JB, Glowacki J. Hemangiomas and vascular malformations in infants and children: a classification based on endothelial characteristics. Plast Reconstr Surg 1982;69(3):412–22.
2. Yang WT, Ahuja A, Metreweli C. Sonographic features of head and neck hemangiomas and vascular malformations: review of 23 patients. J Ultrasound Med 1997;16(1):39–44.
3. Rozylo-Kalinowska I, Brodzisz A, Galkowska E, et al. Application of Doppler ultrasonography in congenital vascular lesions of the head and neck. Dentomaxillofac Radiol 2002;31(1):2–6.
4. Baker LL, Dillon WP, Hieshima GB, et al. Hemangiomas and vascular malformations of the head and neck: MR characterization. AJNR Am J Neuroradiol 1993;14(2):307–14.
5. Parmar H, Ivancevic MK, Dudek N, et al. Dynamic MRA with four-dimensional time-resolved angiography using keyhole at 3 tesla in head and neck vascular lesions. J Neuroophthalmol 2009;29(2): 119–27.
6. Hennedige AA, Quaba AA, Al-Nakib K. Sturge-Weber syndrome and dermatomal facial port-wine stains: incidence, association with glaucoma, and pulsed tunable dye laser treatment effectiveness. Plast Reconstr Surg 2008;121(4):1173–80.
7. Enjolras O, Riche MC, Merland JJ. Facial port-wine stains and Sturge-Weber syndrome. Pediatrics 1985;76(1):48–51.
8. Eivazi B, Fasunla AJ, Hundt W, et al. Low flow vascular malformations of the head and neck: a study on brightness mode, color coded duplex and spectral Doppler sonography. Eur Arch Otorhinolaryngol 2011;268(10):1505–11.
9. Kelly KM, Choi B, McFarlane S, et al. Description and analysis of treatments for port-wine stain birthmarks. Arch Facial Plast Surg 2005;7(5):287–94.
10. Kim Y, Oh SJ, Lee J, et al. Surgical treatment of dermatomal capillary malformations in the adult face. Arch Plast Surg 2012;39(2):126–9.
11. Berenguer B, Burrows PE, Zurakowski D, et al. Sclerotherapy of craniofacial venous malformations: complications and results. Plast Reconstr Surg 1999;104(1):1–11 [discussion: 12–5].
12. Hassanein AH, Mulliken JB, Fishman SJ, et al. Venous malformation: risk of progression during childhood and adolescence. Ann Plast Surg 2012;68(2):198–201.
13. Roh YN, Do YS, Park KB, et al. The results of surgical treatment for patients with venous malformations. Ann Vasc Surg 2012;26(5):665–73.
14. Su L, Fan X, Zheng L, et al. Absolute ethanol sclerotherapy for venous malformations in the face and neck. J Oral Maxillofac Surg 2010;68(7): 1622–7.
15. Gelbert F, Riche MC, Reizine D, et al. MR imaging of head and neck vascular malformations. J Magn Reson Imaging 1991;1(5):579–84.
16. Aspestrand F, Kolbenstvedt A. Vascular mass lesions and hypervascular tumors in the head and neck. Characteristics at CT, MR imaging and angiography. Acta Radiol 1995;36(2):136–41.
17. Trop I, Dubois J, Guibaud L, et al. Soft-tissue venous malformations in pediatric and young adult patients: diagnosis with Doppler US. Radiology 1999;212(3):841–5.
18. Boyd JB, Mulliken JB, Kaban LB, et al. Skeletal changes associated with vascular malformations. Plast Reconstr Surg 1984;74(6):789–97.
19. Salehian S, Fischbein NJ. Association of venous malformation of the head and neck with meningoencephalocele: report of 3 cases. AJNR Am J Neuroradiol 2011;32(4):E65–8.
20. Meyer JS, Hoffer FA, Barnes PD, et al. Biological classification of soft-tissue vascular anomalies: MR correlation. AJR Am J Roentgenol 1991;157(3):559–64.
21. Ziyeh S, Schumacher M, Strecker R, et al. Head and neck vascular malformations: time-resolved MR projection angiography. Neuroradiology 2003; 45(10):681–6.
22. Okazaki T, Iwatani S, Yanai T, et al. Treatment of lymphangioma in children: our experience of 128 cases. J Pediatr Surg 2007;42(2):386–9.
23. Mathur NN, Rana I, Bothra R, et al. Bleomycin sclerotherapy in congenital lymphatic and vascular malformations of head and neck. Int J Pediatr Otorhinolaryngol 2005;69(1):75–80.
24. Fung K, Poenaru D, Soboleski DA, et al. Impact of magnetic resonance imaging on the surgical management of cystic hygromas. J Pediatr Surg 1998; 33(6):839–41.
25. Cahill AM, Nijs E, Ballah D, et al. Percutaneous sclerotherapy in neonatal and infant head and neck lymphatic malformations: a single center experience. J Pediatr Surg 2011;46(11):2083–95.
26. Jamal N, Ahmed S, Miller T, et al. Doxycycline sclerotherapy for pediatric head and neck macrocystic lymphatic malformations: a case series and review of the literature. Int J Pediatr Otorhinolaryngol 2012;76(8):1127–31.
27. Yoo JC, Ahn Y, Lim YS, et al. OK-432 sclerotherapy in head and neck lymphangiomas: long-term follow-up result. Otolaryngol Head Neck Surg 2009;140(1):120–3.
28. Kohout MP, Hansen M, Pribaz JJ, et al. Arteriovenous malformations of the head and neck: natural history and management. Plast Reconstr Surg 1998;102(3):643–54.
29. Kim JY, Kim DI, Do YS, et al. Surgical treatment for congenital arteriovenous malformation: 10 years' experience. Eur J Vasc Endovasc Surg 2006; 32(1):101–6.

30. Seccia A, Salgarello M, Farallo E, et al. Combined radiological and surgical treatment of arteriovenous malformations of the head and neck. Ann Plast Surg 1999;43(4):359–66.
31. Richter GT, Suen JY. Clinical course of arteriovenous malformations of the head and neck: a case series. Otolaryngol Head Neck Surg 2010;142(2):184–90.
32. Chooi WK, Woodhouse N, Coley SC, et al. Pediatric head and neck lesions: assessment of vascularity by MR digital subtraction angiography. AJNR Am J Neuroradiol 2004;25(7):1251–5.
33. Achauer BM, Chang CJ, Vander Kam VM. Management of hemangioma of infancy: review of 245 patients. Plast Reconstr Surg 1997;99(5):1301–8.
34. Salzman R, Buchanan MA, Berman L, et al. Ultrasound-guided core-needle biopsy and magnetic resonance imaging in the accurate diagnosis of intramuscular haemangiomas of the head and neck. J Laryngol Otol 2012;126(4):391–4.
35. Sinno H, Thibaudeau S, Coughlin R, et al. Management of infantile parotid gland hemangiomas: a 40-year experience. Plast Reconstr Surg 2010;125(1): 265–73.
36. Dubois J, Patriquin HB, Garel L, et al. Soft-tissue hemangiomas in infants and children: diagnosis using Doppler sonography. AJR Am J Roentgenol 1998;171(1):247–52.
37. Buckmiller LM, Munson PD, Dyamenahalli U, et al. Propranolol for infantile hemangiomas: early experience at a tertiary vascular anomalies center. Laryngoscope 2010;120(4):676–81.
38. Katona G, Csakanyi Z, Gacs E, et al. Propranolol for infantile haemangioma: striking effect in the first weeks. Int J Pediatr Otorhinolaryngol 2012;76(12): 1746–50.
39. Erickson D, Kudva YC, Ebersold MJ, et al. Benign paragangliomas: clinical presentation and treatment outcomes in 236 patients. J Clin Endocrinol Metab 2001;86(11):5210–6.
40. van Baars F, van den Broek P, Cremers C, et al. Familial non-chromaffinic paragangliomas (glomus tumors): clinical aspects. Laryngoscope 1981; 91(6):988–96.
41. Liapis CD, Evangelidakis EL, Papavassiliou VG, et al. Role of malignancy and preoperative embolization in the management of carotid body tumors. World J Surg 2000;24(12):1526–30.
42. Muhm M, Polterauer P, Gstottner W, et al. Diagnostic and therapeutic approaches to carotid body tumors. Review of 24 patients. Arch Surg 1997;132(3):279–84.
43. Lack EE, Cubilla AL, Woodruff JM, et al. Paragangliomas of the head and neck region: a clinical study of 69 patients. Cancer 1977;39(2):397–409.
44. Olsen WL, Dillon WP, Kelly WM, et al. MR imaging of paragangliomas. AJR Am J Roentgenol 1987; 148(1):201–4.
45. Unlu Y, Becit N, Ceviz M, et al. Management of carotid body tumors and familial paragangliomas: review of 30 years' experience. Ann Vasc Surg 2009;23(5):616–20.
46. Tikkakoski T, Luotonen J, Leinonen S, et al. Preoperative embolization in the management of neck paragangliomas. Laryngoscope 1997;107(6):821–6.
47. Gemmete JJ, Chaudhary N, Pandey A, et al. Usefulness of percutaneously injected ethylene-vinyl alcohol copolymer in conjunction with standard endovascular embolization techniques for preoperative devascularization of hypervascular head and neck tumors: technique, initial experience, and correlation with surgical observations. AJNR Am J Neuroradiol 2010;31(5):961–6.
48. Griauzde J, Gemmete JJ, Chaudhary N, et al. A comparison of particulate and Onyx embolization in preoperative devascularization of carotid body tumors. Neuroradiology 2013;55(9):1113–8.
49. Ramina R, Maniglia JJ, Fernandes YB, et al. Tumors of the jugular foramen: diagnosis and management. Neurosurgery 2005;57(1 Suppl):59–68 [discussion: 59–68].
50. George B. Jugulare foramen paragangliomas. Acta Neurochir (Wien) 1992;118(1–2):20–6.
51. Christie A, Teasdale E. A comparative review of multidetector CT angiography and MRI in the diagnosis of jugular foramen lesions. Clin Radiol 2010; 65(3):213–7.
52. Wilson MA, Hillman TA, Wiggins RH, et al. Jugular foramen schwannomas: diagnosis, management, and outcomes. Laryngoscope 2005;115(8):1486–92.
53. Makiese O, Chibbaro S, Marsella M, et al. Jugular foramen paragangliomas: management, outcome and avoidance of complications in a series of 75 cases. Neurosurg Rev 2012;35(2):185–94 [discussion: 194].
54. Phelps PD, Stansbie JM. Glomus jugulare or tympanicum? The role of CT and MR imaging with gadolinium DTPA. J Laryngol Otol 1988;102(9):766–76.
55. Saringer W, Khayal H, Ertl A, et al. Efficiency of gamma knife radiosurgery in the treatment of glomus jugulare tumors. Minim Invasive Neurosurg 2001;44(3):141–6.
56. Mumber MP, Greven KM. Control of advanced chemodectomas of the head and neck with irradiation. Am J Clin Oncol 1995;18(5):389–91.
57. Midilli R, Karci B, Akyildiz S. Juvenile nasopharyngeal angiofibroma: analysis of 42 cases and important aspects of endoscopic approach. Int J Pediatr Otorhinolaryngol 2009;73(3):401–8.
58. Sessions RB, Wills PI, Alford BR, et al. Juvenile nasopharyngeal angiofibroma: radiographic aspects. Laryngoscope 1976;86(1):2–18.
59. Arslan H, Bozkurt M, Sakarya ME, et al. Power Doppler findings in nasopharingeal angiofibroma. Clin Imaging 1998;22(2):86–8.

60. Lloyd G, Howard D, Phelps P, et al. Juvenile angiofibroma: the lessons of 20 years of modern imaging. J Laryngol Otol 1999;113(2):127–34.
61. Weinstein MA, Levine H, Duchesneau PM, et al. Diagnosis of juvenile angiofibroma by computed tomography. Radiology 1978;126(3):703–5.
62. Levine HL, Weinstein MA, Tucker HM, et al. Diagnosis of juvenile nasopharyngeal angiofibroma by computed tomography. Otolaryngol Head Neck Surg (1979) 1979;87(3):304–10.
63. Thomas RL. Computed tomography in the assessment of patients with juvenile post-nasal angiofibroma. J Otolaryngol 1980;9(4):334–41.
64. Lloyd GA, Lund VJ, Phelps PD, et al. Magnetic resonance imaging in the evaluation of nose and paranasal sinus disease. Br J Radiol 1987; 60(718):957–68.
65. Ardehali MM, Samimi Ardestani SH, Yazdani N, et al. Endoscopic approach for excision of juvenile nasopharyngeal angiofibroma: complications and outcomes. Am J Otolaryngol 2010;31(5): 343–9.
66. Moulin G, Chagnaud C, Gras R, et al. Juvenile nasopharyngeal angiofibroma: comparison of blood loss during removal in embolized group versus nonembolized group. Cardiovasc Intervent Radiol 1995;18(3):158–61.
67. Alvarez FL, Suarez V, Suarez C, et al. Multimodality approach for advanced-stage juvenile nasopharyngeal angiofibromas. Head Neck 2013;35(2): 209–13.
68. Gao M, Gemmete JJ, Chaudhary N, et al. A comparison of particulate and onyx embolization in preoperative devascularization of juvenile nasopharyngeal angiofibromas. Neuroradiology 2013; 55(9):1089–96.
69. Reddy KA, Mendenhall WM, Amdur RJ, et al. Long-term results of radiation therapy for juvenile nasopharyngeal angiofibroma. Am J Otolaryngol 2001; 22(3):172–5.
70. Roche PH, Paris J, Regis J, et al. Management of invasive juvenile nasopharyngeal angiofibromas: the role of a multimodality approach. Neurosurgery 2007;61(4):768–77 [discussion: 777].
71. Sun XC, Wang DH, Yu HP, et al. Analysis of risk factors associated with recurrence of nasopharyngeal angiofibroma. J Otolaryngol Head Neck Surg 2010; 39(1):56–61.

Imaging of Head and Neck Emergencies

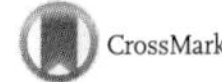

Justin L. Brucker, MD, Lindell R. Gentry, MD*

KEYWORDS

• Emergency radiology • Head and neck infection • Imaging

KEY POINTS

- The anatomy of the head and neck contains very few structures that could be considered expendable and, consequently, is exceptionally intolerant to infection, inflammation, and injury.
- Acute pathologic processes in this body region, therefore, tend to result in significant suffering, functional impairment, or life endangerment if the diagnosis is missed or treatment is delayed.
- Many emergent processes within the cervical region also need to be considered for their possible impact on structures within the head and chest, into which there are many routes for potential communication.
- In the emergent setting, computed tomography (CT) is the favored imaging option because of its rapid image acquisition and superior delineation of the airway and osseous structures.
- On the other hand, MR imaging provides more robust information regarding complex soft tissue structures that may be difficult to distinguish on CT.
- However, any prolonged radiologic examination should only be undertaken in patients who possess a protected airway and are medically stable enough to tolerate the duration of the scan.
- This added step of preimaging clearance should entail a review of the patients' presenting symptoms and past medical history, which will also help to refine the study protocol and provide a clinical context in which to interpret the images.

INTRODUCTION: "CRIMES AGAINST ANATOMY"

If not for the thorough coverage of subject matter provided by the other articles of this book, the authors' one section, dedicated to various medical emergencies of the head and neck, may have read something like an endlessly long police report inspired by an episode of "Head and Neck Imaging's Most Wanted." Admittedly, there are many topics that would have been appropriate to include under this heading; but for the sake of brevity, the authors limits the discussion to the culprits that he found either most offensive or intriguing.

When one sits down to consider what actually constitutes an emergency in this region of the body, any of the following situations may qualify: (1) conditions that are life threatening, (2) conditions that cause loss of function, (3) conditions that incite severe pain or distress, or (4) any situation that can lead to the aforementioned conditions if not identified early or acted on quickly. With that being said, it takes little imagination to see how just about any acquired abnormality of the head or neck has the potential for being declared an emergency on presentation; in reality, this is becoming increasingly more common, according to current fashions in modern clinical practice. It is important to keep in mind that, when dealing with the vital delicate anatomy of the head and neck, even minor violations can lead to serious disability and unnecessary suffering, especially when inaccurately interpreted or missed altogether. It is by the same token that relatively small transgressions may be promoted to the level of heinous criminal activity, should they occur in a sacred and vulnerable location.

Justin L. Brucker is the primary author in this article.
Head and Neck Imaging, Department of Neuroradiology, University of Wisconsin Hospital, University of Wisconsin, E1-311 CSC, 600 Highland Ave, Madison, WI 53792, USA
* Corresponding author.
E-mail address: lgentry@uwhealth.org

Radiol Clin N Am 53 (2015) 215–252
http://dx.doi.org/10.1016/j.rcl.2014.09.007

Take, for example, the act of littering in a nature preserve or smoking cigarettes in the Sistine Chapel (though from a head-and-neck standpoint, too, one should avoid smoking altogether).

In addition to the authors' coverage of head and neck emergencies, this article includes some of the necessary discussion about the relevant anatomy and imaging techniques, though mostly in the context of a specific disease process being presented.

APPROACH TO HEAD AND NECK IMAGING TECHNIQUES

Conventional radiography plays little role in the evaluation of patients with head and neck emergencies. The anatomic information provided is usually insufficient for diagnosing and managing these conditions (**Figs. 1** and **2**). Computed tomography (CT) remains the foremost radiologic tool for imaging the head and neck in the acute setting (see **Figs. 1** and **2**; **Figs. 3–8**), given its many attractive features, which include: fast speed of image acquisition, large field of view (FOV), high spatial resolution, relative insensitivity to patient motion, ability to provide reformatted images from a single data acquisition, wide availability of the technology, and ease of technical use. In the emergent setting, these highly desirable properties should outweigh any concerns one may have about the long-term effects of radiation exposure, especially if one adheres to standard imaging practices and keeps track of CT dose reports (basic radiologic hygiene). Furthermore, the ongoing evolution of widely available low-dose reconstruction algorithms and improvements in detector technology continue to diminish the radiation cost of CT imaging. Of note, we must always take care not to let exuberant dose-limiting practices sacrifice vital diagnostic information from the scan; a safe scan by definition should not facilitate a radiologist in readily missing a critical finding.

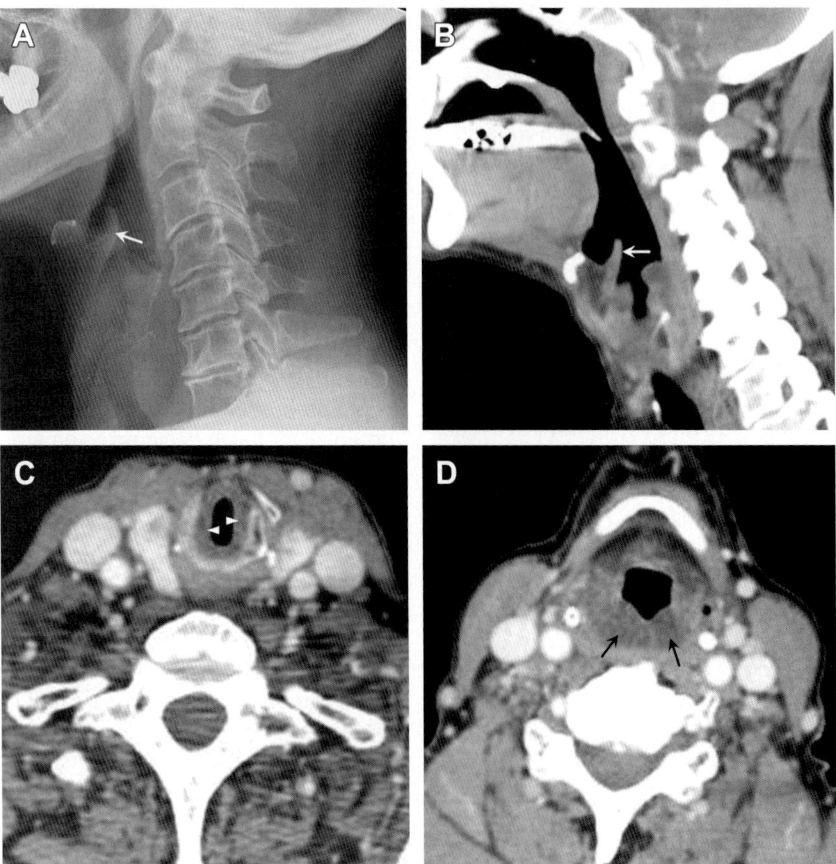

Fig. 1. Acute supraglottitis and laryngitis: (*A*) Lateral radiograph demonstrates enlargement of the suprahyoid and infrahyoid epiglottis (*white arrow*). Sagittal (*B*) and axial (*C, D*) Computed tomography scans also reveal edema of the epiglottis (*white arrow*), aryepiglottic folds (*black arrows*), and mucosal lining of the subglottic larynx (*white arrowheads*).

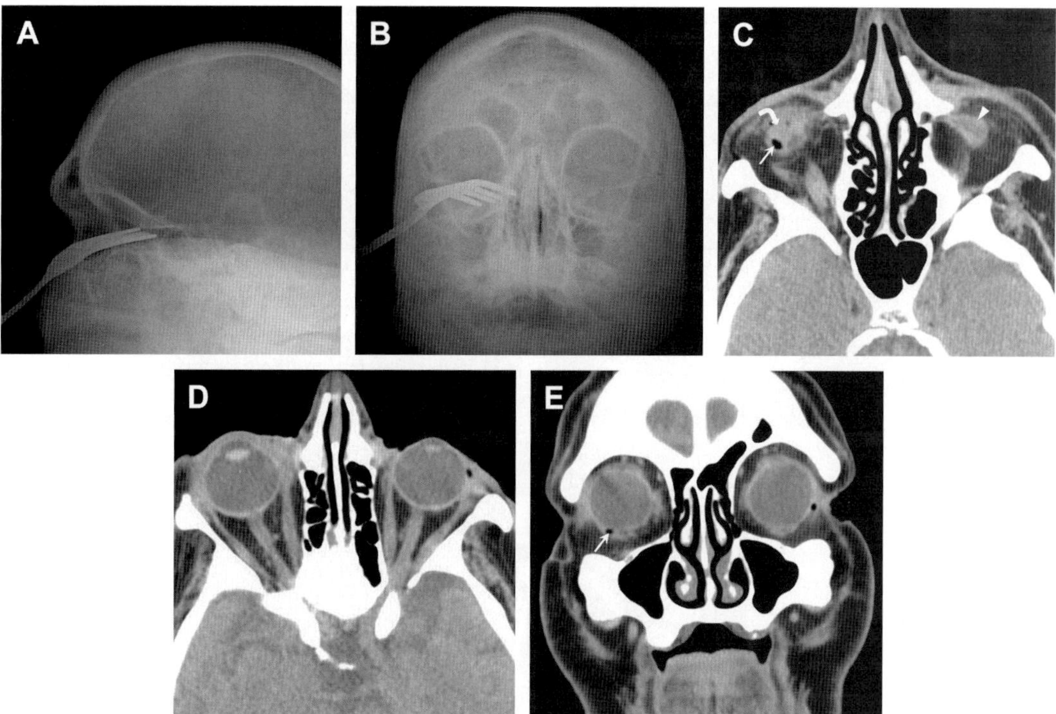

Fig. 2. Penetrating orbital trauma: Male psychiatric patient with a history of visual hallucinations now presenting with blurry vision following self-inflicted penetrating orbital trauma. Lateral (*A*) and anteroposterior (*B*) radiographs demonstrate a penetrating orbital foreign body (fork) extending into the inferior aspect of the right orbit just above the orbital floor. These images do not provide any information about soft tissue injury to the orbital contents. Axial (*C, D*) and coronal (*E*) computed tomography scans reveal a normal appearance of the globe but ill-defined hemorrhage (*curved arrow*) and air (*white arrows*) within the right inferior oblique muscle. Note the normal appearance of the left inferior oblique muscle (*white arrowhead*).

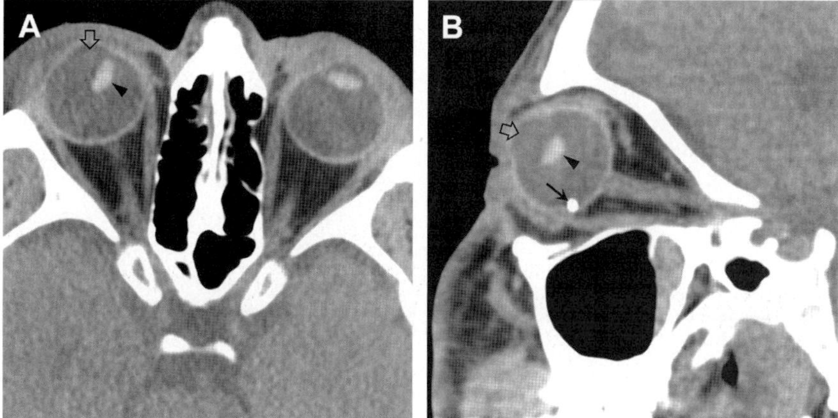

Fig. 3. Penetrating intraocular foreign body, lens dislocation: Axial (*A*) and oblique sagittal (*B*) CT scans demonstrate a metallic foreign body (*black arrow*) near the inferior aspect of the sclera within the globe. There is marked widening of the anterior and posterior chambers of the globe with subtle hemorrhage (hyphema) (*open arrows*) and dislocation of the lens (*black arrowheads*).

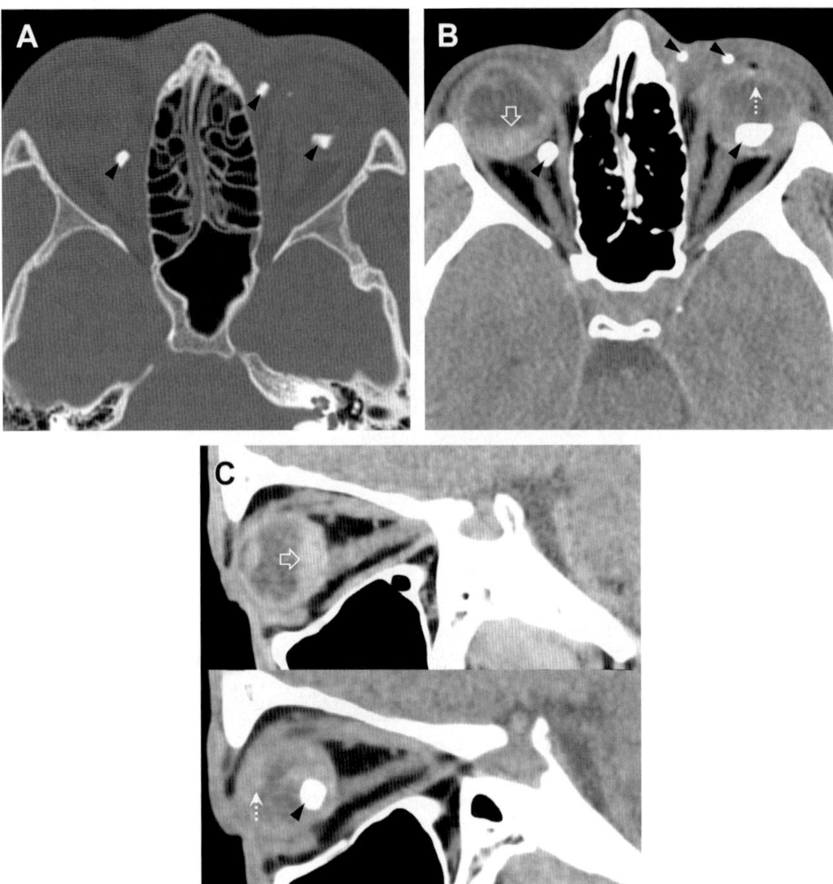

Fig. 4. Penetrating intraocular and intraorbital foreign bodies, intraorbital hemorrhage, lens dislocation: Axial (*A*, *B*) and oblique sagittal (*C*) CT scans demonstrate multiple intraocular and intraorbital glass fragments (*black arrowheads*) in a patient ejected through the windshield of an automobile during a motor vehicle accident. Intravitreal (*open white arrows*) and anterior chamber (hyphema) hemorrhage is present. There is rupture of the left globe as indicated by its abnormally small size. There is traumatic fragmentation of the left lens (*dashed white arrows*).

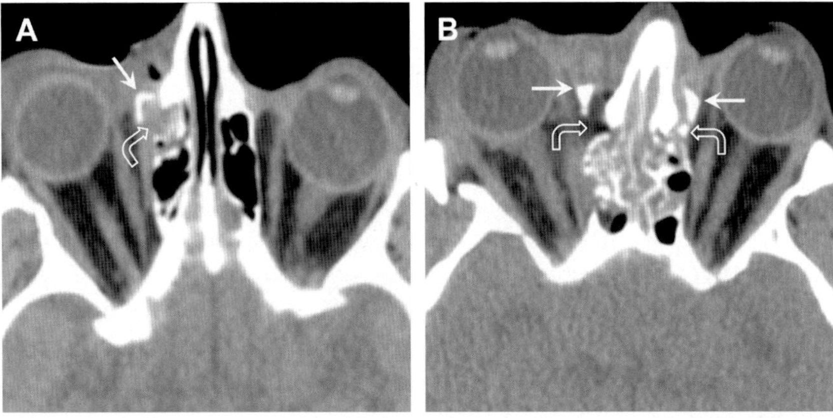

Fig. 5. Blunt central midface trauma with medial canthal ligament disruption, traumatic telecanthus: CT scans (*A*, *B*) of 2 different patients who experienced severe central midface trauma resulting in periorbital contusion, epiphora, and widening of the intrapupillary distance. The scans demonstrate multiple fractures of the central midface including avulsion of the anterior lacrimal crests (*white arrows*) from their attachments indicating disruption of the medial canthal ligament complex. Fractures also involve the lacrimal sac fossa (*curved white open arrows*) explaining the presence of epiphora.

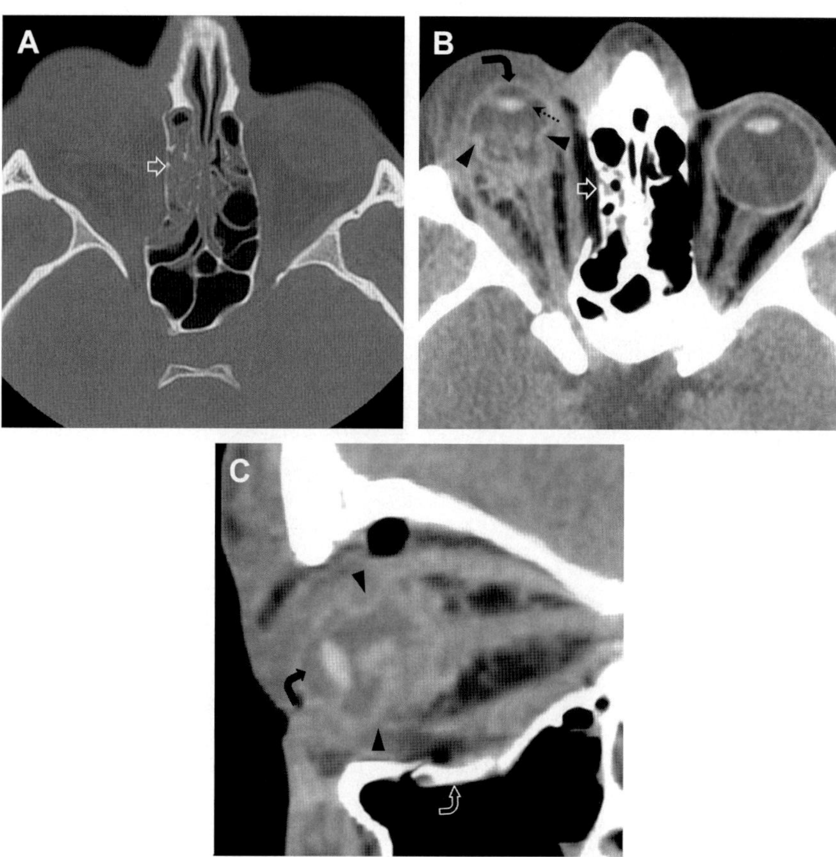

Fig. 6. Medial and inferior orbital wall blowout fractures, ocular rupture: Axial (*A, B*) and oblique sagittal (*C*) CT scans reveal depressed fractures of the medial (*white open arrows*) and inferior (*curved white open arrows*) orbital walls following blunt orbital trauma. There is obvious rupture of the globe indicated by a wrinkled, notched (crenated) appearance (*black arrowheads*) and extensive intravitreal hemorrhage. There is evidence of enlargement and hemorrhage within the anterior chamber of the orbit (hyphema) (*curved black arrows*) as well as slight subluxation of the lens (*dashed black arrow*).

In comparison with CT, MR imaging requires a larger commitment in terms of time, cost, and patient cooperation but continues to play a growing, indispensable role in head and neck imaging. Patients who are either very young, distressed, or presenting with altered levels of consciousness may also require sedation or even general anesthesia in order to successfully complete an MR imaging examination. These patients require close monitoring by dedicated personnel, so this should be kept in mind when planning a potential scan. Before the examination, rigorous screening for metallic foreign bodies or implanted electronic medical devices should be performed to ensure safe, efficacious scanning, so as to prevent injury to patients or damage to sensitive indwelling hardware. At high-magnetic-field strength (3.0 T) MR imaging provides a higher signal-to-noise ratio and improved delineation of soft tissue structures. Higher-field MR imaging may, thus, provide a higher sensitivity for pathologic processes, such as inflammatory and neoplastic lesions (**Figs. 9–13**). The anatomy of the head and neck presents specific challenges for MR imaging evaluation, as the inherent bony anatomy and air interfaces of the head and neck create artifacts related to magnetic field inhomogeneity. Motion from breathing, swallowing, and vascular pulsatility can further degrade image quality. Artifact from physiologic motion can often be minimized by careful saturation band placement, cardiac gating, switching the frequency/phase encoding axes, and effective coaching for breath-holds and cessation of swallowing. Further innovations built around faster pulse sequences, higher temporal resolution, lower specific absorption rates, and precision saturation of fat signal may improve visualization of complex anatomic structures.

Generally speaking, all of the imaging protocols rely on multiplanar images centered over a small

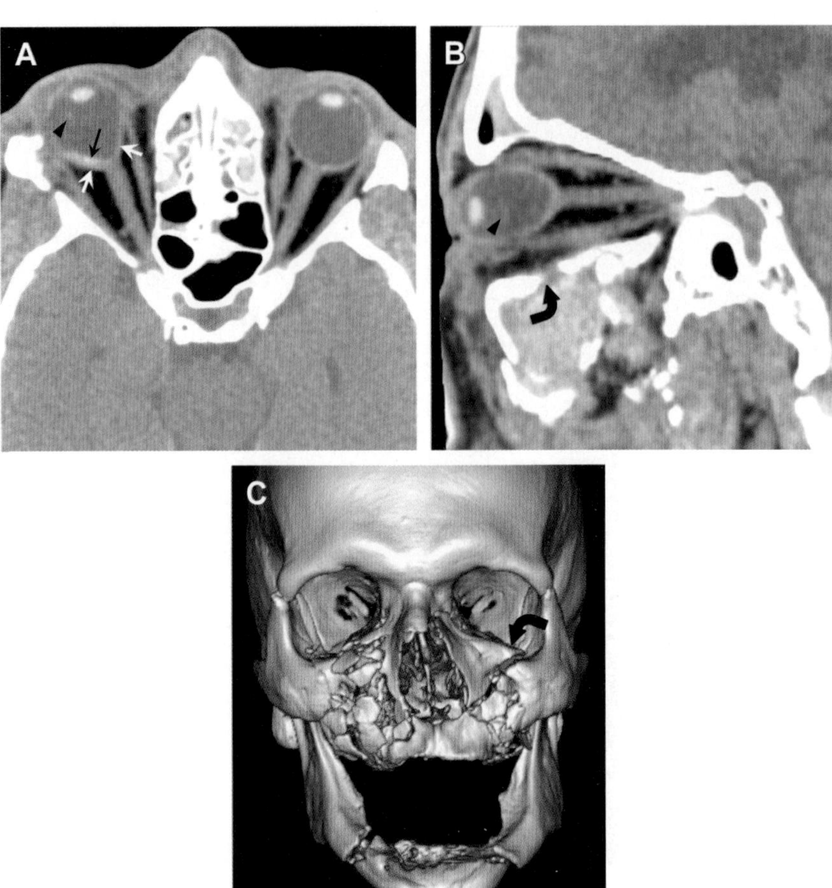

Fig. 7. Bilateral Le Fort I, II and III fractures with posttraumatic retrobulbar mass effect and posterior globe tenting: Axial (*A*), oblique sagittal (*B*), and 3-dimensional (3D) (*C*) CT scans reveal extensive bilateral Le Fort I to III facial fractures. There is evidence of a small amount of intravitreal (*black arrowhead*) and subretinal (*black arrow*) hemorrhage as well as an abnormally elongated right globe. There is flattening (tenting) of the posterior aspect of the globe (*white arrows*) indicating retrobulbar mass effect. The oblique sagittal and 3D CT images reveal upward displacement of the orbital floor (*curved black arrows*) decreasing the volume of the orbit resulting in the mass effect.

FOV with a large matrix. For CT, the authors acquires 0.65-mm axial images and performs thin ($\leq$2 mm) 2-dimensional (2D) reconstructions in the sagittal and coronal planes with both soft tissue and bone reconstruction algorithms. MR imaging protocols are inherently more complicated than their CT counterparts but always include precontrast triplanar T1-weighted images, 2-planar T2-weighted images, and propeller-based fast spin echo diffusion-weighted imaging. Triplanar postcontrast T1-weighted images are then acquired in the same locations as the precontrast T1-weighted images. The variation between individual protocols is driven by the area of anatomic coverage that is needed and the clinical indication. In practice, protocols often need to be tailored to a specific patient's situation. Therefore, the first step to successful head-and-neck imaging is to understand the problem at hand and the clinician's request. Such comprehension will not infrequently require personally reviewing the patient's medical record, familiarizing oneself with their past medical history and presenting issues, and having a brief discussion with the ordering provider.

Teaching point: Successful prescription of a head and neck imaging protocol is always preceded by a review of the patients' medical information.

EMERGENCIES OF THE ORBIT

Very few things inspire a trip to the emergency department as effectively as something unpleasant happening to your eye, which frequently

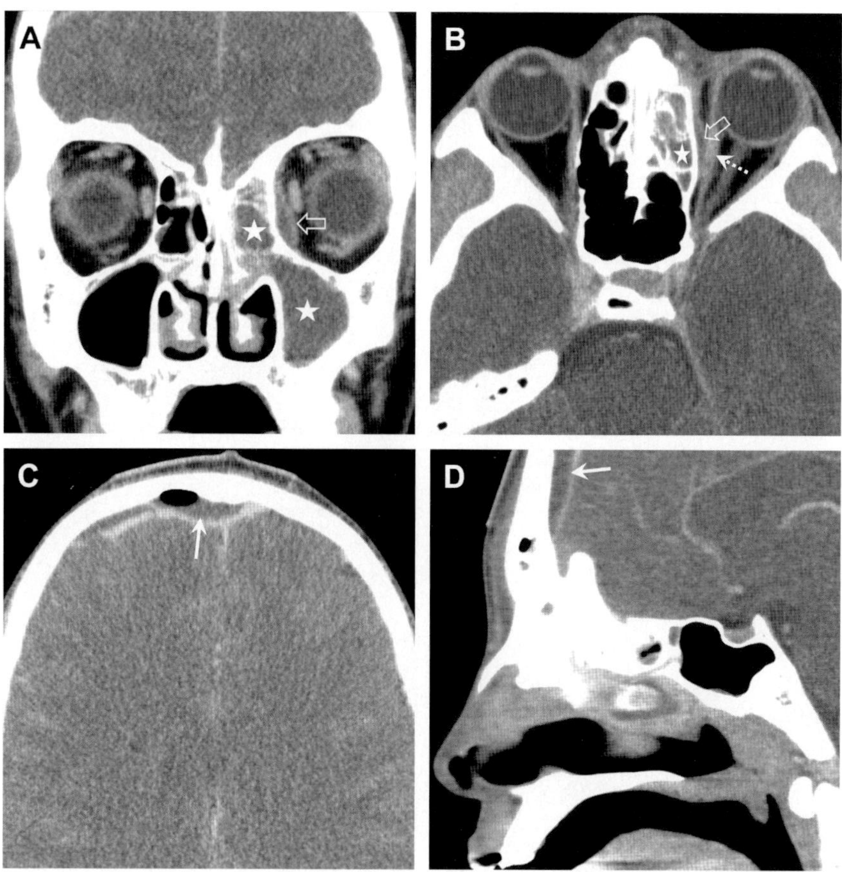

Fig. 8. Ethmoid-maxillary sinusitis, subperiosteal orbital abscess, and epidural abscess: Coronal (*A*), axial (*B*, *C*), and sagittal (*D*) CT images reveal maxillary and ethmoid sinus opacification (*star*) consistent with acute sinusitis. There is a hypodense subperiosteal abscess (*white open arrows*) with peripheral enhancement of the displaced orbital periosteum. Early postseptal orbital cellulitis is indicated by edema of the retro-orbital fat and medial rectus muscle (*dashed white arrow*). One should always carefully look at the intracranial contents in anyone with sinusitis in order to detect intracranial complications, such as this gas-forming epidural abscess (*white arrows*).

occurs in the context of blunt or penetrating craniofacial trauma. Although a great deal of emergent orbital imaging is performed as a part of the workup for facial trauma, the authors limits his discussion to intraorbital emergencies that are not secondary to acute traumatic compromise of the bony orbit. Therefore, the authors focuses on penetrating intraorbital injury (see **Figs. 2–4**), orbital infections (see **Figs. 8–11**), and acute noninfectious inflammatory conditions of the neuro-ocular complex (see **Figs. 12** and **13**).

Penetrating Orbital Injury

It is usually not difficult for the clinician to determine if there has been a penetrating intraorbital event, as there is often obvious disruption to the external soft tissues on examination, with an accompanying complaint of ocular discomfort or vision impairment. Generally speaking, penetrating orbital injury usually implies 2 types of major consequences that require intervention: (1) direct injury to the intraorbital soft tissue structures (see **Fig. 2**) and (2) retention of an intraorbital foreign body (see **Figs. 3** and **4**). During situations in which an obvious foreign body is protruding from the orbit (see **Fig. 2**), attempts at removal should not be performed in the field for risk of exacerbating the injury and inducing intraorbital hematoma. Orbital penetration should be suspected in any patient with a history of high-velocity trauma to the face and orbits. This trauma includes shrapnel from explosions, wood shop mishaps, tree branches snapping back into one's face, poorly caught bridal bouquets, and other tragedies of daily life.

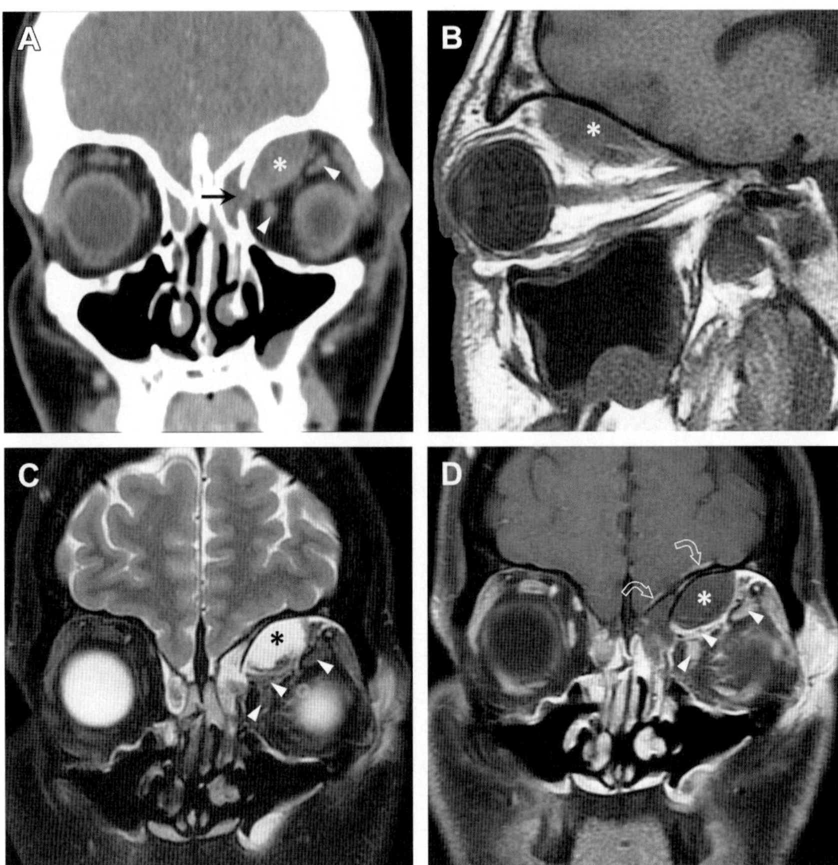

Fig. 9. Subperiosteal orbital abscess: Coronal CT scan (*A*) as well as oblique sagittal T1-weighted (*B*), coronal T2-weighted (*C*), and coronal postcontrast fat-suppressed T1-weighted (*D*) MR images demonstrate a large superomedial subperiosteal orbital abscess (*asterisk*) in this patient who presented with a 2-week history of progressive proptosis and visual loss. The lamina papyracea (*black arrow*) is seen to be eroded on the CT scan. The abscess is lenticular, centrally nonenhancing, and peripherally enhancing and causes marked mass effect on the superomedial group of extraocular muscles. The superior rectus, levator palpebrae superioris, medial rectus, and superior oblique muscles (*white arrowheads*) are inferolaterally displaced. Postseptal orbital cellulitis is manifested by dirty fat on the T2-weighted image, strandlike enhancement of orbital fascia, and poor definition and enhancement of the involved muscles (*white arrowheads*). Pachymeningeal enhancement (*curved white open arrows*) is present indicating early intracranial spread of infection.

One of the strongest imaging signs of a penetrating intraorbital injury is the presence of intraorbital air, particularly if it is seen within the extraocular musculature (see **Fig. 2**) or within the globe itself. In many cases, however, a penetrating object will take the path of least resistance and in doing so glance off of the firmest intraorbital structures, such as the sclera and tendon insertions, and the air will preferentially accumulate within the intraconal and extraconal fat. In these situations, any collection of intraorbital air that is either very focal in distribution, linear in configuration, associated with intraorbital hematoma (see **Figs. 4**, **6** and **7**) or foreign body (see **Figs. 3** and **4**), or seen in the absence of orbital wall fracture should raise suspicion of a penetrating injury. Furthermore, any accumulation of intraorbital air that is large enough to create significant mass effect should be separately discussed and suggested as a possible penetrating event. Excessive trapped retrobulbar air can result in a tension pneumo-orbit in which there is proptosis, stretching of the optic nerve, and tenting of the posterior globe. If overlooked, possible long-term sequelae of tension pneumo-orbit include optic nerve ischemia from compression of the ophthalmic artery or veins, optic nerve injury secondary to mass effect, retinal detachment, and blindness.[1,2]

Other imaging features of orbital injury may be more obvious, such as completely detached

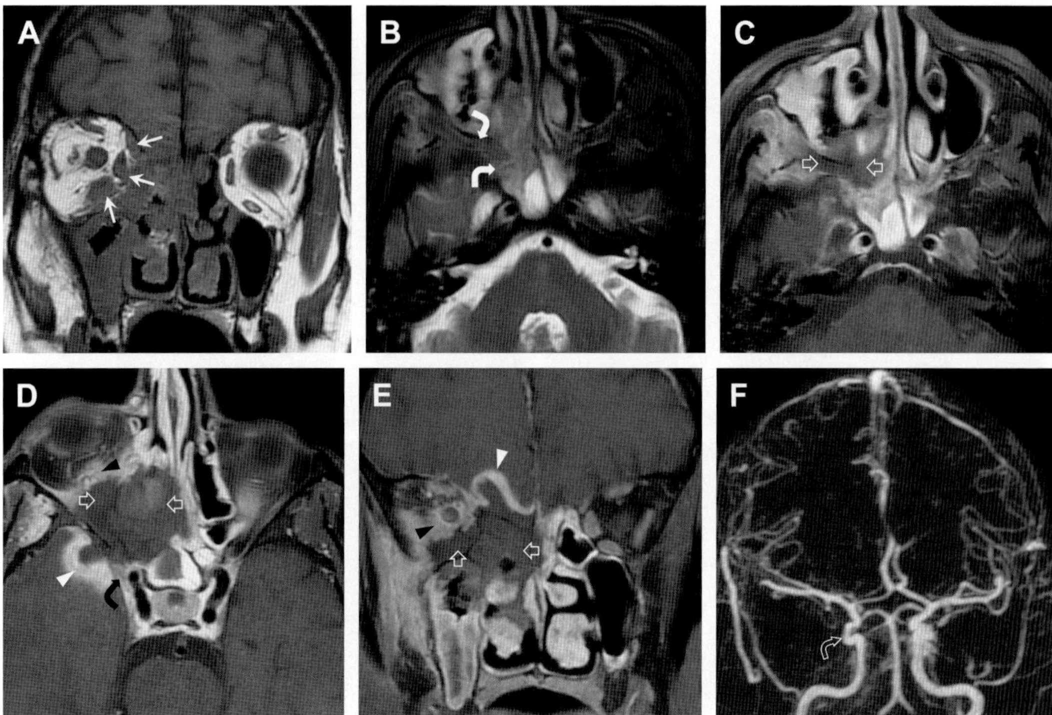

Fig. 10. Orbitorhinocerebral fungal infection (*Aspergillus*): Coronal T1-weighted (*A*), axial T2-weighted (*B*), as well as axial (*C, D*), coronal (*E*) postcontrast fat-suppressed T1-weighted, and contrast-enhanced MR angiographic (*F*) images in this immunocompromised patient demonstrate extensive infection of the sinuses, right orbit, and brain (frontal and temporal lobes). Postseptal orbital cellulitis is revealed by enlargement and peripheral irregularity of several extraocular muscles (*white arrows*). The fungal nature of the infection can be suspected by the T2 hypointense areas of inflammation in the sphenoid sinus and pterygopalatine fossa (*curved white arrows*). Postcontrast images reveal areas of abnormal enhancement (*black arrowheads*) within the orbit indicating orbital cellulitis as well as areas of rindlike enhancement (*white arrowheads*) within the frontal and temporal lobes of the brain consistent with cerebritis. Importantly, however, there are extensive central areas of nonenhancement (*open white arrows*) in the orbit and brain that indicate infected nonperfused necrotic tissue. These areas of necrosis must be surgically removed because the lack of perfusion means antibiotics will not reach these areas. Cavernous sinus thrombophlebitis is revealed by a lack of normal enhancement within the cavernous sinus on MR imaging (*curved black arrow*) and MR angiography (*curved open white arrow*).

extraocular muscles, lens dislocation or disruption (see **Figs. 3** and **4**), severed optic nerve, and deflated globe (see **Figs. 4** and **6**). Several subtle injuries may be missed unless one specifically looks for them. For example, the medial canthus should be inspected for disruption of the medial canthal ligament or avulsion of the bony attachment of this ligament (see **Fig. 5**), injury to the nasolacrimal drainage system (see **Fig. 5**), and hyphema (see **Figs. 4** and **6**). Medial canthal ligament avulsion may manifest as either focal hematoma in that location or lateral subluxation of the globe. Injuries to these structures usually require surgical repair. Similarly, injury to the lateral canthal region should not be overlooked. Inspection of this area should also include evaluation of the lacrimal gland, which is located within the extraconal fat within the anterior superolateral orbit. The lacrimal glands should be symmetric as well as homogeneous in CT attenuation and enhancement pattern. Focal fluid collections or linear hypoenhancing areas within the lacrimal gland are concerning for laceration. Contrast-enhancement may also facilitate the detection of partial-thickness lacerations through the extraocular muscle bellies, which may manifest as linear hypoenhancement extending along the path of injury or irregular margins of the muscle with stranding of the adjacent fat. The presence of a radiopaque foreign body in any of these locations suggests a penetrating injury until proven otherwise.

As mentioned earlier, the presence of intraorbital air can be associated with a retained foreign

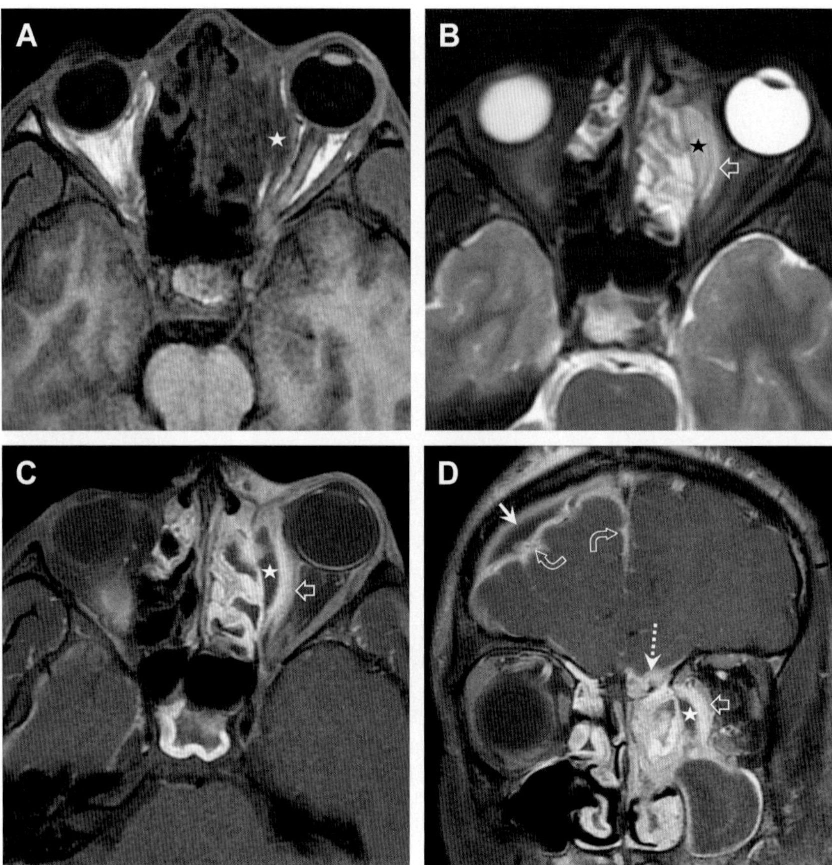

Fig. 11. Subperiosteal orbital abscess, orbital cellulitis, meningitis, subdural empyema: Axial T1-weighted (*A*), axial T2-weighted (*B*), as well as axial (*C*) and coronal (*D*) postcontrast fat-suppressed T1-weighted images demonstrate a subperiosteal orbital abscess (*star*) in this patient with progressive headache, retro-orbital pain, and loss of vision. Postseptal orbital cellulitis is revealed by edema and enhancement of the postseptal orbital fat. Orbital myositis is also present with edema, enlargement, peripheral irregularity, and enhancement of the medial rectus muscle (*open white arrows*). The coronal image reveals extensive intracranial spread of infection with abnormal enhancement of the leptomeninges (*curved open white arrows*), subdural empyema (*white arrow*) and frontal lobe cerebritis (*dashed white arrow*).

body, and the detection of one should prompt a search for the other. Most intraorbital foreign bodies tend to be made of metal or glass, and these materials are characteristically hyperdense on CT (see **Figs. 3** and **4**). MR obviously should be avoided if a ferromagnetic foreign body is suspected. The CT attenuation of glass is variable and ultimately depends on its mineral composition and manufacturing process, ranging anywhere from several thousand Hounsfield units (HU) to minus 200 HU.[3] There is less variability on CT for metallic fragments because most metal will near completely attenuate the x-ray beam. Metallic shavings and splinters are often extremely small but will demonstrate a high level of attenuation that is out of proportion to their size, accounting for their ability to be reliably detected on plain film radiography compared with other types of foreign bodies. In order to increase sensitivity for tiny metallic fragments, it is recommended that one also review images reconstructed with a bone algorithm. It is common for radiopaque foreign bodies to collect along the folds of the eyelids and between eyelashes, representing cutaneous periorbital debris instead of a true retained radiopaque foreign body. In contradistinction, any preseptal densities abutting the surface of the cornea and sclera or lying deep to the eyelid tarsus should raise suspicion of a foreign body either located on or below the conjunctival layer. The diagnosis is clinched by ophthalmologic examination with fluorescein. In addition to persistent eye irritation, retained inorganic foreign bodies can lead to the presence of intraorbital rust deposits as well as

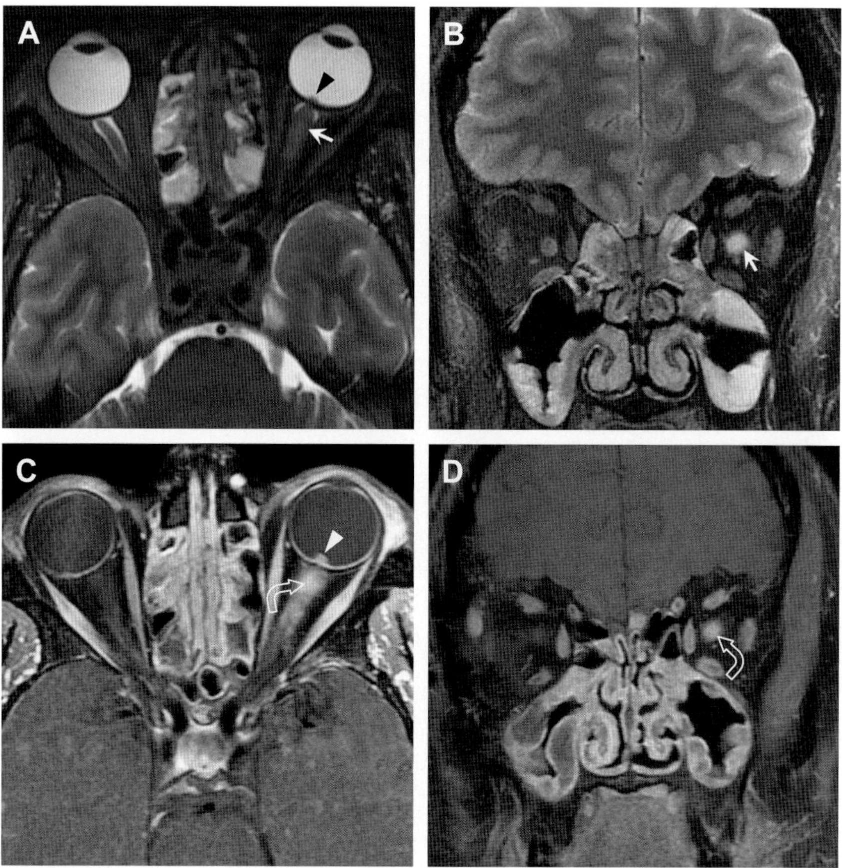

Fig. 12. Optic neuritis (neurosarcoidosis): Axial T2-weighted (*A*), coronal T2-weighted (*B*), as well as axial (*C*) and coronal (*D*) postcontrast fat-suppressed T1-weighted images were obtained in this patient with a 2-week history of retro-orbital pain, loss of vision, and left optic nerve papillitis. The T2-weighted images reveal marked enlargement and edema of the left optic nerve (*white arrows*) as well as marked papilledema (*black arrowhead*). There is a fuzzy appearance of the optic nerve on the coronal T2-weighted image indicating coexistent optic perineuritis. Contrast-enhanced images reveal extensive enhancement (*curved open white arrows*) of the optic nerve, optic sheath, and optic nerve head (*white arrowhead*). The presence of orbital pain, visual loss, and combination of optic neuritis and perineuritis suggest an inflammatory optic neuritis, such as neurosarcoidosis.

reactive aggregations of inflammatory cells. Removal of these foreign bodies is sometimes achieved by microreaming of the surrounding affected tissue.[4]

Although often heralding the presence of a foreign body in some case, intraorbital air may actually impede the identification of foreign bodies composed of wood or certain low-weight plastics. Retained wood products, whether they are fresh or old, are often radiolucent on CT as well as hypointense on most MR sequences, making it difficult to distinguish from air.[5] Although wood often approaches air attenuation on CT, inspecting the orbits with a dedicated lung window may help aid in detection and discrimination of these materials. The presence of an intraorbital wood product has added significance in that organic material is often redolent with bacteria and fungi and can ultimately lead to serious intraorbital infections.

Orbital Cellulitis

Many of the orbital infections leading to emergent imaging are limited to the superficial periorbital soft tissues that are relatively confined to the orbital septum, henceforth distinguished as preseptal cellulitis. It can represent local progression of a preceding skin or eyelid condition, such as blepharitis, furuncles, or other adjacent cutaneous infection. Consistent with its superficial cutaneous roots, *Streptococcus*, *Staphylococcus*, *Pneumococcus*, and *Pseudomonas* are among the most common infecting organisms. Preseptal cellulitis is usually unilateral and presents as marked

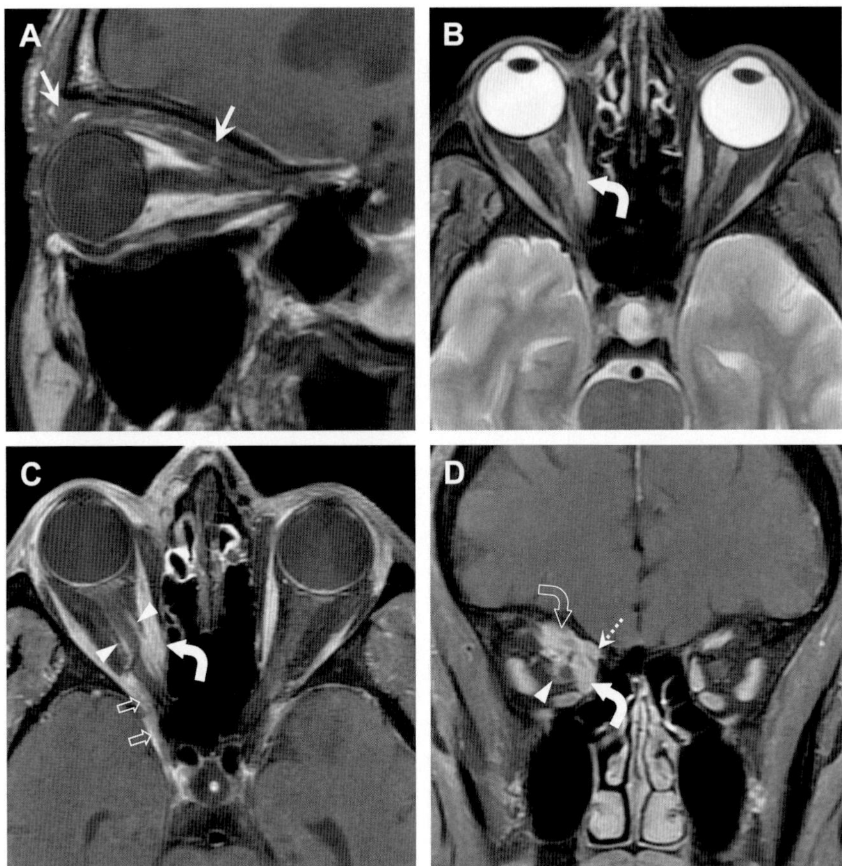

Fig. 13. Idiopathic orbital inflammatory disease: Oblique sagittal T1-weighted (*A*), axial T2-weighted (*B*), as well as axial (*C*) and coronal (*D*) postcontrast fat-suppressed T1-weighted images were obtained in this patient with painful ophthalmoplegia and rapid decrease of vision. There is an extensive ill-defined soft tissue mass (*white arrows*) extending along the superior rectus and levator palpebrae superioris muscle as far anteriorly as the upper eyelid. There is enlargement, edema, and abnormal enhancement of the medial rectus muscle (*curved white arrows*) as well as the superior rectus (*curved white open arrow*) and superior oblique (*dashed white arrow*) muscles. Optic perineuritis is manifested by abnormal enhancement of the optic sheath (*white arrowheads*). The ophthalmoplegia is likely caused by involvement of the cranial nerves 3, 4, and 6 as they traverse the inflammatory mass (*open white arrows*) in the superior orbital fissure and cavernous sinus.

induration, tenderness, and erythema of the eyelid, sometimes seen in association with a stye. Conversely, decreased visual acuity, restricted extraocular movements, exophthalmos, and marked injection and bogginess of the conjunctiva (chemosis) are not expected in preseptal cellulitis and should instead raise concern for an acute process occurring within the postseptal orbit. That being said, it is possible for chemosis to present in more advanced cases of preseptal cellulitis because of local reactive changes. Chemosis secondary to conjunctivitis can also be confused with orbital cellulitis on clinical evaluation, although the inflammatory findings are usually limited to the conjunctival membrane without other discrete signs to suggest postseptal cellulitis. Furthermore, conjunctivitis is often either allergic or viral in origin instead of bacterial; the presentation is, therefore, frequently bilateral.[4,6–8]

Radiology does not typically play a role in the diagnosis of acute conjunctivitis unless it is to exclude the additional presence of preseptal or postseptal cellulitis. In preseptal cellulitis, the radiologic findings will closely follow the clinical presentation, with marked thickening of the eyelid and adjacent superficial soft tissues as well as requisite sparing of the postseptal soft tissues. In severe cases, it may be possible to discern small fluid collections and microabscesses forming within the eyelid, which further secures the diagnosis. When evaluating the orbits, especially if preseptal cellulitis is suspected, close attention should be paid to the paranasal sinuses and nasolacrimal complex because infection and obstruction of these structures may incite edema within the preseptal soft tissues that masquerades as true cellulitis. It can be very difficult to distinguish early preseptal cellulitis from reactive preseptal edema. In fact, both entities may be present at the same time, although unilateral periorbital disease in the setting of bilateral sinusitis may be a clue of a distinct preseptal infection.[6–9] Inflammation and congestion of the preseptal soft tissues can also be secondary to an underlying postseptal infection.

The key imaging feature of postseptal cellulitis is stranding of the intraorbital fat (see **Fig. 9**), which represents a combination of edema, vascular congestion, increased microvascular permeability, and inflammatory infiltrates. As the infection progresses, the stranding may become more coalescent and exhibit increasing intraorbital mass effect. These inflammatory changes may cause stretching of the optic nerve and tenting of the posterior globe, thereby indicating an impending threat to the patients' vision.

Other critical developments in advanced postseptal cellulitis include the development of subperiosteal abscess (see **Figs. 8–11**), extraocular muscle myositis (see **Figs. 8–11**), formation of an intraorbital abscess, and orbital venous thrombophlebitis. Detection of muscular and vascular complications usually requires a contrast-enhanced CT or MR imaging examination, as opposed to the detection of intraorbital fat stranding, which is readily seen on noncontrast examinations. These entities will also necessitate more aggressive management and surveillance. Intraorbital abscesses should appear on CT as isodense to hypodense fluid collections with rim enhancement and perilesional edema. On MR, dedicated T2-weighted images with fat saturation may better delineate tiny fluid pockets scattered throughout the intraorbital soft tissues. Diffusion-weighted imaging also aids in the detection of intraorbital abscesses because these lesions may exhibit restricted diffusion, reflecting the viscous contents of the abscess cavity. This is particularly useful in situations in which contrast cannot be administered. MR imaging can also aid in the diagnosis of orbital thrombophlebitis, which may demonstrate as enlarged, T1-hyperintense veins seen against a background of extensive intraorbital edema. Of note, orbital thrombophlebitis can extend intracranially through valveless veins and result in thrombosis of the cavernous sinus (see **Fig. 10**). This severe complication is associated with high morbidity and mortality. The clinical presentations of cavernous sinus thrombosis and postseptal cellulitis can have tremendous overlap, including extraocular muscle restriction (vs palsy), proptosis, papilledema, headache, fever, and periorbital swelling. Additional palsies involving the V1 or V2 branches of the trigeminal nerve, lateral bowing of the cavernous sinus wall, or hypoenhancement of the cavernous sinuses (see **Figs. 8** and **10**) are, therefore, ominous findings.

As with preseptal cellulitis, the adjacent paranasal sinuses should be part of the search pattern when evaluating postseptal cellulitis. Most postseptal cellulitis cases start as bacterial ethmoid sinusitis (see **Figs. 8–11**) that has gained access to the orbits via foramina and tiny osseous fenestrations. For this same reason, the formation of a subperiosteal abscess between the periorbita and bony orbit often accompanies the diagnosis of postseptal cellulitis. This postseptal cellulitis typically appears as lenticular fluid collections (see **Figs. 8–11**) extending along the lamina papyracea or medial orbital roof, with extrinsic mass effect exerted on the medial conal and extraconal structures. Vision and ocular motility may be compromised as the subperiosteal abscess extends back to the orbital apex with compromise of the optic nerve and cranial nerves III to VI, respectively. In advanced cases, abscess formation can even be directed intracranially (see **Figs. 8** and **10**).[6,8]

Teaching point: Identification of intraorbital disease should prompt the evaluation of the paranasal sinuses for a potential underlying cause.

Noninfectious Orbital Inflammation

In the absence of intraorbital abscess or other clear evidence of orbital infection, inflammatory changes to the postseptal soft tissues are not necessarily specific on imaging.[10] Noninfectious conditions (see **Figs. 12** and **13**) may present with acute loss of vision, orbital pain, or impairment of ocular motility and require urgent evaluation as to the cause of the symptoms. Stranding of the intraorbital fat, proptosis, and periorbital edema is encountered across wide ranges of noninfectious conditions; the diagnosis cannot always be made on an imaging basis alone. Imaging, however, does play a role in identifying the presence of an inflammatory process and helping determine which of the intraorbital structures are involved.

For example, inflammatory changes that are primarily localized to the extraocular muscles and tendons (see **Fig. 13**) usually indicate a diagnosis of orbital myositis. These structures will be enlarged, hyperenhancing, and possess shaggy borders with adjacent fat stranding. Alternatively, inflammatory changes might be limited to the anterior and posteriors margins of the globe (episcleritis), optic nerve head (papillitis), optic sheath (perineuritis), Tenon's capsule (sclerotenonitis), various components of the uveal tract (uveitis), optic nerve sheath (perineuritis), optic nerve (optic neuritis), lacrimal gland (dacryoadenitis), and so forth. Inflammatory changes of the nasolacrimal complex (dacryocystitis) should trigger close inspection of the sinonasal cavity in order to exclude a possible obstructing lesion or infection.[6,11]

Intraorbital inflammatory changes may also encompass a larger set of structures that are related by a shared anatomic region, such as the entire anterior orbit (anterior orbital pseudotumor) and within the orbital apex (orbital apex inflammatory syndrome). All of these orbital inflammatory conditions may be considered part of a larger set of inflammatory diseases, collectively referred to as *idiopathic orbital inflammatory syndrome*, or sometimes *orbital pseudotumor* given their tendency to cause mass effect and non-neoplastic masslike expansion of the native intraorbital structures.[11,12] This inflammation is often idiopathic in that the inciting cause cannot be ascertained. When one encounters any one of these disease entities, one must also consider several systemic conditions, including cytoplasmic antineutrophil cytoplasmic antibody (c-ANCA)–positive granulomatosis with polyangiitis (formerly Wegener granulomatosis), rheumatoid arthritis, Sjögren syndrome, systemic lupus erythematosus, other autoimmune disorders, and sarcoidosis. Lymphoma, pseudolymphoma, and leukemia exist as both potential causes of orbital inflammatory syndrome as well as distinct mimics of the disease. Any of these conditions may manifest as a hypercellular, infiltrative intraorbital soft tissue mass with characteristic enhancement, restricted diffusion, and relative T2-hypointensity. Perusal of the patients' medical records is highly encouraged at this point.

Out of the abovementioned idiopathic inflammatory conditions of the orbit, perineuritis (see **Fig. 12**) of the optic nerve sheath may represent another potential diagnostic pitfall, occasionally being confused with optic neuritis. Clinically, these two diseases may each present as acute-onset intraorbital pain and vision loss, although only optic neuritis represents acute inflammation of the optic nerve fibers instead of the surrounding dural sheath. On CT, both disease entities may demonstrate apparent enlargement of the optic nerve-sheath complex with perineural fat stranding. In these cases, additional involvement of the Tenon's space may help make the diagnosis of perineuritis over optic neuritis, although this differentiating clue is not always available. The specific imaging features of optic neuritis are more readily apparent on MR, presenting as fusiform enlargement, T2 hyperintensity, and hyperenhancement of the affected nerve. Although this presentation may represent acute optic neuritis in isolation, dedicated imaging of the brain and spinal cord is recommended to evaluate for an underlying diagnosis of multiple sclerosis or neuromyelitis optica or other inflammatory and granulomatous conditions affecting the central nervous system (such as sarcoidosis).[6,11,13]

EMERGENCIES OF THE SINONASAL CAVITY

Acute complaints centered on the nasal cavity and paranasal sinuses are frequently encountered in the primary and emergent care settings, largely in thanks to the widespread existence of inflammatory sinus disease, environmental allergies, and the common cold. Although unpleasant in their own right, they rarely require urgent imaging. Urgent imaging of the sinuses may be necessary, however, when patients are immunocompromised, diabetic, or if there is clinical suspicion of orbital or intracranial extension of disease. In these situations, a more sinister process that could pose serious endangerment to patients must be excluded. Of these entities, the authors emphasizes complications of acute bacterial sinusitis, acute invasive fungal sinusitis, and fulminant epistaxis.

Acute Bacterial Sinusitis

Most acute rhinosinusitis cases are viral in cause and, therefore, exhibit a self-limiting course, assuming the absence of comorbid factors. However, persistent or worsening sinonasal symptoms, such as high fever, mucopurulent discharge, orbital pain, and periorbital edema, are concerning for more serious bacterial infections in immunocompetent patients. In particular, unilateral symptoms or symptoms persistent beyond 10 days from onset are worrisome for a bacterial sinusitis, possibly superimposed on a preceding viral infection.[14–16]

Several conditions usually need to be met in order for an acute bacterial sinusitis to develop; impairment of normal sinus drainage provides an opportunity for bacteria to establish themselves within the sinus cavity and is usually the result of multiple factors, including (1) obstructed sinus drainage pathways and ostia, (2) abnormal sinonasal mucosa, (3) decreased mucociliary clearance, and (4) abnormal consistency of sinus secretions. Impaired immune function is an additional risk factor for both bacterial and fungal sinus infections.

Most bacteria are introduced to the sinus cavities via the nasal mucosa and are caused by *Staphylococcus*, *Haemophilus*, *Streptococcus*, and *Moraxella* species. Additionally, several acute bacterial sinusitis cases are dental in origin (odontogenic) and can be caused by anaerobic infections. Therefore, the presence of sinonasal disease should trigger a close examination of the maxillary dentition, and vice versa.[15]

Inflammatory changes of the paranasal sinuses, regardless of their cause, are usually accompanied by enhancement and thickening of the mucosa, with varying degrees of submucosal edema and intraluminal secretions. The severity and pattern of these findings are not entirely specific to acute bacterial infection and can be observed in both chronic and nonbacterial disease. Air-fluid levels are lacking in complete specificity but are regarded as an important sign for identifying acute bacterial sinusitis.[15]

Incompletely treated or otherwise unmitigated acute bacterial sinusitis has the potential to extend beyond its original boundaries, resulting in various complications, usually in the form of subperiosteal abscesses (see **Figs. 8–11**). These complications may present themselves rather suddenly after a protracted course of sinonasal symptoms if the involved sinus cavity is subjected to a rapid increase in sinonasal pressure, such as with forceful nose blowing. For example, in the setting of acute ethmoidal sinusitis, the infection can extend laterally through the lamina papyracea, producing a subperiosteal abscess along the medial and superomedial walls of the orbit. Frontal sinusitis has the option of extending through either the outer or inner cortex of the frontal bone. Permeation through the outer table can result in abscess formation in the superficial soft tissues of the scalp, which will present clinically as a fluctuant inflammatory mass along the forehead (Pott puffy tumor). With further extension of the myofasciitis, there will be involvement of the frontalis muscle. Extension of sinusitis through the inner table of the frontal sinus can result in formation of epidural or subdural empyema, meningitis, or frontal lobe encephalitis. Frontal sinusitis can extend through a pneumatized horizontal plate of the frontal bone directly into the orbit. Complications from acute sphenoid sinusitis can manifest as osteomyelitis of the skull base, cavernous sinus thrombophlebitis (see **Fig. 10**), or abscess formation along the retroclival and paracavernous regions.[14,15]

Teaching point: Identification of sinonasal disease should prompt inspection of the dentition just as identification of intraorbital disease should prompt inspection of the sinuses (the inverse is also true).

Acute Invasive Fungal Sinusitis

There are various forms that fungal infections of the nasal cavity and paranasal sinuses can take; but the most aggressive type, and the one carrying the worst prognosis, is acute invasive (fulminant) fungal sinusitis. This infection is almost exclusively encountered in patients with impaired immune systems (AIDS, organ transplantation, systemic neoplasms, chemotherapy recipients) or other significant systemic metabolic disease (poorly controlled diabetes, renal failure, cirrhosis), so being aware of these major preexisting medical problems beforehand is an important step toward making the diagnosis.

In the immunocompromised patient population, fungal sinonasal infection is usually secondary to *Aspergillus* species (see **Fig. 10**), which are ubiquitous in the environment and gain access to the paranasal sinuses by colonizing the nasal mucosa. Fungi belonging to the Zygomycetes class (*Rhizopus*, *Mucor*) thrive in glucose-rich environments. This fact coincides with the general consensus that severely diabetic patients (for example, those presenting in acute ketoacidosis) are the prototypical target population, although immunocompromised patients are also certainly at high risk. Regardless of the specific fungal species at work or the clinical background, acute fulminant fungal sinusitis is consistent in its characteristic rapid progression and aggressive invasion through the sinus walls and extension along blood vessels into adjacent structures (see **Fig. 10**). Intraorbital or intracranial spread of disease can occur as quickly as within 24 to 72 hours; severe complications include the development of subperiosteal abscess, empyema, meningitis, cerebritis, cerebral infarction, dural and cavernous sinus thrombosis, and often death. Despite rapid intervention with surgical debridement and high-dose intravenous antifungal agents, the overall mortality rate remains extremely high.[14,15,17]

On imaging, acute invasive fungal sinusitis can share features with other forms of sinusitis, including T2 hyperintense mucosa that is thickened and enhancing; but fungal infection should be suspected in the presence of debris that is T2 hypointense and restricts diffusion. Early invasive fungal sinusitis can be primarily a soft tissue infection. Later on, erosive changes to the adjacent sinus wall with transosseous spread are more obvious imaging clues for invasive fungal sinusitis. These changes, however, are not required to make the diagnosis but may only be seen in advanced stages of the disease. Early invasion is often conducted along small traversing vessels of the skull base, allowing unencumbered spread into the intracranial space via natural foramina.[18] It is quite important to look for areas of hypoenhancement on imaging in these patients. These areas usually indicate necrotic nonperfused tissue (see **Fig. 10**) that must be surgically debrided because antibiotics will not be able to penetrate these areas.

Teaching point: Osseous destruction can be a late sign of acute invasive fungal sinusitis. Any sinonasal process associated with T2 hypointensity and restricted diffusion should raise concern for an aggressive disease process, despite apparent intact bony architecture.

Epistaxis: Hemoptysis

The authors admits that nosebleeds are usually a self-limited condition bearing little to no significant clinical consequence. Most cases are associated with irritation or injury to a rich vascular plexus (Kiesselbach plexus) within the anterior nasal septum and easily treated with transient pressure. The eruption of blood from the nasal cavity is often a nonspecific finding but can, on occasion, indicate the presence of a serious underlying condition. In particular, high volume and recurrent epistaxis is more likely to be caused by several worrisome medical conditions, including benign and malignant neoplasms, accidental and iatrogenic trauma, granulomatous disease, vascular malformations (both acquired and hereditary), and acute sinusitis (bacterial or fungal). These conditions can be associated with high morbidity and mortality, so effective and appropriate treatment relies on a timely diagnosis.[19,20]

In theory, epistaxis can be induced by any process that leads to injury or derangement of the normal vasculature. Therefore, the differential for intranasal bleeding is broad. Generally speaking, epistaxis can be categorized by location: anterior versus posterior, lateral versus septal, and internal versus external carotid supply.

The nasal cavity receives blood supply from both the internal carotid (via branches of the ophthalmic artery) and external carotid arteries (via branches of the sphenopalatine and facial arteries). The territories of these arterial branches demonstrate a high degree of overlap, which carries 2 important consequences: (1) It provides a robust network of collateral flow to preserve the viability of delicate soft tissues throughout the nasal cavity. (2) It allows for anastomotic routes between the internal and external arterial circulation. Both scenarios can complicate the management of epistaxis, which may be refractory in some cases or associated with unintentional embolization of the retina or brain in others.

In the region of the anterior nasal cavity, 2 important anastomotic sites should be considered. One is between the dorsal nasal artery (a terminal branch of the ophthalmic artery) and angular artery (a terminal branch of the facial artery) at the level of the medial canthus, sometimes referred to as the *orbital point*. Another is between the superior labial artery (another terminal branch of the facial artery) and the anterior ethmoidal artery, at the level of the columella.[21]

In the posterior nasal cavity, anastomotic connections exist between the branches of the sphenopalatine artery and ethmoidal branches of the ophthalmic artery as well as with the greater palatine artery. The presence and arrangement of these connections tend to be highly variable between individual patients, so they are not described here.[21]

The branches of the anterior and posterior vascular supply intersect at a rich vascular plexus along the anterior nasal septum, also known as *Kiesselbach plexus* or *Little's area*. This site is common for epistaxis, particularly in children, and is often easily treated with tamponade. Treatment of posterior epistaxis can also be attempted with nasal packing but may require more invasive interventions, such as clipping or embolization.[22–24]

Hemoptysis (expectoration of blood, blood-stained sputum) usually has its source lower in the airway (pharynx, larynx, trachea, bronchi, lungs) and is discussed more thoroughly later in the article (**Fig. 14**).

EMERGENCIES OF THE TEMPORAL BONE

When considering the temporal bone, many people think primarily about the part of our anatomy that is chiefly concerned with hearing, whereas, in all fairness, it interfaces with a diverse set of equally important and functionally disparate structures. Therefore, evaluation of the temporal bone should include inspection of more than the ossicles, labyrinth, and internal/external auditory canals. Among other things, the petrous internal carotid canal, sigmoid sinus, jugular foramen, facial nerve, Meckel cave, and cranial fossae are all potential sites of collateral damage in temporal bone disease.

Necrotizing (Malignant) Otitis Externa

Not to be confused with the more frequently encountered swimmer's ear, malignant otitis externa is a severe necrotizing infection of the external ear and subadjacent skull base. It is typically caused by *Pseudomonas aeruginosa* and is seen in patients who are elderly, diabetic, and/or

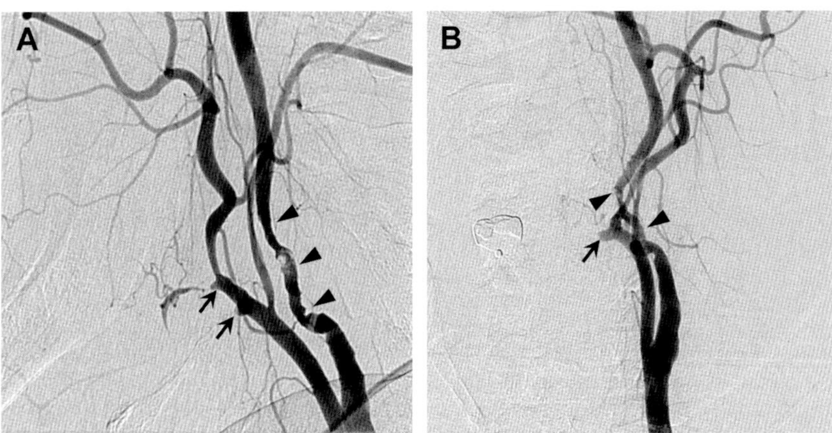

Fig. 14. Hemoptysis, carotid blowout, advanced tonsillar squamous cell carcinoma: Lateral (*A*) and anteroposterior (*B*) carotid angiogram images in a patient presenting with hemoptysis. The patient had a history of recurrent squamous cell carcinoma of the tonsil that was encasing the carotid bifurcation on CT scans (not shown). The angiogram demonstrates narrowing and irregularity of a long segment of the internal carotid artery (*arrowheads*) at the site of carotid encasement. Two focal areas of external carotid artery ulceration (*arrows*) are present at the sites of the carotid blowout.

immunocompromised. Clinically, these patients present with severe otalgia, purulent otorrhea, and inflammatory changes tracking along the external ear and external auditory canal. Radiologically, one may expect to discover an erosive soft tissue mass in this location, with blatant violation of the underlying osseous boundaries. Invasion of the temporomandibular joint, parotid gland mastoid process, middle cranial fossae, and cranial nerves can be features of this disease, so it is not hard to imagine why this particular process has an associated high mortality rate.

Acute Otomastoiditis

Acute bacterial infections of the tympanic cavity and mastoid air cells share several features with acute bacterial infections of the paranasal sinuses. That is, most infections are usually the result of either *Haemophilus* or *Streptococcus* species in the setting of impaired drainage of the mastoid air cells and tympanic spaces. This setup is most notably encountered in younger children, given the more horizontal configuration of the eustachian tubes in early age, although sterile mastoid and tympanic effusions are frequently encountered and often carry no acute clinical significance. However, opacification of the air spaces in a patient with fever, otalgia, middle ear effusion, and postauricular headache are classic signs of acute otomastoiditis. As with acute bacterial sinusitis, the presence of air-fluid levels in the mastoid air cells is very suggestive of acute otomastoiditis.

Also, as seen in acute bacterial sinusitis, acute otomastoiditis can be further complicated by extension beyond the confines of the mastoid process and tympanic space. Externally directed extension in the overlying soft tissues may manifest as subperiosteal abscess formation along the mastoid process surrounded by periauricular cellulitis. A specific form of subperiosteal abscess (Bezold abscess) occurs when the abscess arises along the inferior tip of the mastoid process, around the digastric groove, and extends along the insertion of the sternocleidomastoid muscle (**Fig. 15**). This abscess is most readily identified as a rim-enhancing fluid collection on coronal plane imaging.[14]

Medially directed extension of the infectious process may result in extension through the sigmoid plate into the subdural or epidural spaces of the posterior fossa. As a consequence of this location, the infection may cause sigmoid sinus thrombophlebitis and impairment of sigmoid and transverse sinus venous drainage (**Fig. 16**). This impairment can, in turn, lead to increased intracranial pressure and venous infarctions, often in the distribution of the vein of Labbé. These patients may have additional symptoms of photophobia, retro-orbital headache, dizziness, and nausea. Dedicated imaging of the dural venous sinuses with CT venography (CTV) or MR venography (MRV) may be indicated. On CTV, a hyperdense appearance of the dural sinuses on precontrast imaging, or a hypoenhancing filling defect on postcontrast imaging, are useful clues in making the

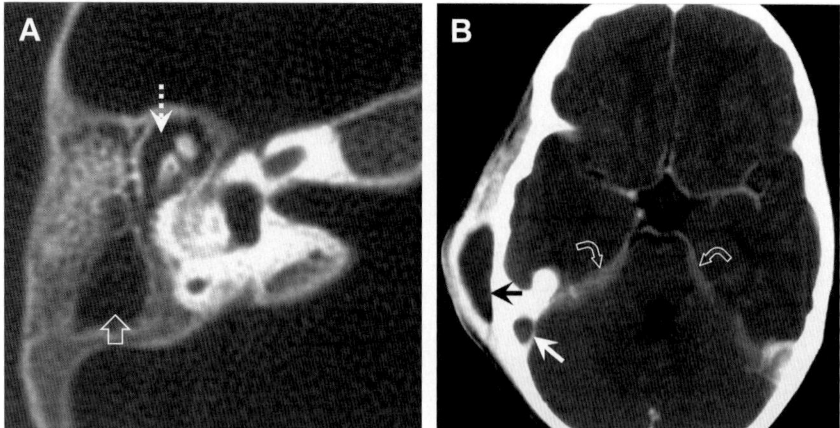

Fig. 15. Acute otomastoiditis, subperiosteal (Bezold) abscess, dural venous thrombophlebitis: A 4-year-old unresponsive child with rapid development of a mass extending along the lateral aspect of the right temporal bone into the upper aspect of the sternocleidomastoid muscle. Contrast-enhanced temporal bone CT scans (*A*, *B*) demonstrate opacification of the tympanic (*dashed white arrow*) and mastoid (*open white arrow*) cavities but no obvious cortical bone erosion. There is a large peripherally enhancing subperiosteal abscess (*black arrow*) lateral to the mastoid and squamous portions of the temporal bone. There is thrombosis of the sigmoid sinus (*white arrow*) and signs of meningitis with abnormal enhancement of the tentorium (curved open *white arrows*).

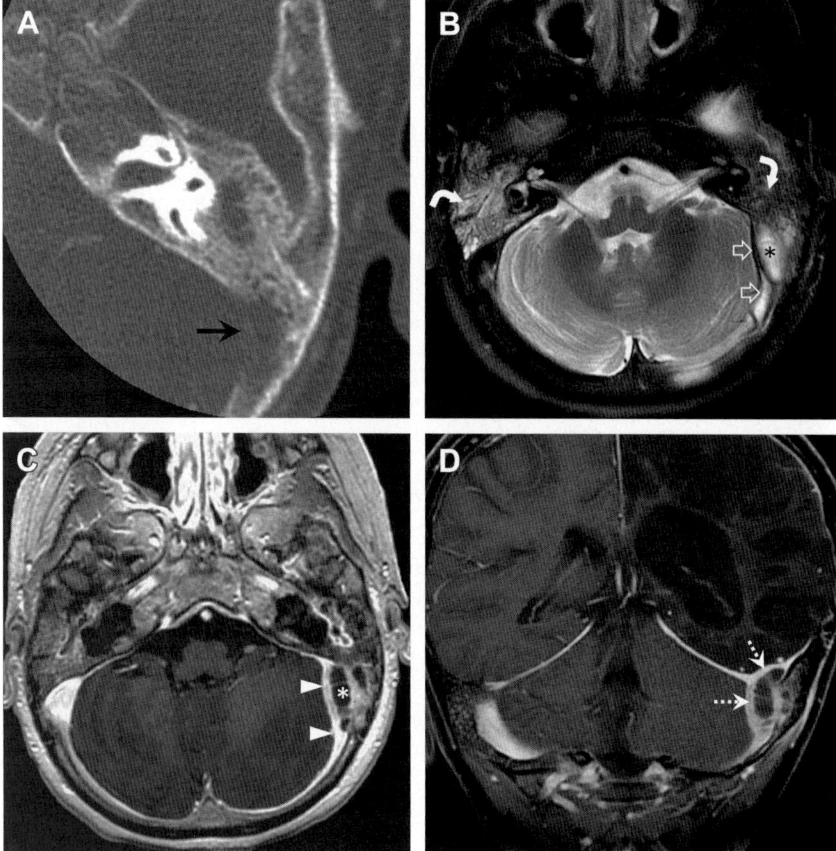

Fig. 16. Acute otomastoiditis, epidural abscess, dural venous thrombophlebitis: A 3-year-old boy who presented 10 days earlier with progressive right hemipareses and unresponsiveness. Contrast-enhanced temporal bone CT (*A*) reveals destruction of bone adjacent to the sigmoid sinus secondary to osteomyelitis (*black arrow*). Noncontrast axial T2-weighted scan (*B*) reveals bilateral tympanomastoid fluid (*curved white arrows*) consistent with acute tympanomastoiditis. The left sigmoid sinus (*open arrows*) is compressed and displaced away from the petrous bone by an epidural abscess (*asterisk*). Contrast-enhanced T1-weighted axial (*C*) and coronal (*D*) scans confirm the presence of the epidural abscess (*asterisk*) as well as severe compression and inflammation of the sigmoid sinus (*white arrowheads*). The epidural location of the abscess is confirmed on the coronal image because of its extension above and below the tentorium (*dashed white arrows*) and displacement of the sigmoid sinus away from the skull. Note the extensive infarction of the left cerebral hemisphere caused by cortical venous and vein of Labbé thrombophlebitis.

diagnosis. Identification of dural venous thrombosis is more complicated on MR imaging–MRV because the signal intensity of thrombus evolves over time with changes of the hemoglobin moiety, cellular integrity, and relative protein/water content over time. For example, subacute thrombus may be indistinguishable from normally opacified sinus on postcontrast T1-weighted imaging as well as hypointense flow voids on T2-weighted imaging (see **Fig. 16**). Therefore, in addition to conventional MR imaging, the authors adds 2D and 3-dimensional phase contrast MRV to the imaging protocols.

Severe otomastoiditis can also progress along the septations of the mastoid process, resulting in their eventual breakdown (coalescent mastoiditis) (see **Figs. 15** and **16**). This breakdown occurs when small microabscesses accumulate under the mucosal layer lining the mastoid air cells leading to bony demineralization induced by local pressure and osteolytic enzymes. Dedicated temporal bone CT is the optimal imaging choice for identifying this particularly aggressive form of acute mastoiditis and will demonstrate either partial or complete absence of the bony septa. The treatment of coalescent mastoiditis usually requires surgical drainage in addition to antibiotic therapy, so the distinction needs to be made from simple acute mastoiditis.[25]

In some cases, acute otomastoiditis may extend anteromedially to involve the petrous portion of the temporal bone. Petrous apicitis is essentially osteomyelitis of the petrous bone and may on occasion present as Gradenigo syndrome, with otorrhea, facial pain or otalgia, and sixth cranial nerve palsy (**Fig. 17**). Associations with V1-branch trigeminal

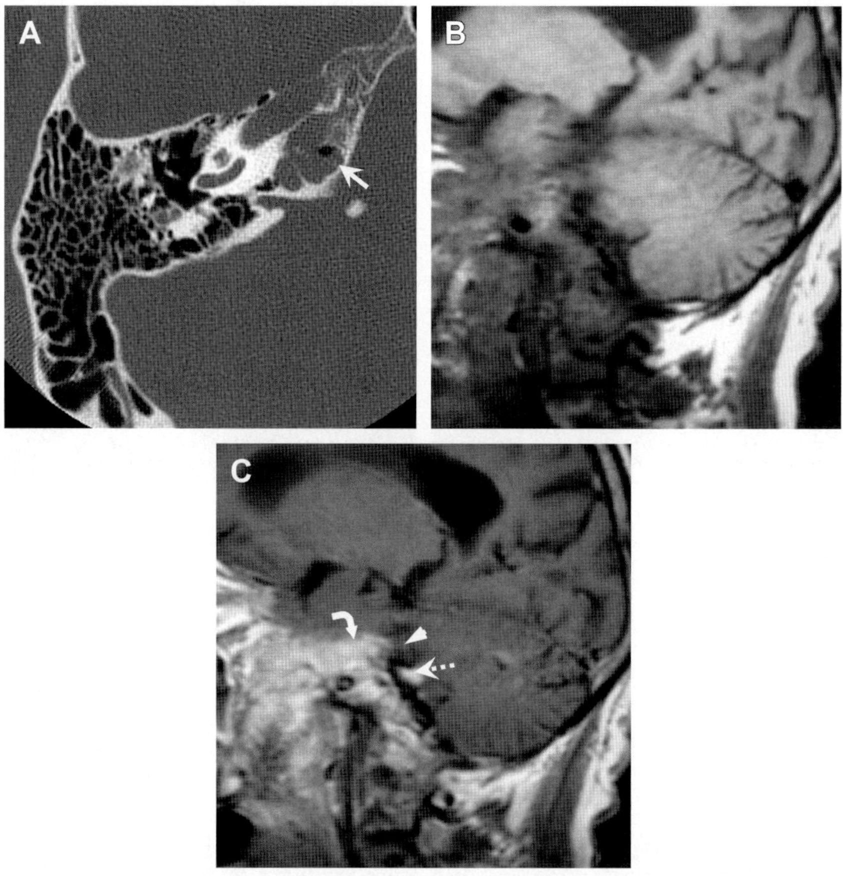

Fig. 17. Gradenigo syndrome: Axial CT (*A*), sagittal noncontrast T1-weighted MR (*B*), and sagittal postcontrast T1-weighted MR (*C*) images in a patient presenting with the triad of unilateral periorbital pain, sixth nerve palsy, and otorrhea. Initial workup of otorrhea by CT revealed extensive petrous apicitis (*white arrow*) that progressed over the next 2 weeks to the full triad of symptoms. Contrast-enhanced T1-weighted MR demonstrates diffuse enhancement of the petrous apex (*curved white arrow*), cranial nerves within the internal auditory canal (*dashed white arrow*), as well as faint enhancement of the preganglionic segment of the trigeminal nerve (*white arrowhead*).

neuralgia and facial nerve palsy have also been reported, given the proximity of the petrous bone to the Meckel cave and the geniculate fossa, respectively.[14,25]

Teaching point: Air-fluid levels anywhere in the head and neck regions should raise suspicion of an acute infection, unless a different explanation can be found.

Labyrinthitis and Facial Neuropathies

The clinical triad of otalgia, sensorineural hearing loss, and vertigo in the acute setting should raise suspicion for inflammation of the inner ear and the seventh and eighth cranial nerve complex. Inflammatory are most readily visualized on MR imaging as abnormal enhancement along the course of the facial nerve and/or membranous labyrinthine structures. Enhancement within the geniculate and mastoid segments of the facial nerve can be seen in normal patients. Enhancement within the labyrinthine, canalicular, and cisternal segments of the facial nerve should always be regarded as abnormal until proven otherwise. In addition to infectious and inflammatory causes of facial nerve or labyrinthine enhancement, do not forget to consider schwannomas, neuromas, ossifying hemangiomas, and perineural tumor spread.

Idiopathic facial nerve palsy (Bell palsy) (**Fig. 18**) is the most common cause of acute peripheral facial nerve dysfunction and is thought to be viral in cause. It has a fairly distinct clinical presentation and course, and imaging is not routinely obtained if the clinical findings are straightforward. MR imaging is useful in atypical cases for excluding other causes of acute facial nerve palsy (neoplasm, infarct, perineural tumor spread). Bell palsy usually causes only minimal enlargement of the nerve, enhances homogeneously, and exhibits no significant nodularity of the nerve. Any nodularity or significant focal enlargement of the

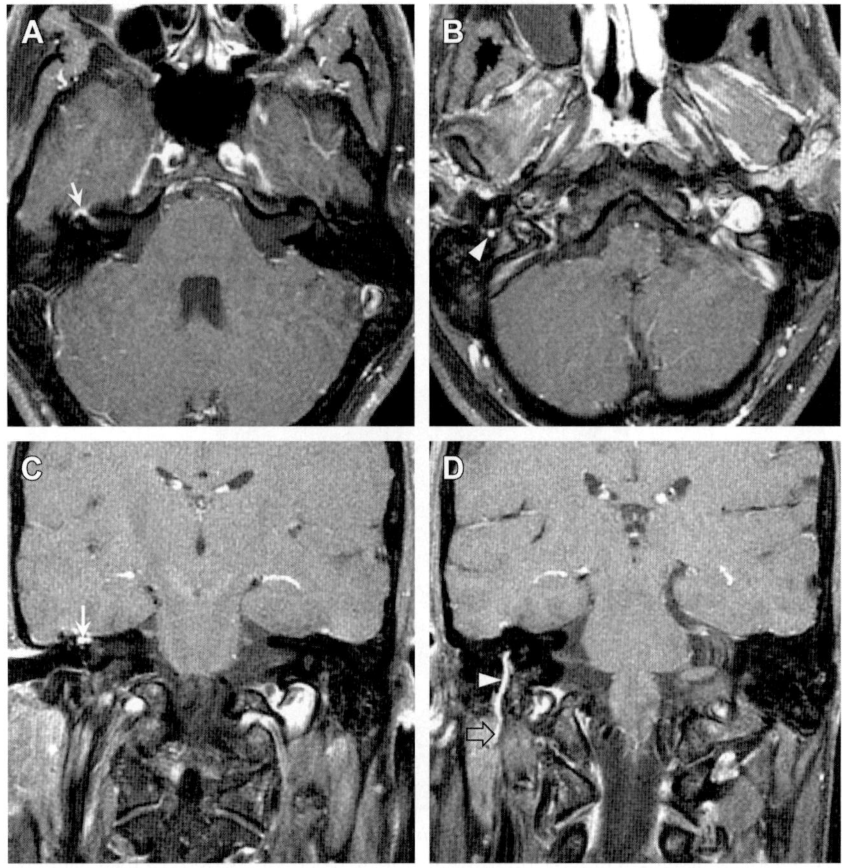

Fig. 18. Bell palsy: Axial (*A, B*) and coronal (*C, D*) contrast-enhanced T1-weighted images were obtained in this patient who presented with a 2-day history of progressive right peripheral facial nerve palsy. The images reveal marked enhancement of the geniculate (*white arrows*), tympanic, mastoid (*white arrowheads*), and parotid (*open black arrow*) segments of the facial nerve. There should be no significant enlargement or nodularity of the nerve in order to confidently make a diagnosis of Bell palsy.

nerve would argue against Bell palsy as a cause (**Fig. 19**).

Another commonly encountered cause of acute inflammatory facial nerve palsy is herpes zoster infection of the external ear and facial nerves. This infection is termed *herpes zoster oticus* or *Ramsay-Hunt syndrome* (**Fig. 20**). Imaging findings may mimic those of Bell palsy, although there is often more cutaneous edema and other cranial nerves may be involved. Ramsay-Hunt syndrome should also be clinically apparent in patients who presents with facial nerve palsy and painful vesicles over the external ear and adjacent facial soft tissues.[25] Sometimes, however, the facial palsy may predate the skin eruptions; the diagnosis may not be immediately obvious, and MR imaging may be required to make the diagnosis in an expeditious manner.

Lyme disease, caused by the spirochete *Borrelia burgdorferi*, is another infectious cause of acute facial nerve palsy, which can be confused with Bell palsy. The diagnosis often depends on a known exposure history in an area that is endemic to the *Ixodes* deer tick, which transmits the spirochete to humans. The clinical presentation may include arthralgias, erythema migrans rash, positive cerebrospinal fluid analysis, and involvement of multiple cranial nerves.

Labyrinthitis refers to any inflammatory or infectious condition that affects the membranous and sensorineural portions of the inner ear. The most common causes are viral and may be preceded by a stereotypical prodrome; but other forms of the disease include autoimmune labyrinthitis, vasculitis (eg, polyarteritis nodosa), and granulomatous disease (eg, granulomatosis with

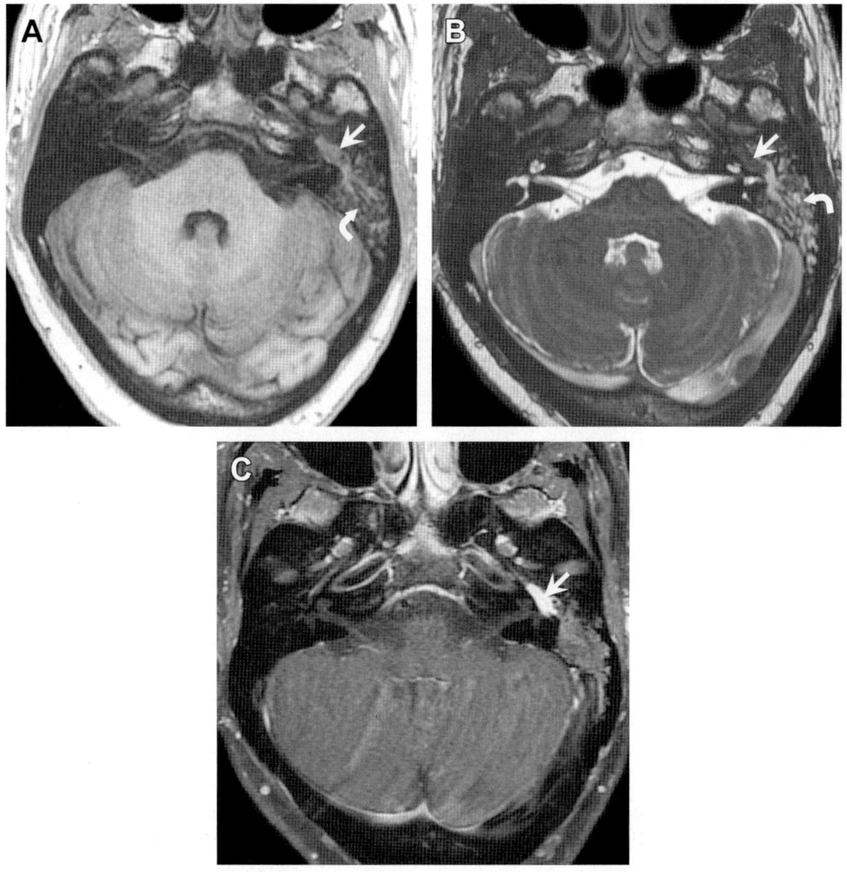

Fig. 19. Bell palsy mimic (ossifying hemangioma): Axial T1-weighted (*A*), T2-weighted (*B*), and postcontrast T1-weighted (*C*) MR images were obtained in this patient who presented with a 1-month history of progressive right facial nerve palsy. The images reveal a T2 hypointense, contrast-enhancing mass in the region of the geniculate ganglion (*white arrows*). The mass is obstructing the hypotympanum resulting in a mastoid effusion (*curved white arrows*). This lesion is inconsistent with Bell palsy because of its masslike nature and prolonged 1-month progression of the facial palsy.

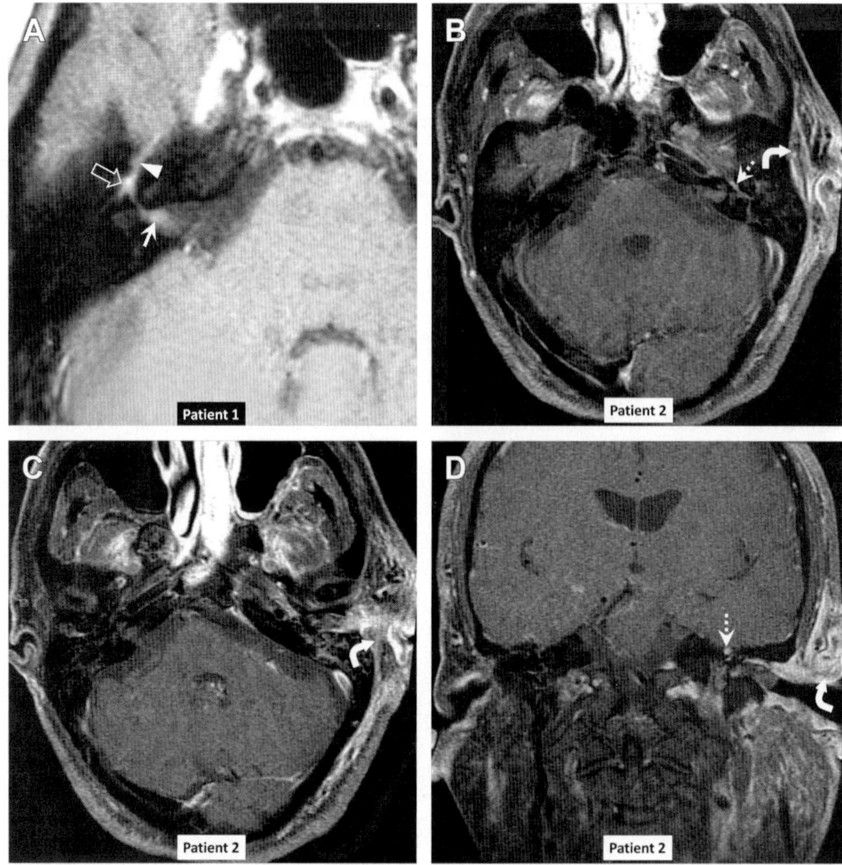

Fig. 20. Ramsay-Hunt syndrome: Two patients with rapid onset of facial nerve palsy, otalgia, and vesicular skin eruption over the ear indicating Ramsay-Hunt syndrome. Patient 1 (*A*): Contrast-enhanced T1-weighted image demonstrates abnormal nonexpansile enhancement of the facial nerve genu (*white open arrow*) and greater superficial petrosal nerve (*white arrowhead*). There is hazy enhancement of the cranial nerves within the internal auditory canal (*white arrow*). The enhancement more consistent with a viral neuritis other than Bell palsy. Patient 2 (*B–D*): Contrast-enhanced T1-weighted axial (*B, C*) and coronal (*D*) MR images reveal very subtle enhancement of the facial nerve genu (*white dashed arrows*). There is marked edema and enhancement of the soft tissues around the left ear (*curved white arrows*) because of the presence of extensive vesicular eruption of the skin. This amount of soft tissue involvement is not associated with Bell palsy and more suggestive of Ramsay-Hunt syndrome.

polyangiitis). Bacterial labyrinthitis is considerably less common but might be encountered in severe cases of prolonged, intractable otomastoiditis. On imaging, abnormally decreased T2 signal intensity of the perilymphatic labyrinthine structures may be seen in addition to postcontrast enhancement.[25,26]

Teaching point: Enhancement of the postgeniculate (postganglionic) segments of the facial nerve can be a normal finding. However, asymmetric enhancement, nodularity, thickening, or extension to the cisternal/canalicular portions of the nerve are suggestive of disease.

EMERGENCIES OF THE GLANDULAR TISSUES

A clinical history of painful neck mass or throat pain will usually prompt the acquisition of a contrast-enhanced CT scan of the neck, typically with the intention of uncovering some acute insult to the salivary glands, tonsils, or lymph nodes. It is important to investigate the patients' relevant clinical history for prior malignancies of the head and neck, prior surgical interventions, autoimmune disorders, or immunosuppression. In the following section, the authors limits the discussion to sialoadenitis and tonsillitis, ranging from the acute inflammatory stage to abscess formation. It should be noted that cervical lymphadenopathy may follow a similar disease course, with features of early inflammation followed by apparent suppuration and cavitation. It is not formally discussed here because lymphadenopathy is often a nonspecific finding, often accompanying other cervical infections caused by reactive changes or, in some cases, malignancy masquerading as infection. In short, abnormal lymph nodes need to be followed to resolution or biopsied if still abnormal after completion of the treatment course.

Acute Sialoadenitis

There is a wide range of pathologic conditions that can lead to acute inflammatory changes of the salivary glands, including various infections, radiation therapy, facial trauma, autoimmune disorders, and ductal obstruction by calculi or neoplasms. Despite the broad differential, patients with acute sialoadenitis usually present with similar symptoms: facial swelling and tenderness, salivary pain that is exacerbated by oral intake, and dry mouth. Acute parotitis, specifically, can be associated with facial paresis and taste disturbances, secondary to inflammatory changes of the facial nerve as it courses through the gland, carrying with it efferent motor and afferent gustatory nerve fibers. Further involvement of parasympathetic fibers within the chorda tympani and lingual nerves may also contribute to submandibular and sublingual gland dysfunction.[14,27–29]

During the acute inflammatory phase, the imaging features of sialoadenitis are potentially nonspecific, usually demonstrating a salivary gland that is enlarged, edematous, and hyperenhancing on both CT and MR imaging (**Fig. 21**). However, there are additional features that may help narrow the differential, such as laterality, precontrast attenuation pattern, evidence of ductal obstruction, and presence of sialoliths.

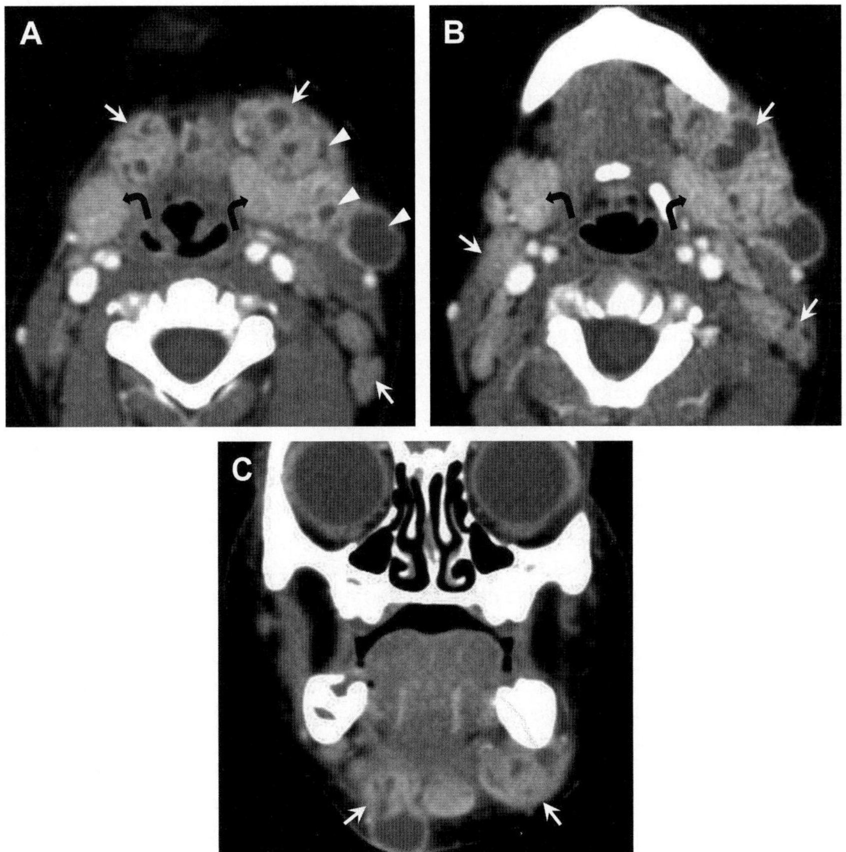

Fig. 21. Atypical mycobacterial sialadenitis and lymphadenitis: A 6-month-old child presenting to the emergency department with fever, progressive neck swelling, and difficulty feeding. Axial (*A, B*) and coronal (*C*) contrast-enhanced CT scans demonstrate extensive submandibular region suppurative lymphadenitis (*white arrows*) with numerous small peripherally enhancing intranodal abscesses (*white arrowheads*). There is abnormal diffuse homogeneous enhancement of the bilateral submandibular glands (*curved black arrows*) consistent with sialadenitis. The epidemiologic evidence suggests that infections like these are acquired from environmental sources, including soil, water, dust, and aerosols. The differential diagnosis is broad and includes lymphadenitis caused by mycobacterium tuberculosis, infectious mononucleosis, cat-scratch disease, brucellosis, actinomycosis, and nocardiosis.

Most unilateral infectious sialoadenitis cases are secondary to bacterial infections, most often involving beta-hemolytic *Streptococcus, Staphylococcus aureus, Streptococcus pneumonia,* and atypical mycobacterial (see **Fig. 21**). Acute sialadenitis is usually seen in the setting of an obstructing sialolith (80%–90% of cases). The submandibular gland is the most commonly involved salivary gland (70%–80% of cases), followed by the parotid gland (10%–20%); the sublingual and minor salivary glands rarely demonstrate primary involvement in acute infectious sialoadenitis but may be secondarily inflamed. The submandibular glands are considered to be most susceptible to intraductal calculus formation and secondary sialoadenitis, owing to the relatively large size of the Wharton duct, small papillary orifice, the ascending course of the duct into the floor of the mouth, higher viscosity of the secretions, and slower salivary flow rate. The opposite can be said about the parotid gland.[14,27–29]

In addition to the nonspecific imaging features of acute inflammation, cases of acute bacterial sialoadenitis can usually be confidently distinguished from other causes of salivary gland disease and not just because it is the statistically most likely choice. Inflammatory changes of the submandibular or parotid gland that are unilateral, associated with dilation and enhancement of the salivary duct, and seen in the presence of a distal obstructing calculus is diagnostic. CT is the optimal modality for identifying calcified sialoliths, which can be easily overlooked on MR imaging. Absence of calculi does not necessarily exclude the diagnosis of obstructive sialoadenitis. Very small calculi may be potentially obscured by dental artifacts or have already passed out of the orifice by the time of the study. However, all cases of sialoadenitis in which an obstructing sialolith is not identified will necessitate further follow-up for any underlying malignant lesions of the oral cavity.[14,27–29]

The treatment of acute bacterial sialoadenitis usually entails a course of antibiotics with broad enough coverage for any potential oral flora, robust hydration, and salivatory promoters (lemons). Small calculi, if present, will often pass on their own, although larger obstructing sialoliths may need to be surgically retrieved. Surgical drainage may also be required in cases of abscess formation. Sometimes gland excision is necessary if there is a history of recurrent/refractory acute/chronic sialoadenitis.

Making the diagnosis of salivary gland abscess can be problematic. The key imaging features are well-circumscribed focus of central low attenuation surrounded by a thin rim of enhancement and inflamed surrounding glandular tissue (see **Fig. 21**). Unfortunately, coalescent edema, nondrainable cellulitis, ductal and acinar dilatation, and preexisting areas of hypoenhancing fibrosis can potentially mimic small abscess formation. Additional pitfalls include the presence of benign cystic structures in the parotid glands, such as lymphoepithelial cysts and first branchial cleft cysts, although these may become secondarily infected to behave like abscesses, after all.

Other patterns of salivary gland inflammation suggest alternative causes of sialoadenitis. For example, bilateral salivary gland involvement is more suggestive of viral infection, radiation-induced sialoadenitis, or an autoimmune disorder (especially Sjögren syndrome). These conditions are not typically associated with enlargement of the extraglandular ducts, although there may be increased conspicuity of the intraglandular ducts secondary to inflammation and ductal obstruction.[14,27–29]

Viral sialoadenitis is still most commonly caused by mumps (*Paramyxovirus*), especially in nonimmunized patients, although cases have been reported with an assortment of viral causes, including *Influenza*, *Coxsackie*, and *Adenovirus*. In these cases, one would expect to see marked pan-sialoadenitis in young patients with fever and other systemic symptoms of illness, without specific evidence of bacterial or obstructive disease. The treatment of these patients is largely supportive because the disease course is usually limited.[14,27–29]

Radiation sialoadenitis should be suspected in any patient who has been administered radioactive iodine therapy (I-131) for thyroid disease or any individual evaluated in the first several months following external beam radiation therapy or head and neck cancer. In the chronic phase, the glands are often small and fibrotic, hyperdense on noncontrast CT, and diffusely hyperenhancing on postcontrast CT. The glands can be swollen, edematous, and hypodense on CT in the acute setting, however. Hyperattenuation of the glands on noncontrast CT is a feature encountered especially within the first days of I-131 administration because of the concentration of the radioiodine within the salivary glands. The inflammatory changes of the salivary glands are otherwise nonspecific and treated with hydration, salivatory stimulants, and antipyretics.[14,27–29]

Sjögren disease is a common autoimmune disorder, characterized by B cell–mediated infiltration and destruction of the lacrimal and salivary glands (particularly the parotid glands). These patients may occasionally present with symptoms and signs of acute sialadenitis. It predominantly affects female patients in the fourth to fifth decades of life. These patients classically present with dry mouth and dry eyes (keratoconjunctivitis sicca) and may have a history of other autoimmune diseases, such as lupus or rheumatoid arthritis, or various forms of interstitial lung disease. Forty percent of Sjögren disease cases are seen in isolation, however.[29] Aside from the patient demographics, early Sjögren disease may be difficult to distinguish from viral sialoadenitis; but long-standing Sjögren disease is usually notable on imaging for atrophic salivary glands with heterogeneous, stippled attenuation, multiple small parotid cysts, and numerous intraglandular sialoliths. In these patients, it is important to be on the lookout for any potential hypercellular masses because there is a reported 44-times increased risk of developing lymphoma. An infiltrative lesion that is hyperenhancing, isoattenuating to hyperattenuating to muscle on CT, or relatively T2 hypointense and restricts diffusion on MR imaging, is concerning for lymphomatous involvement of the gland, although rare cases of chronic sclerosing sialoadenitis can also have this appearance.[27,29]

Teaching point: In the absence of a causative sialolith, cases of sialoadenitis warrant further scrutiny of potential underlying neoplastic disease.

Tonsillitis

Acute tonsillitis is one of the most common infections of the head and neck, particularly among young patients. The most common causes are Epstein-Barr virus in adolescent patients as well as *Staphylococcus aureus* and *Streptococcus* species. The diagnosis is usually clinically apparent in these patients, who present with throat pain, trismus, and tonsillar enlargement and erythema. Imaging is usually required in only the most severe cases in order to evaluate the extent of disease and the presence of abscess.[14]

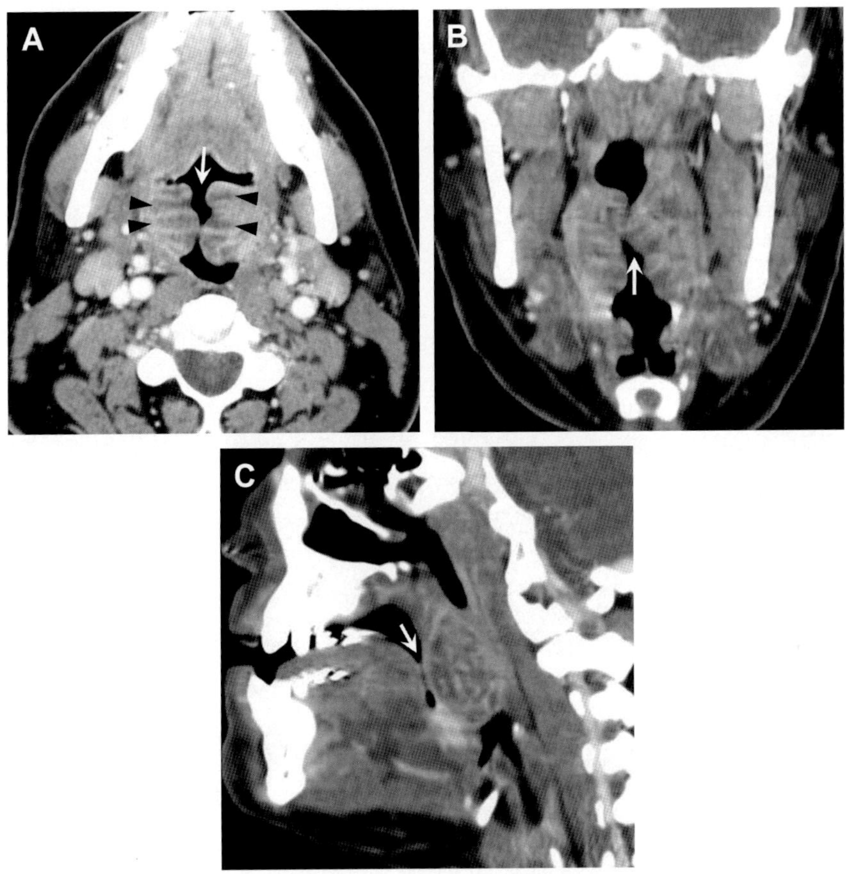

Fig. 22. Acute bilateral tonsillitis: Axial (*A*), coronal (*B*), and sagittal (*C*) contrast-enhanced CT scans demonstrate severe bilateral enlargement of the palatine tonsils with linear streaks of hypodensity (*black arrowheads*) within the tonsils representing pus-filled tonsillar crypts. Note the near-complete compromise of the pharyngeal airway (*white arrows*) by the hypertrophied (kissing) tonsils.

On CT and MR imaging, acute tonsillitis manifests as enlargement, edema, and hyperenhancement of the palatine tonsils, which may touch in the midline oral cavity (kissing). On postcontrast images, tonsillar inflammation may present with a striated enhancement pattern, with parallel streaks of linear hypoenhancement representing areas of edema, trapped fluid, and cellular debris accumulating within the tonsillar crypts (**Fig. 22**). Be careful not to accidentally describe this finding as abscess formation, which would necessitate surgical drainage. Similarly, focal areas of central hypoenhancement within the tonsillar tissues, without discrete peripheral rim enhancement, may represent devitalized nonliquefied suppurated tissue that cannot be drained.[14,30]

Tonsillitis-associated abscess comes in 2 flavors (*sorry, we couldn't resist*): (1) peritonsillar abscess, which is far more common, and (2) true tonsillar abscess formation. With the former, an organized area of inflammatory fluid extends beyond the thin tonsillar capsule into the peritonsillar space (see **Fig. 22**; **Figs. 23** and **24**). This fluid extension can, in turn, result in cellulitis or abscess formation within the parapharyngeal, masticator, and retropharyngeal spaces (see **Fig. 24**). Peritonsillar abscesses may also cause severe midline deviation of the tonsil and airway compromise (see **Fig. 23**). In contrast, a true tonsillar abscess results in an area of liquefaction that is entirely contained by the periphery of the gland and delineated by a thin rim of enhancement. It is important to indicate the size of the abscess, as collections measuring less than 1 cm may be too small to drain. Short-term clinical follow-up with adequate antibiotic and supportive therapy, often as an inpatient, may be the preferred treatment option.[30]

CERVICAL SPACE EMERGENCIES

Not all painful, tender neck masses detected on clinical examination turn out to be solid lesions. The layered arrangement of various fascial planes coursing throughout the neck creates multiple

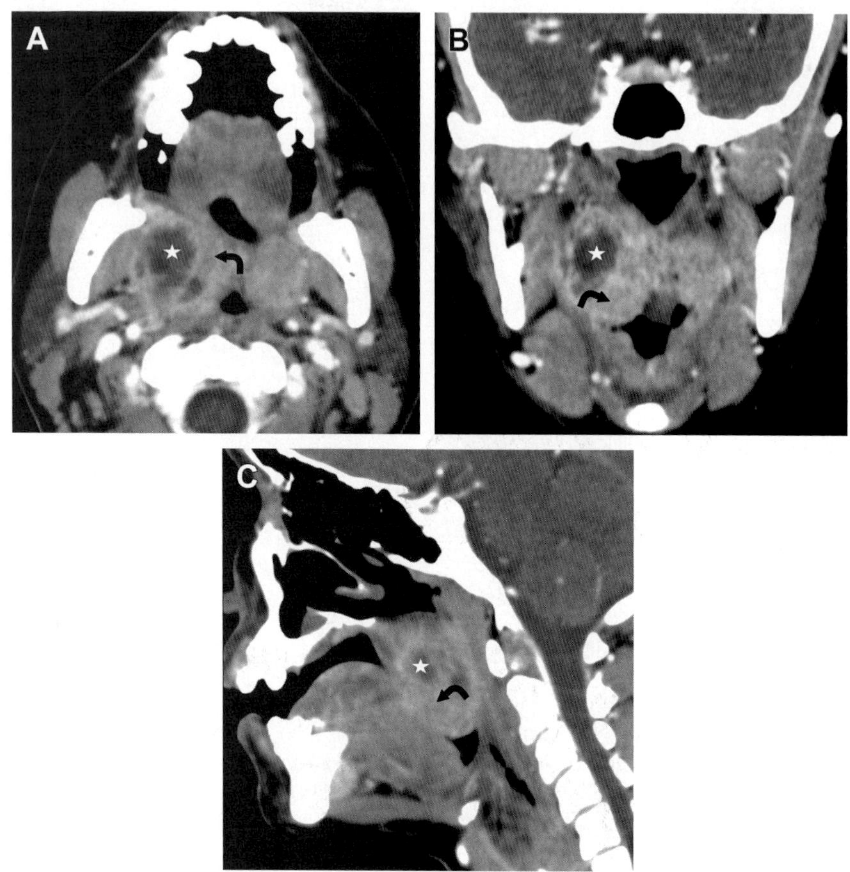

Fig. 23. Peritonsillar-retrotonsillar abscess: Axial (*A*), coronal (*B*), and sagittal (*C*) contrast-enhanced CT scans demonstrate severe bilateral enlargement of the palatine tonsils caused by tonsillitis. There is a large rim-enhancing abscess (*star*) displacing the ipsilateral tonsil (*curved black arrows*) medially and inferiorly.

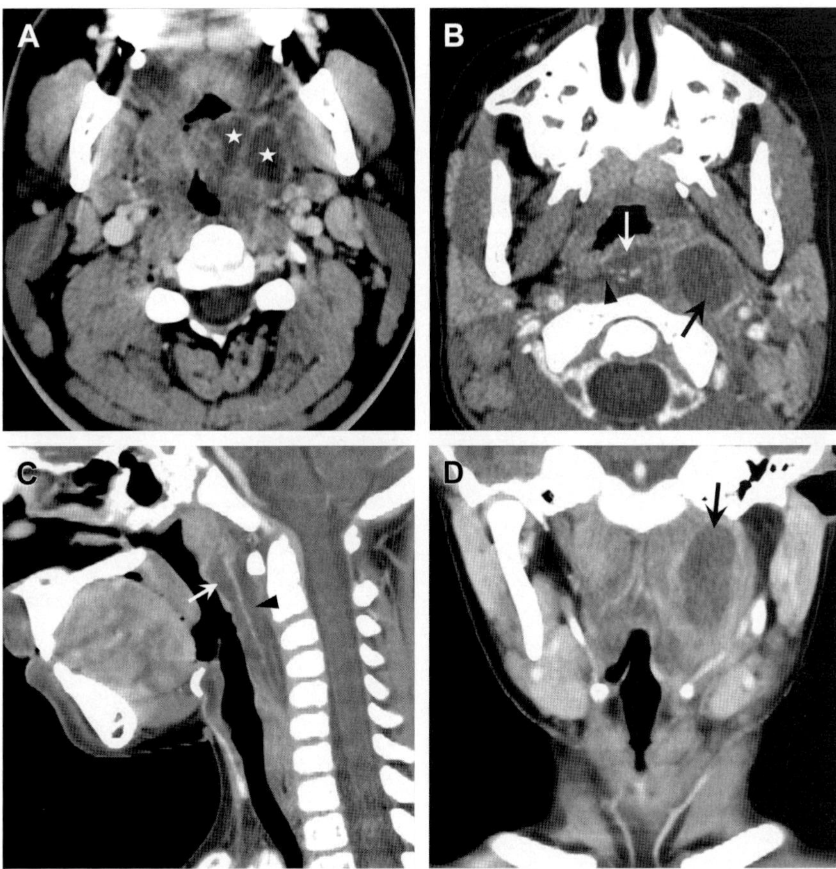

Fig. 24. Peritonsillar, retropharyngeal, and danger space abscesses: Axial (*A*, *B*), sagittal (*C*), and coronal (*D*) contrast-enhanced CT scans demonstrate a multiloculated rim-enhancing peritonsillar abscess (*stars*) as well as a large suppurative lateral retropharyngeal node (*black arrows*). The suppurative lymph node has ruptured into the retropharyngeal space resulting in abscesses within the retropharyngeal (*white arrows*) and danger space (*black arrowheads*) abscesses.

intervening spaces, which can potentially become inoculated by bacteria and progress to severe cellulitis and myofasciitis (**Figs. 25** and **26**). Once established, these infections of the deep cervical spaces are difficult to treat medically and have the potential to affect to the adjacent visceral structures or spread to other spaces within the neck and mediastinum.

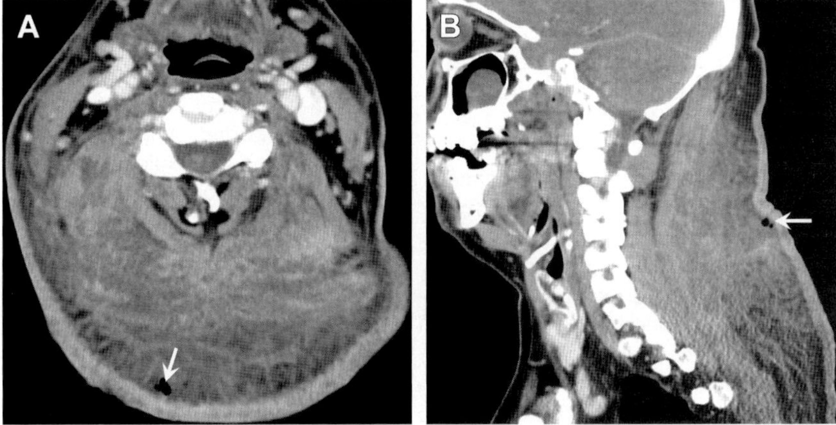

Fig. 25. Posterior cervical space necrotizing myofasciitis: Axial (*A*) and sagittal (*B*) contrast-enhanced CT scans demonstrate extensive edema, skin thickening, gas formation (*arrows*), and abnormal enhancement of the posterior cervical fascial planes and muscles in this patient with *Streptococcus anginosus* necrotizing myofasciitis.

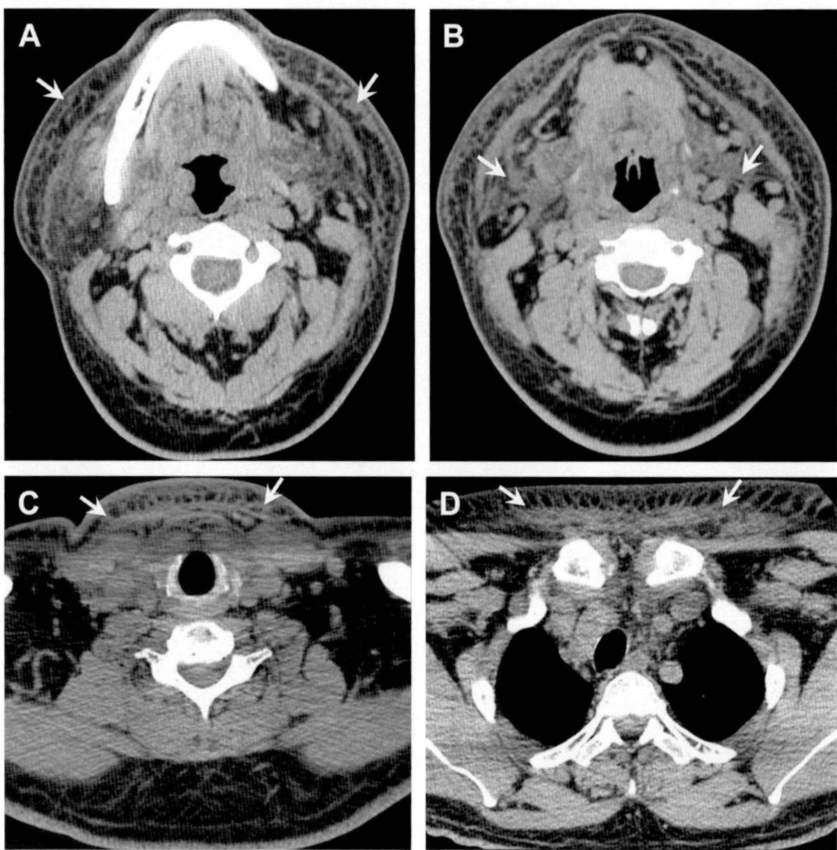

Fig. 26. Necrotizing cervical–mediastinal fasciitis: Axial contrast-enhanced CT scans (*A–D*) reveal rapidly progressive diffuse edema of the fascial planes and muscles in the neck and upper mediastinum (*white arrows*) in this patient with early necrotizing fasciitis.

Floor of Mouth Infections

Most infections arising in the sublingual and submandibular spaces are dental in origin. The 2 spaces are demarcated by the sling of the mylohyoid muscle, which inserts on the mylohyoid line along the lingual margin of the mandible at the approximate level of the mandibular dental roots. Specifically, the roots of the first molar, premolars, and canines terminate above the ridge; dental infections of these teeth are prone to cause sublingual space infections (**Figs. 27** and **28**). The distal roots of the second and third mandibular molar teeth extend below the mylohyoid line. Therefore, submandibular space infections should prompt for inspection of the second or third molar teeth for an odontogenic source. Submandibular space abscesses may also originate from sublingual space infections that spread posterior to the free margin of the mylohyoid muscle (see **Fig. 27**; **Fig. 29**) or directly through small defects in the muscular sling (boutonnière). Other causes include direct extension from contagions of the masticator buccal and parapharyngeal spaces as well as extracapsular extension of complicated submandibular sialoadenitis.[14,31]

With floor-of-mouth abscess formation, as with any other infected fluid collection, one expects to find a nonenhancing low-attenuation fluid collection with peripheral rim enhancement, occasionally containing gas. With odontogenic causes of sublingual or submandibular abscess formation, a subperiosteal abscess may also be seen. This abscess is seen as a sessile rim-enhancing low-attenuation collection with its base oriented longitudinally along the lingual margin of the mandible. This part of the mandibular cortex must be inspected for areas of osseous erosion and dehiscence.

Odontogenic submandibular space abscesses will typically radiate out from the mandibular angle in an inferolateral direction, with subsequent displacement of the submandibular gland and

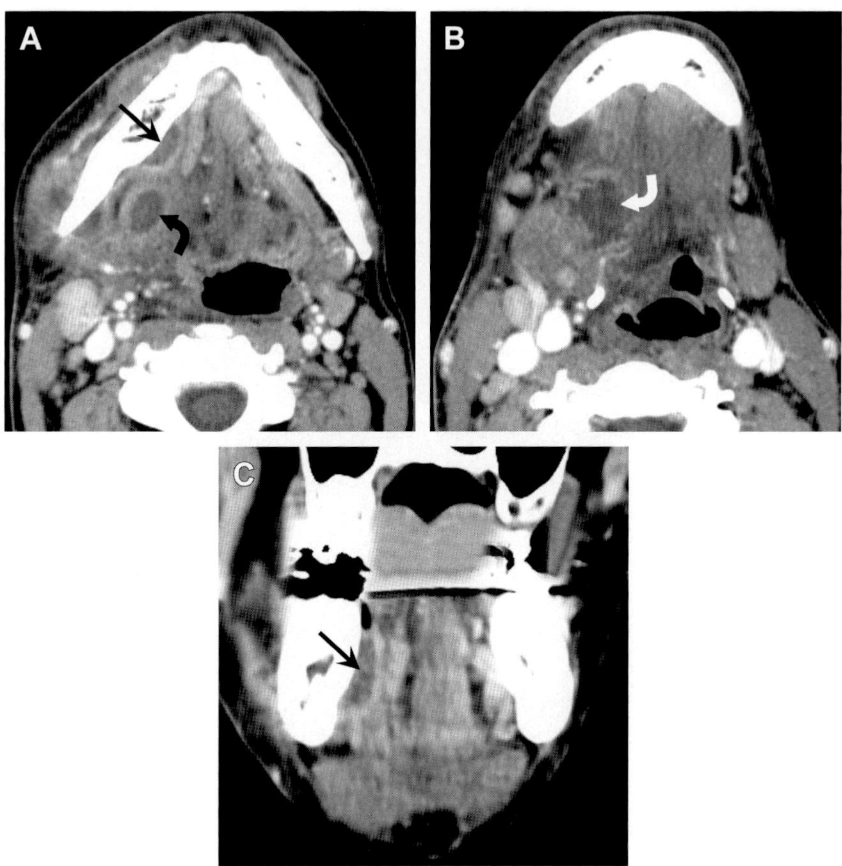

Fig. 27. Subperiosteal mandibular abscess, submandibular and sublingual space abscesses: Axial (*A*, *B*) and coronal (*C*) contrast-enhanced CT scans demonstrate a rim-enhancing abscess abutting the lingual cortex of the mandible (*black arrows*) adjacent to a periapical abscess of tooth 28 (not shown). Additionally seen are similar rim-enhancing abscesses within the posterior portion of the sublingual space (*curved black arrow*) and submandibular space (*curved white arrow*).

stranding of the submandibular fat. The outer margin of the abscess may extend over the buccal and lingual cortical margins of the mandible, potentially involving the mandibular foramen and by association the inferior alveolar nerve. Extension of the abscess to involve the buccal and masticator spaces is common (see **Fig. 28**).

Ludwig angina is a specific type of severe head and neck infection that rapidly progresses throughout the entire floor of the mouth, sublingual space, submandibular space, root of the tongue, and pretracheal soft tissues (**Fig. 30**). These patients present with glossal elevation and protrusion, difficulty controlling oral secretions, and most importantly a threatened upper airway. Although often seen in conjunction with abscess and gas formation, it is technically only defined by the presence of an aggressive cellulitis, which on examination may manifest with painful firmness and distension of the submandibular soft tissues and upper throat.[14,31]

Retropharyngeal Abscess

You will encounter various anatomic descriptions of the retropharyngeal space, which can be a source of confusion when trying to distinguish a retropharyngeal abscess from other infections that have organized in the thin stretches of real estate sandwiched between the pharynx and cervical spine.

The retropharyngeal space is defined anteriorly by the buccopharyngeal fascia (a thin membrane that covers the dorsal margin of the pharyngeal constrictor muscles) and posteriorly by the alar fascia. These two fascial layers and the intervening retropharyngeal space extend superiorly to the base of the skull where they attach separately. The buccopharyngeal and alar fascia fuse

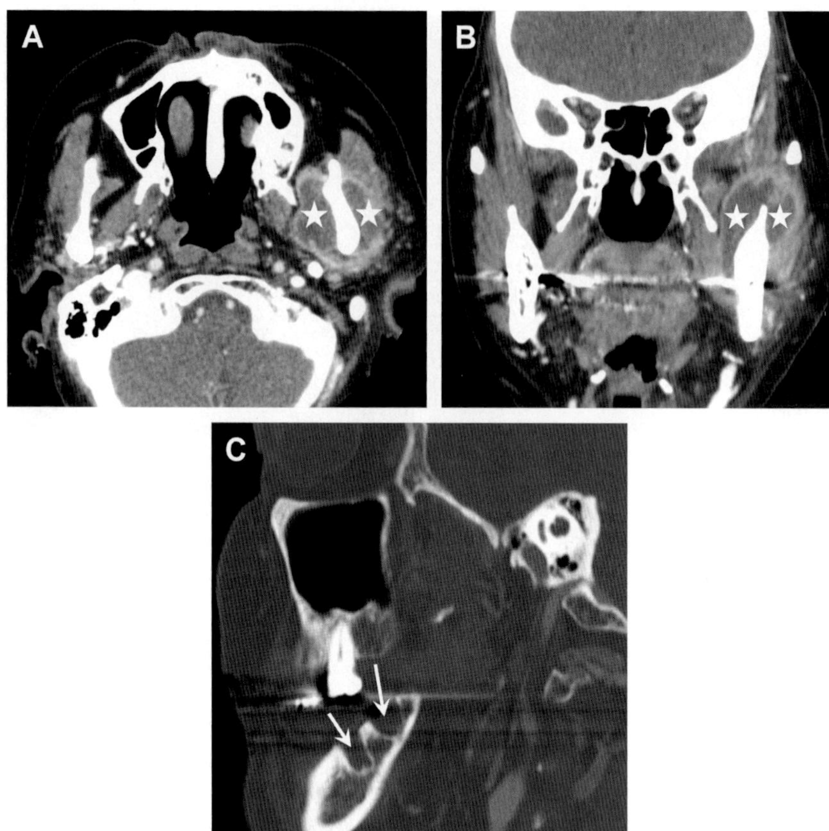

Fig. 28. Masticator space abscess following recent dental extractions: Axial (*A*), coronal (*B*), and sagittal (*C*) contrast-enhanced CT scans demonstrate recent extraction sockets (*white arrows*) of teeth 18 and 19. There is a centrally hypointense rim-enhancing abscess (*stars*) involving the masseter and pterygoid musculature within the masticator space.

inferiorly into a single layer thereby terminating along the posterior margin of the esophagus at the T1-T2 level. At this level, the lower extent of the retropharyngeal space is sometimes referred to as the retrovisceral space and can communicate with the peritracheal space.[14,30] A thin sagittal fibrous band (the median raphe) extends from the midline alar fascia and effectively divides the retropharyngeal spaces into 2 lateral components, each housing its respective half of the retropharyngeal lymphatic drainage system.

The retropharyngeal lymph nodes are responsible for draining the middle ears, eustachian tubes, paranasal sinuses, and upper pharyngeal soft tissues in very young children. The retropharyngeal lymphatic chains usually become mostly obliterated within the first decade of life by repeated pharyngeal infections. In young patients, enlargement of retropharyngeal lymph nodes is rather nonspecific and may be encountered in the setting of any inflammatory process of the upper airway. Severe or prolonged infections, however, can promote bacterial seeding of the retropharyngeal lymph nodes, which can then form intranodal abscesses (suppuration). The rupture of suppurative retropharyngeal lymph nodes is thought to be the pathogenesis of most retropharyngeal abscesses (see **Fig. 24**). Initially the abscess will remain unilateral, bounded medially by the median raphe of the alar fascia. However, the alar fascia is very thin and infection can easily breakthrough to the contralateral retropharyngeal space or posteriorly into the danger space (see **Fig. 24**).[14,30]

Retropharyngeal abscess must be differentiated from acute calcific prevertebral tendinitis (**Fig. 31**), which is a painful inflammatory process that affects the superior inserting fibers of the prevertebral musculature, namely, the longus colli and longus capitis muscles. These muscles course along the anterior margin of the cervical vertebral column and play a role in stabilizing movements

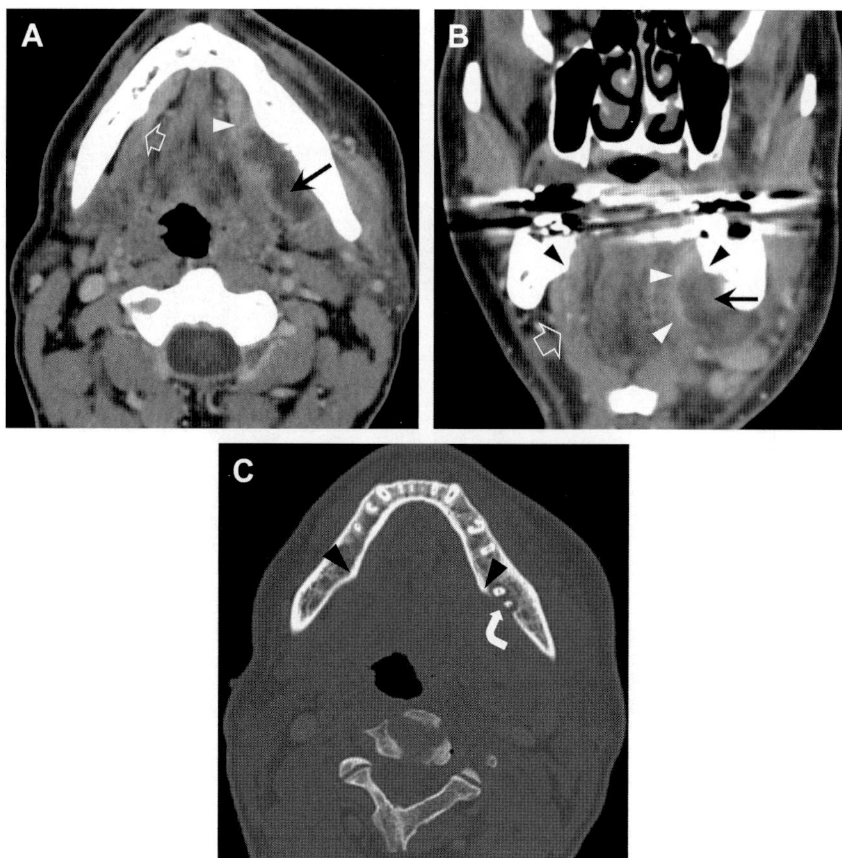

Fig. 29. Masticator space abscess following recent dental extractions: Axial soft tissue (*A*), coronal soft tissue (*B*), and bone (*C*) algorithm images demonstrate a periapical abscess of tooth 18 (*curved white arrow*) that has eroded through the lingual cortex of the mandible. There is an abscess (*black arrows*) located within the submandibular space inferior and lateral to the left mylohyoid muscle (*white arrowheads*). When there is cortical breakthrough of an abscess below the attachment of the mylohyoid muscle to the mylohyoid line of the mandible (*black arrowheads*), the abscess will occur in the submandibular space. The distal roots of the second and third mandibular molar teeth typically extend below this line. Note the attachment of the contralateral mylohyoid muscle (*open white arrows*) to the mylohyoid line.

of the head and neck. The longus colli muscles insert superiorly along the anterior arch of the C1 vertebral body, and the longus capitis muscles insert along the base of the clivus. The inflammatory component of acute calcific prevertebral tendinitis is incited by the presence of hydroxyapatite crystal deposition within the muscle fibers. On imaging, the classic features are a low attenuation effusion within the prevertebral space, without peripheral rim enhancement or loculation, and seen in the presence of calcification among the superior insertions of the prevertebral muscles. The noncalcified portions of these muscles may appear hyperenhancing and edematous, and regional reactive lymphadenopathy can also be seen.

Descending Mediastinitis

The danger space is a potential space that extends from the skull base superiorly down into the retroesophageal mediastinum (see **Fig. 26**). It is defined anteriorly by the alar fascia and posteriorly by the prevertebral fascia, which invests the longus colli and capitis muscles along the anterior margin of the cervical spine. Infections within the retropharyngeal space can permeate the alar fascia and extend directly into the danger space. Danger space infections, with the aid of gravity, can descend unimpeded into the mediastinum resulting in mediastinitis. This condition is potentially life threatening and can be associated with severe sepsis and cardiovascular collapse. Treatment

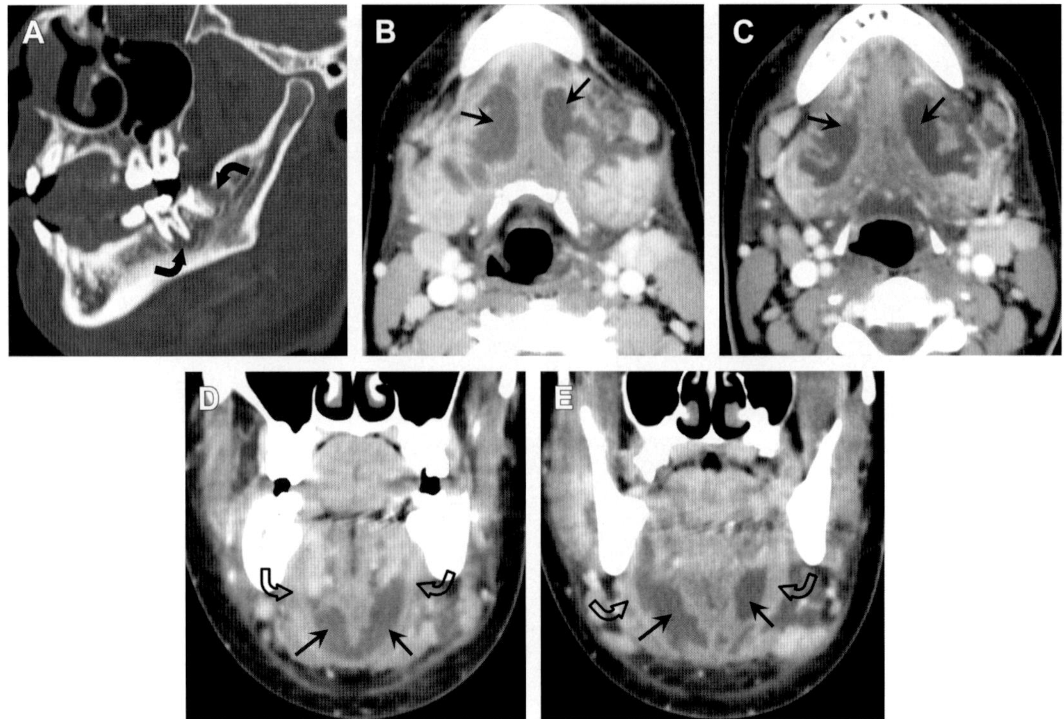

Fig. 30. Ludwig angina: Oblique sagittal (*A*), axial (*B*, *C*), and coronal (*D*, *E*) contrast-enhanced CT scans demonstrate multiple dental caries and periapical abscesses (*curved black closed arrows*) of the molar teeth. There is extensive cellulitis and abnormal enhancement involving the sublingual and submandibular spaces. A crescent-shaped abscess (*straight black arrows*) is present in the sublingual space just superior to the mylohyoid muscle (*curved black open arrows*).

usually includes surgical drainage and intensive care.[14,32,33]

Descending mediastinitis is usually defined by the presence of a preceding infection of the head or neck, as opposed to primary mediastinitis that is secondary to esophageal injury or other direct violation of the mediastinum. Other potential routes for descending cervical infection into the mediastinum (see **Fig. 26**) include the pretracheal space (contiguous with the anterior-superior mediastinum), carotid space (contiguous with the middle mediastinum), and the prevertebral space (contiguous with the posterior mediastinum).[14,32,33]

The prevertebral space is a potential space that runs along the anterior margin of the vertebral column, bordered posteriorly by the anterior longitudinal ligament and anteriorly by the prevertebral fascia. Infections within this space are usually secondary to direct extension from spondylodiscitis. Inflammatory changes within the vertebral bodies, intervertebral disks, and perivertebral musculature can, therefore, help distinguish a prevertebral space infection from an infection in the danger space or retropharyngeal space.[14,32,33] In actuality, any combination of these infections may be present at the same time.

In addition to mediastinal spread, infections that descend along the carotid sheath have the potential of inducing direct injury to the carotid arteries and internal jugular veins. Therefore, the carotid space should be simultaneously evaluated for evidence of venous occlusion secondary to infectious thrombophlebitis (Lemierre syndrome) (**Fig. 32**), arterial occlusion, vasculitis, and mycotic pseudoaneurysm formation. Large pseudoaneurysms may result in actual or semi-contained rupture (carotid blowout injury) and can occur in the setting of carotid space infections, radiation therapy, prior surgery (**Fig. 33**), vasculitis (**Fig. 34**), trauma, and from direct invasion by malignant neoplasms.[34,35] The aftermath of carotid injuries can be catastrophic, possibly leading to embolic phenomena, ischemic infarctions, exsanguination, and death. The course of treatment is determined by the cause of the injury, its extent and location along the vessel, and the presence of intracranial collateral flow. Depending on the situation, endovascular

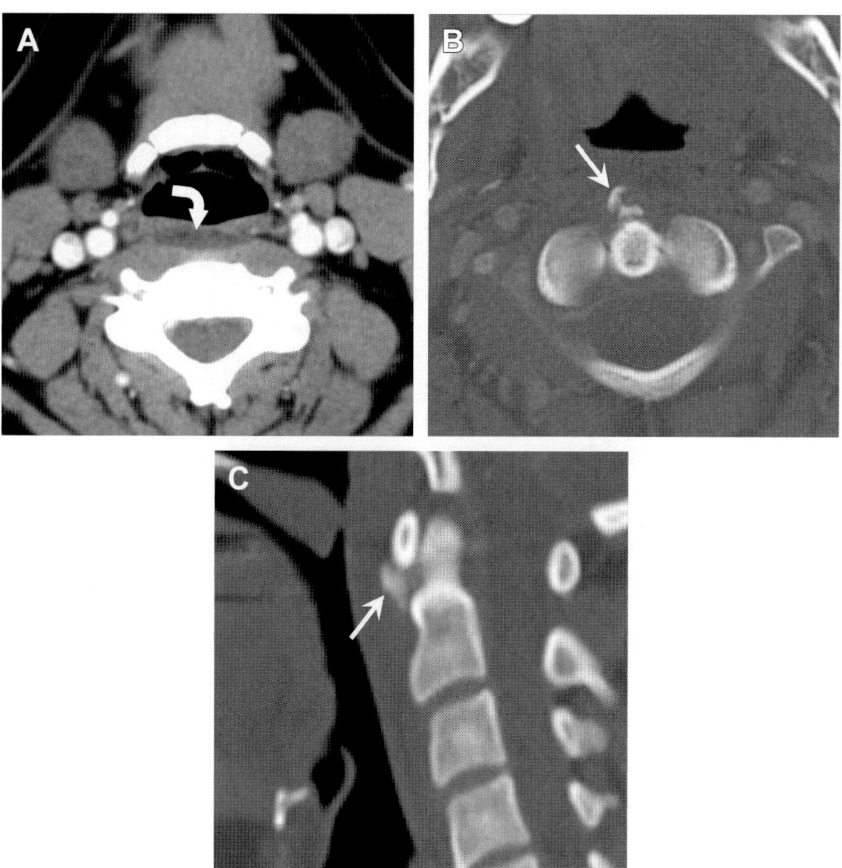

Fig. 31. Calcific prevertebral tendinitis: Axial (*A, B*) and sagittal (*C*) contrast-enhanced CT scans were acquired in this afebrile patient who presented to the emergency department with neck pain. There is evidence of nonenhancing fluid in the retropharyngeal space (*curved white arrow*) raising the possibility of an abscess. Note is made, however, of calcifications (*white arrows*) within the tendinous insertion of the longus coli muscle suggesting that the fluid is likely caused by calcific prevertebral tendinitis rather than a true abscess.

stent-graft repair or surgical sacrifice may be performed.

Teaching point: Infections of the retropharyngeal space, danger space, and prevertebral space need to be evaluated in the sagittal plane. In particular, danger space infections necessitate evaluation of the mediastinum, and prevertebral infections necessitate evaluation of the cervical spine.

AIRWAY EMERGENCIES

Of course, any problem that compromises the airway is a potentially life-threatening emergency. Therefore, patients with an acute upper airway complaint need to have their breathing issues addressed before being transferred to the radiology suite for imaging. Intubation should be considered before any examination that requires patients to be supine (ie, CT and MR imaging), especially if there is any suspicion of anaphylaxis or other difficulties in maintaining oxygen saturation levels. Radiographs and CT examinations offer the advantage of fast scan times, excellent delineation of the airways, and sensitivity for radiopaque foreign bodies. Foreign bodies of the esophagus (**Fig. 35**), hypopharynx, or tracheobronchial tree may also indirectly result in acute or subacute airway compromise if there is secondary aspiration.

Epiglottis

Marked enlargement and edematous changes of the epiglottis and aryepiglottic folds should raise alarm for epiglottitis (see **Fig. 1**), which threatens patency of the laryngeal airway. Infection is usually by *Haemophilus influenzae* or *Streptococcus* species and can be accompanied by

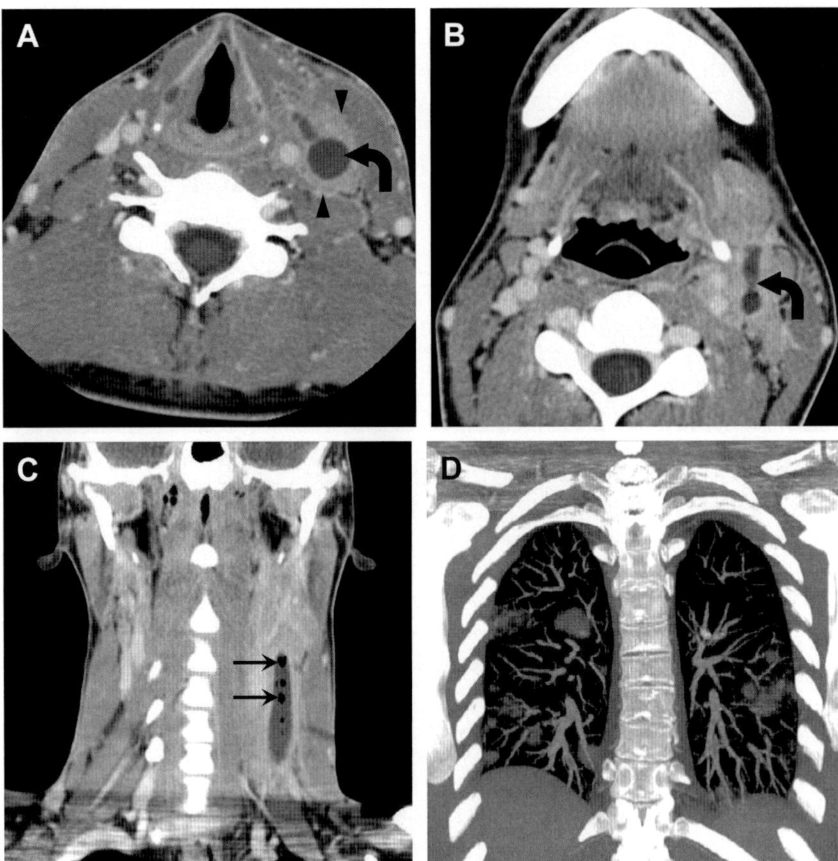

Fig. 32. Internal jugular vein septic thrombophlebitis, Lemierre syndrome (*Fusobacterium necrophorum*): Axial (*A, B*) and coronal (*C*) contrast-enhanced neck CT scans as well as a coronal MIP image of the chest (*D*) were acquired in this patient who presented with fever, headache, and progressive left neck swelling 1 week following an episode of pharyngitis and tonsillitis. The study demonstrates extensive inflammation (*black arrowheads*) surrounding the internal jugular and facial veins (*curved black arrows*). There is a lack of normal enhancement and presence of gas in these veins (*straight black arrows*) consistent with septic venous thrombophlebitis, which was caused by the organism *Fusobacterium Necrophorum* in this case. Lemierre syndrome is caused by suppurative thrombophlebitis of the internal jugular vein and its branches caused by oropharyngeal infections, such as tonsillitis and dental infections. Spread of the infection into the facial venous system leads to septic thrombosis of the jugular vein. This patient also exhibited one of the dreaded complications of this syndrome, numerous septic pulmonary infarcts (*D*).

signs of edema, supraglottic laryngeal swelling, and diffuse cellulitis of the surrounding soft tissues in severe cases. The classic description on lateral radiographs of the neck is the thumb sign, representing bulbous enlargement of the suprahyoid epiglottis. These patients are typically young and present with dyspnea and fever. The treatment is broad-spectrum antibiotic therapy and airway protection, usually achieved via intubation.[14]

Laryngotracheal Angioedema

Generalized inflammatory changes to the mucosa and submucosal soft tissues of the upper airway can lead to varying degrees of luminal airway narrowing and respiratory compromise. The imaging features in these cases are nonspecific but easily recognized: circumferential thickening of the hypopharyngeal, glottic, and/or tracheal soft tissues with subsequent narrowing and deformity of the airway lumen. It should be noted that even relative

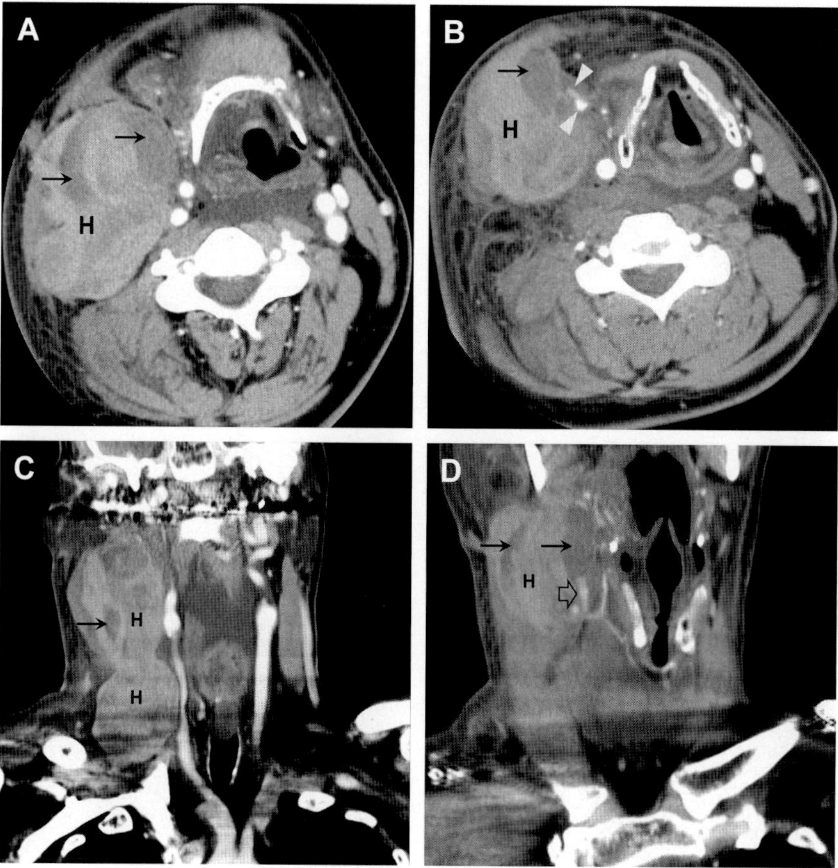

Fig. 33. Enlarging cervical hematoma after neck dissection: Axial (*A, B*) and coronal (*C, D*) contrast-enhanced neck CT scans of the neck performed 6 hours following selective neck for oropharyngeal squamous cell carcinoma. The images demonstrates a huge bilobed, mostly hyperdense cervical hematoma (H). There are areas that are not hyperdense, however, indicating ongoing bleeding and unclotted blood (*black arrows*). There is focal irregularity of external carotid artery branches (*white arrowheads*) and an area of contrast extravasation into an unclotted portion of the hematoma (*black open arrow*).

minor changes in absolute luminal size can result in significant changes in airflow. Luminal resistance increases by a factor that is inversely related to the fourth power of the radius (eg, halving the luminal diameter increases resistance 16-fold). Furthermore, fluid and exudative debris secondary to airway inflammation can further contribute to luminal obstruction.

Significant causes of laryngotracheal angioedema include anaphylaxis, radiation injury, and cellulitis. Treatment is, therefore, directed toward to the underlying disease process, in addition to supportive care and airway protection. Intubation or tracheotomy is often indicated.[14,30]

Teaching point: Inflammatory conditions of the airway have the potential to progress rapidly. Recognition of these conditions needs to be immediately followed by communication to the clinician, with anticipation of the possible need for medical management of the airway.

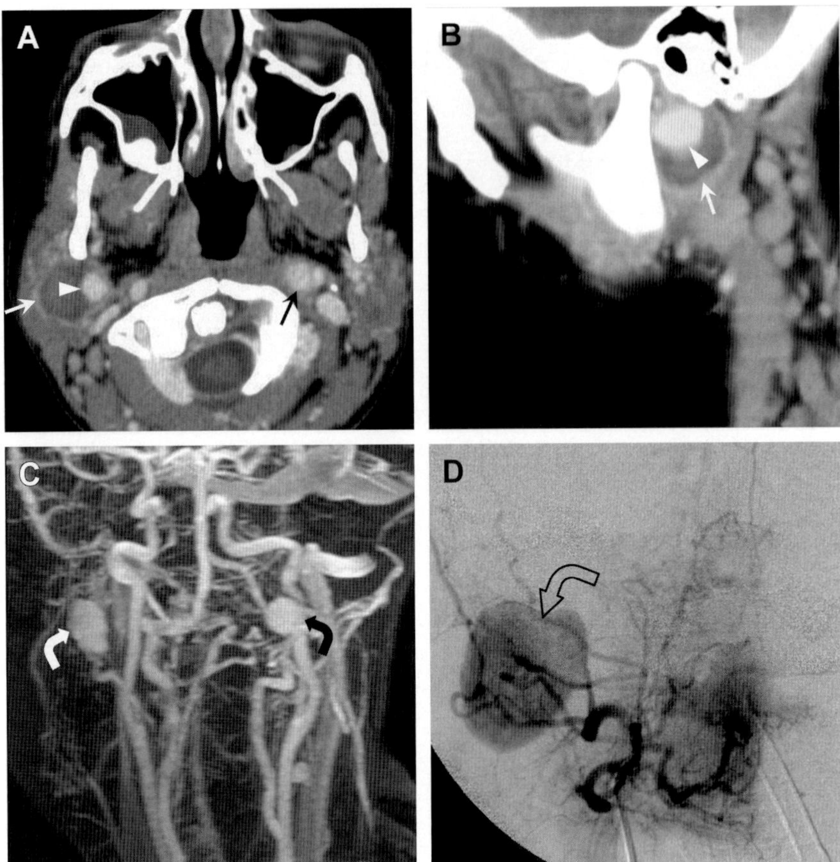

Fig. 34. Multiple external carotid pseudoaneurysms, vasculitis: Axial (*A*) and sagittal (*B*) CT scans of the neck, coronal contrast-enhanced MR angiography (MRA) (*C*), and right external carotid angiogram (ECA) (*D*) were acquired in this patient with acute lymphocytic leukemia and an enlarging right parotid mass. The CT scans demonstrate a ring-enhancing right parotid mass (*white arrows*) with an eccentric area of enhancement (*white arrowheads*) that was not separable from the external carotid artery. An apparent left internal carotid artery dissection and pseudoaneurysm (*black arrow*) is also seen just below the skull base. The contrast-enhanced MRA reveals external (*curved white arrow*) and internal (*curved black arrow*) carotid artery pseudoaneurysms. The ECA angiogram, obtained at the time of embolization, confirms a right ECA pseudoaneurysm (*curved black open arrow*), which was associated with large-vessel vasculitis at pathology.

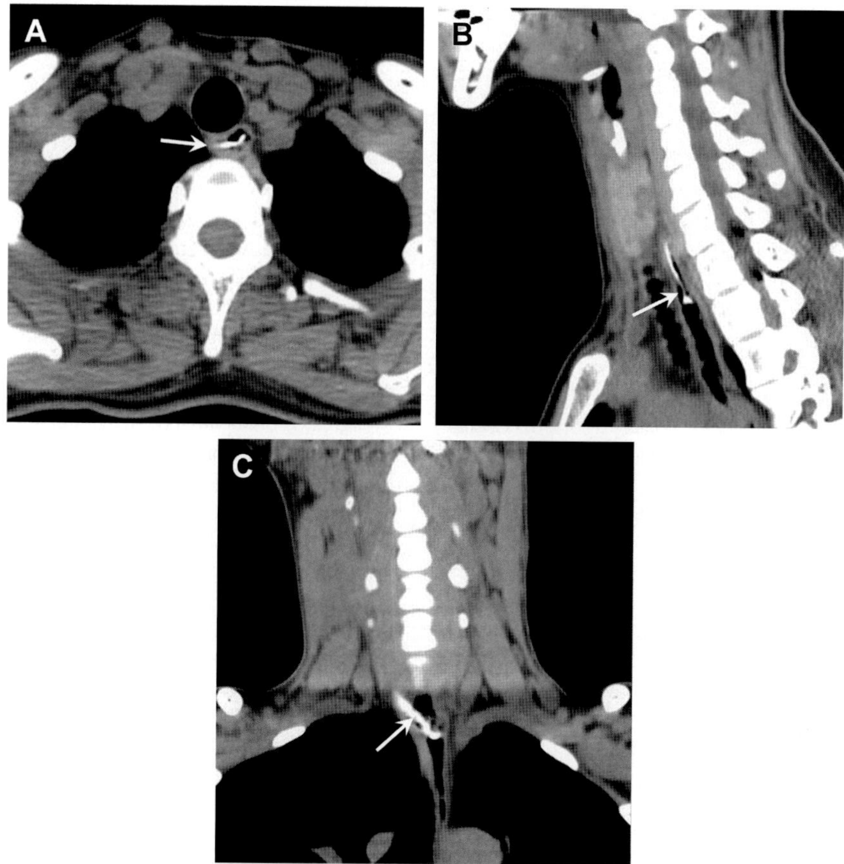

Fig. 35. Esophageal foreign body (chicken bone): Axial (*A*), sagittal (*B*), and coronal (*C*) CT scans of the neck were obtained on this physician who inadvertently swallowed a chicken bone. There is a Y-shaped bone (*white arrows*) in the lumen of the upper esophagus without obvious mucosal penetration.

SUMMARY

The anatomy of the head and neck contains very few structures that could be considered expendable and, consequently, is exceptionally intolerant to infection, inflammation, and injury. Acute pathologic processes in this body region, therefore, tend to result in significant suffering, functional impairment, or life endangerment if the diagnosis is missed or treatment is delayed. Many emergent processes within the cervical region also need to be considered for their possible impact on structures within the head and chest, into which there are many routes for potential communication.

In the emergent setting, CT is the favored imaging option because of its rapid image acquisition and superior delineation of the airway and osseous structures. On the other hand, MR imaging provides more robust information regarding complex soft tissue structures that may be difficult to distinguish on CT. However, any prolonged radiologic examination should only be undertaken in patients who possess a protected airway and are medically stable enough to tolerate the duration of the scan. This added step of preimaging clearance should entail a review of the patients' presenting symptoms and past medical history, which will also help to refine the study protocol and provide a clinical context in which to interpret the images.

REFERENCES

1. Bayar MA, Kokes F, Gokcek C, et al. Post-traumatic tension pneumoorbitus: case report. Turk Neurosurg 1995;5:34–5.
2. Al-Shammari L, Majithia A, Adams A, et al. Tension pneumo-orbit treated by endoscopic, endonasal decompression: case report and literature review. J Laryngol Otol 2008;122:e8.
3. Gor DM, Kirsch CF, Leen J, et al. Radiologic differentiation of intraocular glass: evaluation of imaging techniques, glass types, size, and effect of intraocular hemorrhage. AJR Am J Roentgenol 2001;177:1199–203.
4. Lang GK. Ophthalmology: a pocket textbook atlas. New York: Thieme; 2004.

5. Ho VT, McGuckin JF Jr, Smergel EM. Intraorbital wooden foreign body: CT and MR appearance. AJNR Am J Neuroradiol 1996;17:134–6.
6. Cunnane ME, Sepahdari A, Gardiner M, et al. Pathology of the eye and orbit. In: Som PM, Curtin HD, editors. Head and neck imaging. 5th edition. St Louis (MO): Mosby; 2011. p. 601–3.
7. LeBedis CA, Sakai O. Nontraumatic orbital conditions: diagnosis with CT and MR imaging in the emergent setting. Radiographics 2008;28:1741–53.
8. Sepahdari AR, Aakalu VK, Kapur R, et al. MRI of orbital cellulitis and orbital abscess: the role of diffusion-weighted imaging. AJR Am J Roentgenol 2009;193:W244–50.
9. Tovilla-Canales JL, Nava A, Tovilla y Pomar JL. Orbital and periorbital infections. Curr Opin Ophthalmol 2001;12:335–41.
10. Uehara F, Ohba N. Diagnostic imaging in patients with orbital cellulitis and inflammatory pseudotumor. Int Ophthalmol Clin 2002;42:133–42.
11. Yuen SJ, Rubin PA. Idiopathic orbital inflammation: distribution, clinical features, and treatment outcome. Arch Ophthalmol 2003;121:491–9.
12. Kapur R, Sepahdari AR, Mafee MF, et al. MR imaging of orbital inflammatory syndrome, orbital cellulitis, and orbital lymphoid lesions: the role of diffusion-weighted imaging. AJNR Am J Neuroradiol 2009;30:64–70.
13. Jackson A, Sheppard S, Laitt RD, et al. Optic neuritis: MR imaging with combined fat- and water-suppression techniques. Radiology 1998;206:57–63.
14. Capps EF, Kinsella JJ, Gupta M, et al. Emergency imaging assessment of acute, nontraumatic conditions of the head and neck. Radiographics 2010;30:1335–52.
15. Som PM, Brandwein MS, Wang BY. Inflammatory disease of the sinonasal cavities. In: Som PM, Curtin HD, editors. Head and neck imaging. 5th edition. St Louis (MO): Mosby; 2011. p. 167–72.
16. Piccirillo JF. Clinical practice. Acute bacterial sinusitis. N Engl J Med 2004;351:902–10.
17. Aribandi M, McCoy VA, Bazan C 3rd. Imaging features of invasive and noninvasive fungal sinusitis: a review. Radiographics 2007;27:1283–96.
18. Momeni AK, Roberts CC, Chew FS. Imaging of chronic and exotic sinonasal disease: review. AJR Am J Roentgenol 2007;189:S35–45.
19. Kasperek ZA, Pollock GF. Epistaxis: an overview. Emerg Med Clin North Am 2013;31:443–54.
20. Pallin DJ, Chng YM, McKay MP, et al. Epidemiology of epistaxis in US emergency departments, 1992 to 2001. Ann Emerg Med 2005;46:77–81.
21. Geibprasert S, Pongpech S, Armstrong D, et al. Dangerous extracranial-intracranial anastomoses and supply to the cranial nerves: vessels the neurointerventionalist needs to know. AJNR Am J Neuroradiol 2009;30:1459–68.
22. Cohen JE, Moscovici S, Gomori JM, et al. Selective endovascular embolization for refractory idiopathic epistaxis is a safe and effective therapeutic option: technique, complications, and outcomes. J Clin Neurosci 2012;19:687–90.
23. Mahadevia AA, Murphy KJ, Obray R, et al. Embolization for intractable epistaxis. Tech Vasc Interv Radiol 2005;8:134–8.
24. Pope LE, Hobbs CG. Epistaxis: an update on current management. Postgrad Med J 2005;81:309–14.
25. Swartz JD, Hagiwara M. Inflammatory diseases of the temporal bone. In: Som PM, Curtin HD, editors. Head and neck imaging. 5th edition. St Louis (MO): Mosby; 2011. p. 1183–224.
26. Lemmerling MM, De Foer B, Verbist BM, et al. Imaging of inflammatory and infectious diseases in the temporal bone. Neuroimaging Clin N Am 2009;19:321–37.
27. Kaneda T, Minami M, Ozawa K, et al. MR of the submandibular gland: normal and pathologic states. AJNR Am J Neuroradiol 1996;17:1575–81.
28. Silvers AR, Som PM. Salivary glands. Radiol Clin North Am 1998;36:941–66, vi.
29. Som PM, Brandwein-Gensler MS. Anatomy and pathology of the salivary glands. In: Som PM, Curtin HD, editors. Head and neck imaging. 5th edition. St Louis (MO): Mosby; 2011. p. 2482–523.
30. Wesolowski JR, MSK. Pathology of the pharynx. In: Som PM, Curtin HD, editors. Head and neck imaging. 5th edition. St Louis (MO): Mosby; 2011. p. 1781–95.
31. Forghani R, Smoker WRK, Curtin HD. Pathology of the oral region. In: Som PM, Curtin HD, editors. Head and neck imaging. 5th edition. St Louis (MO): Mosby; 2011. p. 1705–15.
32. Ridder GJ, Maier W, Kinzer S, et al. Descending necrotizing mediastinitis: contemporary trends in etiology, diagnosis, management, and outcome. Ann Surg 2010;251:528–34.
33. Scaglione M, Pinto A, Giovine S, et al. CT features of descending necrotizing mediastinitis–a pictorial essay. Emerg Radiol 2007;14:77–81.
34. Chaloupka JC, Putman CM, Citardi MJ, et al. Endovascular therapy for the carotid blowout syndrome in head and neck surgical patients: diagnostic and managerial considerations. AJNR Am J Neuroradiol 1996;17:843–52.
35. Chang FC, Lirng JF, Luo CB, et al. Carotid blowout syndrome in patients with head-and-neck cancers: reconstructive management by self-expandable stent-grafts. AJNR Am J Neuroradiol 2007;28:181–8.

Index

Note: Page numbers of article titles are in **boldface** type.

Radiol Clin N Am 53 (2015) 253–260
http://dx.doi.org/10.1016/S0033-8389(14)00176-6

S

T

U

V

W